T0272034

Pain Management in Small Animal Medicine

Steven M Fox
MS, DVM, MBA, PhD
Surgical Specialist: New Zealand VMA
Independent Consultant, Clive, Iowa USA
Adjunct Assistant Professor, College of Veterinary Medicine, University of Illinois
Adjunct Associate Professor, Massey University NZ
Program Chairman (2000-02), President (2004), Veterinary Orthopedic Society

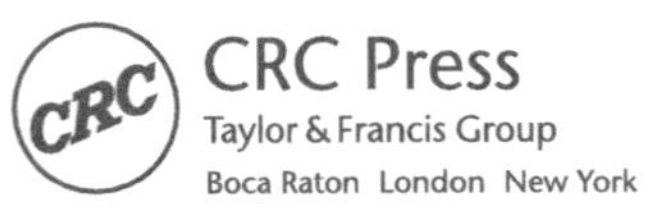
CRC Press
Taylor & Francis Group
Boca Raton London New York

CRC Press is an imprint of the
Taylor & Francis Group, an **informa** business

CRC Press
Taylor & Francis Group
6000 Broken Sound Parkway NW, Suite 300
Boca Raton, FL 33487-2742

Printed on acid-free paper
Version Date: 20130731
International Standard Book Number-13: 978-1-84076-183-2 (Hardback)

Visit the Taylor & Francis Web site at
http://www.taylorandfrancis.com

and the CRC Press Web site at
http://www.crcpress.com

Cover image: Nerve cell, computer artwork, courtesy of Sciepro/Science Photo Library

CONTENTS

DISCLAIMER

FOREWORD

Thank you for your interest in this text.
In 2010, Manson published the forerunner to this text, *Chronic Pain in Small Animal Medicine*. That text was ground-breaking for a couple of reasons. Firstly, it was pre-eminent in companion animal practice as a focus to the challenging conditions of chronic pain. Secondly, it was a unique attempt to present not only treatment suggestions, but also the neurobiologic mechanisms responsible for pain. In his book *Why We Hurt: the Natural History of Pain*, the distinguished neurosurgeon Dr. Frank Vertosick states, "When treating pain, knowledge is still the best weapon" (Harcourt, London, 2000, p.14).

Pain has become the 5th cardinal sign in human medicine and the 4th cardinal sign in many veterinary practices. The increased interest in managing pain has several drivers, including: compassion for animals, pet owner demand, commercial growth opportunities, educational focus, and research insights. At the same time, many agents with human analgesic features have been adapted 'off-label' for veterinary use. This can present a bit of a 'Catch 22': more agents are becoming available, but they do not have regulatory agency (Food and Drug Administration [FDA]) approval for veterinary patients. I suggest many of these agents will never gain approval for our patients due to the resource constraints of pursuing such approval. Therefore, it is incumbent upon the licensed veterinarian to understand the mechanisms of a patient's pain as well as to understand the drug's mode of action (including potential side-effects), and then make a benefit:risk assessment before administering the agent 'off label'. Only by understanding the mechanism of a patient's pain, can advancement be made in a patient's treatment.

Chronic Pain in Small Animal Medicine was well received and ran out of print. After consultation with the professional team at Manson Publishing, it was agreed that our readership would be best served with an 'expansion' of the chronic pain text rather than a second edition. Accordingly, this text, *Pain Management in Small Animal Medicine*, is an endeavor to retain the best from the Chronic Pain text but expand content with inclusion of areas beyond chronic pain. There are, of course, real world constraints, so a number of graphics have been reproduced from the Chronic Pain text, particularly to illustrate the core theme of 'mechanism base'.

This text was created for the veterinary healthcare professional seeking a greater depth of knowledge in mechanisms of pain and potential targets for treatment. It aspires to meet the needs as a quick reference, but more importantly, to go beyond the 'cookbook protocols' found in many offerings, by providing contemporary understandings of 'why and how to treat'. There will always be 'holes' in the evidence-based literature regarding areas of pain management for veterinary patients. Herein, it is informative to explore data obtained from different species and this text cites many such references. The caveat comes in weighing 'species specificity' vs. 'one science' in the clinical decision making. The author is also hopeful that this text will well serve those pursuing advanced credentials in the discipline of pain management.

We are all fleetingly placed on this planet so as to learn how to get along and love unselfishly. Dogs already know how to do that, so they don't need to stay as long.

ACKNOWLEDGEMENTS

I want to thank Manson Publishing for their recognition of contemporary veterinary issues, servicing their readers' interests with quality resources, and providing a congenial framework for collaboration. Special recognition is given to Jill Northcott, Commissioning Editor, and to Mike Manson himself, who has been so receptive to exploring new frontiers. The team at Manson Publishing is exceedingly helpful and give meaning to the term 'professionalism'.

Thank you to the visionaries who have created and grown the International Veterinary Academy of Pain Management (IVAPM) and the International Association for the Study of Pain: Non-human Special Interest Group (IASP-SIG). These associations have provided a framework through which we can all advance the science and practice of pain management. Thanks also to associations' membership who have recognized a forum for the promotion of our common, compassionate interests.

Many of my colleagues have encouraged me to create compositions such as this, where broad reaches of information can be found in a single volume. Thanks to them for their support and their individual research commitments.

Again, thanks to my supportive wife, Pam, who dusts around the stacks of reprints, keeps the coffee warm, and encourages my effort to raise the standards of pain management for both our beloved pets and yours.

'The best doctor in the world is the veterinarian,
He can't ask his patients what is the matter –
he's got to just know.'
Will Rogers

ABBREVIATIONS

5-HT	5-hydroxytryptamine
AA	arachidonic acid
AAFP	American Association of Feline Practitioners
AAHA	American Animal Hospital Association
ACE	angiotensin-converting enzyme
ACh	acetylcholine
ACL	anterior cruciate ligament
ACVA	American College of Veterinary Anesthesiologists
ADE	adverse drug event
ADH	antidiuretic hormone (arginine vasopressin)
AD-MSC	adipose-derived mesenchymal stem cell
ADP	adenosine diphosphate
AHCPR	Agency for Health Care Policy and Research
AHT	animal health technician
ALA	alpha-linolenic acid
ALP	alkaline phosphatase
ALT	alanine aminotransferase
AL-TENS	acupuncture-like TENS
AM	alternative medicine
AMA	American Medical Association
(c)AMP	(cyclic) adenosine monophosphate
AMPA	alpha-amino-3-hydroxy-5-methyl-isoxazole-4-propionic-acid
APS	American Pain Society
ARS	acute radiation score
ASA	acetyl salicylic acid (aspirin)
ASU	avocado/soybean unsaponifiable
ATL	aspirin-triggered lipoxin
ATP	adenosine triphosphate
BSA	body surface area
BUN	blood urea nitrogen
CBPI	canine brief pain inventory
CCK	cholecystokinin
CGRP	calcitonin gene-related peptide
CIPN	chemotherapy-induced peripheral neuropathy
CMPS	composite measure pain scale
CNS	central nervous system
CODI	Cincinnati Orthopedic Disability Index
COX	cyclo-oxygenase
CRI	constant rate infusion
CSF	cerebrospinal fluid
CSUVMC	Colorado State University Veterinary Medical Center
DA	dopamine
DAT	dopamine transporter
DEA	Drug Enforcement Administration
DHA	docosahexaenoic acid
DJD	degenerative joint disease
DMOAA	disease-modifying osteoarthritic agent
DMOAD	disease-modifying osteoarthritic drug
DRG	dorsal root ganglion
EBVM	evidence-based veterinary medicine
ELISA	enzyme-linked immunosorbent assay
EPA	eicosapentaenoic acid
ESWT	extracorporeal shock wave therapy
ET	endothelin
EVA	elk velvet antler
FDA	Food and Drug Administration
GABA	γ-aminobutyric acid
GAG	glycosaminoglycan
GCMPS	Glasgow composite measure of pain scale, short form
GDNF	glial-derived neurotrophic factor
GI	gastrointestinal
GLM	green lipped mussel
GS/CS	glucosamine and chondroitin sulfate
HCN	hyperpolarization-activated cyclic nucleotide-gated channel
HCPI	Helsinki Chronic Pain Index
HCP-Zeel	homeopathic combination preparation-Zeel
HETE	hydroxyeicosatetraenoic acid
HFT	high frequency TENS
HIV	human immunodeficiency virus
HRQL	health-related quality of life
IASP-SIG	International Association for the Study of Pain: Non-human Special Interest Group
IBS	irritable bowel syndrome
IC	interstitial cystitis
ICU	intensive care unit
IFN	interferon
IL	interleukin
ISFM	International Society of Feline Medicine
IVAPM	International Veterinary Academy of Pain Management
IVD	intervertebral disk
JCAHO	Joint Commission on Accreditation of Health Care Organization

JHP joint health product
LFT low frequency TENS
LLLT low-level laser therapy
LOX lipoxygenase
LSD lysergic acid diethylamide
LT leukotriene
MAC minimum alveolar concentration
MAOI monoamine oxidase inhibitor
MDMA 3,4-methylenedioxy-methanamphetamine
MEC minimum effective concentration
MED minimum effective dose
MFPS multifactorial pain scale
MMP matrix metalloproteinase
MSC mesenchymal stem cell
NA noradrenaline
NAASM National Alliance of Animal Supplement Manufacturers and Marketers
NAPQI N-acetyl-para-benzoquinoneimine
NASC National Animal Supplement Council
NAVNA North American Veterinary Nutraceutical Association
NCCAM National Center of Complementary and Alternative Medicine
NE norepinephrine
NET norepinephrine transporter
NF nuclear factor
NGF nerve growth factor
NIH National Institutes of Health
NK neurokinin
NMDA N-methyl-D-aspartate
NMES neuromuscular electrical stimulation
NNH number-needed-to-harm
NNT number-needed-to-treat
NO nitric oxide
(i)NOS (inducible) nitric oxide synthase
NRS numeric rating scale
NS nociceptive-specific
NSAID nonsteroidal anti-inflammatory drug
OA osteoarthritis
OCD osteochondrosis dissecans
OHE ovariohysterectomy
OIH opioid-induced hyperalgesia
OTC over-the-counter
OTM oral transmucosal
P2X ionotropic purinoceptor (subtype of ATP receptor)
P54FP tumeric extract
PAG periaqueductal gray
PCA patient-controlled analgesia
PCP phencyclidine
PG prostaglandin
PGI prostacyclin
PHN postherpetic neuralgia
PKC protein kinase C
PMN polymorphonuclear leukocyte (neutrophil)
PNS peripheral nervous system
PPOP persistent postoperative pain
PPS pentosan polysulfate
PSGAG polysulfated glycosaminoglycan
PVF peak vertical force
QOL quality of life
R&D research and development
RBW relative body weight
RCT randomized controlled trial
RER rough endoplasmic reticulum
RNA ribonucleic acid
ROM range of motion
RVM rostral ventromedial medulla
SAMe S-adenosylmethionine
SAP serum alkaline phosphatase
SDS simple descriptive scale
SE serotonin
SERT serotonin transporter
SG substantia gelatinosa
SHT spinohypothalamic tract
SMF static magnet field
SMPC special milk protein concentrate
SNRI serotonin and norepinephrine reuptake inhibitor
sP substance P
SRI serotonin (5-HT) reuptake inhibitor
SRT spinoreticular tract
SSRI selective serotonin reuptake inhibitor
STT spinothalamic tract
TCA tricyclic antidepressant
TCM traditional Chinese medicine
TDF transdermal fentanyl
TDPS transdermal patch delivery system
TENS transcutaneous electrical nerve stimulation
TGF transforming growth factor
TIMP tissue inhibiting metalloproteinase
TNF tumor necrosis factor
TRP transient receptor potential
TTX tetrodotoxin
TX thromboxane
US ultrasound
VAS visual analog scale
VGCC voltage-gated calcium channel
VRS verbal rating scale
VTP Veterinary Thermoplastic
WBC white blood cell
WDR wide dynamic range
WHO World Health Organization

Chapter 1

Background for Pain Management in Small Animal Medicine

INTRODUCTION

The Veterinarian's Oath declares the use of scientific knowledge and skills for 'the relief of animal suffering'. Such commitment is more than a trivial pledge to join a fraternity. In essence, this oath declares a life-long obligation (and privilege) to act as advocates for the well-being of animals. We cannot expect to resolve all pain, but there is no excuse for suffering! In human medicine, the most common reason for patients seeing a physician is because of pain. Comparatively speaking, the physician has a jump-start on treating their patients because most of their patients are able to describe their pain. As the USA humorist and showman, Will Rogers, is noted for stating, "The best doctor in the world is the veterinarian. He can't ask his patients what is the matter – he's got to just know."

'Just knowing' is the *art* of veterinary medicine. And, the art of veterinary medicine is an integration of knowledge with clinical practice. The new graduate has the knowledge base, but lacks the clinical 'practice' to implement 'best medicine'. Accordingly, he/she initiates clinical practice with a 'standard of care'. Two points are to be made here: 1) our knowledge is never complete, and knowledge is our best weapon to fight disease/pain; and 2) as the athlete will attest, you must practice, practice, practice! Over the past couple of decades there has been exponential growth of scientific information regarding pain mechanisms and management as well as therapeutic modalities. It is unrealistic to believe we can practice 'best medicine' without the continued pursuit of current knowledge. Further, we will never develop the 'art' of veterinary medicine unless we practice (implement/observe/implement) pain management for our patients – which they need and deserve.

Pain management in small animal practice can actually be extrapolated to be a reflection of our cultural values. Questionnaire responses from pet owners validate that pets play a major role in our lives. Some owners state that their pet is as important to them as family members; many state that cost is not an issue in treating their pet; and many report that they share the same bed with their pet(s). Considering the physical and emotional role pets play in our lives, there is an expectation that we would make every effort to minimize the pain and suffering of 'man's best friend'.

CLINICAL USE OF ANALGESICS OVER THE PAST 25 YEARS

In 1996, Dohoo and Dohoo[1] reported on factors influencing the postoperative use of analgesics (pain relievers) in dogs and cats by Canadian veterinarians. Data analysis identified gender and the presence of an animal health technician (AHT) in the practice as the two factors that influence pain perception by veterinarians (**Fig. 1**). Unquestionably, AHTs have a marked impact on the well-being of veterinary patients.

Within a 'sister-paper'[2] the same authors revealed that 77% of Canadian veterinarians considered their knowledge of issues related to the recognition and control of postoperative pain to be inadequate, again emphasizing the importance of the AHT within the pain management team.

From a historical perspective (15 years ago), several observations made by Dohoo and Dohoo provide a benchmark by which we can assess our progress in managing patient pain. Firstly, these surveys identified opioids as the postoperative drug of choice, with butorphanol being the most commonly used in both dogs and cats. This is not surprising since for many years it was not a 'controlled' substance. However, butorphanol is a weak opioid, relatively expensive, and has a short duration of analgesic effect (about 40 minutes in the dog). Most notably, butorphanol's sedative effect is much stronger than its pain relieving effect. Accordingly, it is quite easy to misinterpret sedation for analgesia (pain relief), i.e. the animal is still in pain but does not appear so. It is also worth noting that Dohoo and Dohoo identified a 100-fold range in dose reported for the use of butorphanol in dogs following orthopedic surgery, with a 50-fold range reported in cats. This is noteworthy because butorphanol is recognized to be an agent with a 'ceiling effect' in dogs: with the addition of more drug more sedation is noted (dysphoria frequently noted in cats[3]), but not more pain relief.

Secondly, the reluctance to use potent opioid analgesics is likely explained by concerns associated with the administration of these drugs in the postoperative period. The majority of veterinarians had at least one concern in which the risk outweighed the benefit. The three issues that were perceived to pose the greatest risk in dogs were respiratory depression, bradycardia (slow heart rate), and sedation. In cats, the three major risks were perceived as excitement, respiratory depression, and bradycardia (*Table 1*). The concern for use of these agents in cats is regrettable, since these analgesics are effective and do not cause excitement in cats when appropriate

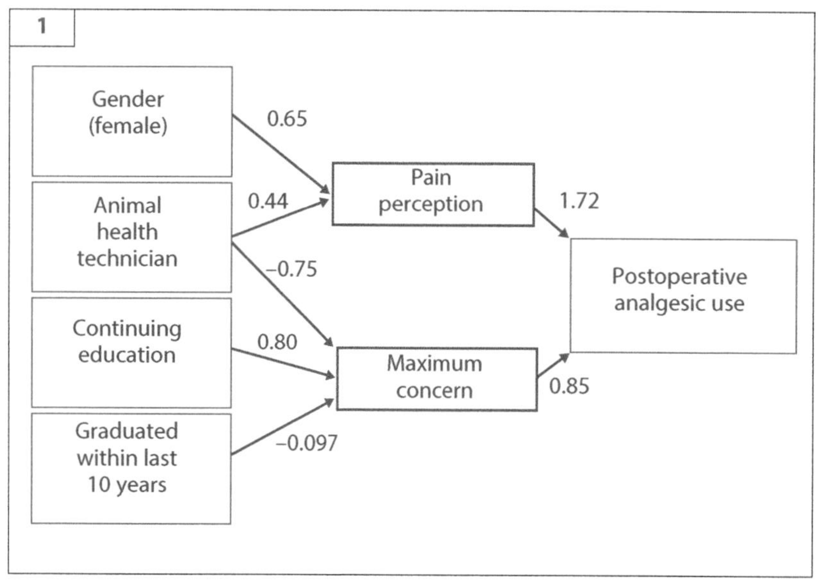

Fig. 1 Path diagram showing the relationship among factors that influence postoperative analgesic use by Canadian veterinarians. Coefficients on arrows leading to pain perception and maximum concern are linear regression coefficients, while those on arrows leading to postoperative analgesic use are odds ratios[3].

TABLE 1: Ranking of the concerns associated with the use of potent opioid agonists in the postoperative period for dogs and cats[2]

	Dogs		Cats	
Concern	Mean	s[b]	Mean	s[b]
Sedation (dog)	3.7	2.2		
Excitement (cat)			5.3	2.7
Respiratory depression	4.4	2.2	4.7	2.4
Bradycardia	4.2	2.2	4.4	2.3
Cost of drugs	2.7	2.1	2.7	2.2
Record keeping	3.1	2.7	3.1	2.7
Human abuse potential	3.4	2.8	3.5	2.9
Damage to surgery site	3.3	2.3	3.5	2.6

[a]Ranking done on a scale where: 1 = disagree completely that the risk outweighs the benefits, 10 = agree completely that the risk out-weighs the benefits.
[b]Standard deviation.

doses are used[4,5]. Finally, the 'need' for postoperative analgesia was influenced by the veterinarians' perception of pain associated with the procedure. Extrapolation from the human experience combined with clinical observation suggests that pain relief is required for at least 12 to 48 hours following surgical procedures[6,7].

Clinical implication: postoperative analgesia should be continued for a minimum of 48 hours. Mechanical hyperalgesia lasts approximately 2–3 days, while thermal hyperalgesia from inflammation lasts approximately 6–7 days.

REASONS FOR UNDER-DOSING ANALGESICS

Evidence suggests that at the turn of the century (2000) as many as 96% of human trauma and surgical intensive care unit (ICU) patients received doses of analgesics lower than those prescribed[8–11]. During this same timeframe (nearly 10 years after the Dohoo studies were published[1,2]), Armitage *et al.*[12] reported on the evaluation of compliance among nursing staff in administration of prescribed analgesic drugs to critically ill dogs and cats. In this study, 22% of dogs and 35% of cats hospitalized in the ICU received decreased analgesics, compared with prescribed orders. The difference in analgesic treatment of cats and dogs was speculated to reflect poor recognition of pain in cats, suggesting the need for additional research in cats. Nevertheless, when a reason for decreasing an analgesic dose was recorded the most common was concern about adverse effects of opioids (e.g. sedation, hypotension, and hypothermia). Interestingly, opioids were the only drugs that were decreased in dosing, supporting the conclusion that concerns relating to adverse effects of opioid drugs was the major reason for dosing changes. Similar concerns have been cited for veterinary patients[2,13] as for human patients[11] in opioid use.

Given the relatively high number of patients in which changes in analgesic dosing is observed, education of clinicians regarding most effective techniques of analgesia is a logical step toward improving efficacy and safety of pain management. Another important factor that has improved analgesic dosing compliance in human patients is education of nursing staff[14].

It is often left to the responsibility of the nursing staff to ensure that opioids are appropriately titrated to achieve pain control without causing excessive sedation or cardiorespiratory depression. In the course of deciding whether to administer analgesics as prescribed, avoidance of these adverse effects may have been prioritized over recognition of signs, of pain in the Armitage study[12], where nursing staff in the ICU used behavioral signs, such as restlessness, vocalization, and an unwillingness to lie down, in assessment of pain intensity. These observations suggest that education in pain management and determination of the significance of adverse effects will improve compliance, providing the care our patients need and deserve.

While pain in veterinary patients is inevitable in the face of surgery, trauma, injury, osteoarthritis, and so on (*Table 2*), suffering is not. It is well established that uncontrolled pain is not only ethically problematic, but physiologically damaging[15]. In recent years pain management modalities have been developed in human medicine to address the evolving understanding of the complexities of the pain experience. Many of these pain treatment strategies have been adopted by veterinary medicine. Pain and suffering should be sought out, the cause identified to the greatest degree possible, and alleviated when feasible.

PAIN AS THE FOURTH CARDINAL SIGN

The American College of Veterinary Anesthesiologists (ACVA) published a position paper on the treatment of pain in animals in the 1998 September issue of the *Journal of the American Veterinary Medical Association*[16]. They stated that animal pain and suffering are clinically important conditions that adversely affect an animal's quality of life, either in the short or long term. Further, the ACVA endorses a philosophy that promotes prevention and alleviation of animal pain and suffering as an important and reasonable therapeutic goal. This is in keeping with the Veterinarian's Oath, pledging to '...use my scientific knowledge and skills for the benefit of society through... the relief of animal suffering...'

The World Health Organization (WHO), International Association of the Study of Pain (IASP), Agency for Health Care Policy and Research (AHCPR), and American Pain Society (APS) are key organizations that have established

TABLE 2: Pain ranking[a] by veterinarians following selected surgical procedures[2]

	Dogs		Cats	
Surgery	**Mean**	**s^b**	**Mean**	**s^b**
Orthopedic[c]	8.18	1.45	8.03	1.59
Cruciate	7.06	1.70	N/A	N/A
Declaw	N/A	N/A	6.58	2.01
Abdominal (non-ovariohysterectomy)[c]	5.46	1.55	5.33	1.57
Ovariohysterectomy[c]	4.20	1.54	4.05	1.63
Castration[c]	3.38	1.40	2.91	1.40
Dentistry[c]	5.07	2.05	4.89	2.10

[a]Ranking done on a scale where: 1 = no pain at all in the first 12 hours following surgery, 10 = the worst pain imaginable.
[b]Standard deviation.
[c]Difference between dogs and cats significant ($P < 0.05$) based on Wilcoxon signed rank test.

standards by which to benchmark pain management efficacy in human medicine. In 2001, the Joint Commission on Accreditation of Health Care Organization (JCAHO) implemented standards for compliance in pain management for human patients. JCAHO required accredited facilities and organizations to develop policies and procedures that formalize their obligation in assessing and managing pain. This mandate included hospitals, long-term-care facilities, home health care agencies, outpatient clinics, and managed-care organizations. Under the JCAHO standards, healthcare providers are expected to be knowledgeable about pain assessment and management, and facilities are expected to promulgate policies and procedures supporting the appropriate use of analgesics and other pain control therapies. All this added up to a heightened awareness of pain as the 'fifth vital sign' (as originally designated by the Department of Veterans Affairs) that should be monitored with the same vigilance as blood pressure, pulse, temperature, and respiratory rate. Among the new requirements, human medical facilities must ask their patients if they are experiencing pain, rate their level of pain, and the results must be documented.

Implementation of the JCAHO standards in human medicine gave a huge boost to awareness of pain in veterinary patients, subsequent to which many institutions have adopted the concept of pain as a fourth cardinal sign (in addition to temperature, pulse, and respiration)[17]. (In contrast to human medicine, blood pressure is seldom considered a cardinal sign in veterinary medicine.) However, changing habits or creating new protocols is often analogous to 'herding cats' and implementing JCAHO standards was seen by many as a 'pain in the assessment'[18]. Building an institutional commitment to pain management is as challenging in veterinary hospitals as it is in human hospitals. Lessons learned in establishing and implementing new standards emphasizes the need for support from all aspects of the hospital (administrative, professional and periprofessionals), as well as simultaneous education for maximum benefit to the patient and minimal frustration for professionals[19].

COMMITTING TO PAIN MANAGEMENT

The following is an eight-step process suggested for institutionalizing a commitment to pain management: The Commitment Strategy[20].

Step 1

Develop an interdisciplinary work group:

- Clarify team goals.
- Create improvement plan.
- Clearly define roles.
- Establish clear communications.
- Note beneficial team behaviors.
- Design well-defined decision making procedures.
- Encourage balanced participation.
- Establish ground rules.
- Build awareness of group process.
- Use a scientific approach.

Step 2

Analyze current pain management practices in your present setting:

- Plan a needs assessment to collect information about pain management in your setting.
- Look for root causes of inadequate pain management in your setting.
- Plan to obtain baseline data for future comparisons and evidence of progress.
- Differentiate the purposes of data collection for quality improvement, external performance measures, and research.

Step 3

Articulate and implement a standard of practice:

- Keep in mind that standards articulate a minimum level of practice to which clinicians can be held legally accountable; guidelines assist practitioners to prevent, diagnose, treat, and manage clinical conditions.
- Use every avenue possible to integrate principles of pain management into the system of care.

Step 4

Establish accountability for pain management:

- A lack of accountability for pain management is one of the major barriers to good pain control.

- Clarify lines of responsibility for pain management among caregivers.
- Embed accountability for pain management in existing systems, such as practice standards, position descriptions, policies and procedure competency statements, and performance reviews.

Step 5
Provide information about pharmacologic and nonpharmacologic interventions to clinicians to facilitate order writing and interpretation and implementation of orders:
- Bring information and education to the wards where clinicians need it most.
- Provide guidelines to help clinicians and pet owners make decisions about treatment of pain.
- Give practitioners tools for change.

Step 6
Promise pet owners a quick response to reports of pain:
- Create consumer demand for quality pain management as an effective way to influence practice patterns.
- Make pain education materials readily available to pet owners.
- Set up a system to inform pet owners that pain relief is an important part of their pets' treatment.

Step 7
Provide education for staff:
- Education requires careful planning.
- Utilize adult learning principles and competency-based education.
- Education should support the process of institutionalizing pain management, not replacing it.

Step 8
Continually evaluate and work to improve the quality of pain management:
- Maintain consistency in your outcome measures.
- Utilize recommendations for outcome monitoring and pet owner surveys.

The (human) APS suggests that every care-providing organization have a pain care committee to study and improve systematically the processes involved in pain management. Experience reveals that this is the most efficient and effective method for building institutional commitment to improving pain management. Whereas such a committee may feel overwhelmed in creating a needs assessment to identify pain management strengths and weaknesses in an institution, the following listing can be used to prioritize the activities of the committee as it gets started and to ensure that important needs are not overlooked.

PERSONALIZING A PAIN MANAGEMENT PLAN

Institutional needs assessment tool: an example of institutional pain management needs assessment, which helps to determine strengths and weaknesses and provides direction for pain management improvement efforts.

An interdisciplinary work group examines and re-examines issues and practices of pain management:
- Is there a process to gain administrative support to develop a pain management improvement work group and carry out a work plan?
- Are there other work groups or committees already in existence that might be able to support the change efforts?
- Can you identify and recruit individuals from a variety of disciplines (e.g. surgeons, interns, AHTs, receptionists) who are interested in improving pain management?
- Can you identify individuals to co-ordinate and lead the interdisciplinary work group?
- Is there hospital experience or training opportunities in continuous quality improvement?

A standard for pain assessment and documentation ensures that pain is recognized and treated promptly:
- Do current AHT documentation forms screen for pain and provide for the ongoing recording of assessment, interventions, and trends of pain relief?

- Is there a written standard of practice that articulates the method and frequency for documenting pain assessments?
- Does your method for pain documentation place pain in a highly visible and prominent position that encourages regular review by all disciplines?
- Are there standards or guidelines that define the maximum acceptable pain intensity that will trigger a change in the pain management plan or consultation?
- Does your system ensure communication of the pain management plan as patients move across settings (e.g. ICU to recovery ward)?
- Do staff have access to a variety of pain assessment tools for populations that are at particular risk for under-treatment of pain (e.g. puppies/kittens, geriatrics, trauma patients)?
- Are there written protocols or do the clinicians' orders include alternatives when pain is unrelieved by the initial patient orders (e.g. titrating with supplemental doses or increasing the dose)?

Explicit policies and procedures guide the use of specialized techniques for analgesic administration:

- Are there policies to govern the use of all available specialized techniques, such as IV analgesia, transdermal drugs, and oxygen cage use?
- Do these policies differentiate roles and responsibilities and describe a mechanism for competency monitoring for all staff involved?
- Do these policies define appropriate indications and contraindications and the acceptable level of patient monitoring?
- Are the necessary medications available in the formulary for specialized analgesic techniques?

Accountability for pain management is clearly defined:

- Is evaluation of pain management performance integrated into annual staff evaluations?
- Are there accountability clauses for pain management in existing policies that address procedures known to cause pain (e.g. invasive procedures)?
- Is there a clear line of consultation for difficult pain problems?
- Is there a competency-based system for orientation and evaluation of staff performance related to the management of pain?
- Do policies and procedures that address pain assessment, documentation, and treatment, and analgesic technology clearly define the role and responsibilities of all healthcare providers involved?

Information about analgesics and nonpharmacologic interventions is readily available to clinicians:

- Are equi-analgesic charts available in all clinical areas where orders and prescriptions are written (i.e. charts showing equivalent results from different drugs)?
- Do staff have easy access to clinical practice guidelines for pain assessment and management, such as the American Animal Hospital Association (AAHA) guidelines and institution-specific guidelines?
- Are there tools to help clinicians select and dose analgesics, such as algorithms, protocols, formulary guidelines, or preprinted orders?
- Are there quick reference materials available to address pain assessment and treatment, such as pocket reference cards or computer help screens?
- Are there 'experts' in pain management that are readily available to staff?
- Is there an easily accessible mechanism that informs staff who they can consult for pain issues?
- Can staff readily provide nondrug interventions (e.g. massage, cold/heat therapy)?

Pet owners informed about the importance of pain relief:

- Are all pet owners informed verbally and in an electronic or printed format that effective pain relief is an important part of their pets' treatment, and that staff will respond promptly to their report of a pet's painful state?
- Is pain management addressed in your 'Patients' Bill of Rights' or organization's mission statement?
- Is information about pain integrated in existing classes or educational materials for pet owners?
- Does each unit maintain a supply of institutional-specific brochures on pain management or pet owner guides for acute, osteoarthritis, and cancer pain or any other pain patient-related materials?
- Are there opportunities for pet owners to learn about pain management at support group meetings?

Staff has ongoing educational opportunities in pain management:

- Has your hospital surveyed its clinicians, AHTs, and receptionists assessing prevalent knowledge and attitudes about pain management?
- Are there ongoing opportunities for case presentations or teaching rounds on patients with pain problems?
- Does your hospital offer a variety of resources on pain management, such as self-directed learning programs, videos, websites, and printed materials?
- Is information about pain management incorporated in employee orientation programs?
- Is there a budget committed to staff education about pain management?

An ongoing process evaluates the outcomes and works to improve the quality of pain management:

- Are pain assessment and management outcomes monitored and reported through a quality assessment and improvement process?
- Does outcome monitoring involve periodic surveys of patients, including questions about pain intensity, expectations and goals, impact of pain, and satisfaction with staff?
- Is staff compliance with documentation standards evaluated?
- Are there ongoing, frequent opportunities to provide staff with feedback about improvements in pain and/or areas for future focus?
- Can you use drug utilization reviews to monitor prescribing practices?
- Are there avenues to analyze cost issues related to unrelieved pain, such as extended length of stay, client satisfaction, rates of revisits for pain?

Defining and changing outdated, obstructive practices takes time and requires an individualized approach as well as support from upper-level management. Not all systems within an institution require change; some can simply be modified slightly to support improvements in pain management. This suggests that some departments and disciplines may merely have to expand their current responsibilities, while others will assume entirely new responsibilities. No matter what the refocus, the AHT must be the driver for improvement and the instrument of implementation.

The American Animal Hospital Association has established a credible 'pain management guidelines for dogs and cats' and is among several sources for guidance (*Table 3*).

TABLE 3: Useful URL links for pain management in dogs and cats

URL	Content
The American Animal Hospital Association www.aahanet.org	Pain management standards
American Association of Feline Practitioners www.catvets.com	Feline behavior guidelines, feeding tips, environmental issues
International Academy of Veterinary Pain Management www.cvmbs.colostate.edu/ivapm/	Professional and pet owner information
Cornell University, College of Veterinary Medicine, Feline Health Center www.felinevideos.vet.cornell.edu	Medicating cats, other feline issues
International Association for the Study of Pain www.iasp-pain.org	Nonhuman special interest group, terminology
Center for Veterinary Medicine, Food and Drug Administration www.fda.gov/cvm	Information about specific approved drugs
United States Pharmacopoeia www.usp.org	Drug information, including modes of action and potential adverse effects
Veterinary Anesthesia and Analgesia Support Group www.vasg.org	Information about specific drugs, protocols and videos of drugs and effects
International Society of Feline Medicine Isfm.net	A feline focus for the veterinary profession
European Medicines Agency (EMA) www.ema.europa.eu/	European Union's FDA equivalent
CATalyst council Catalystcouncil.org	Focus is to ensure that cats receive the proper care and attention they need and deserve

Chapter 2

Communications in Small Animal Medicine Pain Management

ANIMAL HEALTH TECHNICIAN

Animal health technicians (AHTs) are recognized by a number of titles including veterinary technician and veterinary nurse. They are asked to do a variety of tasks within the veterinary hospital and comprise the largest segment of the hospital's total staff. Results of regression analysis in an economic survey of USA veterinarians suggested that the typical veterinarian's gross income increases by $93,311 per year for each additional credentialed veterinary technician per veterinarian in the practice[1]. Given the realities of veterinary practice, practice management, client consultations, and diagnostic/surgical procedures usually consume most of the veterinarian's time. Animal observation, treatment, and assessment in the wards are mainly the responsibility of AHTs. AHTs are in the best position to assess animals both pre- and postoperatively, and they are patient advocates when it comes to managing pain. In an unpublished survey[2] from four teaching hospitals, when veterinarians were asked 'How do you know when your patient is in pain?' the most consistent response was 'because my technician tells me', which is not surprising, given the technicians' role. Additionally, technicians in the intensive care unit observe patients closely for extended periods and are usually the first to notice changes in a patient's status.

'Credentialed' veterinary technicians include those that are recognized through an accredited veterinary technician program.

AHT OPPORTUNITIES IN A CLIENT COMMUNICATIONS ROLE

In the majority of veterinary practices, the AHT conducts preadmission assessments, administers hospitalization patient management, and discharges patients. It is the AHT who has the greatest contact time with both the pet owner and the pet. In most circumstances, the pet owner feels more comfortable in discussions with the AHT than with the attending veterinarian. It is important for the AHT to set the groundwork for professional–client communication in companion animal practice. Accordingly, the AHT plays an important role in establishing the image of the hospital and gaining confidence of the clientele as well as ensuring well-being of the patient.

Following the lead of Dohoo and others[3–9], Vaisanen *et al.*[10] reported on opinions of (Finnish) small animal owners about surgery and pain management in small animals (**Fig. 2**). Overall, owners responded to treatment of animal pain favorably, postoperative analgesia in particular (*Tables 4–6*). Owners' concern over ovariohysterectomy was a major issue and the study pointed out the value for veterinary surgeons to acknowledge these owner concerns.

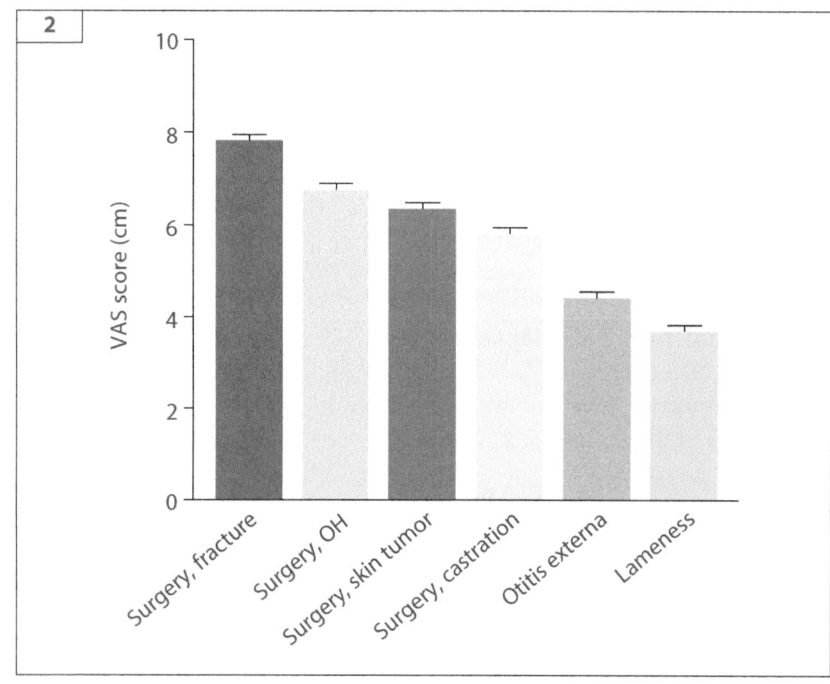

Fig. 2 Owner responses of the perceived pain in various conditions. OH: ovariohysterectomy; VAS: visual analogue scale[8].

TABLE 4: Owner responses to attitude statements

Statement	Owner agreement with statement (%)				
	Agree	Partly	Partly disagree	Disagree	Uncertain
Cost of analgesics is not a problem	77	15	5	2	1
Small animals experience pain like human beings do	71	19	4	2	4
Analgesics are effective in small animals	52	14	1	1	32
Use of analgesics hastens recovery	47	32	8	4	9
Pain after surgery can be an advantage	21	48	13	15	3
Adverse effects of analgesics are rare	17	27	26	12	18
I have enough information on how to manage animal pain	8	25	31	35	1
Pain in small animals is easy to recognize	5	37	37	20	1

TABLE 5: Owner responses to the importance of preoperative information[10]

Information	Owner ratings for importance of information (%)				
	Very important	Somewhat important	Not so important	Not at all important	Information not wanted
Who to contact during animal's postoperative recovery	93	6	1	0	0
Milestones for postoperative recovery	91	6	1	0	0
The most severe risks associated with anesthesia and surgery	83	15	1	0	1
Treatment of my animal's pain	78	20	2	0	0
All the procedures performed on my animal	67	24	7	2	0
All the possible risks associated with anesthesia and surgery	63	30	6	0	1
Monitoring of my animal during anesthesia and hospitalization	60	31	7	1	1
Costs of anesthesia and surgery	26	45	23	6	0

Owners of dogs and cats (n_{tot} = 482) were asked to indicate the importance of selected pieces of information that they could receive if anesthesia and surgery were to be performed on their own animal.

TABLE 6: Owner preferences for use of analgesics[10]

Clinical scenario	Owner preferences (%)			
	Always needed	Likely to be needed, should administer	Not likely to be needed	Not needed
Surgery, fracture repair	81	18	1	0
Surgery, OH	64	29	6	1
Surgery, skin tumour excision	60	35	5	0
Surgery, castration	45	38	14	3
Otitis externa	13	48	34	5
Lameness	9	48	36	7

Owners of dogs and cats (n_{tot} = 482) were asked to indicate whether they would use analgesics in their animal with the presented condition assuming that no pain-alleviating drugs had been administered. With surgery, the use of analgesics referred to their use at home, after the operation. OH: Ovariohysterectomy.

The two items of greatest pet owner concern regarding potential preoperative issues were animal fear or anxiety during hospitalization and postoperative pain (**Fig. 3**). Owners indicated higher levels of concern over the possible negative emotional experiences in their animal than they did over professional aspects of patient care.

Among human surgical patients and parents of children, surgery-related fears have included not only pain, but also concerns over the receipt of kind treatment by healthcare professionals[11] and the qualifications of the anesthesiologist[12]. In Vaisanen *et al.*'s study[10], over 90% of owners deemed the information on relevant milestones for the animal's recovery and information on whom they could contact during recovery as 'very important', emphasizing the valuable role support staff and AHTs can play to ensure client satisfaction.

INFORMED CONSENT AND COMMUNICATIONS

In veterinary medicine, the importance placed on the quality of communication between veterinarians and clients has been emphasized in several studies within the past 10 years[13]. Within the healthcare field, consumer perception is often considered the gold standard for evaluating how effectively we have communicated, and whether the client was fully informed.

Information from the human medicine database has revealed that the manner in which clinicians interact with patients has a major effect on a number of healthcare outcomes, including malpractice risk, satisfaction, compliance with treatment recommendations, and diagnostic accuracy[14]. Unfortunately, the task of communication training in clinical care has traditionally been considered a 'soft skill' in medical education.

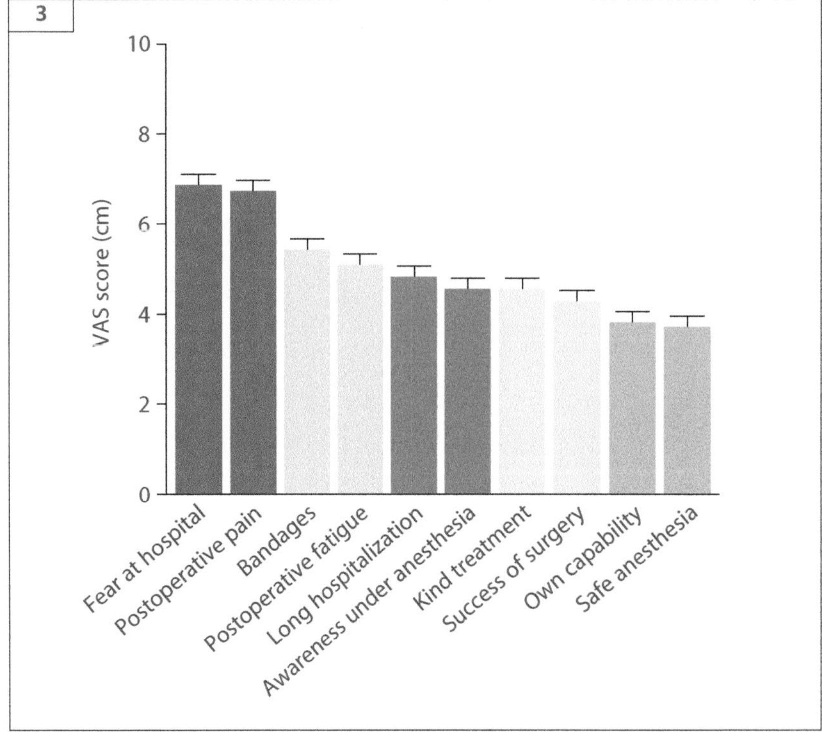

Fig. 3 Owner responses of surgery-related worries. VAS: visual analogue scale[8].

Yet, it is estimated that 75–95% of the information needed by physicians to make a correct diagnosis comes from the medical history reported by the patient, requiring thorough interviewing and communication skills[15]. Dr. Jerome Groopman, in his popular book, *How Doctors Think*[16], preaches the concept of listening as the foundation of diagnostic accuracy, and how straying from this foundation leads to misdirected diagnostics. Beckman *et al.*[17] noted that the major reason behind a patient's decision to pursue litigation against a physician is a perceived lack of caring by the physician. Further, 25% of plaintiffs report poor delivery of medical information and poor listening by the physician. For practitioners, malpractice suits can lead to financial strife, emotional burnout, defensive-medicine practices, and abandonment of practice.

According to Braddock *et al.*[18], true informed consent involves the following:

- Discussion of clinical issues.
- Discussion of options, including 'pros and cons'.
- Discussion of uncertainties of the decision, such as side-effects and after care.
- Assessment of client understanding.
- Exploration of client preferences.

Less than 50% of human visits to the physician included more than one of these elements.

Veterinarians often overlook true informed consent because of the perception that it requires lengthy discussions or because they feel explaining complex procedures may overwhelm clients; yet, most people agree that veterinarians must do more than just give their clients a consent form to sign. Without question, informed consent requires an active conversation between the client and the veterinarian/AHT.

Bonvicini and Cornell[19] suggest the *ask-tell-ask* technique as a tool for client communications. This approach is based on the notion that client education required identifying what the client already knows and building on that knowledge, closing the loop to assess the client's comprehension of the information exchanged. This technique also utilizes the 'chunk and check' approach of giving a portion of the information and then checking with the client to see how well it is understood. Information is provided in short, digestible chunks: perhaps no more than three pieces of information at a time. This process allows assessment of the client's level of knowledge, emotional state, and degree of education. The use of visual information (e.g. diagrams, charts, software programs, drawings, and other client-education tools) is helpful in the 'telling' step.

The final step in the informed consent process is asking the client to restate the conversation exchange in their words, as if they were summarizing for a family member, and then documenting in writing that the consent conversation occurred: what was discussed, who was present, and when and where it took place.

'Owner release forms'

Perhaps this is an opportune time to comment on 'owner release' forms, a term commonly used to describe written consent from the pet owner to administer pain relief associated with a surgical/medical procedure (thereby releasing the veterinarian from making the decision). Such forms are discouraged for two primary reasons: 1) all surgical procedures are painful, and it is inappropriate to perform them without analgesia; 2) such practice takes the standard of care away from the hospital staff and places it at the discretion of the pet owner; the pet owner is now dictating the standard of care!

Cost is most often the driving force for utilizing 'release forms'; however, the cost of pain relief is actually a moot point since most patients can be provided with pain relief for less than USA$3.00/day. More importantly, these release forms project to the public the standard of care, suggesting that pain relief is an optional issue. Perhaps it would be appropriate to replace the 'release form' with a document stating something to the effect: 'It is the ethical standard of our hospital that we administer medications for the relief of pain as we feel is appropriate for the best interest of your pet'. Thereafter, the pet owner renders a signature. This approach serves two objectives: 1) it places the decision for administration of pain relief in the hands of the medical staff, where it should be; and 2) serves as a practice builder by 'advertising' that pain relief is a priority within the hospital. Further, the cost of the analgesics can be 'buried' into other areas of the invoice whereas pain relief can be invoiced as free, allowing the veterinarian to emphasize the importance of pain relief. At the time of patient discharge it can be emphasized that pain relief is included in the 'Best Medicine standard of care'. Alternatively, pain relief can be itemized separately to demonstrate that it was indeed administered.

MEETING CLIENT EXPECTATIONS

Research suggests that veterinarians' perceptions of their clients' needs and expectations, with respect to veterinary healthcare, may differ from what those clients actually need or expect when they bring their animals in for care[20–22]. In human medicine, unmet patient expectations have been shown to contribute to patient dissatisfaction, poor compliance, malpractice litigation, and lower physician satisfaction[23]. Meeting client expectations is the foundation of success in a veterinary practice and, through client communications, the AHT plays a key role. Client communication in companion animal practice was the subject of a special report in the October 1, 2008 issue of the *Journal of the American Veterinary Medical Association*[24].

Five themes relating to client communication were identified (**Fig. 4**):

1. Educating clients:
    - Explaining important information, providing information 'up front', and providing information in various forms.
    - Pet owners want information related to the 'medical' process, diagnosis, treatment, and cost to be presented 'up front'.

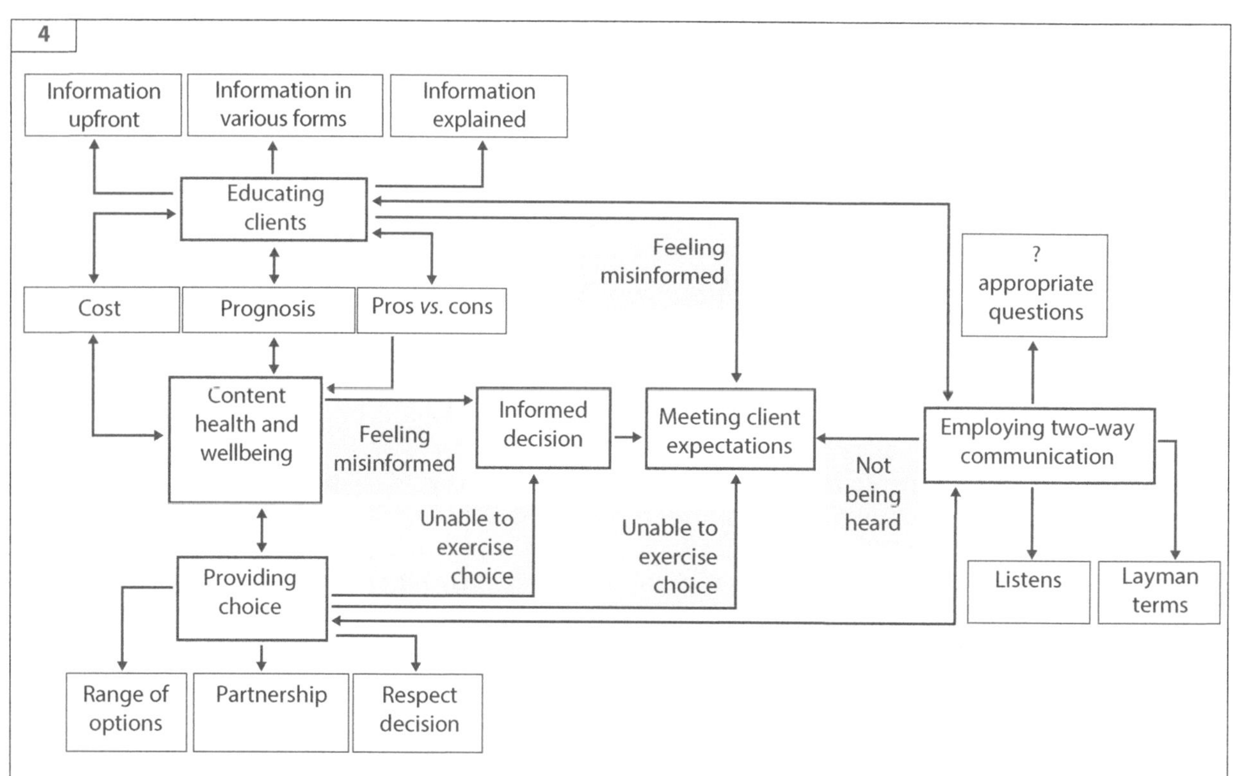

Fig. 4 A conceptual map of the relationships among themes and sub-themes in veterinarian–client communication, and where breakdowns in communication can have an adverse effect on meeting client expectations[22].

- Pet owners expect the provision of additional information in the form of written discharge instructions, handouts, pamphlets, and information packs as well as the cost of care, insurance coverage, and emergency contact information.
- AHTs should be well informed regarding their inventory of client education materials and should take the initiative to offer these materials to pet owners.

2. Providing choice:
   - Providing pet owners with a range of options, being respectful of owners' decisions, and working in partnership with owners.
   - Pet owners feel it is their right to know their options and be presented with the information they need to make informed decisions in terms of potential outcomes for their pets, given the situation and the cost.
   - Pet owners do not want to be pressured or made to feel guilty when making difficult decisions relating to their pets' care.
   - Because pet owners usually feel more relaxed (sometimes less intimidated) when talking with AHTs, clients will often ask their advice, such as 'what would you do if this were your pet?' Under such circumstances the AHT can endorse the veterinarian's recommendation(s) and make the pet owner more comfortable with their decision.

3. Using two-way communication:
   - Using language clients understand, listening to what clients have to say, and asking the right questions.
   - Pet owners expect veterinarians to be able to communicate information in lay terms, and it can be condescending when the veterinarian presents information outside the client's understanding. This is a difficult task for many veterinarians and clients seldom tell veterinarians they don't understand their 'lingo'. This is an area where AHTs prove to be invaluable – as interpreters! AHTs tend to 'walk the talk' of clients and should ensure that the technical jargon used by veterinarians is understood by the pet owner. It has been suggested that clients be provided with small segments of information at a time and then inquire into the client's interpretation and understanding before proceeding ('chunking and checking')[25]. Clients desire easily understood terms and the use of shorter words and sentences to increase their understanding. Illustrations are also helpful for understanding.
   - Listening to clients demonstrates respect, caring, and interest in both the client and pet. Research in human medicine emphasizes the importance of listening in clinical interactions, having found that physicians on average interrupt patients within 12–23 seconds after patients begin their opening statement[26–28].
   - Veterinarians and staff predominantly use a closed-ended questioning style: they ask questions that prompt a simple yes or no response. Including more well-phrased, open-ended, and fewer specific, closed-ended questions reveals more relevant medical information more efficiently and provides a deeper appreciation and understanding of individual clients and their pets.
   - Listening and communicating takes time and many veterinarians operate under the strategy that 'time is money', thereby compromising these issues of importance to the client. Again, here is where the AHT can bridge the gap, providing explanation of technical jargon so that it is easily understood by the client.

4. Breakdowns in communications that affect the clients' experience:
   - Owners feeling that they had been misinformed, that they had not been given all the options, and that their concerns had not been heard.
   - Pet owners tend to 'confide' in AHTs, who they believe will 'guarantee' their interests and the well-being of their pet.

5. Challenging communications:
   - Monetary issues, client misinformation (as might be obtained on the internet or from breeders), involvement of more than one owner, and time limitations.
   - Understandably, veterinarians are under time constraints, and eliciting all of a client's concerns, building client rapport, and involving clients in decision making takes time.
   - Efficient use of AHT time and strengths can make her/him an integral part of the patient management team, analogous to the ward nurse in a human hospital. The AHT can manage many of these communication issues with the advice of their veterinarian, allowing the veterinarian more time to administer her/his trained skills of diagnosis and treatment.

THE AHT AS THE SURROGATE PET OWNER

The AHT can play an integral role in a successful veterinary practice and is often the driving force behind effective pain management. Because of their innate passion for the well-being of animals, they are often considered by clients as surrogate 'parents' for their pets while they are under 'professional' medical care. To be effective in the hospital, the AHT must present two sets of information concerning the animal's well-being: 1) what the patient is doing that might suggest a painful state; and 2) reviewing corrective measures that have already been taken and considered inadequate. This proactive approach delivers necessary patient information in order to gain the veterinarian's confidence in the technician's assessment skills and knowledge of the case, and establishes the 'team' approach to ensure the patient receives the attention and care it needs and deserves.

Chapter 3

Pain Assessment in Small Animal Medicine

THE CHALLENGES OF PAIN ASSESSMENT

The ability to recognize and quantify the signs of pain is important to the development of effective pain relieving strategies. The International Association for the Study of Pain has defined pain as an unpleasant sensory and emotional experience associated with actual or potential tissue damage or described in terms of such damage[1], from which has been extrapolated the following definition for animals: 'Pain in animals is an aversive sensory and emotional experience (a perception), which elicits protective motor actions, results in learned avoidance, and may modify species-specific traits of behavior, including social behavior'. Pain depends on the activation of a discrete set of receptors and neural pathways and is usually or potentially noxious (that is, harmful, damaging to tissue)[2]. Pain is a complex phenomenon involving pathophysiologic and psychological components that are commonly difficult to recognize and interpret in animals. In human patients, pain is what the patient says it is; in animals, pain is what the observer says it is (**Fig. 5**)!

Clinical impression: someone must accept the role as an animal's advocate!

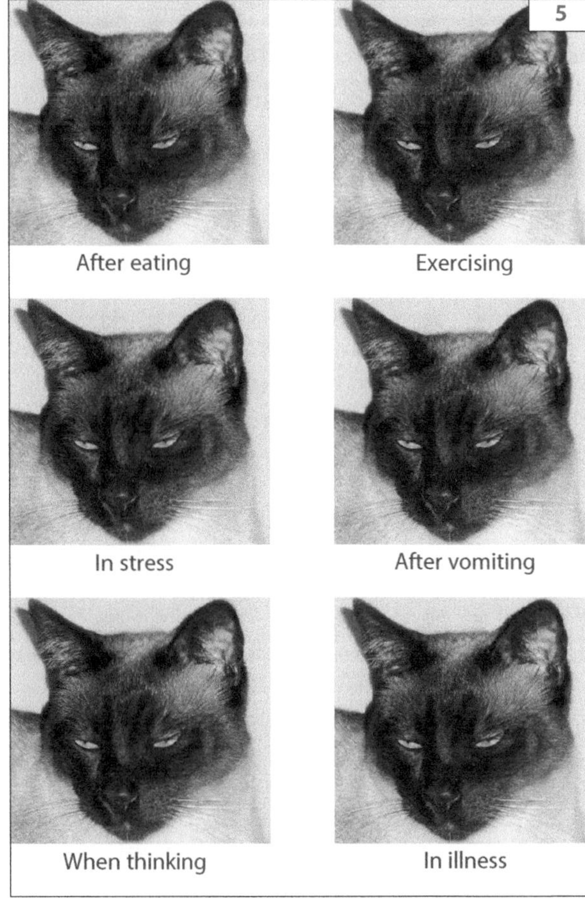

Fig. 5 When is a cat lethargic? (Inspired by Larson's 'How to recognize the moods of an Irish setter'.)

NOCICEPTION

Pain is a sensory and emotional response to a noxious or deleterious stimuli that is unique to the individual; an animal may or may not experience pain in response to nociception. In this respect, the interpretation of pain is analogous to the perception of beauty – it is in the eyes of the beholder. Although the terms 'pain' and 'nociception' are sometimes used interchangeably, they should not be. Nociception is the detection, transduction, and transmission of noxious stimuli (*Table 7*). Think of nociception as the physiologic processes involved in transmitting a pin-prick from the finger to the brain for a subsequent interpretive response.

When nociceptors (free nerve endings) are stimulated by thermal, mechanical, or chemical tissue damage, they send impulses to the central nervous system for modulation and adjustments: the impulse either lives or dies. Thereafter, the impulse is processed in the brain by the conscious animal to be interpreted as pain. An important point to note here is that an animal must be conscious in order for it to sense the nociceptive signals as pain.

Is an ovariohysterectomy a painful procedure?

This can be appreciated by noting plasma cortisol concentrations observed during an ovariohysterectomy[3] (**Fig. 6**). Plasma cortisol level is a physiologic response to 'stress' from the spay. In this report, during the anesthesia time (34–91 minutes) the animals were under a surgical plane of anesthesia (unconscious and showing no behavioral response to the surgery); however, the nociceptive process gave rise to elevated plasma cortisol concentrations during this time. Following extubation (at 91 minutes) and the return to consciousness, there was a continued rise in plasma cortisol concentrations due to a combination of conscious interpretation (cognition) of the nociceptive signaling, sensing a relative hypothermia from anesthesia, and recognition of a 'strange environment'. At this point the subjects demonstrated behavioral changes consistent with pain. The point being made here is that although there was sufficient nociceptive signaling during the anesthesia period to incite the pain state, technically the patient was not in a state of pain because it was unable to interpret signaling because its brain was in a state of unconsciousness.

Variability in the pain response

An individual's response to pain varies with many factors, including age (e.g. young animals generally have a lower tolerance to acute pain, but are less sensitive to emotional stress or anxiety associated with an anticipated painful procedure), gender (females tend to be more sensitive to pain), health status (e.g. ill animals are less capable of tolerating pain than are healthy individuals; severely debilitated animals still experience pain but may not be able to respond), species variation (e.g. cows tend to be 'stoic' [although the adverse effects of pain may be no less] whereas cats are more excitable), breed differences (e.g. working breeds of dogs tend to be more tolerant of pain than toy breeds), and environment (e.g. distractions, such as the presence of people, will alter an animal's behavior). Because of these variables, the fact that animals cannot speak, and the observation that the physiologic process of pain is similar in animals as in humans, it is generally assumed that

TABLE 7: Pain recognition processes

Physiological process	Definition
Transduction	Conversion of energy from a noxious stimulus (mechanical, thermal, or chemical) into nerve impulses by sensory receptors (nociceptors)
Transmission	Transference of neural signals from the site of transduction (periphery) to the CNS (spinal cord and brain)
Modulation	Alterations of ascending signals initially in the dorsal horn and continues throughout the CNS. This includes descending inhibitory and facilitatory input from the brain that influences (modulates) nociceptive transmission at the level of the spinal cord
Perception	Receipt and cognitive appreciation of signals arriving at higher CNS structures as pain

CNS: central nervous system.

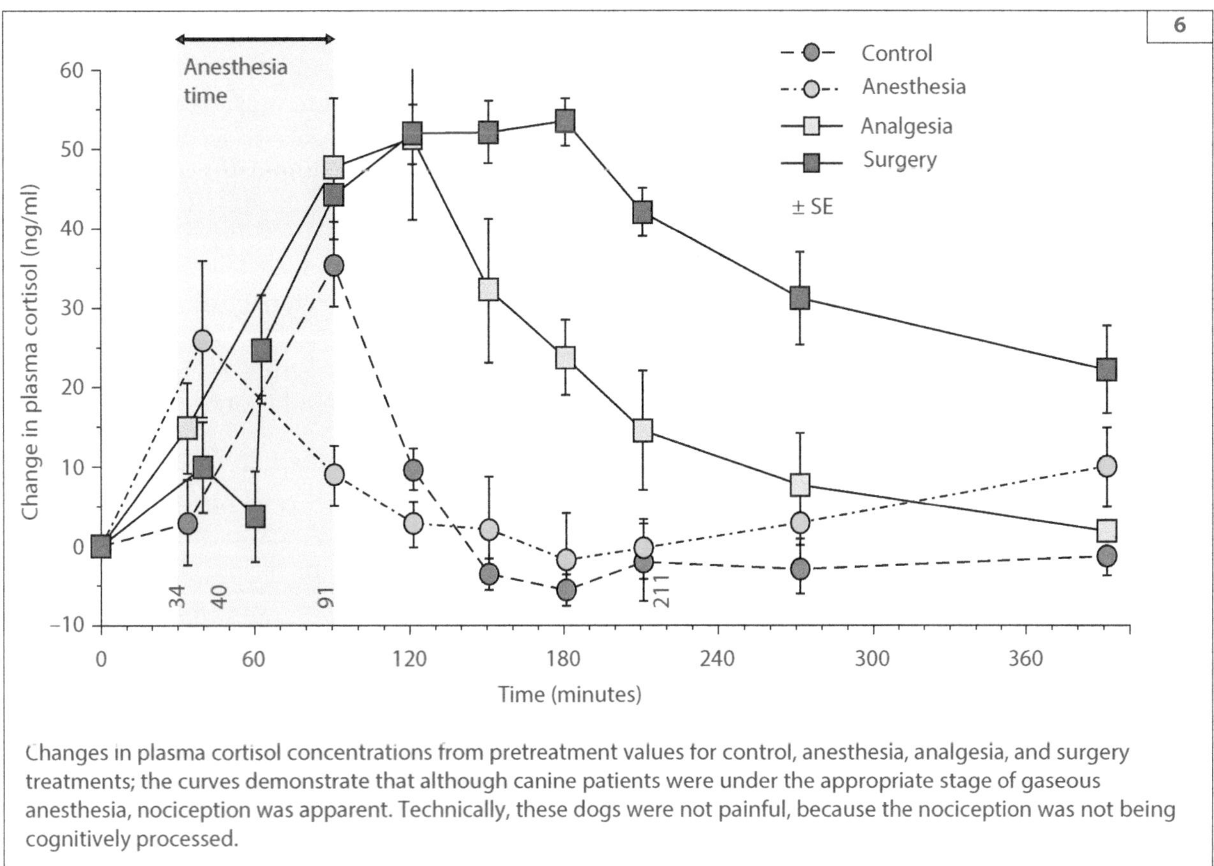

Changes in plasma cortisol concentrations from pretreatment values for control, anesthesia, analgesia, and surgery treatments; the curves demonstrate that although canine patients were under the appropriate stage of gaseous anesthesia, nociception was apparent. Technically, these dogs were not painful, because the nociception was not being cognitively processed.

Fig. 6 Plasma cortisol concentrations during the course of an ovariohysterectomy[3].

if a procedure is painful in humans, then it must also be painful in animals. This is termed the anthropomorphic approach.

Anthropomorphism – attributing human characteristics to animals.

It can be legitimately argued that the key to successful pain management is not necessarily new drugs or high-tech delivery systems, but appropriate use of existing therapies and education about the importance of pain recognition and management[4]. Teaching animal health technicians (AHTs), as well as veterinary students, how to recognize, evaluate, and treat pain in dogs and cats is a challenging task. The 'practice' of veterinary medicine has often been described as the integration of science and art. Graduate AHTs and veterinarians have the science; however, only after considerable participation do these professionals have the experience necessary to develop the 'art' of practice, and in no area of veterinary practice is this more true than pain management.

Identifying pain

Scaling is a common approach to pain assessment. Regardless of the scale used, it is important that the caregiver recognizes the limitations of the scale used and the purpose for which the scale was designed. Points to note: 1) pain scales should be used in conjunction with a thorough physical examination and history to assess every patient; 2) recognize that all pain scales have limitations; 3) individual patient behavior may dictate prompt pain relief, regardless of the pain score; and 4) caregivers should strive for low pain scores in a comfortable appearing patient.

Further, in formal 'scientific' training we are conditioned to recognize the importance of data in terms of a 'mean±standard deviation'. This represents the most common finding or outcome within a population of subjects. We must rethink our approach regarding pain management. Considering the entire population of pets we might treat for pain, we want to ensure that all patients within the population are given the benefit of pain relief that they might need and deserve. Avoid simply targeting the 'mean' responders, because even the so-called 'wimp' should be included, therefore, when in doubt, treat.

Anticipating pain

The pre-emptive scaling of pain 'front ends' effective pain management. This involves a 'best guess' of how invasive a procedure might be for the patient. In general, the more invasive the procedure, the more pain the patient will experience. Pre-emptive scaling is a valuable aid in planning perioperative analgesic strategies, the most impactful focus of postoperative pain management.

Anticipated levels of pain associated with surgical procedures, illness or injuries have been suggested[5]:

Severe to excruciating:

- Neuropathic pain, including nerve entrapment, cervical intervertebral disk herniation, and inflammation (e.g. bacterial, chemical, impingement).
- Extensive inflammation (e.g. peritonitis, fascilitis [especially streptococcal], cellulitis)
- Postsurgical pain when extensive tissue injury or inflammation exists (e.g. triple pelvic osteotomy, tibial plateau leveling osteotomy).
- Multiple fracture repair when extensive soft tissue injury exists (tissue manipulation intraoperatively to be considered) or there is impingement or orthopedic implants on neural tissue.
- Necrotizing pancreatitis.
- Necrotizing cholecystitis.
- Pathologic fractures (often a result of bone cancer).
- Bone cancer (especially following biopsy).
- Meningitis.

Moderate-to-severe and severe (varies with degree of illness or injury):

- Osteoarthritis, acute polyarthritis.
- Intra-articular surgical procedures (e.g. large dogs, extensive manipulation).
- Fracture repair.
- Limb amputation.
- Onychectomy (declaw).
- Peritonitis (e.g. bacterial, urine, bile, pancreatic).
- Capsular pain as a result of organ distention (e.g. pyelonephritis, hepatitis, splenitis, splenic torsion).
- Hollow organ distention.
- Mysenteric, gastric, testicular or other torsions.
- Ureteral, urethral or biliary obstruction.
- After thoracotomy.
- After laparotomy.
- Pleuritis (inflammation of the chest cavity).
- Traumatic diaphragmatic hernia repair (associated with organ and extensive tissue injury).
- Trauma (e.g. orthopedic, extensive soft tissue, head).
- Thoracolumbar disk disease.
- Total ear canal ablation.
- Rewarming after accidental hypothermia.
- Frostbite.
- Cancer pain.
- Mucositis after radiation therapy.
- Thrombosis or ischemia (arterial or venous), aortic saddle thrombosis.
- Hypertrophic osteodystrophy.
- Panosteitis (inflammation within the bone cavity).
- Corneal abrasion or ulceration.
- Glaucoma.
- Uveitis.
- Whelping or queening.
- Mastitis.

Moderate:

- Extracapsular (articular) cruciate repair.
- Minimally invasive orthopedic procedures (e.g. external fixator, tail amputation).
- Laparotomy (i.e. short procedure with minimal manipulation and no inflammation).
- Inguinal hernia repair.

- Diaphragmatic hernia repair (acute, simple with no organ injury).
- Mass removal (depends on location, size, and structures involved; if extensive, pain should be upgraded).
- Early or resolving pancreatitis.
- Soft tissue injuries (e.g. less severe than those previously mentioned).
- Urethral obstruction.
- Ovariohysterectomy (i.e. older obese animals and more extensive procedure).
- Castration (some animals).
- Some dental procedures.
- Eye enucleation.

Mild-to-moderate:
- Ovariohsterectomy (young animals).
- Castration (some animals).
- Lump removal.
- Some ophthalmic surgical procedures.
- Some dental procedures.
- Some lacerations.
- Cystitis.
- Otitis.
- Chest drains.

Mild:
- Early, resolving, or simple involvement of conditions mentioned previously.

It is helpful to have knowledge of a surgical procedure, so as to anticipate more accurately the pain associated with recovery (*Table 8*). The head and face of animals are highly innervated and surgeries involving the eye, periorbital structures, ears, nose, and teeth are painful. Following

TABLE 8: The American Animal Hospital Association/American Association of Feline Practitioners pain management guidelines for dogs and cats further recognizes frequently overlooked causes of pain (www.aahanet.org)

System	Condition
Cardiopulmonary	Congestive heart failure (pulmonary edema and pleural effusion); pleuritis, cerebral vascular accident, thromboembolism (clot)
Oncology	Any/all cancers
Dermatology	Otitis, severe pruritus, burns, chronic wounds; abscess, cellulitis, clipper burns, urine scalding, severe chin acne
Dental	Oral tumors, feline oral resorptive lesions ('neck' lesions), fractures (no matter how small), tooth abscess, ulcers, stomatitis
Gastrointestinal	Constipation, obstipation, obstruction, megacolon; anal sac impaction, hemorrhagic gastroenteritis, pancreatitis, gastric dilatation/volvulus, foreign body
Musculoskeletal	Most often overlooked in cats. Muscular soreness, arthritis, degenerative joint disease, tendon or ligament injury, intervertebral disk disease, facet pain of spondylosis, osteodystrophy, dislocations
Ocular	Corneal disease and ulcers, glaucoma, uveitis
Urogenital	Uroliths, ureteroliths, queening/whelping, feline lower urinary tract disease/interstitial cystitis, acute renal failure, enlarged kidneys, lower urinary tract infections, urinary obstruction. Vaginitis (especially in obese cats)
Hospital	Restraint (examination, obtaining blood procedures and urine samples, radiographs, and ultrasound; even gentle handling and hard surfaces can increase pain in an already painful animal). Urinary/IV catheterization, bandaging, surgery, thoracocentesis, chest tube placement and drainage procedures, abdominocentesis. Manual extraction of stool and anal sac expression (especially in cats)
Surgical	Ovariohysterectomy, castration, declaw (regardless of method used), growth removal, and all other surgical procedures
Neurologic	Diabetic neuropathy

anesthesia recovery, animals may shake their heads excessively, rub or paw at the surgical site, and vocalize. Orthopedic procedures are generally painful because of trauma to large muscle masses, and amputation, especially high on the limb, induce severe pain. Thoracotomy induces severe pain and because respiration continues to move structures at the surgical site well after the surgery is completed, these patients need postoperative pain relief for an extended period of time. Surgeries involving the cervical vertebrae tend to be more painful than procedures involving the thoracic or lumbar vertebrae. Perirectal procedures (i.e. perianal fistulas, anal sacculectomy and rectal strictures) are generally painful and animals often rub and scoot their buttocks in response to pain.

Species-specific and individual responses to pain are quite varied; therefore, it is important for those staff evaluating animals for pain to have a thorough understanding of typical species-specific and individual behaviors. An important part of determining whether an animal is in pain is the ability to recognize departure from normal. Herein, it is important to appreciate owner/handler observations, because they may be able to recognize subtle behaviors indicative of pain that would otherwise go unnoticed.

PATIENTS' EXPRESSION OF PAIN

The behavioral and physiologic characteristics associated with pain in cats and dogs are listed below[5,6]. (These signs may not be consistently present in painful states and some may be present in an animal simply anxious or excited.)

Abnormal posture:

- Hunched up guarding or splinting of the abdomen.
- 'Praying' position (forequarters on the ground, hindquarters in the air).
- Sitting or lying in an abnormal position.
- Not resting in a normal position (e.g. sternal or curled up).

Abnormal gait:

- Stiff.
- No-to-partial weight bearing on an injured limb.
- Slight to obvious limp.

Abnormal movement:

- Thrashing.
- Restless.
- No movement when not sleeping.
- Vocalization (dogs tend to whine or whimper; cats hiss or growl).
- Screaming.
- Whining (intermittent, constant, or when touched).

Miscellaneous:

- Looking, licking, or chewing at the painful area (behaviors can lead to self-mutilation).
- Hyperesthesia or hyperalgesia.
- Allodynia ('painful' response to 'nonpainful' stimulus, e.g. light touch).
- Change in personality or attitude (normally quiet and docile animal suddenly becomes aggressive, or an aggressive animal becomes quiet).
- Change in facial expression (eyes become dull, and pupils may be dilated). Pinning of the ears, grimacing, and sleepy or photophobic (sensitive to light) appearance.
- Behavioral characteristics associated with pain in cats and dogs, but may also be associated with poor general health (medical problems).
- Restless or agitated.
- Trembling or shaking.
- Tachypnea or panting.
- Weak tail wag.
- Low carriage of tail.
- Depressed or poor response to caregiver.
- Head hangs down.
- Not grooming (ruffled fur, a greasy appearance indicative of a lack of grooming, and piloerection [hair standing up] may indicate pain).
- Appetite decreased, picky, or absent.
- Dull.
- Lying quietly and not moving for hours and does not dream.
- Stuporous (diminished response to stimulation).
- Urinates or defecates and makes no attempt to move.
- Recumbent and unaware of surroundings.
- Unwilling or unable to walk.
- Bites or attempts to bite caregiver.

May also be associated with apprehension or anxiety:
- Restless or agitated.
- Trembling or shaking.
- Tachypnea or panting.
- Weak tail wag.
- Low tail carriage.
- Slow to rise.
- Depressed (poor response to caregiver).
- Not grooming.
- Bites or attempts to bite caregiver.
- Ears pulled back.
- Restless.
- Barking or growling (intermittent, constant, or when approached by caregiver).
- Growling or hissing (intermittent, constant, or when approached by caregiver).
- Sitting in the back of the cage or hiding under a blanket (cat).

May be normal behavior:
- Reluctant to move head (eye movement only).
- Stretching all four legs when abdomen touched.
- Penile prolapse.
- Cleaning (licking a wound or incision).

Physiologic signs that can be associated with pain:
- Tachypnea or panting.
- Tachycardia (mild, moderate, or severe).
- Dilated pupils.
- Hypertension.
- Increased serum cortisol and epinephrine (adrenaline).

Dogs in pain tend:
- Not to yawn.
- Not to 'wet dog shake'.
- To exhibit restlessness.
- To want to sit rather than lay down and hold their head in a hanging position ('hang sit') position.

Physiologic parameters, including heart rate, respiratory rate, blood pressure, and temperature, are not consistent or reliable indicators of pain[6–9]. Further, pain is usually accentuated in the presence of infection.

Although many different 'tools' have been used in human medicine to assess pain, few have been used in veterinary medicine and currently there is no suitable tool to assess pain accurately in animals. The most effective 'litmus test' for pain is a response to analgesia. If the administration of pain relief returns the animal to normal behavior, including eating, sleeping, dreaming, yawning, normal stretching, grooming, and general appearance of well-being, then the relief was needed because the animal was in pain! With this in mind, analgesics can serve as diagnostic tools as well as treatment medications.

Behavioral change as a pain response

Most pain assessment schemes use behavior as an indicator. When pain is assessed in animals, the patient cannot convey the sensory and emotional experience by any means other than its behavior. The advantage of using behavioral indicators is that changes in behavior are immediate in their appearance, while physiologic indices, such as cortisol, take time to quantify[10]. In addition, it has been revealed that changes in behavioral patterns correspond with physiologic signs of distress under clinical circumstances such as ovariohysterectomy[6,11]. The presence of more than one behavioral indicator of pain (posture, facial expression, specific movements, and vocalization) helps to increase confidence in identifying pain. A drawback of behavior assessment is that only levels of pain that cause the animal to alter its behavior in some way can be conveyed to the observer.

Vocalization is considered an important indicator of pain in different species, but is often over-emphasized, especially by pet owners. Animals may vocalize for a variety of reasons (pain, attention getting, anxiety, stress). Vocalization tends to be an insensitive and nonspecific indicator of pain and should not be relied on as the sole criterion for determining whether an animal requires treatment for pain. On the other hand, pet owners may not think their pet is in pain if it is not vocalizing. Frequently animals are presented to the hospital three-legged lame (using only three of their four legs). When asked if their pet is in pain, a common response is 'I don't think so'. This response is usually based upon the animal's absence of vocalization. In truth, animals refuse to use a limb either because they cannot (musculoskeletal restraints such as contracted muscles, congenital or developmental defects) or because they will not (due to pain). Pain is the most common reason for guarding a limb, yet because the pet is not vocalizing, the pet owner tends to think their pet is not in pain.

Pain scales

Various acute pain assessment measures have been used by researchers to quantify pain. These include verbal rating scales (VRSs), simple descriptive scales (SDSs), numeric rating scales (NRSs), and visual analog scales (VASs), all of which have their limitations. The VRS and SDS schemes appear simple to use, rating pain as none, mild, moderate, or severe; however, these schemes lack sensitivity due to the limited number of categories, thereby limiting discrimination between the different levels of pain. A study investigating the number of response levels needed to assess pain intensity in human chronic pain patients reported that a 10- to 20-level scale was needed to provide sufficient levels of discrimination for differentiating pain intensity[12]. Using the NRS scheme, the observer assigns a numerical score (typically on a 0 to 10 scale) of pain intensity for a given listing of traits indicating pain. This can be problematic for several reasons:

1. Selection of traits indicative of pain are often arbitrary and not validated. When authors cite that their NRS scale has been 'validated', arguably, this simply means that the scale has been used before. There are several forms of validity, including content, criterion, construct, and so on. The simplest form of content validity is face validity, which is founded on expert opinion to establish whether, 'on the face of it', the items appear relevant to, and encompassing of, the test attribute[13].
2. The cut-off total added score, above which indicates a pain state dictating pain relief, is totally arbitrary.
3. 'Weighting' of the different traits is seldom present (i.e. a lack of specificity). It is likely that all changes from normal behavior are not of equal importance as indicators of pain. For example, vocalization can contribute to a high total pain score if the observer considers it to be one of the highest signs of pain. Further, a dilemma: is the quiet animal in the rear of the cage comfortable and without pain or is it in so much pain that it refuses to move?

The VAS has proved to be sensitive, reproducible, and feasible in human studies of evaluating pain[14] and has been used in veterinary practice[15,16]. Potential drawbacks are that observers must be experienced in assessing pain and trained in the use of the VAS. The VAS is a ruler (usually 100 mm in length) with only a description of the limits of pain placed at either end of the scale such that 0 represents no pain and 100 represents the worst pain possible. The observer (or human patient) is asked to mark anywhere along the scale were the perceived (or experienced) pain would fall. VAS is one of the easiest pain scoring systems to implement into the hospital setting, and although it is liable to have a higher amount of observer variation, it is often considered to be more sensitive than NRS or SDS because defined categories are not used[17]. In contrast, criticism levied against the VAS is that it can give a false impression of increased sensitivity, appreciating that a person scoring their own pain can only differentiate between a maximum of 39 distinct levels of pain[18,19].

Multidimensional scales

Historical limitations of scales used to assess pain have been the assessment of pain on intensity alone. Such limitations have led to development of multidimensional scales. The McGill pain questionnaire[20] was developed in human medicine to provide a quantitative measure of clinical pain that could be treated statistically and would also take account of the sensory and affective quantities of pain in addition to intensity. Adopting the same broad protocols, in 2001 Holton *et al*. developed a composite measure pain scale (CMPS) in dogs[21]. The prototype CMPS was based on seven behavioral categories: posture, comfort, vocalization, attention to wound, demeanor, mobility, and response to touch (each containing several expressions describing the dog's behavior). This instrument takes the form of a questionnaire completed by the observer during a prescribed examination procedure, which includes observation of spontaneous behavior and assessment of interactive behavior at rest and during specified movements.

The CMPS was actually preceded by the University of Melbourne pain scale, reported by Firth and Haldane in 1999, which is based upon both behavioral and physiologic measurements (7 *overleaf*)[17]. Six categories were derived from a review of the pain measurement literature in dogs: physiologic variables, response to palpation, activity, mental status, posture and vocalization; weights are assigned to each item subjectively according to the developers' perception of how much pain it implied. Assessment of the animal's mental status, heart rate, and respiratory rate are based on the change from its presurgery status, which limits the scale's use to circumstances in which measurements can be made before surgery. Details on how item selection was determined, especially physiologic signs (as well as pupil dilation), which inconsistently show a relationship to pain intensity, and proof of content validity have been questioned[22].

Maturation of the CMPS gave rise to the 'Glasgow Composite Measure Pain Scale'[21], a multidimensional scheme made up of a number of sections (**Fig**. **8** *page 37*). Although it is detailed, its on-going refinement may result in increased utilization. Clear and specific definitions of each word or expression used in a scale are considered to be necessary to ensure that it is used consistently.

The Glasgow short form Composite Measure Pain Scale (CMPS-SF) can be applied quickly and reliably in a clinical setting and has been designed as a clinical decision making tool which was developed for dogs in acute pain (**Fig**. **9**)[23]. It includes 30 descriptor options within six behavioral categories, including mobility. Within each category, the descriptors are ranked numerically according to their associated pain severity, and the person carrying out the assessment chooses the descriptor within each category which best fits the dog's behavior/condition.

The Glasgow Pain Scales are copyrighted, requiring approval for reproduction and use.

The Colorado State University Veterinary Medical Center (CSUVMC) has developed acute pain scales for both the canine and feline that integrate many features of previously described scales (**Fig**. **10, Fig**. **11** *pages 40, 41*). These scales are single-page, user-friendly, very practical, and incorporate multidimensional expressions of pain. They can be down loaded from:

http://www.manageanimalpain.com/ivapm/attachments/102_Feline%20Acute%20Pain%20Scale.pdf

http://www.manageanimalpain.com/ivapm/attachments/102_Canine%20Acute%20Pain%20Scale.pdf.

The CSUVMC scales include psychological and behavioral signs of pain and palpation responses. They also evaluate body tension as an additional parameter. A VAS (0–4, rather than a 100 mm scale) and color-coding of the different scalings is integrated into the scheme. For the five levels of pain depicted on the scales, there are artist's suggestions of the animals' characteristic posturing and expressions.

7

CATEGORY	DESCRIPTOR	SCORE
Physiologic data		
a)	Physiologic data within reference range	0
b)	Dilated pupils	
c) *Choose only one*	Percentage increase in heart rate relative to preprocedural rate	
	> 20%	1
	> 50%	2
	> 100%	3
d) *Choose only one*	Percentage increase in respiratory rate relative to preprocedural rate	
	> 20%	1
	> 50%	2
	> 100%	3
e)	Rectal temperature exceeds reference range	1
f)	Salivation	2
Response to palpation		
Choose only one	No change from preprocedural behavior	0
	Guards/reacts* when touched	2
	Guards/reacts* before touched	3
Activity		
Choose only one	At rest-sleeping	0
	- semiconscious	0
	- awake	1
	Eating	0
	Restless (pacing continuously, getting up and down)	2
	Rolling, thrashing	3
Mental status		
Choose only one	Submissive	0
	Overtly friendly	1
	Wary	2
	Aggressive	3
Posture		
a)	Guarding or protecting affected area (includes fetal position)	2
b) *Choose only one*	Lateral recumbency	0
	Sternal recumbency	1
	Sitting or standing, head up	1
	Standing, head hanging down	2
	Moving	1
	Abnormal posture (e.g. prayer position, hunched back)	2
Vocalization†		
Choose only one	Not vocalizing	0
	Vocalizing when touched	2
	Intermittent vocalization	2
	Continuous vocalization	3

The pain scale includes 6 categories. Each category contains descriptors of various behaviors that are assigned numeric values. The assessor examines the descriptors in each category and decides whether a descriptor approximates the dog's behavior. If so, the value for that descriptor is added to the patient's pain score. Certain descriptors are mutually exclusive (e.g. a dog cannot be in sternal recumbency and standing up at the same time). These mutually exclusive descriptors are grouped together with the notation 'choose only one'. For mental status, the assessor must have completed a preprocedural assessment of the dog's dominant/aggressive behavior to establish a baseline score. The mental status score is the absolute difference between preprocedural and postprocedural scores. The minimum possible total pain score is 0 points, the maximum possible total pain score is 27 points.

*Includes turning head toward affected area; biting, licking, or scratching at the wound; snapping at the handler; or tense muscles and a protective (guarding) posture. †Does not include alert barking.

Fig. 7 University of Melbourne Pain Scale for dogs[17].

8

First, approach the kennel (not wearing 'surgical greens' or a laboratory coat).
While approaching, look at the dog's behavior and reactions.

Look at the dog's posture. Does it seem:

Rigid ☐ Neither of these ☐

Hunched or tense ☐

Does the dog see to be:

Restless ☐ Comfortable ☐

If the dog is vocalizing, is it:

Crying or whimpering ☐ Screaming ☐

Groaning ☐ Not vocalizing/none of these ☐

If the dog is paying attention to its wound, is it:

Chewing ☐ Ignoring the wound ☐

Licking, looking, or rubbing ☐

Approaching the kennel door, call the dog's name. Then open the door and encourage the dog to come. Assess the dog's character as you observe the dog's response.

Does the dog seem to be:

Aggressive ☐ Quiet or indifferent ☐

Depressed ☐ Happy and content ☐

Disinterested ☐ Happy and bouncy ☐

Nervous, anxious, or fearful ☐

During this procedure, did the dog seem to be:

Stiff ☐ None of these ☐

Slow or reluctant to rise or sit ☐ Assessment not carried out ☐

Lame ☐

Next, assess the dog's response to touch. If the animal has a wound, apply gentle pressure to the wound using two fingers in an area approximately 2 inches (5 cm) around the wound. If the position of the wound is such that it is impossible to touch, then apply the pressure to the closest point to the wound. If there is no wound, apply the same pressure to the stifle and surrounding area.

When touched, did the dog:

Cry ☐ Growl or guard wound ☐

Flinch ☐ None of these ☐

Snap ☐

Fig. 8 Glasgow Composite Measure Pain Scale[21]. *(continued)*

***Terms used in the Glasgow scale*:**

Posture
Rigid: Animal lying in lateral recumbency, legs extended or partially extended in a fixed position.
Hunched: When animal is standing, its back forms a convex shape with abdomen tucked up, or, back in a concave shape with shoulders and front legs lower than hips.
Tense: Animal appears frightened or reluctant to move, overall impression of tight muscles; animal can be in any body position.
Normal body posture: Animal may be in any position, appears comfortable, muscles relaxed

Activity
Restless: Moving body position, circling, pacing, shifting body parts, unsettled.
Comfortable: Animal resting and relaxed, no avoidance or abnormal body position evident, or settled, remains in same body position, at ease.

Vocalization
Crying: Extension of the whimpering noise, louder and with open mouth.
Whimpering: Often quiet, short, high pitched sound, frequently closed mouth (whining).
Groaning: Low moaning or grunting deep sound, intermittent.
Screaming: Animal making a continual high pitched noise, inconsolable, mouth wide open.

Wound attention
Chewing: Using mouth and teeth on wound area, pulling stitches.
Licking: Using tongue to stroke area of wound.
Looking: Turning head in direction of area of wound.
Rubbing: Using paw or kennel floor, etc. to stroke wound area.
Ignoring: Paying no attention to wound area.

Demeanor
Aggressive: Mouth open or lip curled showing teeth, snarling, growling, snapping or barking.
Depressed: Dull demeanor, not responsive, shows reluctance to interact.
Disinterested: Cannot be stimulated to wag tail or interact with observer.
Nervous: Eyes in continual movement, often head and body movement, jumpy.
Anxious: Worried expression, eyes wide with white showing, wrinkled forehead.
Fearful: Cowering away, guarding body and head.
Quiet: Sitting or lying still, no noise, will look when spoken to, but not respond.
Indifferent: Not responsive to surroundings or observer.
Content: Interested in surroundings, has positive interaction with observer, responsive and alert.
Bouncy: Tail wagging, jumping in kennel often vocalizing with a happy and excited noise.

Mobility
Stiff: Stilted gait, slow to rise or sit, may be reluctant to move.
Slow to rise or sit: Slow to get up or sit down but not stilted in movement.
Reluctant to rise or sit: Needs encouragement to get up or sit down.
Lame: Irregular gait, uneven weight bearing when walking.
Normal mobility: Gets up and lies down with no alteration from normal.

Touch response
Cry: A short vocal response; looks at area and opens mouth, emits a brief sound.
Flinch: Painful area is quickly moved away from stimulus either before or in response to touch.
Snap: Tries to bite observer before or in response to touch.
Growl: Emits a low prolonged warning sound before or in response to touch.
Guard: Pulls painful area away from stimulus or tenses local muscles in order to protect from stimulus.
None: Accepts firm pressure on wound with no reaction.

9

SHORT FORM OF THE GLASGOW COMPOSITE PAIN SCALE

Dog's name ____________________

Hospital Number ___________ Date / / Time

Surgery Yes/No (delete as appropriate)

Procedure or Condition ____

In the sections below please circle the appropriate score in each list and sum these to give the total score.

A. Look at dog in kennel

Is the dog?

(i)		(ii)	
Quiet	0	Ignoring any wound or painful area	0
Crying or whimpering	1	Looking at wound or painful area	1
Groaning	2	Licking wound or painful area	2
Screaming	3	Rubbing wound or painful area	3
		Chewing wound or painful area	4

In the case of spinal, pelvic or multiple limb fractures, or where assistance is required to aid locomotion do not carry out section **B** and proceed to **C**. *Please tick if this is the case* ☐ then proceed to C.

B. Put lead on dog and lead out of the kennel.

When the dog rises/walks is it?

(iii)	
Normal	0
Lame	1
Slow or reluctant	2
Stiff	3
It refuses to move	4

C. If it has a wound or painful area, including abdomen, apply gentle pressure 2 inches round the site.

Does it?

(iv)	
Do nothing	0
Look round	1
Flinch	2
Growl or guard area	3
Snap	4
Cry	5

D. Overall

Is the dog? (v)		*Is the dog?* (vi)	
Happy and content or happy and bouncy	0	Comfortable	0
Quiet	1	Unsettled	1
Indifferent or non-responsive to surroundings	2	Restless	2
Nervous or anxious or fearful	3	Hunched or tense	3
Depressed or non-responsive to stimulation	4	Rigid	4

Total Score (i+ii+iii+iv+v+vi) = ____________

Fig. 9 Short form of the Glasgow Composite Pain Scale[23].

10

Colorado State University
Veterinary Medical Center

Feline Acute Pain Scale

Date ____________________

Time ____________________

Rescore when awake

□ Animal is sleeping, but can be aroused – Not evaluated for pain
□ Animal can't be aroused, check vital signs, assess therapy

Pain Score	Example	Psychological & Behavioral	Response to Palpation	Body Tension
0	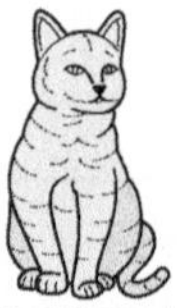	□ **Content and quiet** when unattended □ **Comfortable** when resting □ Interested in or **curious** about surroundings	□ **Not bothered** by palpation of wound or surgery site, or to palpation elsewhere	Minimal
1	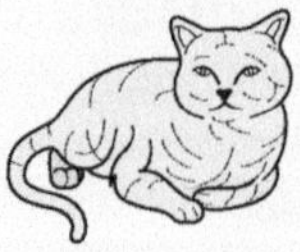	□ **Signs are often subtle and not easily detected in the hospital** setting; more likely to be detected by the owner(s) at home □ Earliest signs at home may be **withdrawal from surroundings or change in normal routine** □ In the hospital, may be content or slightly unsettled □ **Less interested** in surroundings but will look around to see what is going on	□ May or may not react to palpation or wound or surgery site	Mild
2	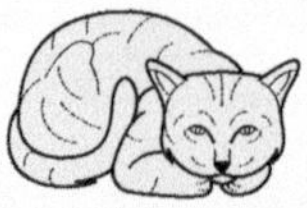	□ Decreased responsiveness, **seeks solitude** □ **Quiet,** loss of brightness in eyes □ **Lays curled up or sits tucked up** (all four feet under body, shoulders hunched, head held slightly lower than shoulders, tail curled tightly around body) with eyes partially or mostly closed □ **Hair coat appears rough** or fluffed up □ May intensively groom an area that is painful or irritating □ Decreased appetite, **not interested in food**	□ **Responds aggressively or tries to escape** if painful area is palpated or approached □ Tolerates attention, may even perk up when petted as long as painful area is avoided	Mild to Moderate **Reassess analgesic plan**
3	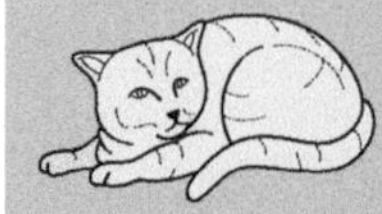	□ Constantly **yowling, growling, or hissing** when unattended □ May bite or chew at wound, but **unlikely to move** if left alone	□ **Growls or hisses at non-painful palpation** (may be experiencing allodynia, wind-up, or fearful that pain could be made worse) □ **Reacts aggressively** to palpation, **adamantly pulls away** to avoid any contact	Moderate **Reassess analgesic plan**
4	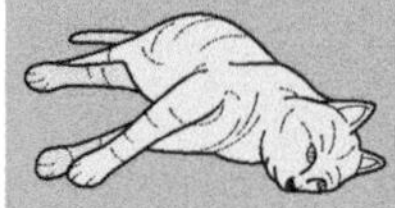	□ Prostrate □ Potentially **unresponsive** to or unaware of surroundings, difficult to distract from pain □ Receptive to care (even mean or wild cats will be more tolerant of contact)	□ **May not respond** to palpation □ **May be rigid to avoid painful movement**	Moderate to Severe **May be rigid to avoid painful movement** **Reassess analgesic plan**

Right

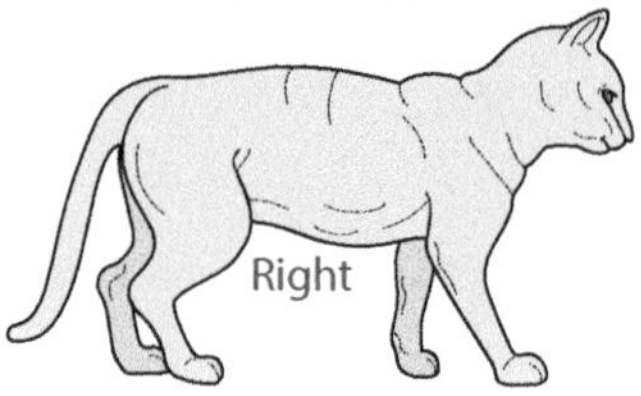

○ Tender to palpation
× Warm
■ Tense

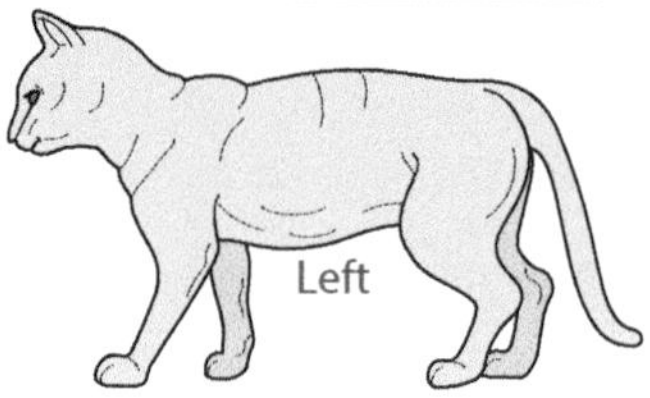

Left

Comments ____________________

Fig. 10 Colorado State University Veterinary Medical Center Feline Acute Pain Scale.

11

Colorado State University
Veterinary Medical Center

Canine Acute Pain Scale

Date ______________________

Time ______________________

Rescore when awake
☐ Animal is sleeping, but can be aroused – Not evaluated for pain
☐ Animal can't be aroused, check vital signs, assess therapy

Pain Score	Example	Psychological & Behavioral	Response to Palpation	Body Tension
0		☐ **Comfortable** when resting ☐ **Happy, content** ☐ Not bothered by wound or surgery site ☐ Interested in or curious about surroundings	☐ **Not tender** to palpation of wound or surgery site, or to palpation elsewhere	Minimal
1		☐ **Content to slightly unsettled** or restless ☐ **Distracted easily** by surroundings	☐ **Reacts to palpation** of wound, surgery site, or other body part by **looking around, flinching,** or **whimpering**	Mild
2		☐ Look **uncomfortable** when resting ☐ May **whimper** or cry and may **lick or rub wound** or surgery site when unattended ☐ Droopy ears, **worried facial expression** (arched eye brows, darting eyes) ☐ **Reluctant to respond** when beckoned ☐ **Not eager to interact** with people or surroundings but will look around to see what is going on	☐ Flinches, whimpers cries, or guards/pulls away	Mild to Moderate **Reassess analgesic plan**
3		☐ **Unsettled, crying, groaning, biting or chewing** wound when unattended ☐ **Guards or protects** wound or surgery site by altering weight distribution (limping, shifting body position) ☐ **May be unwilling to move** all or part body	☐ May be **subtle** (shifting eyes or increased respiratory rate) if dog is too painful to move or is stoic ☐ May be **dramatic**, such as a sharp cry, growl, bite or bite threat, and/or pulling away	Moderate **Reassess analgesic plan**
4		☐ **Constantly groaning or screaming** when unattended ☐ May bite or chew at wound, but unlikely to move ☐ **Potentially unresponsive** to surroundings ☐ **Difficult to distract** from pain	☐ **Cries at non-painful palpation** (may be experiencing allodynia, wind-up, or fearful that pain could be made worse) ☐ May react aggressively to palpation	Moderate to Severe **May be rigid to avoid painful movement** **Reassess analgesic plan**

Right

○ Tender to palpation

× Warm

■ Tense

Left

Comments ____

Fig. 11 Colorado State University Veterinary Medical Center Canine Acute Pain Scale.

QUALITY OF LIFE

Currently, there are no validated 'scales' to assess maladaptive pain. Several investigators have suggested exploring this area of interest through the creation of novel questionnaires as an instrument for measuring maladaptive pain in dogs from its impact on health-related quality of life (HRQL)[24–27].

In 2000, Franklin McMillan published a treatise on quality of life (QOL) in animals[26]. It was noted that although the term QOL was being used in the veterinary literature, it was not defined; authors typically assume that individuals assessing QOL know what it means and leave evaluators to define the term in their own way. Criteria for assessing or measuring QOL are rarely provided; QOL is equated to health status, so that assessments of QOL are assessments of health status; QOL is being used as an outcome objective and to compare efficacy of treatments; and QOL is being used to make decisions regarding euthanasia of animals. McMillan's treatise proposed the following definition: 'Quality of Life is a multidimensional, experiential continuum. It comprises an array of affective states, broadly classifiable as comfort–discomfort and pleasure states. In general, the greater the pleasant and lesser the unpleasant effects, the higher the QOL. Quality of life is a uniquely individual experience and should be measured from the perspective of the individual'.

Most QOL questionnaires incorporate at least three broad domains taken from the human model: physical, psychological, and social functioning. Physical functioning involves symptoms associated with the disease itself and its treatment, as well as the ability to perform daily living activities. Psychological functioning ranges from severe psychological distress to a positive sense of well-being, and may also encompass cognitive functioning. Social functioning refers to quantitative and qualitative aspects of social relationships, social interactions, and societal integrations.

QOL assessments from neonates, infants, mentally disabled patients, and patients who are severely ill are difficult. Therefore, investigators have devised means for acquiring QOL information from other sources, such as parents, spouses, partners, caregivers, siblings, and healthcare providers. These individuals are termed proxy informants. Any assessments of animal QOL must come indirectly from a proxy informant. For pets, the best proxy informant is likely to be the person most familiar with the pet, which in most instances would be its owner.

Using the human model, Yazbek and Fontana[28] propose a simple questionnaire, useful in assessing HRQL in dogs with pain secondary to cancer (**Fig. 12**). These investigators maintain that dogs with pain secondary to cancer often have important changes in their emotional behavior, physical status, and their relationship with their owner that can be demonstrated with a HRQL scale; however, the owner must have a true knowledge of all of the dog's activities during the day for questionnaire answers to be reliable. The mean HRQL score for dogs with cancer in this study was 20.7, suggesting that they had a decreased QOL compared with healthy dogs for which the mean HRQL score was 34. The conclusion of this study was that pain in the dogs with cancer adversely affected the dogs' QOL.

Brown *et al.*[29] at the University of Pennsylvania, have developed a Canine Brief Pain Inventory (CBPI) for reliably obtaining quantifiable assessments from owners regarding the severity and impact of maladaptive pain and its treatment on dogs with osteoarthritis (**Fig. 13** *overleaf*). The CBPI is a questionnaire with two dimensions, severity and interference. The severity dimension consists of a four-question 0–10 numerical rating scale assessment of the severity of pain (at its worst, least, average, and right now). The responses from those four questions can be averaged to obtain a severity score for the dog. The interference dimension consists of a six-question 0–10 numerical rating scale assessment of how the pain interferes with the dog's normal functioning. The responses from those six questions can be averaged to obtain an interference score. In addition there is a one-question 'Likert scale' global assessment of the dog's overall QOL, which gives the owner the opportunity to address the relative importance of the pain.

12

Questionnaire for evaluating health-related quality of life in dogs with signs of pain secondary to cancer.

How much do you think the disease is disturbing your dog's quality of life?
Very much [0]
Much [1]
A little [2]
Not at all [3]

Does your dog still do what it likes (e.g. play or go for a walk)?
No [0]
Rarely [1]
Frequently [2]
In a normal way [3]

How is your dog's mood?
Totally altered [0]
Some episodes of alteration [1]
Changed a little bit (2)
Normal [3]

Does your dog keep its hygienic habits (i.e. does your dog clean itself)?
No [0]
Rarely [1]
Less than before [2]
Yes (3)

How often do you think that your dog feels pain?
All the time [0]
Frequently [1]
Rarely [2]
Never [3]

Does your dog have an appetite?
No [0]
Only eats when forced; will eat more of what it likes [1]
Little [2]
Normal [3]

Does your dog get tired easily?
Yes, always [0]
Frequently [1]
Rarely [2]
No [3]

How is your dog sleeping?
Very badly; not sleeping at all [0]
Badly [1]
Almost normally [2]
Normally [3]

How often does your dog vomit?
Always [0]
Frequently [1]
Rarely [2]
Never [3]

How are the intestines of your dog functioning?
Very badly [0]
Badly [1]
Almost normally [2]
Normally [3]

Is your dog able to position itself to defecate and urinate?
Never positions itself to urinate or defecate [0]
Rarely positions itself to urinate or defecate [1]
Sometimes positions itself to urinate or defecate [2]
Urinates and defecates normally [3]

How much attention is your dog giving to the family?
Indifferent [0]
Little attention [1]
Increased attention: the dog is needy [2]
Has not changed [3]

Scores (values in parentheses) for all 12 questions are summed to determine the health-related quality-of-life score. Possible scores ranged from 0 to 36.

Fig. 12 Questionnaire for evaluating health-related quality (HRQL) of life in dogs with signs of pain secondary to cancer[28].

13

Today's Date ☐☐ / ☐☐ / ☐☐
Month Day Year

Patient/Study ID ______________

Canine Brief Pain Inventory (CBPI)

Description of Pain:

Rate your dog's pain.

1. Fill in the oval next to the **one number** that best describes the pain at its worst in the last 7 days.
   ○0 ○1 ○2 ○3 ○4 ○5 ○6 ○7 ○8 ○9 ○10
   No Pain Extreme Pain
2. Fill in the oval next to the **one number** that best describes the pain at its least in the last 7 days.
   ○0 ○1 ○2 ○3 ○4 ○5 ○6 ○7 ○8 ○9 ○10
   No Pain Extreme Pain
3. Fill in the oval next to the **one number** that best describes the pain at its average in the last 7 days.
   ○0 ○1 ○2 ○3 ○4 ○5 ○6 ○7 ○8 ○9 ○10
   No Pain Extreme Pain
4. Fill in the oval next to the **one number** that best describes the pain at its right in the last 7 days.
   ○0 ○1 ○2 ○3 ○4 ○5 ○6 ○7 ○8 ○9 ○10
   No Pain Extreme Pain

Description of function:

Fill in the oval next to the **one number** that describes how during the past 7 days pain has interfered with your dog's:

5. General activity
   ○0 ○1 ○2 ○3 ○4 ○5 ○6 ○7 ○8 ○9 ○10
   Does not interfere Completely interferes
6. Enjoyment of life
   ○0 ○1 ○2 ○3 ○4 ○5 ○6 ○7 ○8 ○9 ○10
   Does not interfere Completely interferes
7. Ability to rise to standing from lying down
   ○0 ○1 ○2 ○3 ○4 ○5 ○6 ○7 ○8 ○9 ○10
   Does not interfere Completely interferes
8. Ability to walk
   ○0 ○1 ○2 ○3 ○4 ○5 ○6 ○7 ○8 ○9 ○10
   Does not interfere Completely interferes
9. Ability to run
   ○0 ○1 ○2 ○3 ○4 ○5 ○6 ○7 ○8 ○9 ○10
   Does not interfere Completely interferes
10. Ability to climb up (for example stairs or curbs)
    ○0 ○1 ○2 ○3 ○4 ○5 ○6 ○7 ○8 ○9 ○10
    Does not interfere Completely interferes

Overall Impression:

11. Fill in the oval next to the one response that best describes your dog's over all quality of life over the last 7 days.
    ○Poor ○Fair ○Good ○Very Good ○Excellent

Fig. 13 University of Pennsylvania Canine Brief Pain Inventory, used to assess osteoarthritis-related pain[29].

In 2009, Hielm-Bjorkman *et al.*[30] reported that their 11 question, Finnish version of the Helsinki Chronic Pain Index provided a valid, reliable, and responsive tool for assessment of response to treatment in dogs with osteoarthritis, that is, maladaptive pain.

Owner assessment

Expanding on the value of owner assessment, a client-specific outcome measures scheme (Cincinnati Orthopedic Disability Index questionnaire) was developed for evaluating nutraceuticals in dogs by Gingerich and Strobel[31]. In this scheme, five very specific problems related to osteoarthritis were identified, which are recorded, and the intensity of the problem is monitored as treatment progresses. Because the questions are very specific to the individual animal in its environment, this measurement system appears to be very sensitive.

A similar, very sensitive questionnaire used at North Carolina State University Comparative Pain Research Laboratory to assess pain associated with clinical osteoarthritis in cats is presented in **Fig. 14**. Activity or behavior that is suspected to have become altered as a result of the pain and specific to the animal and its home environment are defined. Activities are graded at the start of treatment and after analgesic treatment is started. A left shift corresponds to pain relief.

An overview of pain scales is more than an exercise in the history of pain. Several certifying organizations, such as the American Animal Hospital Association, insist that medical records include some scheme for assessing a patient's pain. This raises the question of what is considered to be the best scheme for a given hospital to adopt. To help hospital staff to make this decision, a review of the various 'pros and cons' for various choices is worthwhile.

The importance of implementing an accurate pain scoring system is paramount in the identification of pain and its alleviation. Accuracy is less important in the clinical setting. Regardless of the scheme of pain assessment chosen, simply implementing a printed pain assessment form will elevate the hospital's collective standard of care[32]. A question here would be, 'Do you wish to practice best medicine, or simply practice the 'standard of care'?" There is no fault in the latter; however, the former will provide the best quality of care for the patient, generate a sense of pride among the hospital staff, instill confidence within the pet owner, and grow business.

14

Problems in mobility related to osteoarthritis in your cat	No problem	A little problematic	Quite problematic	Severely problematic	Impossible
1. Jumping onto sofa		▽	✓		
2. Jumping onto kitchen counter			▽		✓
3. Walking up steps on back deck	▽		✓		
4. Jumping on bed	▽				✓
5. Using litter tray	▽	✓			

✓ Start of treatment ▽ After treatment

Fig. 14 North Carolina State University Comparative Pain Research Laboratory Client Specific Outcome Measures – Activity, used to assess pain associated with clinical osteoarthritis in cats.

Chapter 4

Functional Physiology of Pain

MALADAPTIVE PAIN

Pain is both a good and a potentially very bad phenomenon. From an advantageous perspective, pain is an early warning sign that we should avoid potential tissue damage. It is the 'fight or flight' stimulus. From a negative perspective, pain can lead to stress, distress, and suffering. Our goal should not be to abolish all pain, which is likely not possible in the conscious animal, but rather to control maladaptive pain so as to maintain as near normal physiologic functions as is possible and to prevent suffering.

Adaptive pain protects the body from injury and promotes healing by inhibiting activity when injury has occurred.
Maladaptive pain reflects pathologic activity of the nervous system – the result of complex processes of neuronal plasticity: pain as a disease state.

The notion that pain-induced restricted activity is a benefit (i.e. pain is good for a postoperative orthopedic patient) is an inappropriate rationalization! This is a position taken by some, particularly following orthopedic surgical repairs. In fact, a fundamental tenant of internal orthopedic fixation is to allow patients earlier activity. As a result of this earlier activity, there is increased vascularization to the injured area, and subsequently earlier fracture healing. For such patients, we have many options to restrict exercise. Pain as an imposed activity restraint has no place in current veterinary practice.

Maladaptive pain is never beneficial! Pain, particularly that associated with severe trauma or extensive surgical procedures, produces a series of behavioral, neurophysiologic, endocrine (**Fig. 15**), metabolic, and cellular responses that initiate, maintain, and amplify the release of noxious and inflammatory mediators. Pain can adversely affect nearly every system in the body (**Fig. 16**, *Table 9*).

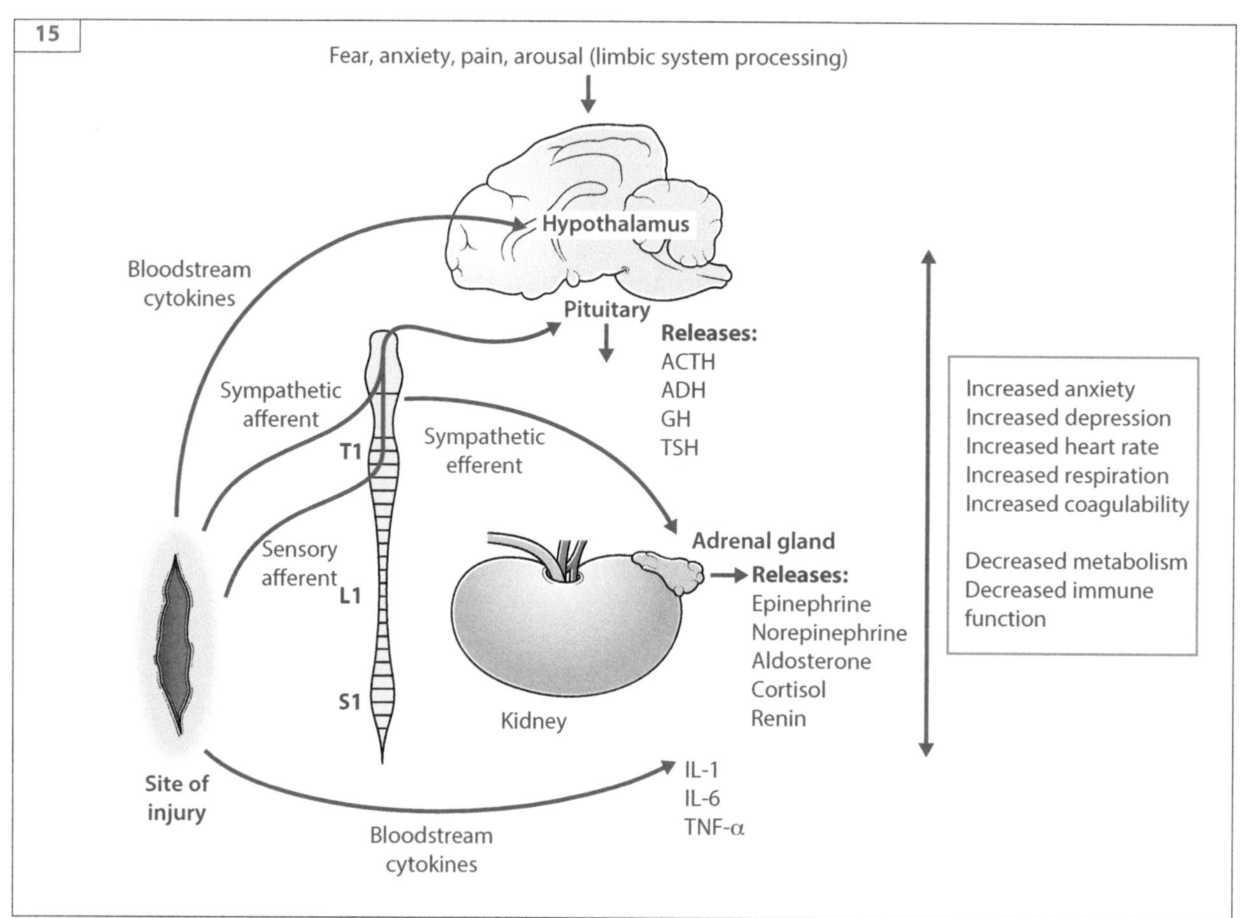

Fig. 15 Diagram of the neuroendocrine axis that plays an integral role in the pain/stress response. ACTH: Adrenocorticotrophic hormone; ADH: antidiuretic hormone; GH: growth hormone; IL: interleukin; L1: first lumbar (vertebra); S1: first sacral (vertebra); T1: first thoracic (vertebra); TNF-α: tumor necrosis factor-α; TSH: thyroid-stimulating hormone.

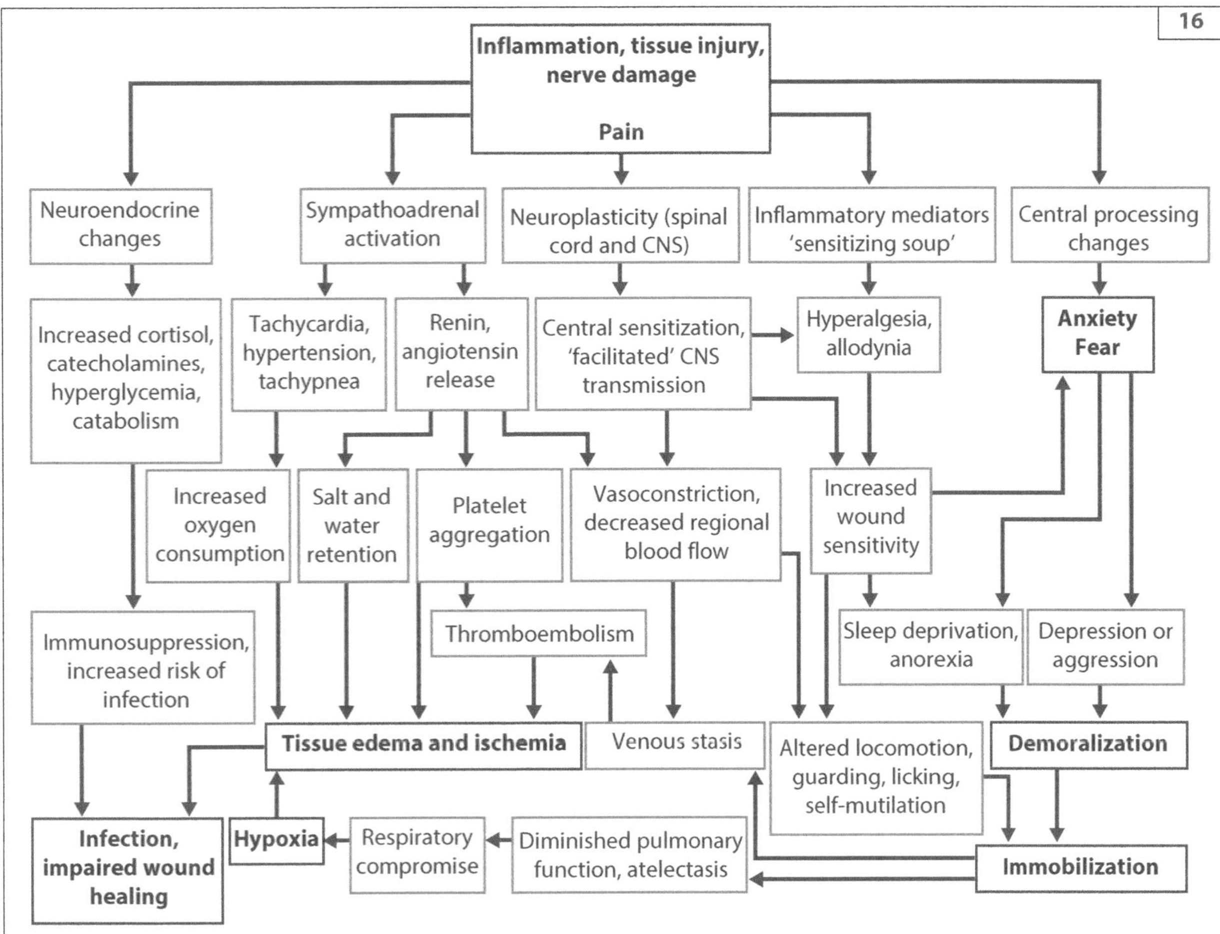

Fig. 16 Consequences of maladaptive pain. (After Reference 1.) CNS: central nervous system.

TABLE 9: Consequences of maladaptive pain

Body system	Pain-induced change	Consequences
Cardiovascular	Increased heart rate, blood pressure, cardiac output, and risk of arrhythmia	Impaired cardiovascular function
Gastrointestinal	Increased intestinal secretions, and paralytic ileum	Vomition, anorexia, increased risk of gastric ulceration, and intestinal pain
Immune system	Impaired immune function	Increased risk of infection and sepsis, enhanced metastatic tumor spread, and increased risk of tumor recurrence
Metabolism	Increased metabolism and oxygen consumption; breakdown of muscle, fat and glucose stores	Delayed wound healing, weight loss, and and increased tissue breakdown
Nervous system	Increased sensitization	Hyperalgesia and allodynia, chronic pain
Respiration	Increased respiratory rate, and reduced ventilation	Hypoxemia, hypercapnia, acidosis, increased risk of atelectasis and pneumonia
Urinary	Urinary retention; water and sodium retention	Electrolyte imbalances

FROM NOCICEPTION TO PAIN

There is no 'pain pathway'! There are no 'pain fibers'! Adaptive pain is a good thing!

Nociceptive pathway

A good way to understand the physiology of pain is to follow the nociceptive signal tracks from the periphery (transduction) to the brain (perception), with a focus on the integration and modulation of the nociceptive signal at different steps within the central nervous system (CNS) (**Fig. 17, Fig. 18**). Further, it is helpful to define various terms and concepts along the way.

Nociception (synonym: nocioception or nociperception) is defined as 'the neural processes of encoding and processing noxious stimuli'. It is the incoming activity produced in the peripheral and central nervous system by stimuli that have the potential to damage tissue. This activity is initiated by **nociceptors** (also called pain receptors), that can detect mechanical, thermal, or chemical changes above a set threshold.

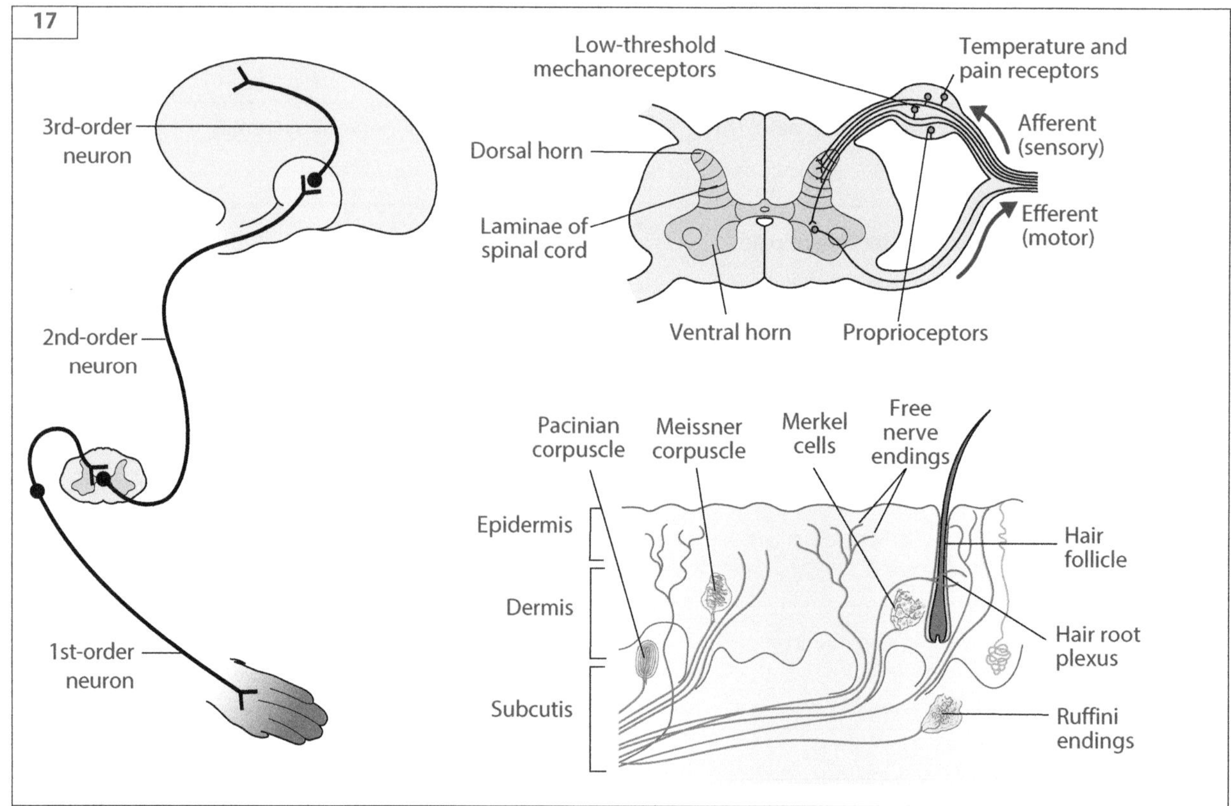

Fig. 17 Pathway from insult to perception of pain.

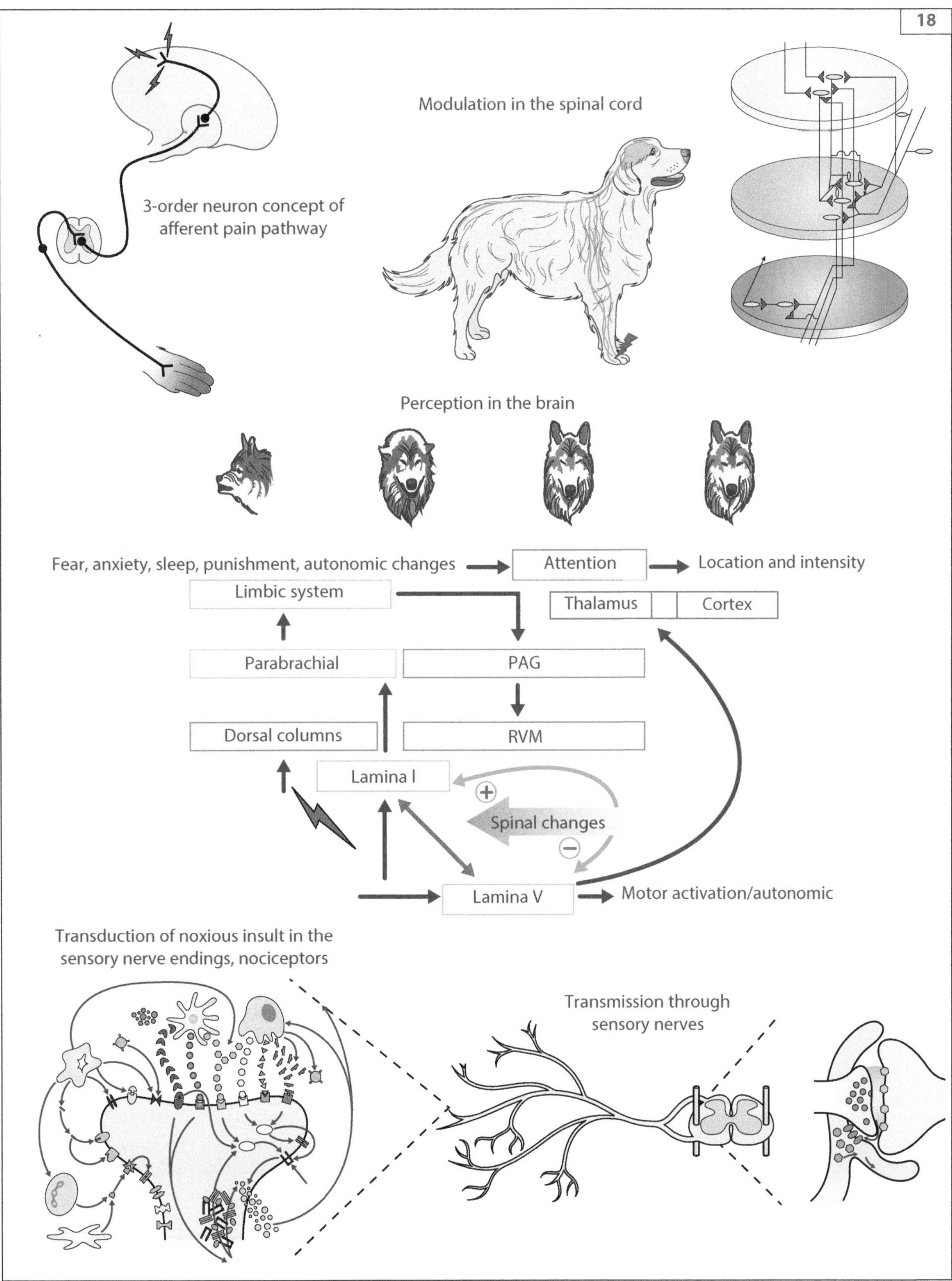

Fig. 18 The nociceptive pathway is complex, with networks of activities in each of the physiologic processes of transduction, transmission, modulation, and perception. PAG: periaqueductal gray; RVM: rostral ventromedial medulla.

To paraphrase Albert Einstein, 'some things can be made simple, but only so much so before they lose meaning'. So it is that the 3-order-neuron 'pain pathway' provides an easy to understand image of the nociceptive signal pathway to pain; however, each component of this pathway is extremely complex. In some respects this complexity is a good thing (i.e. many targets are available for suppression). As we begin to discover different mechanisms of action within the track of nociception, so comes identification of new targets for the development of innovative agents to alleviate or modify the pain response.

Peripheral nervous system

The peripheral nervous system (PNS) comprises nervous tissue outside the spinal canal and brain. Nociception first undergoes change in the PNS, followed by dynamic changes in the dorsal horn of the spinal cord, where it is determined if the signal lives or dies. Peripheral receptors (specialized nerve cell terminals in skin) transduce (converts one physical quantity to another, e.g. pressure or temperature to an electrical signal) nociceptive and proprioceptive events for processing by first-order sensory neurons in the segmental dorsal root ganglion (DRG), whose extension terminates in the dorsal horn of the spinal cord (**Fig. 19**).

The PNS includes cranial nerves, spinal nerves with their roots and branches (rami), peripheral components of the autonomic nervous system, and peripheral nerves whose primary sensory neurons are located in the associated DRG, also a part of the PNS. Axons are extensions of the cell body and contain a continuous channel of nerve cell cytoplasm.

Transmission of information: receptors and action potential

Membrane potentials are employed by nerve fibers to transmit nerve impulses, which is the means by which informational signals are transmitted from one part of the nervous system

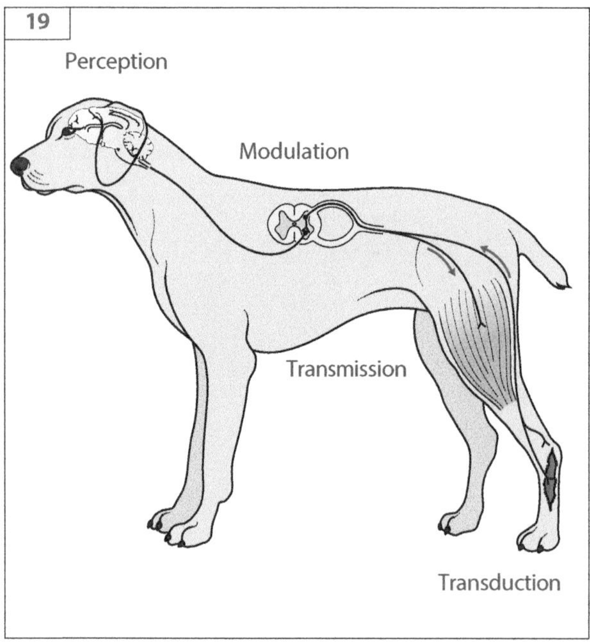

Fig. 19 Nociceptive pathway. Release of a variety of inflammatory mediators (e.g. prostaglandins, bradykinin, serotonin) at the site of insult results in receptor excitation that transduces or translates specific forms of energy into action potentials. Such action potentials become the nociceptive messengers for pain. The nociceptive pathways from the periphery conduct to the brain after two synaptic relays. The first-order Aδ- and C-fibers make their first synapse with the projection neurons in the dorsal horn of the spinal cord. The second-order neurons branch immediately in the spinal cord and conduct to the thalamic nuclei where they make the second synaptic contact. Finally, the third-order neurons project to the somatosensory cortices for the sensory-discriminative component of pain and to limbic structures for the motivational component of pain.

to another. This is achieved by means of action potentials, which are abrupt, pulse-like changes in the membrane potential, lasting a few ten thousandths to a few thousandths of a second. These action potentials move along the length of the nerve, giving rise to the 'nerve signals'.

Receptors

An action potential can be elicited in a nerve fiber by almost any factor that suddenly increases the permeability (infiltration) of the nerve membrane to sodium ions. Such factors include electrical stimulation, mechanical compression of the fiber, application of chemicals to the membrane, or almost any other event that disturbs the normal resting state of the membrane. Several of the more complex receptors include Merkel's disks, the tactile hairs, Pacinian corpuscles, Meissner's corpuscles, Krause's corpuscles, and Ruffini's end-organs (**Fig. 20**, *Table 10*). In the skin these receptors detect the tactile sensations of touch, pressure, and vibration. In the deep tissues, they detect stretch, deep pressure, or any other type of tissue deformation, including the stretch of joint capsules and ligaments to determine the angulation of a joint.

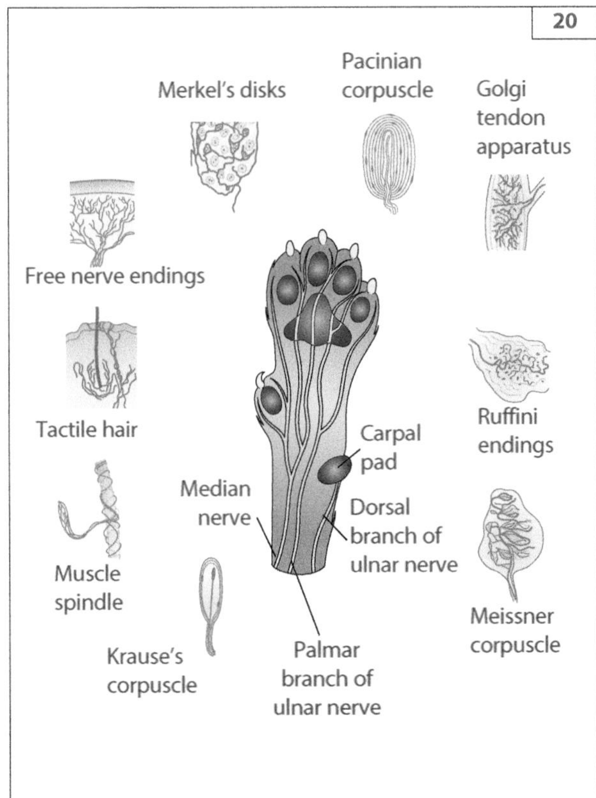

Fig. 20 Afferent receptors are widely dispersed and serve different functions, allowing the animal to sense its environment. Stimulation of these receptors can initiate signals in the nervous system.

TABLE 10: Common receptors in somatic sensation

Receptor	Modality	Nerve fiber type
Nociceptors	**Pain**	
Mechanical	Sharp, pricking	Aδ
Thermal-mechanical	Burning, freezing	Aδ, C
Polymodal	Slow burning	C
Cutaneous and subcutaneous	**Touch**	
Pacini	Vibration	Aα, β
Ruffini	Skin stretch	Aα, β
Merkel	Pressure	Aα, β
Meissner	Stroking	Aα, β
Thermal	**Temperature**	
Heat nociceptors	Hot temperature	Aδ
Cold nociceptors	Cold temperature	C
Muscle and skeletal mechanoreceptors	**Limb proprioception**	
Muscle spindles	Muscle length and stretch	Aα, β
Golgi tendon	Muscle contraction	Aα
Joint capsule	Joint angle	Aβ
Stretch	Excessive stretch	Aδ

The Golgi tendon apparatus detects degree of tension in tendons, and the muscle spindle detects relative change in muscle length. Free nerve endings are found in all parts of the body and contain a plethora of receptors, which can generate action potentials (**Fig. 21**).

Cytokines are a heterogeneous group of polypeptides that activate the immune system and mediate inflammatory responses, acting on a variety of tissues, including the peripheral and central nervous systems. Cytokines act at hormonal concentrations, but in contrast to circulating endocrine hormones, they exert their effects on nearby cells over short extracellular distances at low concentrations, and thus serum levels may not reliably reflect local activation. Models of painful nerve injury reveal changes in cytokine expression in the injured nerve itself, in the dorsal root ganglion, in the spinal cord dorsal horn, and in the central nervous system.

Chemokines are a family of small cytokines, or proteins secreted by cells. Their name is derived from their ability to induce directed chemotaxis in nearby responsive cells; they are chemotactic cytokines. These proteins exert their biologic effects by interacting with G-protein-linked transmembrane receptors called chemokine receptors, that are selectively found on the surfaces of their target cells. Some chemokines are considered proinflammatory, while others are considered homeostatic, involved in controlling the migration of cells during normal processes of tissue maintenance or development.

Resting nerve membrane potential

Nerve cell membranes contain sodium–potassium pumps, three sodium ions being pumped to the exterior for each two potassium ions pumped to the interior. The resting nerve membrane is normally 50–100 times as permeable to potassium as to sodium. Therefore, potassium diffuses with relative ease through the resting membrane, whereas sodium diffuses with difficulty. Inside the nerve fiber are large numbers of anions (negatively charged) that cannot diffuse through the nerve membrane at all or that diffuse very poorly. Such ions include organic phosphate ions, sulfate ions, and protein ions. These points considered, the nerve reaches a resting membrane potential. Firstly, sodium is pumped to the outside of the fiber, while potassium is pumped to the inside. But, since three sodium ions are pumped out of the fiber for every two potassium ions pumped in, more positive ions are continually being pumped out of the fiber than into it. Since most of the negatively charged anions inside the nerve fiber are nondiffusible, the negative charges remain inside the nerve fiber, so that the inside of the fiber becomes electronegative, while the outside becomes electropositive: the resting state. Once the sodium and potassium concentration differences have been created across the cell membrane, the occurrence of action potentials does not depend upon operation of the sodium–potassium pump.

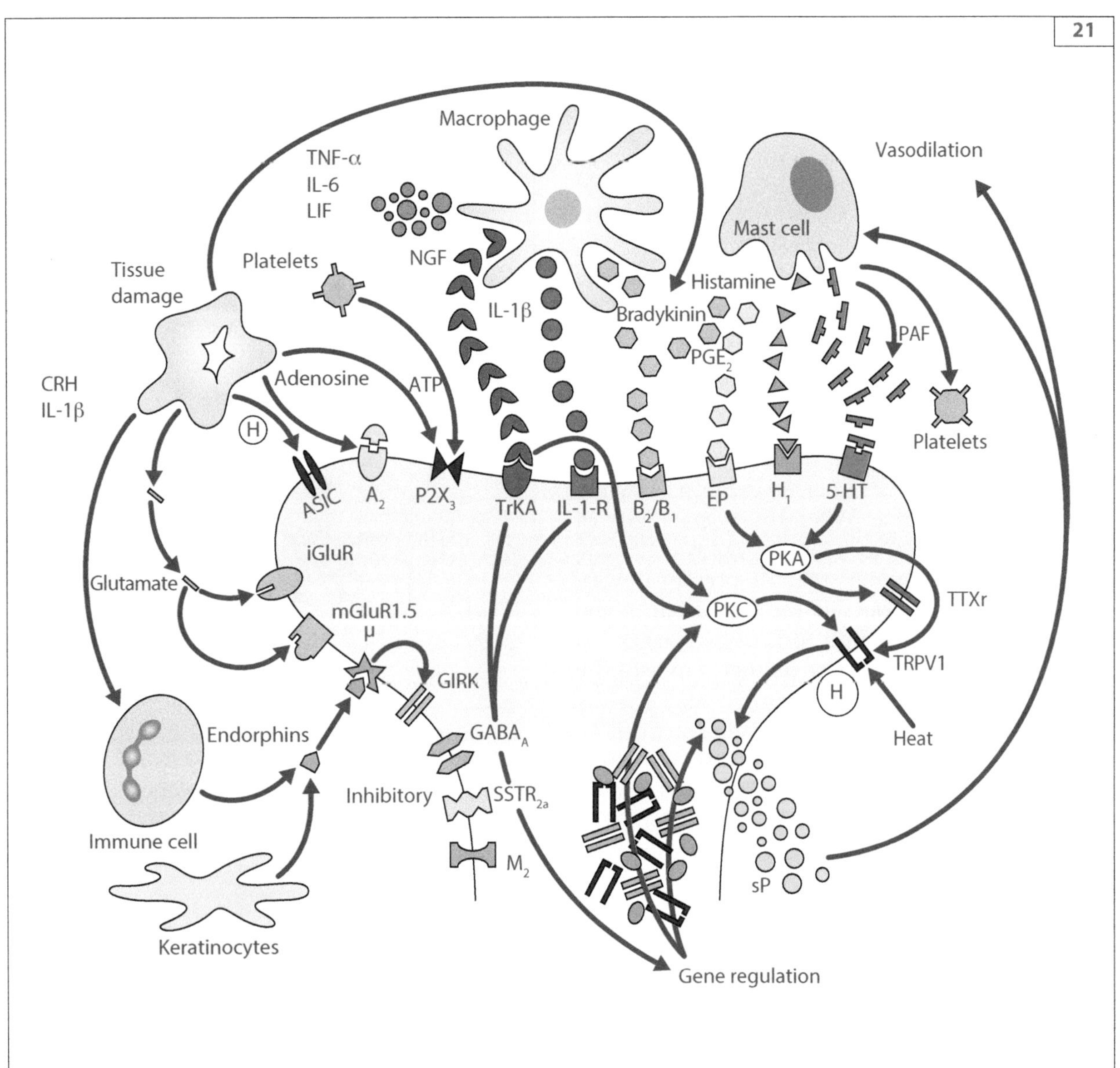

Fig. 21 Receptors on primary afferent terminals. Action potentials can be generated by receptors located on free nerve endings. These receptors are varied and plentiful. Further, their response to stimulation can be influenced by various cytokines and chemokines in the surrounding area. 5-HT: 5-hydroxytryptamine; A_2: adenosine receptor; ASIC: acid-sensing ion channel; ATP: adenosine triphosphate; B_2/B_1: bradykinin B_2/B_1 receptors; CRH: corticotrophin-releasing hormone; EP: prostaglandin E_2 receptor; GABA: γ-aminobutyric acid; GIRK: G protein-coupled inwardly-rectifying potassium channel; H: hydrogen ion; H_1: histamine receptor; iGluR: ionotropic glutamate receptor; IL: interleukin; IL-R: interleukin receptor; LIF: leukemia inhibitory factor; M_2; muscarinic receptor; mGluR1.5: metabotropic glutamate receptor 1.5; NGF: nerve growth factor; PAF: platelet-activating factor; PGE: prostaglandin E; PKA: protein kinase A; PKC: protein kinase C; $P2X_3$: ATP receptor; sP: substance P; SSTR: somatostatin receptor; TNF: tumor necrosis factor; TrKA: tyrosine kinase A; TRPV1: transient receptor potential vanilloid V1; TTXr: tetrodotoxin-resistant sodium channel.

Action potential

The action potential results from rapid changes in membrane permeability to sodium and potassium ions; the sodium permeability increases about 5,000-fold at the onset of the action potential, followed instantaneously by return of the sodium permeability to normal, and then the potassium permeability increases greatly. As a result, the membrane potential changes rapidly from its normal negative value to an instantaneous positive value, then equally rapidly back to its negative value (**Fig. 22**).

The action potential occurs in two separate stages called membrane depolarization and membrane repolarization. In the resting state the inside of the nerve fiber is negative, while the outside is positive. When the permeability of the membrane to sodium ions suddenly increases, many of the sodium ions that are present in very high concentration outside the fiber rush to the inside, carrying enough positive charges to the inside to cause complete disappearance of the normal negative resting potential, and usually enough charges actually to develop a positive state inside the fiber. This sudden loss of normal negative potential inside the fiber is called depolarization. The positive potential that develops momentarily inside the fiber is called the reversal potential.

Almost immediately after depolarization takes place, the pores of the membrane again become almost impermeable to sodium ions, but at the same time considerably more permeable than normal to potassium ions. Therefore, sodium ions stop moving to the inside of the fiber, and instead, potassium ions move to the outside because of the high potassium concentration on the inside. Because the potassium ions are positively charged, the excess positive charges inside the fiber are transferred back out of the fiber, and the normal negative resting membrane potential returns. This is called repolarization. An action potential elicited at any one point on an excitable membrane usually excites adjacent portions of the membrane, resulting in propagation of the action potential in both directions away from the stimulus, along all branches of the nerve fiber, until the entire membrane has become depolarized.

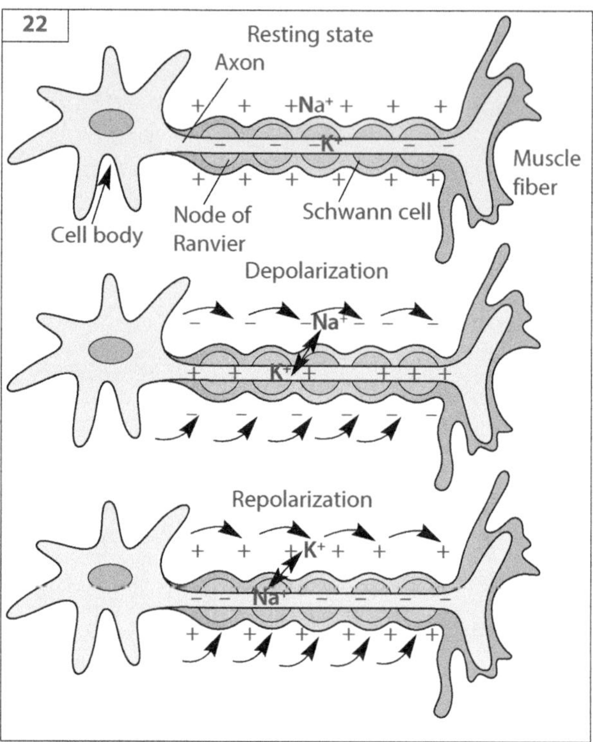

Fig. 22 Action potentials transmit information in the nervous system.

Neurotransmitters

Neurotransmitters are endogenous chemicals that transmit signals from a neuron to a target cell across a synapse. Neurotransmitters are packaged into clusters beneath the membrane on the presynaptic side of a synapse, and are released into the synaptic cleft, where they bind to receptors in the membrane on the postsynaptic side of the synapse. Release of neurotransmitters usually follows arrival of an action potential at the synapse, but may also follow graded electrical potentials. Low level 'baseline' release also occurs without electrical stimulation. Neurotransmitters are synthesized from plentiful and simple precursors, such as amino acids, which are readily available from the diet and which require only a small number of biosynthetic steps for conversion.

There are many different ways to classify neurotransmitters; dividing them into amino acids, peptides, and monoamines is historical.
Major neurotransmitters:
- Amino acids: glumate, aspartate, D-serine, γ-aminobutyric acid (GABA), glycine.
- Monoamines and other biogenic amines: dopamine (DA), norepinephrine (NE; noradrenaline, NA), epinephrine (adrenaline), histamine, serotonin (SE; 5-hydroxytryptamine, 5-HT).

Others:
- Acetylcholine (ACh).
- Adenosine.
- Anandamine.
- Nitric oxide (NO).

Some neurotransmitters are commonly described as 'excitatory' or 'inhibitory'. The only direct effect of a neurotransmitter is to activate one or more types of receptor. The effect on the postsynaptic cell depends, therefore, entirely on the properties of those receptors. It happens that for some neurotransmitters (for example, glutamate), the most influential receptors all have excitatory effects: that is, they increase the probability that the target cell will fire an action potential. For other neurotransmitters, such as GABA, the most important receptors all have inhibitory effects (although there is evidence that GABA is excitatory during early brain development). There are, however, other neurotransmitters, such as ACh, for which both excitatory and inhibitory receptors exist; there are also some types of receptors that activate complex metabolic pathways in the postsynaptic cell to produce effects that cannot appropriately be called either excitatory or inhibitory. Thus, it is an oversimplification to call a neurotransmitter excitatory or inhibitory. Nevertheless, it is so convenient to call glutamate excitatory and GABA inhibitory that this usage is seen frequently.

Examples of important neurotransmitter actions:
- Glutamate is used at the great majority of fast excitatory synapses in the brain and spinal cord. It is also used at most synapses that are 'modifiable' (i.e. capable of increasing or decreasing in strength). Modifiable synapses are thought to be the main memory-storage elements in the brain. Excessive glutamate release can lead to excitotoxicity, causing cell death.
- GABA is used at the great majority of fast inhibitory synapses in virtually every part of the brain. Many sedative/tranquilizing drugs act by enhancing the effects of GABA. Correspondingly, glycine is the inhibitory transmitter in the spinal cord.
- ACh is distinguished as the transmitter at the neuromuscular junction connecting motor nerves to muscles. The paralytic arrow-poison, curare, acts by blocking transmission at these synapses. ACh also operates in many regions of the brain, but using different types of receptor.
- DA has a number of important functions in the brain. It plays a critical role in the reward system, but dysfunction of the DA system is also implicated in Parkinson's disease and schizophrenia.
- SE (5-HT) is a monoamine neurotransmitter. Most is produced by, and found in, the intestine (human: approximately 90%), and the remainder in CNS neurons. It functions to regulate appetite, sleep, memory and learning, temperature, mood, behavior, muscle contraction, and function of the cardiovascular and endocrine systems. It is speculated to have a role in (human) depression, as some depressed patients have lower concentrations of metabolites of SE in their cerebrospinal fluid and brain tissue.
- Substance P (sP) is an undecapeptide (11 peptide chain) responsible for transmission of pain from certain sensory neurons to the CNS.

Small-molecule neurotransmitters are synthesized at nerve terminals (**Fig. 23A**). The enzymes necessary for neurotransmitter synthesis are made in the cell body of the presynaptic cell (1) and are transported down the axon by slow axonal transport (2). Precursors are taken up into the terminals by specific transporters, and neurotransmitter synthesis and packaging takes place within the nerve endings (3). After vesicle fusion and release (4), the neurotransmitter may be enzymatically degraded. The reuptake of the neurotransmitter (or its metabolites) starts another cycle of synthesis, packaging, release, and removal (5).

Peptide neurotransmitters, as well as the enzymes that modify their precursors, are synthesized in the cell body (1). Enzymes and prepeptides are packaged into vesicles in the Golgi apparatus. During fast axonal transport of these vesicles to the nerve terminals (2), the enzymes modify the prepeptides to produce one or more neurotransmitter peptides (3). After vesicle fusion and exocytosis, the peptides diffuse away and are degraded by proteolytic enzymes(4) (**Fig. 23B**).

Small neurotransmitters (such as NO) are synthesized at the presynaptic terminals of a neuron using enzymes manufactured in the cell body. Neurotransmitter precursors are pulled into the cell at the synaptic terminal and used to create neurotransmitter molecules that will be loaded into vesicles before being dumped into the synapse.

In contrast, larger polypeptide neurotransmitters, such as ACh and SE, tend to be synthesized in the cell body of the neuron by the rough endoplasmic reticulum before being packaged into vesicles by the Golgi apparatus. These peptide neurotransmitters may undergo further processing inside the vesicles as well.

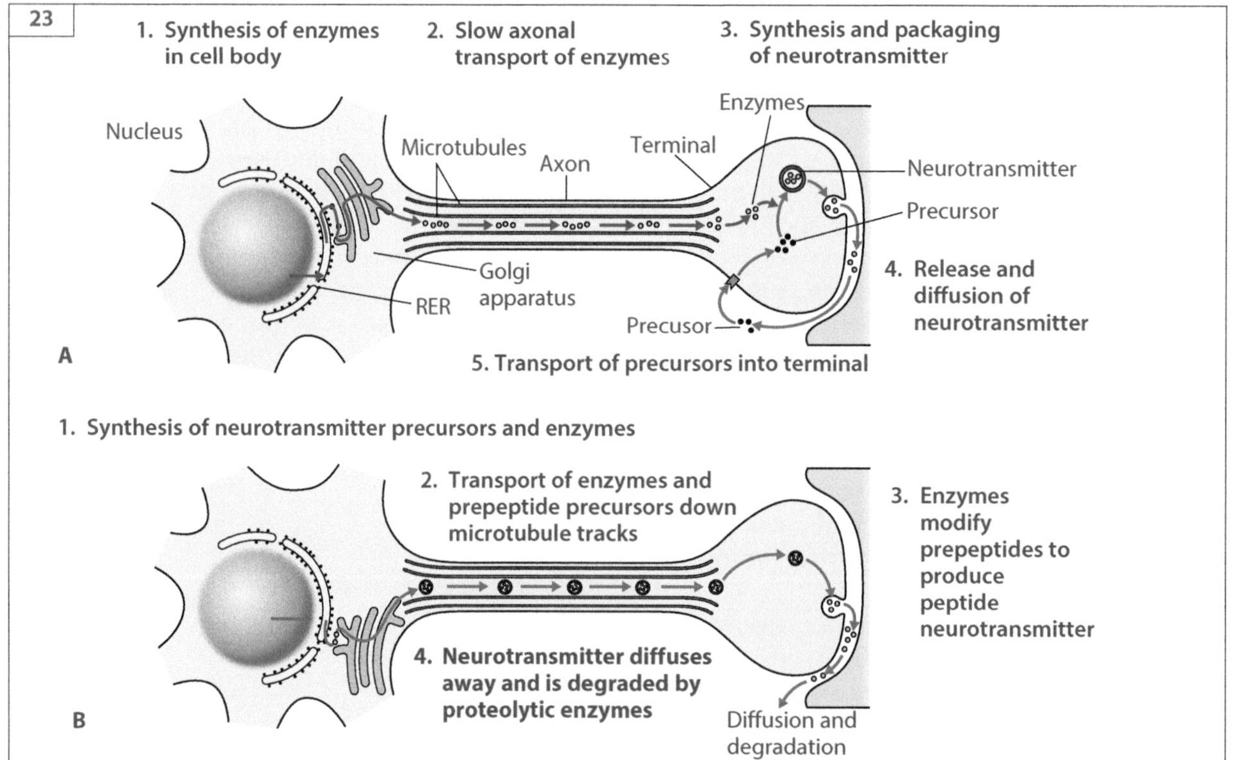

Fig. 23 Creation and packaging of small neurotransmitters (**A**), and large polypeptide neurotransmitters (**B**). RER: rough endoplasmic reticulum.

Fast axonal transport allows vesicles to travel as fast as 400 mm/day (as opposed to ~5 mm/day for the slow axonal transport that carries enzymes to the axon terminus). In this fast mode of transport, vesicles are moved along long microtubule 'tracks' by adenosine triphosphate (ATP)-driven 'motor' proteins.

Once the vesicle holding a neurotransmitter merges with the presynaptic terminal membrane of the neuron, the neurotransmitter molecules are released into the synapse. They then diffuse across the synaptic cleft and bind with receptors on the postsynaptic membrane, opening specific ion channels there. After release, neurotransmitter molecules may diffuse away from the synapse, may be broken down by an enzyme (e.g. acetylcholinesterase), or may be taken up by a neuron via a membrane protein transporter. In any case, the effect of the neurotransmitter is brief as quick, prompt removal of the neurotransmitter terminates signal transmission.

Nerve cell synapses

Transmission up and down chains of linked nerves is primarily via synapses, where one nerve contacts another and neurotransmission occurs as follows: (1) an action potential reaches the presynaptic terminal; (2) depolarization of the presynaptic terminal opens ion channels allowing calcium (Ca++) into the cell; (3) intracellular calcium triggers release of neurotransmitters from storage vesicles; (4) neurotransmitters within the synaptic cleft bind to receptor sites on postsynaptic membranes; (5) activated receptor sites on postsynaptic membranes cause opening and closing of postsynaptic (effector cell) ion channels, that causes changes in the membrane potential; (6) what follows is an action potential that is now propagated through the second neuron; and finally, (7) neurotransmitters are inactivated or transported back into the presynaptic terminal of the first neuron (**Fig. 24**).

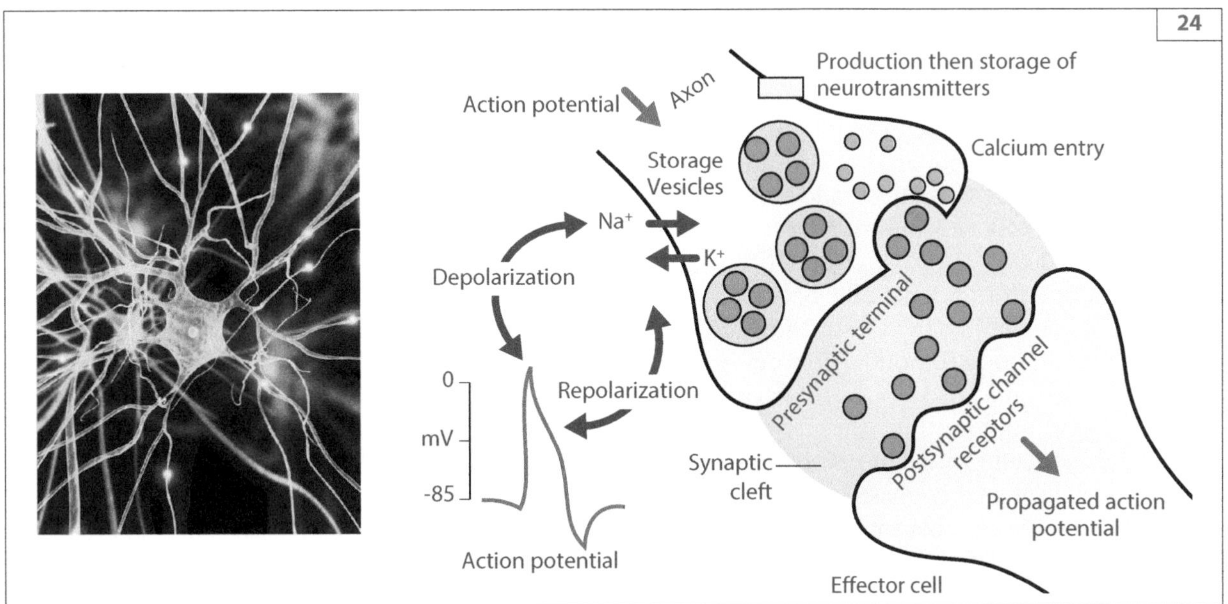

Fig. 24 Chains of nerves conduct information via neurotransmitters across synaptic clefts. Action potentials generate the release of these neurotransmitters, which in turn generate action potentials in the effector cell.

Size matters!

As a theory of electrical engineering, there is a relationship between nerve fiber size and conduction velocity; however, conduction velocity may be enhanced by Schwann cell activity or reduced by pathology (*Table 11*, **Fig. 25**).

Nearly all large-diameter, myelinated Aβ-fibers normally conduct non-noxious stimuli (e.g. touch, joint position, muscle contraction) applied to the skin, joints, and muscles, and thus these large sensory neurons usually do not conduct noxious stimuli[2]. In contrast, most small-diameter sensory fibers – nonmyelinated C-fibers and finely myelinated A-fibers – are specialized sensory neurons known as nociceptors, whose major function is to detect environmental stimuli that are perceived as harmful, and convert (transduce) them into electrochemical signals that are then transmitted to the CNS.

Schwann cell

The term 'nerve fiber' refers to the combination of the nerve's axon and Schwann cell as a functional unit. The Schwann cell (the oligodendrocyte is the corresponding CNS cell) significantly accelerates the speed of action potential propagation and acts as a first-line phagocyte (a cell that ingests micro-organisms or foreign material). It also plays a major role in nerve regeneration and axonal maintenance. All peripheral nerve axons are surrounded by segmental Schwann cells, although only some Schwann cells produce myelin – a lipid-rich insulating covering. Myelin is formed by serial wrapping of Schwann cell cytoplasm around an axon; sequential myelinated Schwann cells are separated by nodes of Ranvier, a location of high sodium channel concentration. Nodes of Ranvier provide rapid axon 'saltatory conduction'–where the conduction does not actually occur down the nerve axon, but rather by a faster mechanism of 'jumping' from node to node. After nerve injury, new axonal sprouts arise from a node of Ranvier. In the region surrounding these nodes of the axon, high concentrations of potassium channels are exposed during early phases of demyelination, which facilitate repolarization.

Gate theory

In 1954 Rexed demonstrated that the gray matter of the spinal cord could be divided into distinct laminae, or layers, based on cellular architecture[3]. The apex of the dorsal horn is capped by an area called the substantia gelatinosa (SG). The SG is one point where first-order neurons of the spinothalamic tract synapse. Many μ- and κ-opioid receptors, both pre- and postsynaptic, are found on these nerve cells. C-fibers and some Aδ-fibers also terminate in the SG (**Fig. 26**).

The aforementioned physiology is relevant in order to understand one of the earliest and fundamental theories of how the CNS modulates nociceptive transmission: the Gate Theory. The existence of a specific pain modulatory system was first clearly described in 1965 by Melzack and Wall[4] in the Gate Control Theory of pain. This was the first theory to propose that the CNS controls nociception. The basic premises of the theory are that activity in large (non-nociceptive) fibers can inhibit the perception of activity in small (nociceptive) fibers, and that descending activity from the brain also can inhibit that perception: interneurons of the SG regulate the input of large and small fibers to lamina V cells, serving as a gating mechanism.

Most simplistically, the Gate Theory states that fast moving action potentials in myelinated fibers activate inhibitor neurons that shut down second-order neurons before slower arriving signals reach the inhibitor neurons via nonmyelinated fibers. These signals from nonmyelinated fibers would normally shut down inhibitor neurons, thereby allowing further transmission through second-order neurons (**Fig. 27**).

With the Gate Theory, Melzack and Wall[4] formalized observations that encoding of high-intensity afferent input was subject to modulation. Although their concept was accurate, details of their explanation have since been more accurately modified.

As an example, transcutaneous electrical nerve stimulation (TENS) therapy is a clinical implementation of the Gate Theory. Systematic reviews and meta-analysis show that TENS is effective (in humans) for osteoarthritis, rheumatoid arthritis, postoperative pain, and chronic musculoskeletal pain[5–7]. TENS is thought to act by preferential stimulation of peripheral somatosensory fibers, which conduct more rapidly than nociceptive fibers. This results in a stimulation of inhibitory interneurons in the

TABLE 11: Relationship between fiber size and conduction velocity

Cutaneous nerve	Muscle nerve	Conduction velocity in the cat (m/sec)	Diameter (μm)
	Group I	72–130	12–22
Aαβ		35–108	6–18
	Group II	36–72	6–12
Aδ	Group III	3–30	3–7
C	Group IV	0.2–2	0.25–1.35

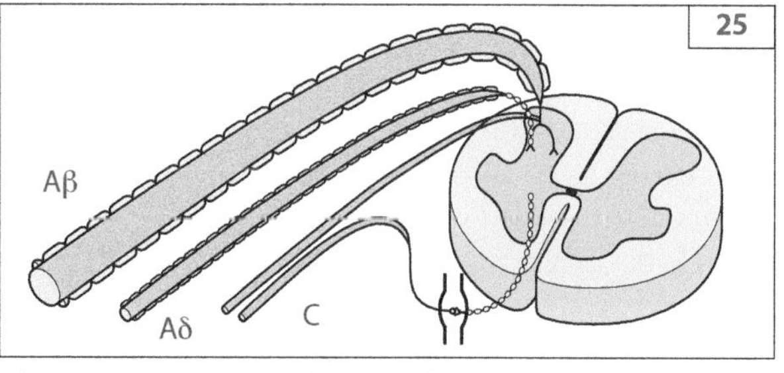

Fig. 25 Nociceptive afferent fibers can be separated according to their physical characteristics as well as their conduction velocity. (Yellow ellipses represent myelination.)

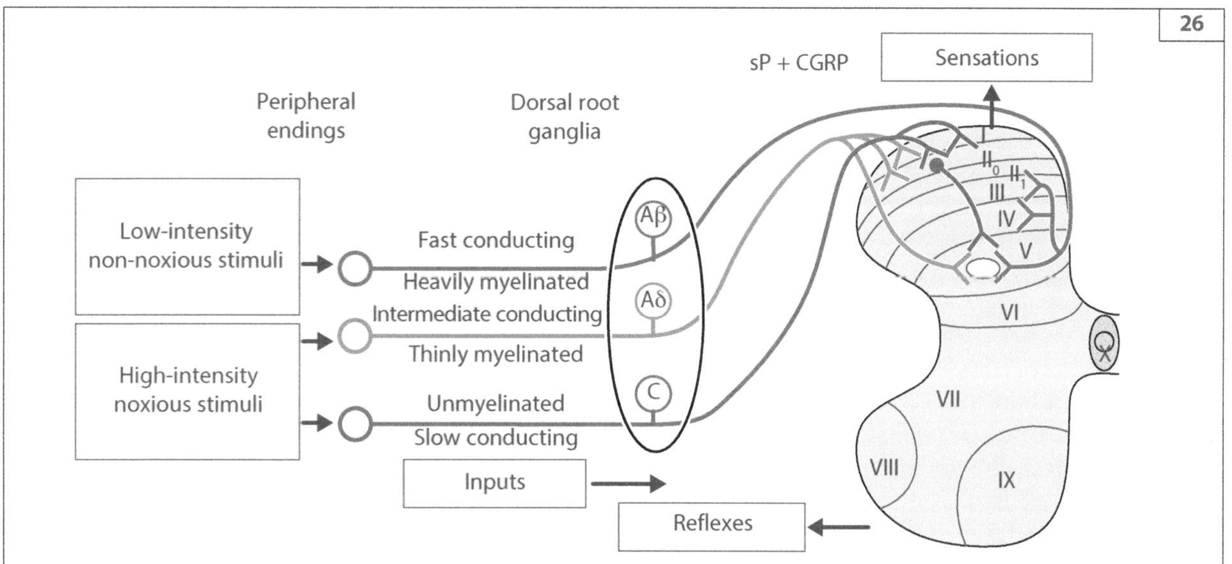

Fig. 26 Pathway for noxious stimuli through the substantia gelatinosa in the dorsal horn. CGRP: calcitonin gene-related peptide; sP: substance P.

Fig. 27 Melzack and Wall's Gate Theory of pain. Signals conducted through the fast-transmitting myelinated fiber reach the inhibitor neuron faster than signals from the slow-transmitting unmyelinated fiber. The inhibitor neuron then shuts down the transmitter neuron, rendering the signal from the slow-transmitting unmyelinated fiber ineffective.

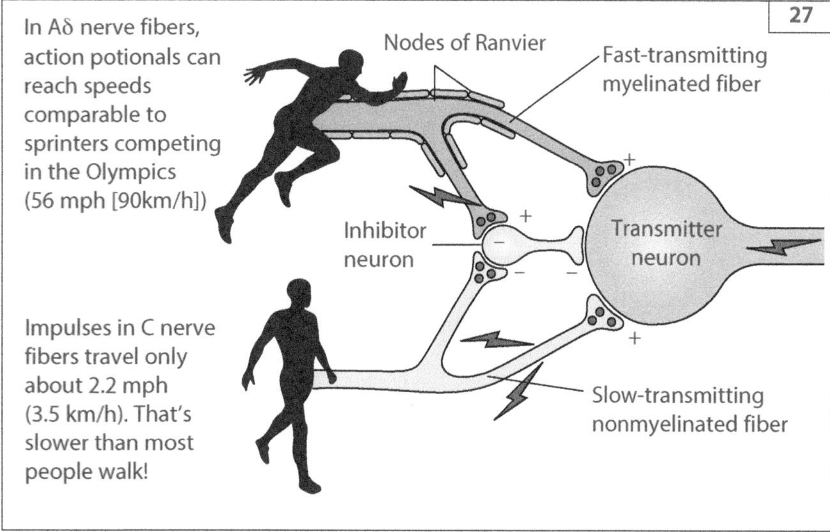

second lamina of the posterior horn (SG) that effectively blocks nociception at the spinal cord level. Additionally, TENS utilizes central opioid receptors to produce analgesia in a frequency-dependent manner, and analgesic tolerance develops after repeated use of TENS due to chronic activation of opioid receptors. This tolerance can be modulated by the administration of low doses of cholecystokinin receptor antagonist[8]. The release of endogenous opioids following high-frequency TENS application has also been proposed as a possible mechanism of action[9,10]. In 2010, Leonard *et al.* showed that high-, but not low-dose naloxone blocked high-frequency TENS analgesia, hence providing the first evidence that the analgesia induced by high-frequency TENS in humans is mediated by opioid receptors[11]. The Gate Theory may explain why some people feel a decrease in pain intensity when skin near the pain region is rubbed with a hand ('rubbing it better'). An additional example would be the shaking of a burned hand, an action that predominantly activates large nerve fibers.

Clinical implication: you can 'desensitize' an area of skin before inserting a needle by scratching the skin with your fingernail.

Signaling plasticity

The classic Cartesian view of pain stemmed from René Descartes (1596–1650), who proposed that 'pain' was transmitted from the periphery to a higher center through tubes of transfer (**Fig. 28**), and that there was a fixed relationship between the magnitude of stimulus and subsequent sensation (i.e. the greater the injury, the greater the pain). Studying World War II injuries, Henry Beecher observed that some soldiers with horrendous injuries often felt no pain, while soldiers with minor injuries sometimes had severe pain. Beecher concluded that Descartes' theory was wrong: there is no linear relationship between injury and the perception of pain.

It is now appreciated that there exists a plasticity or variable options of pain encoding. A diminished response (as with the administration of the analgesic morphine) to a given noxious stimulus can give rise to <u>hypo</u>algesia (analgesia).

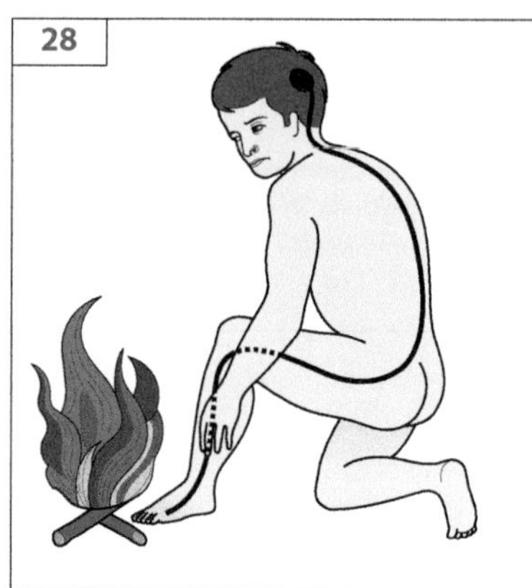

Fig. 28 In the early 1600s, pain was believed to be transmitted through 'tubes of transfer'.

On the other hand, local injury can shift the stimulus–response curve to the left, giving rise to the same pain report with a lower stimulus: <u>hyper</u>algesia. If the curve is shifted such that a non-noxious stimulus becomes noxious, the state is referred to as allodynia (**Fig. 29**). Allodynia is sometimes seen in dogs which 'scream with pain' at the lightest touch. Dogs with a herniated intervertebral disk can show this behavior. This left-shift of the stimulus–response curve is due in part to local effects on the peripheral nerve fibers, altered by the release of inflammatory mediators, cytokines (e.g. interleukins [ILs], tumor necrosis factors [TNFs], interferons, and others) and chemokines (factors that attract immune cells to sites of inflammation, infection, or trauma).

Hyperalgesia to both heat and mechanical stimuli that occur at the site of an injury is due to sensitization of primary afferent nociceptors[12,13]. Mechanisms of the phenomena have been studied in various tissues, including the joint, cornea, testicle, gastrointestinal tract, and bladder. Hyperalgesia at the site of injury is termed primary hyperalgesia, while hyperalgesia in the uninjured tissue surrounding the injury is termed secondary hyperalgesia.

Central hyperalgesia is a phenomenon that refers to sensitization that occurs within the CNS. Repeated recruitment of C-fibers after an injury will produce central sensitization by changing the response properties of the membrane of secondary neurons. Such change will result in an increase in firing rate, a phenomenon known as wind-up[14]. This will induce an increase in perceived pain, even if the intensity of the stimulation remains constant. This central sensitization at the spinal level sometimes lasts for only a few minutes, but can also persist for hours and even days[15]. This neuronal plasticity of the secondary neuron will result in a reduced recruitment threshold or the spontaneous activity of these neurons in the spinal cord, and can produce hyperalgesic and allodynic responses that may persist even after the healing of the injury. To address this, an aggressive and early treatment plan will help in preventing ongoing chronic pain.

Remember: threshold is the level at which a signal is generated.

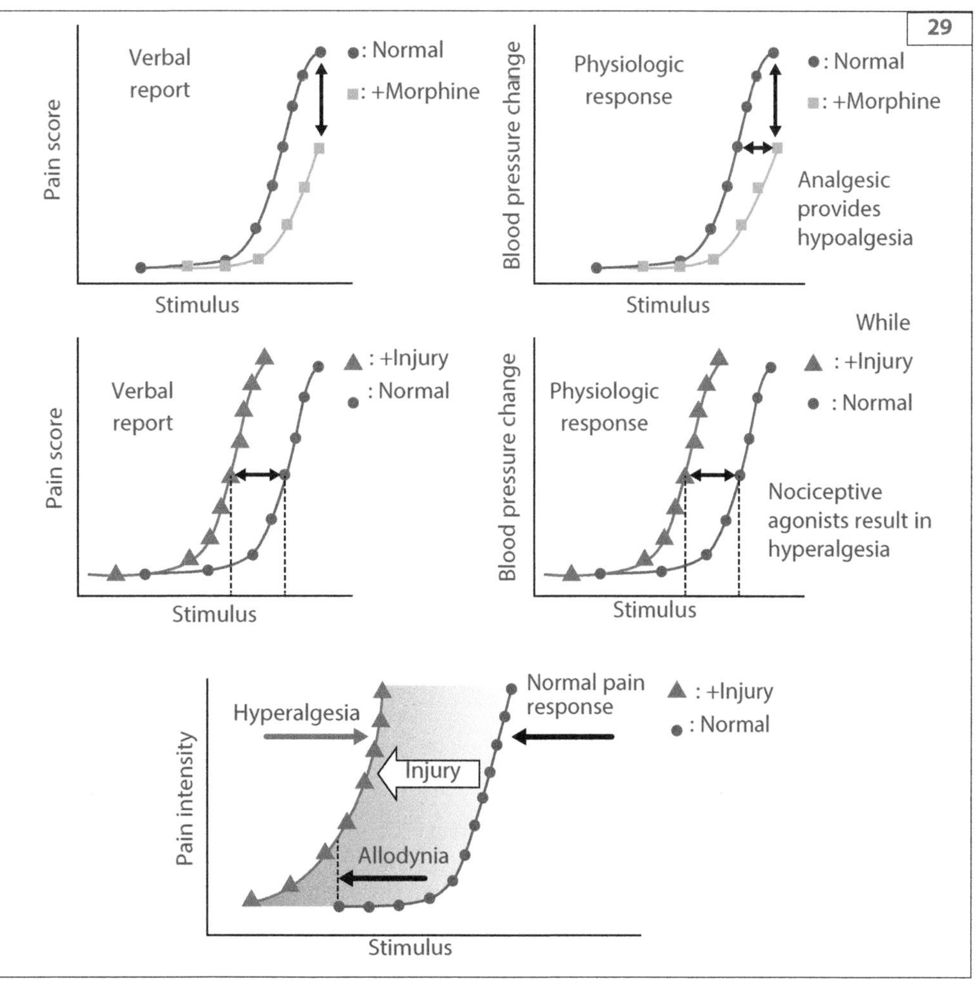

Fig. 29 Pain encoding is 'plastic' (i.e. it can be varied). Top tracings: under the influence of the analgesic morphine, the same stimulus results in a lower pain score and blood pressure than without the morphine (normal). Middle tracings: the influence of inflammatory mediators from injury yield a higher pain score and blood pressure for the same stimulus than in the normal subject. As injury causes the stimulus–response curve to shift to the left (where a smaller noxious stimulus is required to yield the same pain response), a point can be reached where a normally inocuous stimulus (i.e. simply touching the hair follicles) is perceived as painful, a state referred to as allodynia.

Wind-up

Wind-up is a form of activity-dependent plasticity that is characterized by a progressive increase in action potential output from dorsal horn neurons elicited during the course of a train of repeated low-frequency C-fiber or nociceptor stimuli[16]. Repetitive discharge of primary afferent nociceptors results in a co-release with glutamate of neuromodulators, such as sP and calcitonin generelated peptide (CGRP), from the nociceptor central terminals. Release of these neuropeptides activates postsynaptic G-protein-coupled receptors, which leads to slow postsynaptic depolarizations lasting tens of seconds. A behavioral correlate of wind-up can be produced in humans by repeated peripheral noxious heat or mechanical stimuli, where the pain increases with each successive stimulus, even though the stimulus intensity does not change.

A low intensity stimulus acting via low-threshold afferents can thus generate pain, the phenomenon of allodynia, and noxious inputs result in a pain response that is augmented in amplitude (hyperalgesia) and duration (hyperpathia). Dynamic increases in excitability (central sensitization) occur as a result of both local change in the spinal cord and in response to increased facilitation input from the brainstem.

Central sensitization needs to be differentiated from peripheral sensitization, a change in the transduction properties of the peripheral terminals of high-threshold (nociceptor) primary afferents, reducing their threshold, which contributes to pain hypersensitivity at the site of tissue injury or inflammation. Central sensitization in the dorsal horn typically results in tactile allodynia (e.g. brush-evoked pain) and a spread of pain hypersensitivity beyond an area of tissue damage (secondary hyperalgesia).

Wind-up has been a key milestone to the understanding of sensory processing in the spinal cord. Wind-up can lead to central sensitization; however, central sensitization can occur without wind-up. Wind-up can initiate central sensitization because it produces an elevation of intracellular calcium, not because of the progressive increase in action potential discharge. In other words, if intracellular calcium is elevated without any associated change in action potential firing, central sensitization can still occur. Such elevations in intracellular calcium may occur in a number of different ways.

What therefore is the association between wind-up and central sensitization? Central sensitization is the expression of an increase in excitability of neurons in the spinal cord[17]. This occurs at the single cell level as a change in receptive field properties with a reduction in threshold, and an increase in responsiveness and area involved as well as the recruitment of novel inputs. Behaviorally, it appears as abnormal or heightened sensitivity with a spread of hypersensitivity to uninjured sites (secondary hyperalgesia), and the generation of pain by low threshold Aβ mechanoreceptors (allodynia)[18]. More commonly, central sensitization is triggered by impulse traffic entering the CNS from the periphery as a result of normal nociceptive input (nociceptive pain), exaggerated nociceptive input due to inflammation, or peripheral neuropathy (neuropathic pain). Tenderness to touch (tactile allodynia) in both inflammatory pain and neuropathologic pain is due to central amplification of sensory input from normal Aβ touch afferents. Because of the central sensitization, light touch is felt as painful. The 'bottom line' is that wind-up is an initiator of central sensitization.

Clinical implication: perioperative analgesia should be planned to avoid excessive trauma leading to a state of wind-up.

NMDA receptor and wind-up

The most involved receptor in the sensation of acute pain, alpha-amino-3-hydroxy-5-methyl-isoxazole-4-propionic-acid (AMPA), is always exposed on afferent nerve terminals. In contrast, those most involved in the sensation of chronic pain, N-methyl-D-aspartate (NMDA) receptors, are not functional unless there has been a persistent or large-scale release of the transmitter glutamate.

Remember: afferents are incoming signals to the central nervous system.

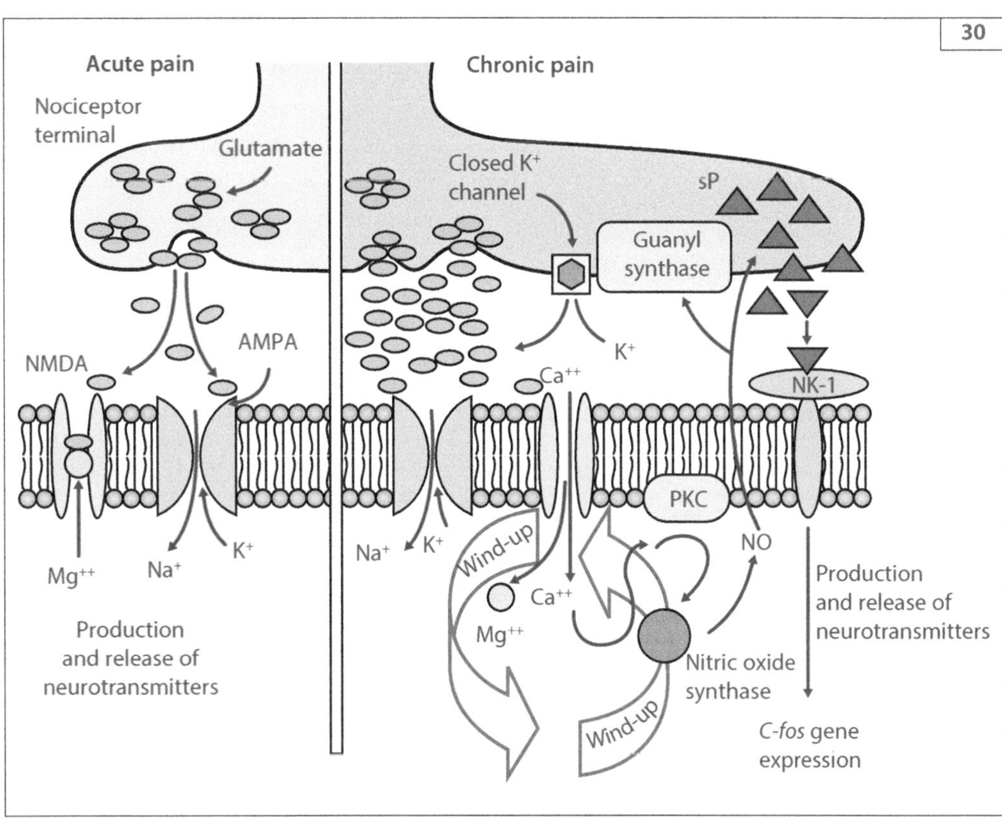

Fig. 30 Chronic pain often involves wind-up. In wind-up the cell membrane becomes permeable to calcium. Once the intracellular concentration of calcium is sufficient, a sequence of events follows that intensifies the propagation of nociception signaling, and renders opioids less efficient. Further, the intracellular calcium magnifies the release of neurotransmitters produced in, and released from, the cell membrane. AMPA: alpha-amino-3-hydroxy-5-methyl-isoxazole-4-propionic-acid; NK-1: neurokinin-1; NMDA: N-methyl-D-aspartate; NO: nitric oxide; PKC: protein kinase C; sP: substance P.

Repeated activation of AMPA receptors dislodges magnesium ions that act like 'stoppers' in transmembrane sodium and calcium channels of the NMDA receptor complex. Calcium flowing into the cell activates protein kinase C, the enzyme needed for nitrous oxide (NO) synthase production of NO. NO diffuses through the dorsal cell membrane and synaptic cleft into the nociceptor nerve and stimulates guanyl synthase-induced closure of potassium channels. Since endorphins and enkephalins inhibit pain by opening these channels, closure renders opioids less effective (see section on opioid mode of action in Chapter 5). NO also stimulates the release of sP, which by binding to neurokinin-1 receptors in the dorsal horn membrane promotes neural remodeling and hypersensitization. Accompanying this wind-up, less glutamate is required to transmit the pain signal and more antinociceptive input (drug) is required for analgesia (**Fig. 30**). Endorphins cannot keep up with the demand and essentially lose their effectiveness. The clinical implications are under-appreciated: *inadequately treated pain is a much more important cause of opioid tolerance than use of opioids themselves*. NMDA activation can also cause neural cells to sprout new connective endings[19], which then generates more possible sources for stimulation.

Endorphins and **enkephalins** are neurohormones naturally found in the brain, which have analgesic features similar to morphine.

Clinical implication: in the patient who appears to need increasing opioid for pain control, the state of wind-up may be suppressing the desired effect of the opioid.

It is important to note that NMDA-associated wind-up is a process where 'normal' underlying nociceptive signaling (much of which occurs in the spinothalamic tract) is *facilitated* by activity of the NMDA receptor. When this *facilitation* is blocked by an NMDA-antagonist, the underlying nociception signaling remains, which must be treated with other analgesics. For this reason, NMDA antagonists best serve as *adjuncts* in a multimodal analgesic protocol (**Fig. 31**).

Clinical implication: a N-methyl-D-aspartate antagonist would be a drug of choice for the patient in a state of wind-up-facilitated pain.

Transmission

Nociceptor neurons are considered the first-order neurons (**Fig.17**) of the nociceptive pathway. Their cell bodies extend axons into the gray matter of the dorsal horn of the spinal cord and synapse with second-order neurons (**Figs. 24, 30**). Second-order neurons are of varying types and have various different functions:

- Interneurons are both excitatory and inhibitory; involved in local processing and modulation of nociception messaging.
- Neurons extending over multiple spinal segments that comprise reflex arcs. These neurons stimulate efferent fibers that cause muscle contraction, producing simple motor withdrawal responses.

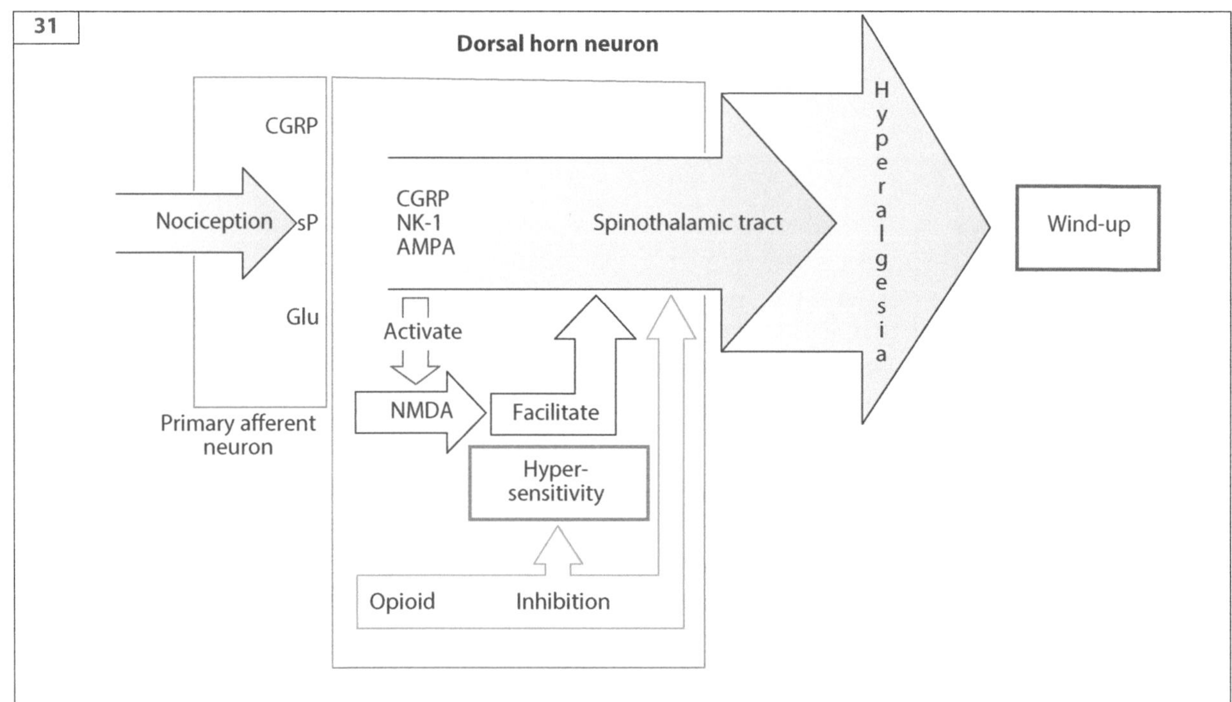

Fig. 31 NMDA-mediated wind-up facilitates the underlying nociceptive signaling, resulting in a state of hyperalgesia. Therefore, for optimal results, NMDA antagonists are administered as 'adjuncts' to a baseline protocol. AMPA: alpha-amino-3-hydroxy-5-methyl-isoxazole-4-propionic-acid; CGRP: calcitonin gene-related peptide; Glu: glutamate; NK-1: neurokinin-1; NMDA: N-methyl-D-aspartate; sP: substance P.

- Interneurons projecting to sympathetic reflex arcs surrounding the injury site that lead to release of NE and local cardiovascular changes, such as vasoconstriction.
- Projection neurons with axons ascending up the spinal cord into the fore- and midbrain.
- Nociceptive-specific neurons which receive input from Aδ and C nociceptor fibers only, therefore activated by noxious stimuli only.
- Wide dynamic range neurons that receive input from Aδ- and C-fibers and also Aβ-fibers – mechanoreceptors.
- Complex neurons, which receive and integrate inputs from both somatic and visceral tissues.

All types of second order neurons interact, and are involved in the modulation, processing and integration of nociceptive information that contributes to the animal's overall cognitive pain response (**Fig. 32**). Projection neurons that ascend within the spinal cord to the brain form several tracts: the most noted being the spinothalamic, (STT) spinoreticular (SRT), and spinohypothalamic (SHT).

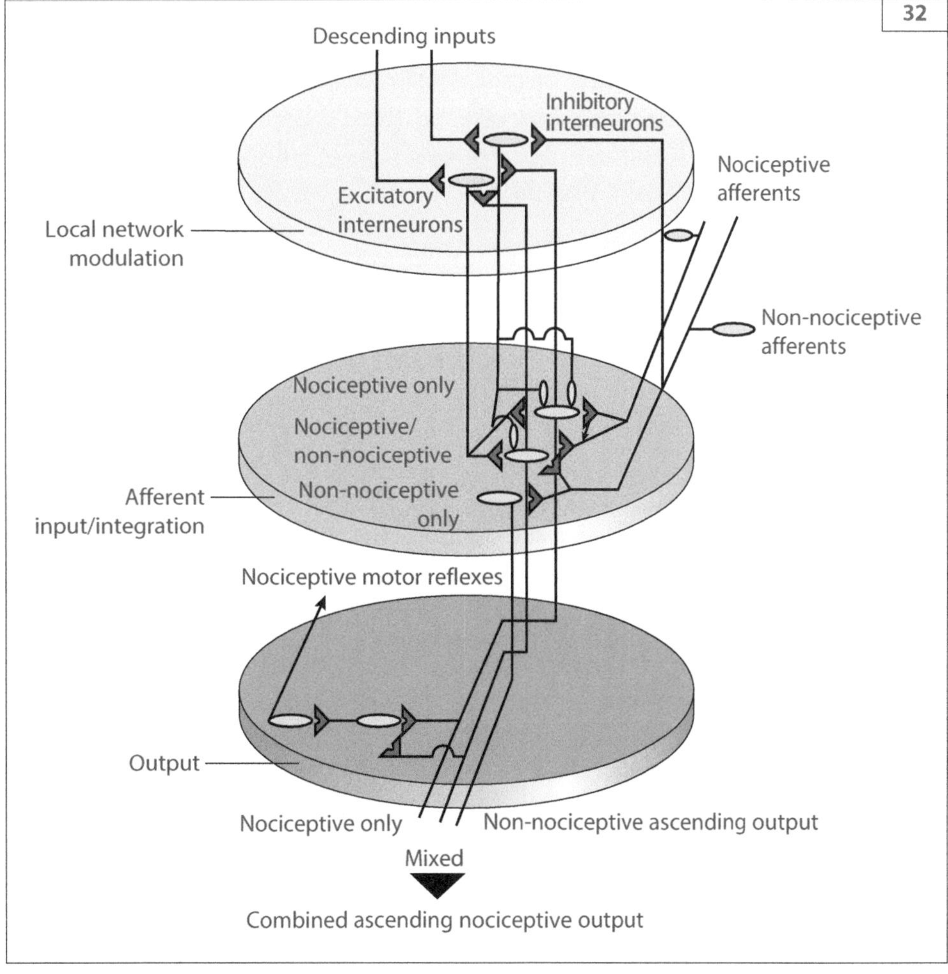

Fig. 32 Dorsal horn neurons consist of projecting neurons, propriospinal neurons, and local interneurons.

The STT ascends to the thalamus in the forebrain. A subset of these neurons is thought to be involved in the conscious localization and characterization of noxious stimuli. Another subset is apparently involved in the emotional reaction to the pain and overall response (behavioral changes). Klop *et al.*[20] have shown that in the cat it appears that a total of 12,000 cells in the spinal cord project to the thalamus.

Neurons in the SRT reach the reticular formation in the brainstem and some reach the thalamus. These neurons are implicated in the perception of pain that leads to emotional reactions, such as depression, anxiety, and suffering. The reticular formation is also thought to be responsible for levels of sleep and consciousness.

Clinical implication: excessive reticular formation stimulation from noxious stimuli can over-ride sleep and cause 'anesthetic arousal'.

The SHT is less frequently recognized, but contains neurons projecting directly to the hypothalamus of the forebrain. Accordingly, it is associated with the neuroendocrine and autonomic changes that are associated with the stress response. Katter *et al.*[21] estimated the number of SHT neurons in the cat to be approximately 900.

Descending inhibitory systems

As important as the ascending pathways, are fibers that descend from the brainstem to the spinal cord which modulate the incoming signals (**Fig. 33**). It has been commonly considered that brainstem–spinal pathways predominantly inhibit pain. Notable neurotransmitters mediating this antinociceptive effect include NE, especially in the locus ceruleus section of the brain, and SE in the raphe nuclei of the brain.

The **locus ceruleus** is an area in the brainstem involved with physiologic responses to stress, depression, and anxiety. Some antidepressant medications are believed to act on neurons in this area.

The **raphe nucleus** is a moderate sized cluster of nuclei found in the brainstem. Its main function is the release of serotonin to the rest of the brain. Selective serotonin reuptake inhibitor antidepressants are believed to act in these nuclei, as well as at their targets.

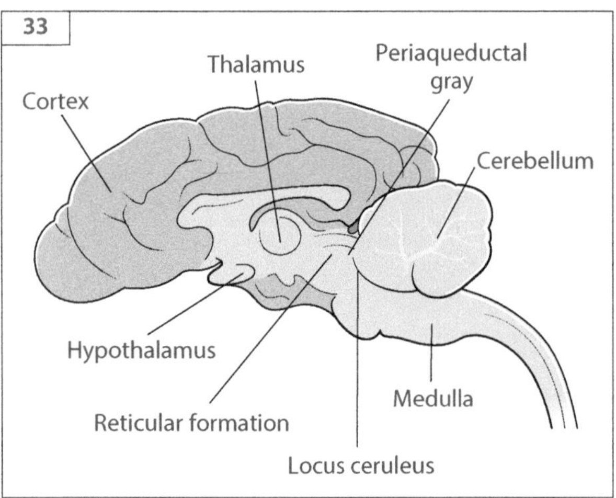

Fig. 33 Regions of the brain that are linked to the descending inhibitory systems.

Descending pain inhibitory pathways originate in, or relay through, a number of brainstem nuclei, and each pathway has a different neurochemistry and different neuroanatomical connection. Some of the brainstem nuclei are involved not only in descending but also ascending inhibition of pain-related responses. With advanced age, the function of descending pain inhibition is impaired and this is associated with a loss of noradrenergic and serotoninergic fibers in the spinal dorsal horn[22]. Additionally, there appears to be a gender difference, where activated descending pain modulatory pathways have a weaker pain suppressive effect in females than in males[23].

Clinical implications: these data suggest that older (particularly female) patients are less tolerant of pain than younger patients, because of changes within their own neuroanatomy.

Primary projection pathways conducting information between the dorsal horn of the spinal cord and 'supraspinal' locations in the brain are: STT, SRT, spinomesencephalic tract, and SHT. Such tracts are named based upon the origin and destination of the tract (e.g. the STT originates from the dorsal horn of the spine [Laminae I and IV to VII] en route to the thalamus). The STT is the most prominent ascending nociceptive pathway, where the thalamus plays an integral role as part of the limbic system. The limbic system integrates information associated with behavior, emotion, fear, anxiety, memory, arousal, vigilance, and sympathetic autonomic activity. The caudal extension of the limbic system, the periaqueductal gray (PAG), receives descending information from various supraspinal centers (in the brain and brainstem), as well as the spinal cord. The PAG is considered to be an important relay for descending facilitative and inhibitory modulation of nociceptive input. Further, the PAG connects with the rostral ventromedial medulla (RVM) from which NE- and SE-releasing fibers descend to the dorsal horn of the spinal cord, inducing inhibitory or analgesic effects. Stimulation of the PAG matter of the midbrain activates enkephalin-releasing neurons that project to the raphe nuclei in the brainstem. SE released from the raphe nuclei descends to the dorsal horn of the spinal cord where it forms excitatory connections with the 'inhibitor interneurons' located in the dorsal horn. When activated, these interneurons release either enkephalin or dynorphin (endogenous opioid neurotransmitters), which bind to mu (μ) opioid receptors on axons of incoming nociceptors. The activation of the μ-opioid receptor inhibits release of sP from these incoming first-order neurons and, in turn, inhibits the activation of the second-order neuron that is responsible for transmitting the pain signal up the STT to the thalamus, that is, the nociceptive signal is inhibited before it is able to reach the cortical areas that interpret the signal as 'pain'. This is sometimes referred to as the Gate Control Theory of Pain, resulting in immediate and profound analgesia.

There are three well-characterized families of endogenous opioid peptides: **enkephalins**, **endorphins**, and **dynorphins**. They are internally derived. The receptors for enkephalin are the δ opioid receptors.

Superficial laminae of the spinal dorsal horn have a population of interneurons containing inhibitory neurotransmitters, such as γ-aminobutyric acid (GABA), glycine, and enkephalin[24]. GABA is the chief inhibitory neurotransmitter in the mammalian CNS. Its binding to transmembrane receptors causes the opening of ion channels to allow the flow of either negatively charged chloride ions into the cell or positively charged potassium ions out of the cell. Whether this chloride flow is excitatory/depolarizing (makes the voltage across the cell's membrane less negative), shunting (has no effect on the cell's membrane), or inhibitory/hyperpolarizing (makes the cell's membrane more negative) depends on the direction of the flow of chloride ions. Neurons that produce GABA as their output are called GABAergic neurons, and have chiefly inhibitory action at their receptors.

The magnitude of the ascending nociceptive signal and the consequent pain sensation can be greatly influenced by descending pathways originating in the brainstem and terminating in the spinal dorsal horn. In conditions that cause persistent pain, such as inflammation or injury, the function of descending pathways may change to enhance the efficacy of descending inhibition. Alternatively, depending on a number of factors, injury and inflammation may result in a decrease of descending inhibition or an increase of descending facilitation of pain. Additionally, disorders of neurotransmitter systems *per se* potentially lead to hypofunction of descending pain inhibition and, consequently, to chronic pain. It is noteworthy that many of the neural structures involved in descending pain inhibition also have other functions, such as control of vigilance, motor behavior, circulation, and respiration. Bottom line: *the brain 'talks' to the spinal cord* (**Fig. 34**).

Preventive analgesia (pre-emptive analgesia)

Pain memories imprinted within the CNS, mediated by NMDA receptors, produce hyperalgesia and contribute to allodynia. In several animal experiments, central sensitization and wind-up do not occur if nociceptive blockade is applied prior to the nociceptive event. Such findings suggest that presurgical blockade of nociception may prevent postsurgical wound pain or pain hypersensitivity following surgery (i.e. pre-emptive analgesia), as advocated by the eminent pain physiologist, Professor Patrick Wall[25]. Recent trends suggest abandoning the term 'pre-emptive analgesia' for 'preventive analgesia'[26].

Successful preventive analgesia must meet three criteria: 1) intense enough to block all nociception; 2) wide enough to cover the entire surgical area; and 3) prolonged enough to last throughout surgery and even into the postoperative period.

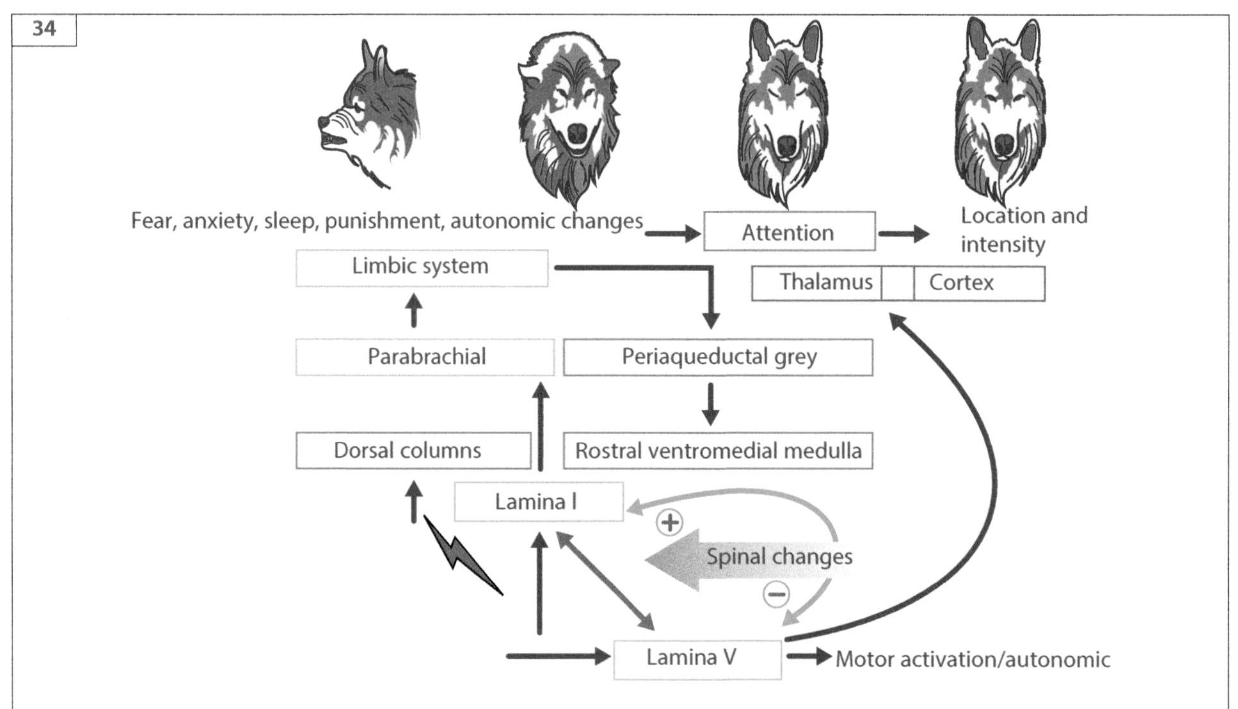

Fig. 34 The descending inhibitory pathway plays a major role in the plasticity of the central nervous system, where the brain 'talks back' to the spinal cord.

It is important to note that adequate levels of general anesthesia with a volatile drug, such as isoflurane, do not prevent central sensitization. The potential for central sensitization exists even in unconscious patients who are unresponsive to surgical stimuli. This has been demonstrated in the dog[27,28], where ('pain-induced distress') cortisol spikes occurred in response to the noxious stimulus of ovariohysterectomy during the anesthetic period, demonstrating the link between surgical stimulus and neural responsiveness during anesthetic-induced unconsciousness.

In 1988, Professor Patrick Wall introduced the concept of pre-emptive analgesia to clinicians with his editorial in the journal *Pain*[25]. The emphasis of preventive analgesia is to prevent sensitization of the nervous system throughout the perioperative period. Pain is to be expected from all surgeries as well as the hypersensitivity that subsequently develops. Analgesia administered after sensitization may decrease pain somewhat, but has little long-term benefit in addressing the pain resultant from postsurgical inflammation. Analgesia administered before surgery limits inflammatory pain and decreases subsequent hypersensitivity. The most effective preventive analgesic regimen occurs when initiated before surgery and continued throughout the postoperative period (**Fig. 35**).

Remember: the best prevention of wind-up is blocking nociceptive entry into the central nervous system.

A review of preventive analgesia, with inclusion of suggested drugs (available in 2001) and dosage has been provided elsewhere[29]. A logical preventive, synergistic drug protocol would include an opioid, α_2-agonist, ±NMDA antagonist[30], and a nonsteroidal anti-inflammatory drug (NSAID)[31]. The implementation of perioperative NSAIDs is controversial based upon their antiprostaglandin effect, which in the face of hypotension, might enhance the potential for acute renal failure. This is why perioperative fluid support is such an important consideration.

Inhalant anesthetics can cause a decreased perfusion of the renal tissues. When renal perfusion becomes dangerously low, the body releases prostaglandins to cause vasodilation, bringing increased blood flow to the renal tissues. Since nonsteroidal anti-inflammatory drugs act as antiprostaglandins, they block this physiologic response.

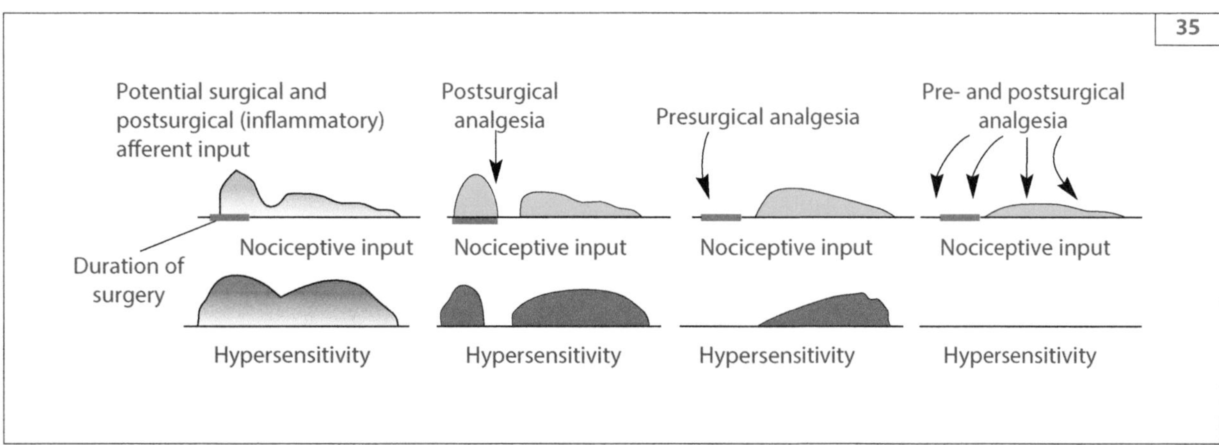

Fig. 35 Simply administering analgesics before surgery is not as effective as the continued administration of analgesics throughout the perioperative period. This is because most postoperative pain is due to inflammation, which persists for some time after the actual surgery.

However, anti-inflammatory drugs play a substantial role in perioperative pain management[32], because surgery cannot be performed without subsequent inflammation. Reducing the inflammatory response in the periphery, and thereby decreasing sensitization of the peripheral nociceptors, should attenuate central sensitization[33]. It has also been recognized for some time that NSAIDs synergistically interact with both μ-opioid and α_2-adrenoceptor agonists[34–37]. In human medicine, the use of perioperative NSAIDs has reduced the use of patient-controlled analgesic morphine by 40–60%[38,39].

Synergism is a response greater than the additive effect.

Adaptive pain (acute pain)

Everyday adaptive pain, or 'nociceptive pain', occurs when a strong noxious (harmful) stimulus (mechanical, thermal, or chemical) impacts the skin or deep tissue. Nociceptors, a special class of primary sensory nerve fibers, fire impulses in response to these stimuli, which travel along the peripheral nerves, past the sensory cell bodies in the DRG, through the dorsal roots, and into the spinal cord (or brainstem). Thereafter, the conscious brain interprets these transmissions from populations of second- and third-order neurons of the CNS.

Adaptive pain is purposeful. It protects against potentially severe tissue injury as a result of noxious insults from everyday activities. Adaptive pain is also short-acting, and relatively easy to treat (**Fig. 36**).

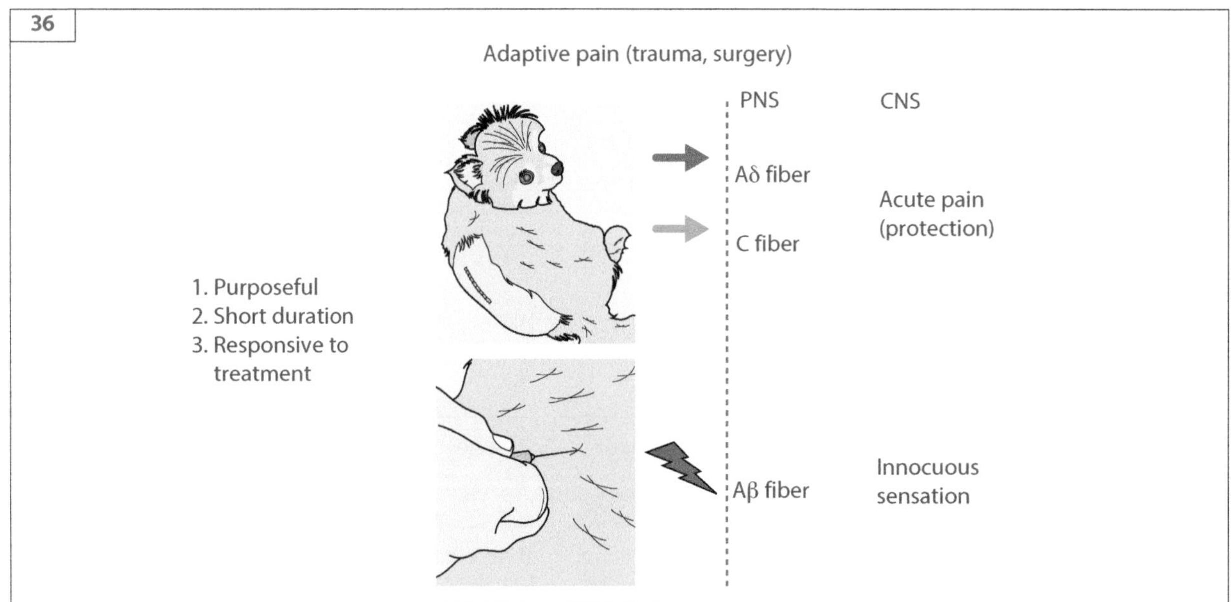

Fig. 36 Adaptive (acute) pain is purposeful, of short duration, and usually responsive to treatment. Aδ- and C nerve fibers transmit responses from noxious insults to the central nervous system (CNS), where they are processed as pain. Aβ-fibers can also be 'recruited' to send such signals, but are usually involved in the transmission of innocuous information, such as touch, joint position, and so on. PNS: peripheral nervous system.

Physiologic pain, a term synonymous with nociceptive pain, occurs after most types of noxious stimulus, and is usually protective. This type of pain plays an adaptive role as part of the body's normal defensive mechanisms, warning of contact with potentially damaging environmental insults, and it initiates responses of avoidance – fight or flight. Dr. Frank Vertosick states, 'Pain is a teacher, the headmaster of nature's survival school'[40]. This protective system relies on a sophisticated network of nociceptors and sensory neurons that encode insult intensity, duration, quality, and location. Physiologic pain is rarely a clinical entity for treatment, but rather a state to avoid, for example, a sharp object. Pathologic pain, inferring that tissue damage is present, is not transient, and may be associated with significant tissue inflammation and nerve injury. It is often further classified into inflammatory pain, neuropathic pain, or maladaptive pain. From the perspective of duration, recent pathologic pain can be considered a symptom, whereas maladaptive pain can be considered a disease.

A **nociceptor** is a sensory receptor that reacts to potentially damaging stimuli by sending nerve signals to the spinal cord and brain. This process, called **nociception**, usually causes the perception of pain.

Inflammatory pain

Inflammatory pain, often categorized along with adaptive pain as 'nociceptive,' refers to pain and tenderness felt when the skin or other tissue is inflamed, hot, red, and swollen. The inflammatory process is mediated and facilitated by the local release of numerous chemicals, including bradykinin, prostaglandins (PGs), leukotrienes (LTs), SE, histamine, sP, thromboxanes, platelet-activating factor, adenosine and ATP, protons, and free radicals. Cytokines such as ILs and TNF, and neurotropins, especially nerve growth factor, are also generated during inflammation. Most of these chemical 'messengers' are referred to as cytokines or chemokines.

When there is tissue injury and inflammation, the firing threshold of Aδ and C nociceptive afferents in response to heating of the skin is lowered into the non-noxious range. This is a result of PG production and release into the local area of inflammation. Threshold lowering occurs for thermal but not electrical stimuli.

Afferents are incoming signals to the central nervous system.

Postoperative, incisional pain is a specific and common form of adaptive pain. Studies in rodents have characterized the primary hyperalgesia to mechanical and thermal (from inflammation) stimuli[41]. *Primary hyperalgesia from mechanical stimuli (such as tissue movement) lasts for 2–3 days, while hyperalgesia to heat lasts longer, 6 or 7 days*. Secondary hyperalgesia in surrounding tissues is attributable only to mechanical, not thermal stimuli[42].

Clinical implication: for routine noxious procedures, a minimum of 3–7 days of take-home analgesics is warranted.

In humans, acute postoperative pain is followed by persistent pain in 10–50% of patients after common operations. Since maladaptive pain can be severe in about 2–10% of these patients, persistent postoperative pain (PPOP) represents a major, largely unrecognized clinical problem[43]. Such discomfort lasts for more than 3–6 months after surgery. PPOP is the consequence either of ongoing inflammation or, more commonly, a manifestation of neuropathic pain, resulting from surgical injury to major peripheral nerves. Consequently, surgical techniques that avoid nerve damage should be applied whenever possible. Also, early therapy for postoperative pain, such as cold compression therapy[44], should be implemented, since the intensity of acute postoperative pain correlates with the risk of developing a persistent pain state.

Neurogenic inflammation

Release of sP and NGF into the periphery causes a tissue reaction termed neurogenic inflammation. Neurogenic inflammation is driven by events in the CNS and does not depend on granulocytes or lymphocytes as with the classic inflammatory response to tissue trauma or immune-mediated cell damage. Cells in the dorsal horn release chemicals that cause action potentials to fire backwards down the nociceptors. The result of this dorsal root reflex is that nociceptive dendrites release sP and CGRP into peripheral tissues, causing degranulation of mast cells and changing vascular endothelial cell characteristics. The resultant outpouring of potent inflammatory and vasodilating agents causes edema and potentiates transmission of nociceptive signals from the periphery (**Fig. 37**).

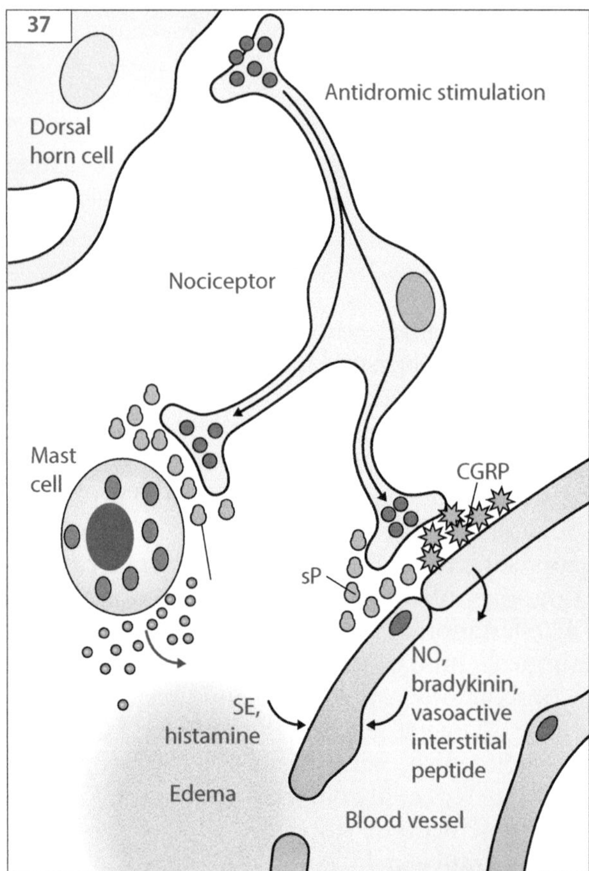

Fig. 37 Neurogenic inflammation varies from the classic inflammatory response as it is driven by events in the central nervous system. CGRP: calcitonin gene-related peptide; NO: nitric oxide; SE: seretonin; sP: substance P.

Neuropathic pain

The International Association for the Study of Pain defines neurogenic (neuropathic) pain as 'pain initiated or caused by a primary lesion or dysfunction or transitory perturbation in the peripheral or central nervous system'[45]. Simplistically, neuropathic pain can be identified as pain due to a primary lesion or malfunction of the PNS or CNS. There is vagueness in identifying neuropathic diseases and currently no tests are available that can unequivocally diagnose neuropathic pain. Nevertheless, a large body of evidence validates the physiologic process underlying neuropathic pain. Neurogenic pain, deafferentiation pain, and dysesthetic pain are all terms used to describe this entity. The word 'neuropathic' is preferred because it encompasses changes in function as well as damage to a nerve as possible causes of pain.

Primary sensory neurons are able to signal specific sensory experiences because they respond with electrical impulses to specific types of stimuli (touch, pinch, heat, cold, vibration), and because they communicate with second-order sensory neurons in the spinal cord via specific synaptic connectivity using specific neurotransmitters. Maintaining these settings requires a complex biologic process. If there has been nerve injury, the electrical properties, neurochemistry, and central connectivity of these neurons can change, bringing havoc on normal sensory processing, and sometimes inducing severe maladaptive neuropathic pain.

Many kinds of nerve injury can induce electrical changes: trauma, viral or bacterial infection, poor nutrition, toxins, autoimmune events, and so on. Axon and myelin damage are known to cause a number of key changes in the functioning (phenotype) of sensory neurons, some of which lead to ectopic spontaneous discharge.

The relative role of peripheral and central mechanisms in neuropathic pain is not well understood and likely reflects different disease states and genetic differences; however, the abnormal input of neural activity from nociceptor afferents plays a dynamic and ongoing role in maintaining the pain state. Two key concepts are critical to an understanding of neuropathic pain: 1) inappropriate activity in nociceptive fibers (injured and uninjured); and 2) central changes occur in sensory processing that arise from these abnormalities (**Fig. 38**).

Two major consequences for pain in neuropathy result from central sensitization. Input from residual uninjured Aβ touch afferents is rendered painful, whereas they are not normally painful. More than amplification, this is a change in modality; from touch to pain. Secondly, central sensitization may recruit Aβ-fiber activity that now augments the painful response.

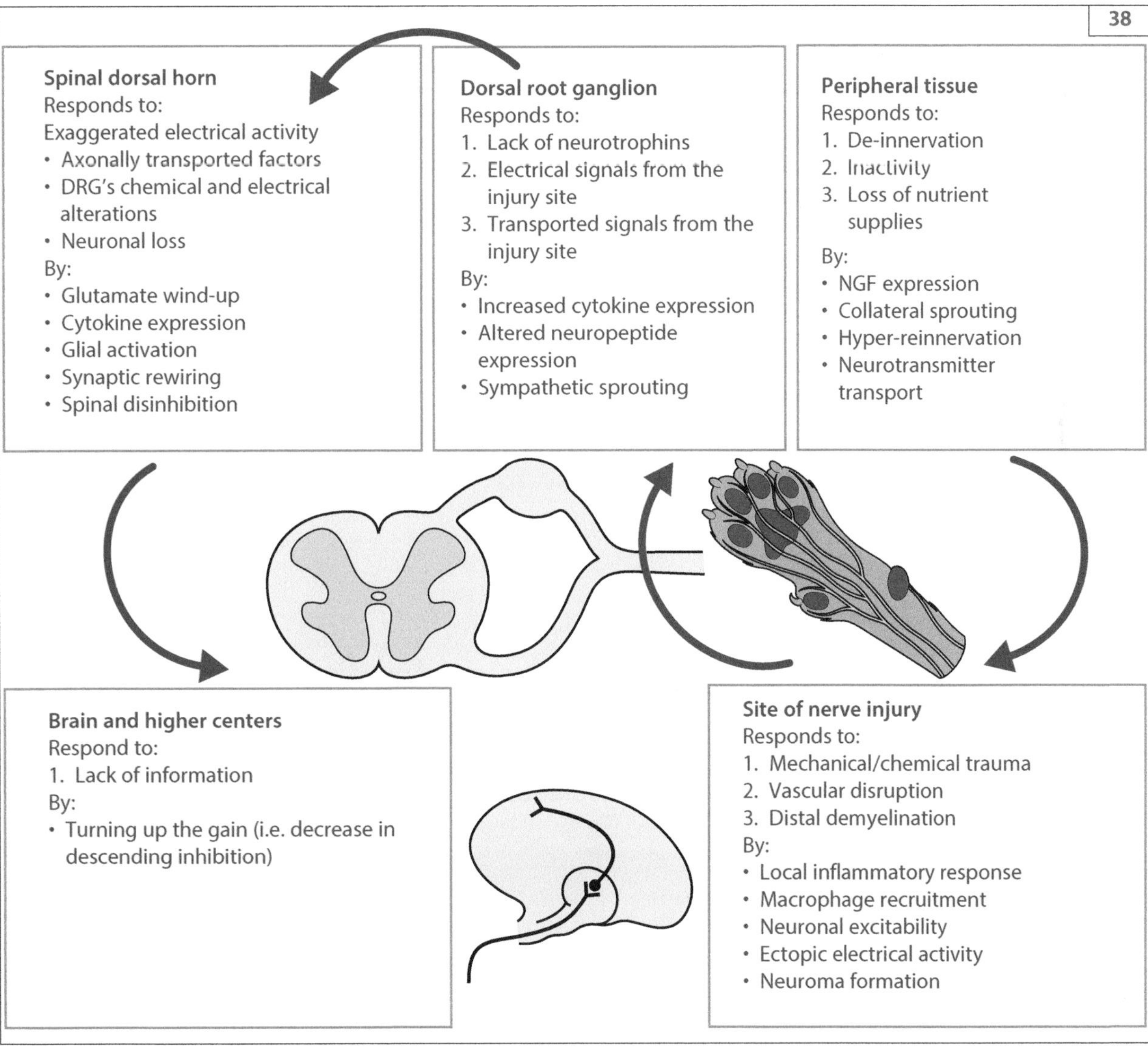

Fig. 38 Possible sites for the generation of neuropathic pain. DRG: dorsal root ganglion; NGF: nerve growth factor.

An understanding of neuropathic pain is increasing with the realization that the nervous system is not a 'hard-wired, line-labeled system', but one that demonstrates 'plasticity', in that function and structure of the system alters with continuing development, experience, or consequences of injury. That is to say, the nervous system is not like a light switch, where an input (turning the switch on) consistently gives a predictable response (there is light). Instead, the nervous system is more like a 'smart computer' where data are entered, but depending on the software, the response can vary. Targets for the control of neuropathic pain are shown in *Table 12*.

Maladaptive pain (chronic pain)

In contrast to adaptive pain, where the pain stops quickly after the noxious stimulus has been removed, the pain and tenderness of inflammation may last for hours, days, months, and years. Recognition of the potential mediators of peripheral sensitization after inflammation gives insight as to the complexity of this process. Persistent, or maladaptive, pain is often neuropathic pain, which arises from injury to the PNS or CNS. Maladaptive pain appears to have no purpose, is characterized by extended duration, and is frequently difficult to treat, but may respond to certain anticonvulsants, tricyclic antidepressants, and antiarrhythmics.

TABLE 12: Mechanisms of neuropathic pain with corresponding drug targets

Mechanism	Target	Drug (human use)
Peripheral sensitization	TRPV1 receptors	Capsaicin
Altered expression, distribution, and function of ion channels	Voltage-gated K^+ channels	-
	Voltage-gated Na^+ channels	Local anesthetics, e.g. lidocaine; antiepileptics, e.g. carbamazepine, lacosamide, lamotrigine; antiarrhythmic agents, e.g. mexiletine
	HCN channels	-
	P2X-receptor-gated channels	-
	Voltage-gated Ca^{2+} channels	Ziconotide, gabapentin, pregabalin
Increased central excitation	NMDA receptors	Ketamine, ifenprodil
	NK-1 receptors	-
Reduced spinal inhibition	Opioid receptors	Morphine, oxycodone, tramadol
	GABA receptors	Baclofen
	Glycine receptors	-
Deregulated supraspinal control	Monoamines	Tricyclic antidepressants, e.g. amitryptiline, nortriptyline; serotonin and norepinephrine reuptake inhibitors, e.g. duloxetine, tramadol
Immune system involvement	Cytokines	NSAIDs
	TNF-α	-
	Microglia	-
Schwann cell dedifferentiation	Growth factors	-

GABA: γ-aminobutyric acid; HCN: hyperpolarization-activated cyclic nucleotide-gated channel; NK-1: neurokinin-1; NMDA: N-methyl-D-aspartate; NSAID: nonsteroidal anti-inflammatory drugs; P2X: subtype of adenosine triphosphate receptor; TNF-α-: tumor necrosis factor-α; TRPV1: transient receptor potential V1.

Local anesthetics applied systemically, topically, or to block nerves may also be effective in maladaptive pain. The separation between inflammatory and neuropathic pain does not exclude inflammatory components in neuropathic pain or neuropathic components in inflammatory pain. There are no systematic studies in neuropathic pain patients on the correlation between the intensity of the symptoms and the nature and severity of the nerve injury.

Maladaptive pain can result from sustained noxious stimuli, such as ongoing inflammation, or it may be independent of the inciting cause (**Fig. 39**). Regardless of its origin, maladaptive pain offers no useful biologic function or survival advantage. The nervous system itself actually becomes the focus of the pathology and contributes to patient morbidity. Effective treatment for maladaptive pain can be a frustrating challenge. A number of studies have shown that the longer a pain lingers, the harder it is to eradicate. This is because pain can reconfigure the architecture of the nervous system it invades.

Clinical implication: treat pain early and aggressively.

Chronic pain was traditionally defined as pain lasting more than 3 or 6 months, depending on the source of the definition[46,47]. More recently, chronic pain has been defined as 'maladaptive pain that extends beyond the period of tissue healing and/or with low levels of identified pathology that are insufficient to explain the presence and /or extent of pain'[48]. There is no general consensus on the definition of maladaptive pain. In clinical practice it is often difficult to determine when adaptive pain has become maladaptive.

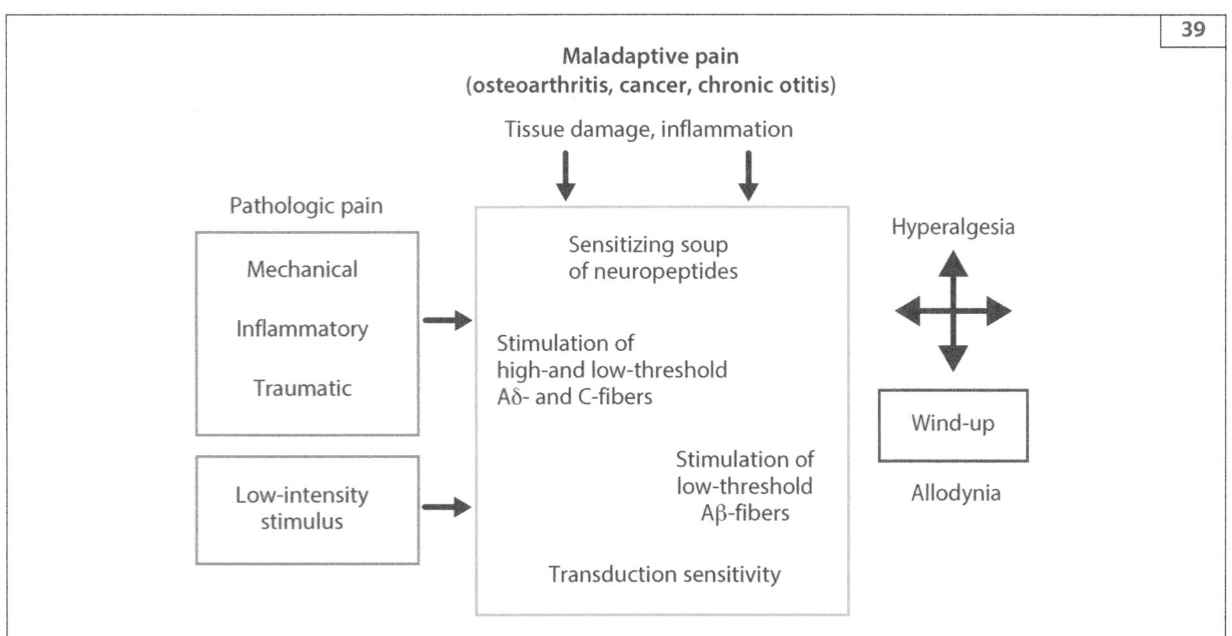

Fig. 39 Osteoarthritis, cancer and long-standing otitis can often be the origin of maladaptive pain. In the process of transduction (conversion of noxious stimulus into nerve impulses), nociception is influenced by a 'sensitizing soup' of cytokines and chemokines (e.g. bradykinin, histamine, eicosanoids, hydrogen ions), Aβ-fibers are recruited to carry 'painful signals', and the result is hyperalgesia, often associated with wind-up and potentially a state of allodynia.

Adaptive to maladaptive pain

Normally, a steady state is maintained in which there is a close correlation between injury and pain. Yet, long-lasting or very intense nociceptive input or the removal of a portion of the normal input can distort the nociceptive system to such an extent that the close correlation between injury and pain can be lost. A progression from adaptive to maladaptive pain might be considered as three major stages or phases of pain, proposing that different neurophysiologic mechanisms are involved, depending on the nature and time course of the originating stimulus[49]. These three phases include: 1) the processing of a brief noxious stimulus; 2) the consequences of prolonged noxious stimulation, leading to tissue damage and peripheral inflammation; and 3) the consequences of neurologic damage, including peripheral neuropathies and central pain states (**Fig. 40**).

Phase 1: Adaptive pain (physiologic pain)

Mechanisms underlying the processing of brief noxious stimuli are fairly simple, with a direct route of transmission centrally toward the brain resulting in the conscious perception of pain, with the possibility for modulation occurring at synaptic relays along the way. It is reasonably easy to construct logical and detailed neuronal circuits to explain the features of phase 1 pain.

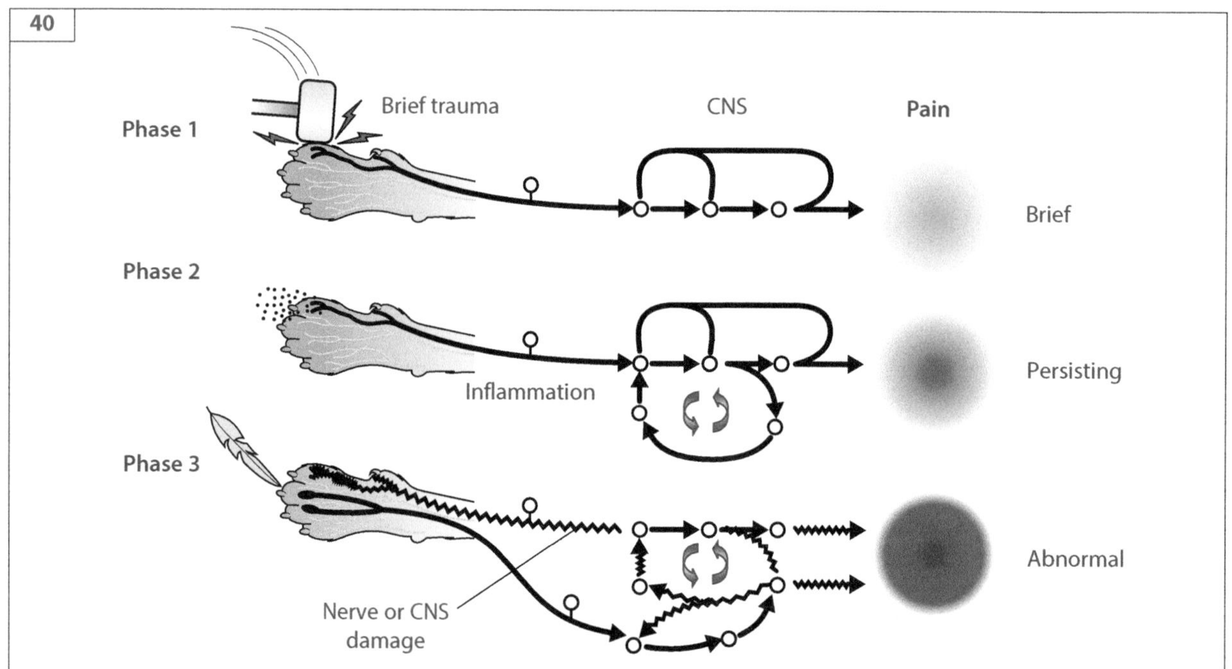

Fig. 40 Progression of adaptive to maladaptive pain can be considered as three phases of pain: brief (acute nociceptive), persisting (inflammatory), and abnormal (neuropathic). CNS: central nervous system.

Phase 2: Inflammatory pain

If a noxious stimulus is very intense, or prolonged, leading to tissue damage and inflammation, it might be considered phase 2 pain, as influenced by the response properties of various components of the nociceptive system changing. These changes note that the CNS has moved to a new, more excitable state as a result of the noxious input generated by tissue injury and inflammation. Phase 2 is characterized by its central drive, a drive that is triggered and maintained by peripheral inputs. Patients experience spontaneous pain and sensation changes resulting from stimulation of the injured and surrounding area. This change is known as hyperalgesia – a leftward shift of the stimulus–response curve (**Fig. 29**).

Remember: hyperalgesia in the area of injury is termed primary hyperalgesia, and in the areas of normal tissue surrounding the injury site, as secondary hyperalgesia.

Phase 3: Neuropathic pain

Phase 3 pain is abnormal pain, generally the consequence of either damage or altered neuroprocessing within peripheral nerves or within the CNS itself, characterized by a lack of correlation between injury and pain. Clinically, phase 1 and 2 pains are symptoms of peripheral injury, whereas phase 3 pain is a symptom of neurologic disease. These pains are spontaneous, triggered by innocuous stimuli, or are exaggerated responses to minor noxious stimuli.

Particular combinations of mechanisms responsible for each of the pain states is likely unique to the individual disease, or to a particular subgroup of patients. Phase 3 pain may involve genetic, interpretive, or other brain processing that has yet to be identified. Activation of these mechanisms may be abnormally prolonged or intense due to abnormal input from damaged neurons, or simply because the regenerative properties of neurons are very poor or 'misdirected'. Healing may never occur. Finally, there are many mixed nociceptive–neuropathic pains, not only in cancerous disease, but also in conditions such as herniated intervertebral disk and postamputation (phantom) limb pain. Because of these changes, maladaptive pain is often considered a disease *per se*, rather than a symptom.

Visceral pain

Healthy viscera are insensate (not consciously sensed) or, at best, minimally sensate. Such observation dates back to 1628 when Sir William Harvey exposed the heart of a patient, and with pinching and pricking determined that the patient could not reliably identify the stimulus[50]. This is in contrast to the body surface (somatic tissues), which is always sensate. Injury to the surface of the body initiates the reflex response of fight or flight, whereas visceral pain tends to invoke immobility. In general, there is a poor correlation between the amount of visceral pathology and intensity of visceral pain. Traditional 'clinical wisdom' has it that: 1) viscera are minimally sensate, whereas body surfaces are always highly sensate; 2) visceral pain has poorer localization than superficial pain; and 3) visceral pain is more strongly linked to emotion than superficial pain.

In this context, the term **viscera** refers to organs within the abdomen, e.g. gastrointestinal tract, bladder, kidney, and so on.

Dogs are nonverbal, therefore unable to state their origin of discomfort; yet depression, despondency, dullness, or 'ain't doin' right' are common presentation concerns of pet owners. This might suggest that visceral pain is more common than is appreciated. With the intent of being most thorough in our work-up of differential diagnoses, it is important to understand why visceral pain is different from somatic pain.

The neuroanatomy of canine viscera (**Fig. 41**) suggests their unique pain response. Yet, a separate pathway for transmitting visceral input from the site of origin to the brain does not exist. Every cell that has visceral input has somatic input: 'visceral–somatic convergence'. There are cells that receive somatic input only, but there are no cells that receive visceral input only. During normal activities, information is conducted from somatic origin, such as skin, through the STT in the spinal cord, to CNS areas for interpretation of nociception. With myocardial infarct/angina, for example, the same STT cells are activated as with a somatic peripheral nociceptive input, and theory has it that the STT may have become 'conditioned' to the everyday somatic responses; so it now 'presumes' it is sensing a somatic afferent signal rather than a visceral afferent signal.

A suggested mechanism for referred pain is that visceral and somatic primary neurons converge onto common spinal neurons. This is the convergence–projection theory (**Fig. 42**), which has considerable supporting experimental evidence[51].

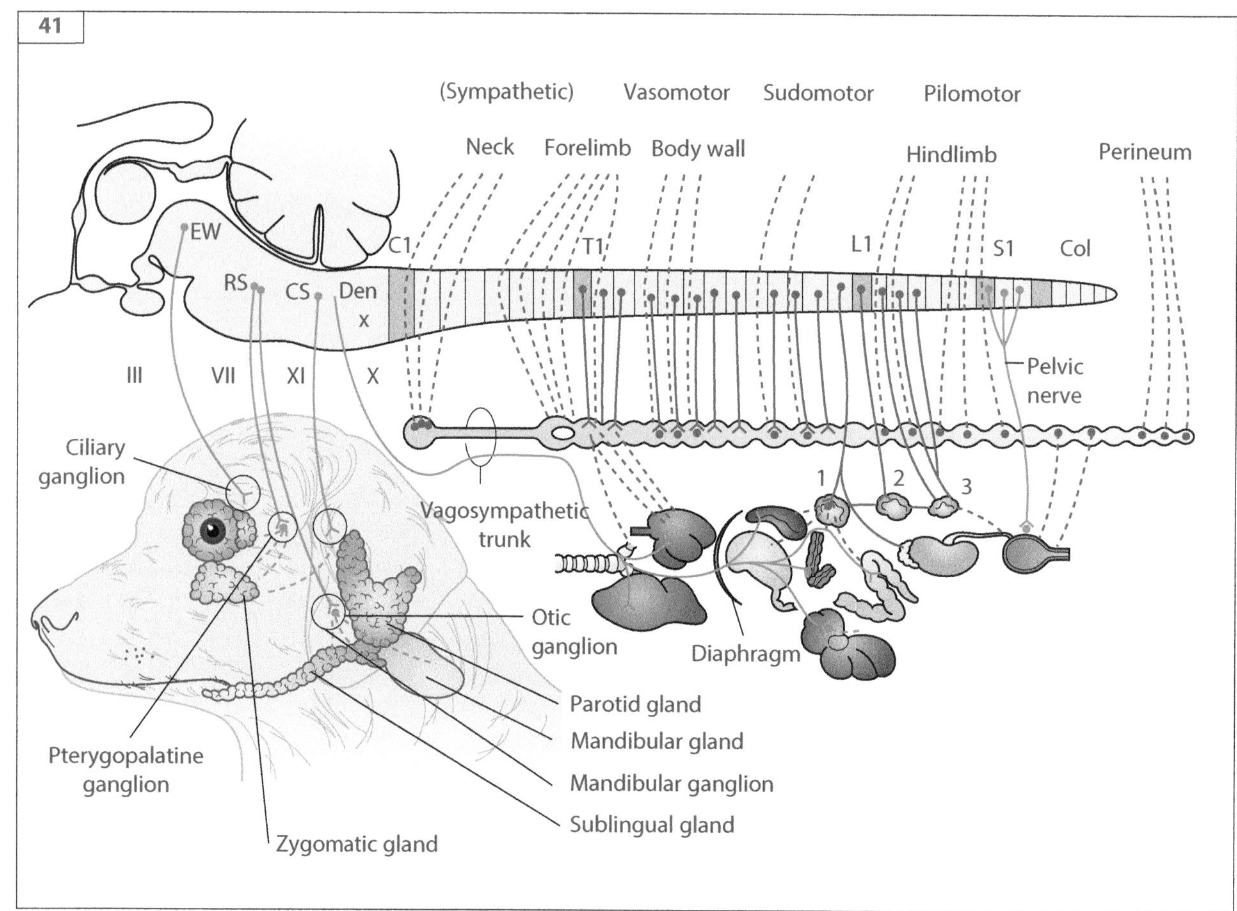

Fig. 41 Neuroanatomy of canine viscera. C1: first cervical vertebra; Col: coccygeal 1; CS: caudal salivatory nucleus; Den: dorsal efferent nucleus of the vagus; EW: Edinger-Westphal nucleus; L1: first lumbar vertebra; RS: rostral salivatory nucleus; S1: first sacral vertebra; T1: first thoracic vertebra; 1–3 denote that visceral pain is more unpleasant, diffuse and variable than cutaneous pain of similar intensity, independent of the duration of the presented stimulus.

A lack of sensitivity in viscera at baseline may relate to the sparse population of visceral afferents themselves, which are quantitatively fewer per unit area than cutaneous afferents. This may suggest that increased activity is required to cross a threshold for visceral perception. The large proportion of silent afferents in viscera also helps to explain the variation of sensitization. Silent afferents have been frequently noted in visceral structures to form up to 50% of the neuronal sample[52].

Fine sensory nerve fibers have been detected that are not excited by physiologic stimuli, even at potentially tissue damaging intensities. These silent afferents are known to supply knee joint, skin, and viscera; in the last case, silent afferents seem to be particularly numerous. When an artificial inflammation is induced, many silent afferents develop spike activity, others remain quiet. Silent afferents that do respond probably have a nociceptive sensory function. Under inflammatory conditions some silent afferents are sensitized to physiologic stimuli, others are probably chemospecific. Normal conduction in silent afferents may sum spatially and temporally in second-order neurons with other nociceptive information, and may thereby contribute to different pain states. Furthermore, there is evidence that the activation of chemospecific silent afferents may lead to sensitization of nociceptive dorsal horn neurons. Some silent afferents probably contain neuropeptides that may be released under pathophysiologic conditions, such as inflammation. Whether certain pathologic states can be exclusively attributed to the activation of silent afferents or whether silent afferents sustain the functions of 'conventional' nociceptors is unclear.

The mucosa, muscle, and serosa of hollow organs as well as the mesentery, but not the parenchyma of solid organs, contain visceral receptors[53]. Inflammation will lower nociceptor firing thresholds, resulting in sensitization to lower distention pressures. As mentioned, inflammation also recruits 'silent' nociceptors (Aβ-fibers), which fire at lower thresholds or become sensitized by hypoxemia (low oxygen) and ischemia (low blood supply)[54]. Acute pain is the sum of high threshold nociceptors activated at high pressures, where chronic noxious stimuli recruit previously unresponsive or silent nociceptors through hypoxemia or inflammation. Pain sensations correlate with generated intracolonic or small bowel pressures and increased wall tension rather than intraluminal volume[55]. Accordingly, patients may have ileus without pain.

Parenchyma refers to the functional elements of an organ, as contrasted to its framework or stroma.

Ileus is failure of contents to move down the bowel.

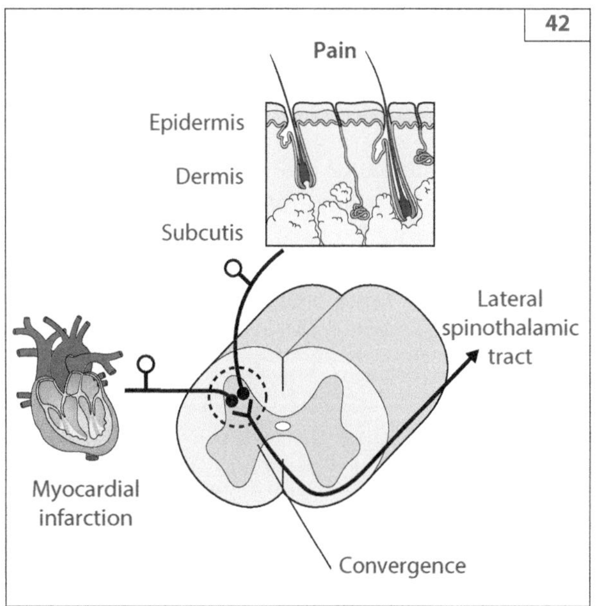

Fig. 42 Convergence of first-order neurons from both somatic and visceral origins onto second-order neurons renders the second-order neuron (e.g. spinothalamic tract) unable to determine the actual origin of nociception.

To explain better 'referred pain with somatic hyperalgesia', two theories have been proposed. The convergence–facilitation theory proposes that abnormal visceral input would produce an irritable focus in the relative spinal cord segment, thus facilitating messages from somatic structures. The second postulates that the visceral afferent barrage induces the activation of a reflex arc, the afferent branch of which is represented by visceral afferent fibers and the efferent branch by somatic efferents and sympathetic efferents toward the somatic structures (muscle, subcutis, and skin). The efferent impulses toward the periphery would then sensitize nociceptors in the parietal tissues (organ walls) of the referred area, thus resulting in the phenomenon of somatic hyperalgesia.

Efferent refers to conduction **away** from a center (central nervous system), as contrasted to **afferent**, which refers to conduction **toward** a center.

Visceral pain is also processed differently. Although primary afferents serving visceral, cutaneous, and muscle pain are mostly distinct, at the dorsal horn there is considerable convergence of these pathways so that the STT, SRT, and spinomesencephalic tract all contain neurons that respond to both somatic and visceral stimuli[56].

Gender and visceral pain

A review of the human literature[57] suggests that women are more likely than men to experience a variety of recurrent and visceral pains. Generally, women report more severe levels of pain, more frequent pain, and pain of longer duration than do men. Reports of visceral pain in veterinary patients are sparse. A report of veterinary outpatients visiting the Ohio State University showed that in the year 2002, 1,153 dogs and 652 cats were presented[58]. Twenty percent of dogs and 14% of the cats were diagnosed as in pain, with approximately half of each species being diagnosed with visceral pain. No differences were noted related to gender; however, most animals presented were neutered or spayed. Studies in rats show that visceral hypersensitivity varies over the estrous cycle, where rats are more sensitive during proestrus, and proestrus rats are more hypersensitive than male rats[59]. Kamp *et al.*[60] have shown that female mice are more sensitive to visceral pain than males in a colorectal distention model, but have also shown that response varies with the strain of mouse. There is a stunning over-representation of male subjects in the study of pain (approximately 20:1)[61], perhaps reflecting the concern of experimental variability with female subjects, supporting the case for inclusion of more female subjects in basic science studies of pain.

Visceral pain models

A number of visceral pain models exist from which information can be used to generate a higher index of suspicion for clinical expression of disease. Distention of hollow organs is a common model. Distention of the distal gastrointestinal tract (colon, rectum) has been used to evoke respiratory, cardiovascular, visceromotor, behavioral, and neurophysiologic responses in multiple species, including horse, dog, cat, rabbit, and rat. Contemporary thinking is that viscera are not insensate, but are minimally sensate in the healthy state and can become very sensitive following pathology that up-regulates sensation from a subconscious state to the conscious state.

Strigo *et al.*[62] have used psychophysical measures to compare directly visceral and cutaneous pain and sensitivity (**Fig. 43**). Healthy human subjects evaluated perceptions evoked by balloon distention of the distal esophagus compared to contact heat on the upper chest. For esophageal distention, the threshold for pain intensity was higher than that observed for unpleasantness, whereas for contact heat, pain and unpleasantness thresholds did not differ for either phasic or tonic stimulus application. Results suggest that visceral pain is more unpleasant, diffuse, and variable than cutaneous pain of similar intensity, independent of the duration of the presented stimuli.

Poor localization of visceral pain

Much of our knowledge surrounding the poor localization of visceral pain comes from clinical practice in humans. Visceral pain is not normally perceived as localized to a given organ, but to somatic structures that receive afferent inputs at the same spinal segments as visceral afferent entry.

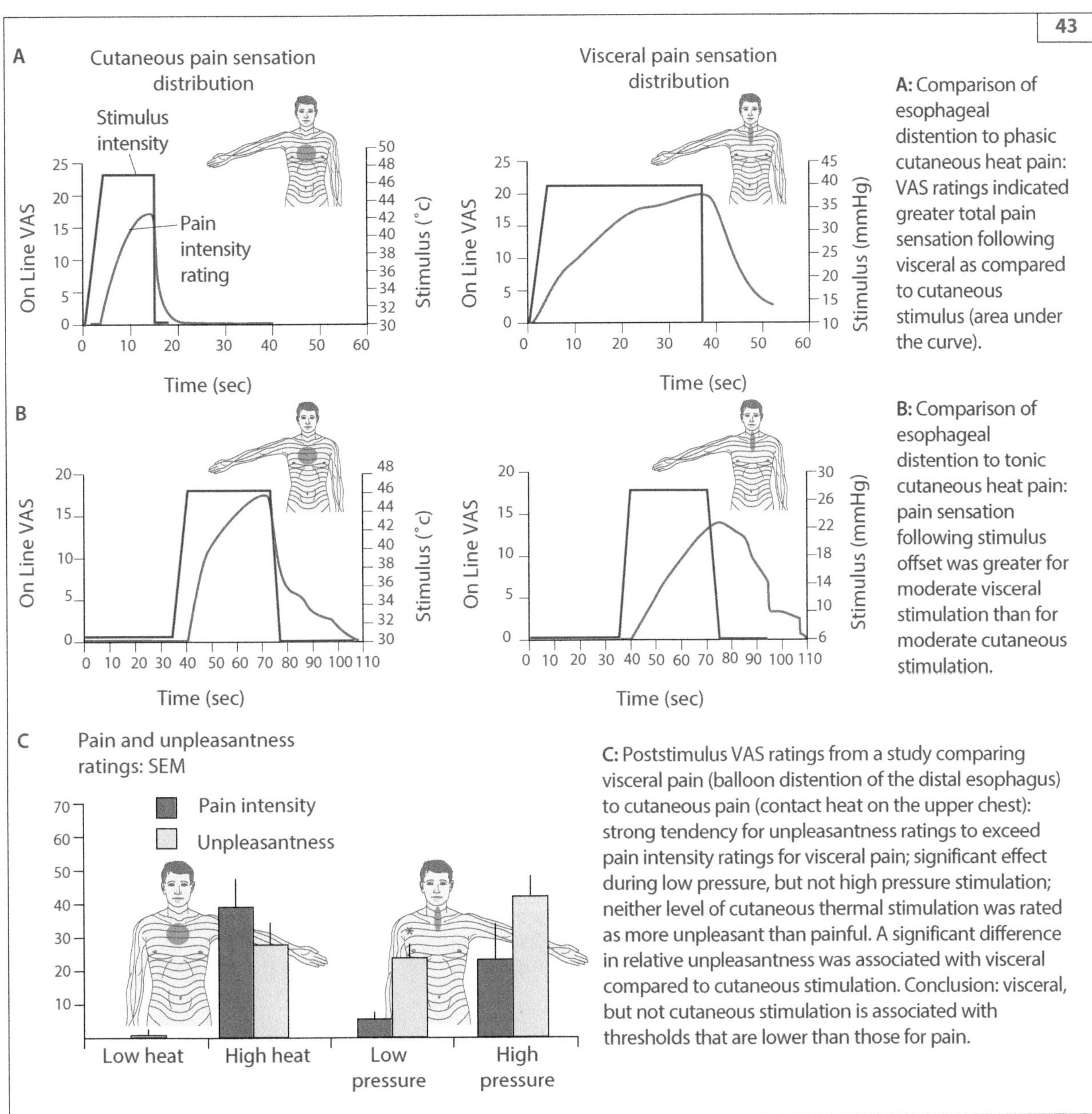

Fig. 43 Comparison of visceral and cutaneous pain and sensitivity in humans. Visceral pain is more unpleasant, diffuse, and variable than cutaneous pain of similar intensity. VAS: Visual Analog Scale.

The actual source of the visceral pain may only be localized when the manipulation of physical examination might stimulate the painful organ. Classically, visceral pain is considered either wholly unlocalized pain or as referred pain, with two separate components: 1) the diseased viscera sensation is transferred to another site (e.g. ischemic myocardium felt in the neck and arm); or, 2) hypersensitivity at other sites from inputs directly applied to those other sites (e.g. flank muscle becoming sensitive to palpation concurrent with urolithiasis), a phenomenon called secondary somatic hyperalgesia.

The very neuroanatomy of viscera suggests its unique pain response. The pattern of distribution for visceral primary afferents differs markedly from cutaneous primary afferents (**Fig. 44**). Visceral sensory pathways tend to follow perivascular routes that are diffuse in nature. Visceral afferent pathways have peripheral sites of neuronal synaptic contact that occur with the cell bodies of prevertebral ganglia, such as the celiac ganglion, mesenteric ganglion, and pelvic ganglion. This architecture can lead to alterations in local visceral function outside central control. The gut is probably an extreme example, where it functions by its own 'independent brain' that regulates the complex activities of digestion and absorption.

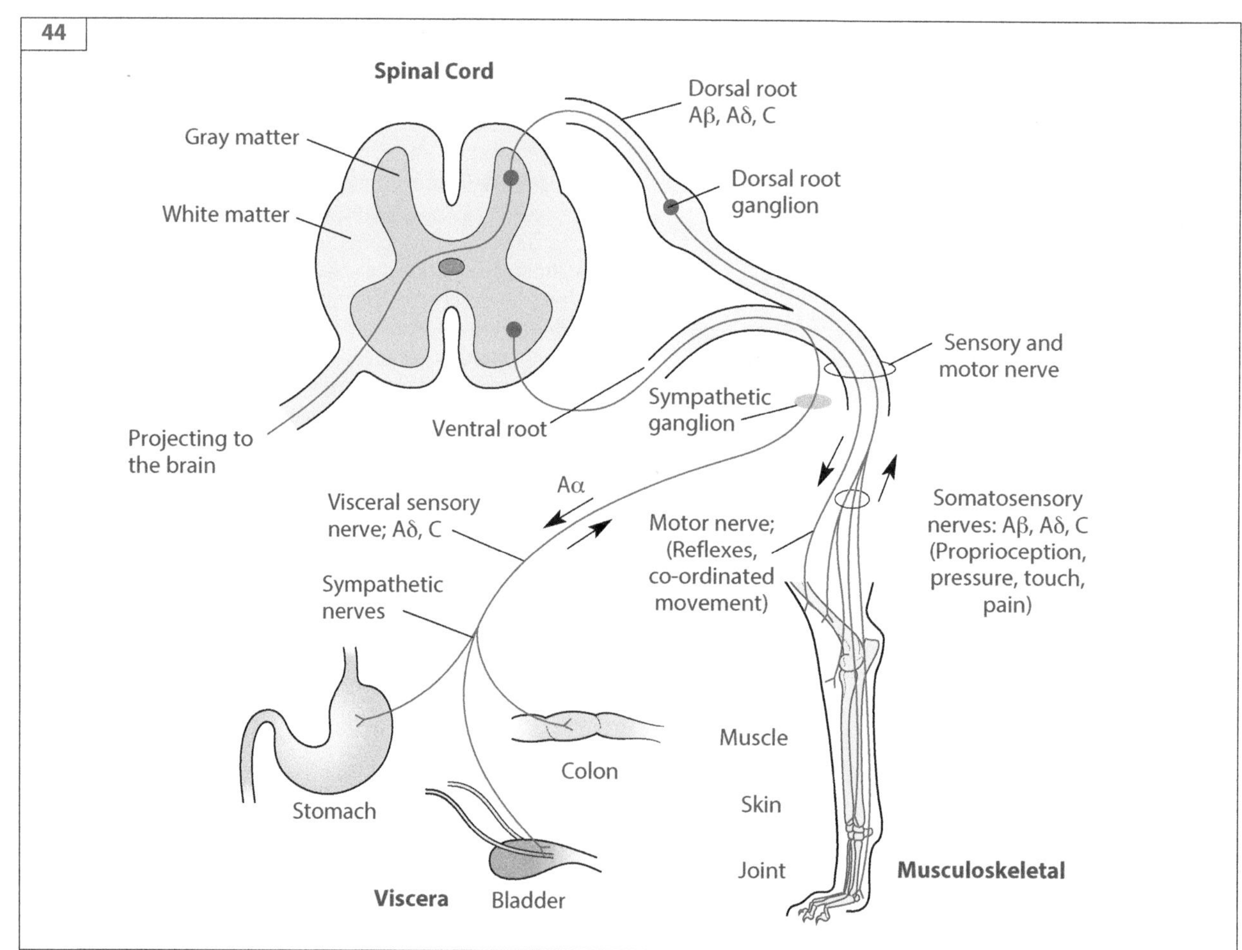

Fig. 44 Different nerve fibers conduct information to and from the brain via the spinal cord. Many of the fibers innervating the viscera travel with sympathetic nerves, passing through the sympathetic ganglion before reaching the dorsal root ganglia.

DRG neurons innervating the viscera tend to follow the original location of structural precursors of the viscera during embryological development. Afferents of a given organ may have cell bodies in the DRG at 10 or more spinal levels, bilaterally distributed. Further, individual visceroceptive afferent fibers branch once they enter the spinal cord and may spread over 12 or more spinal segments, interacting with neurons in at least five different dorsal horn laminae located bilaterally in the spinal cord[63]. Upon further examination, spinal dorsal horn neurons with visceral inputs have multiple inputs, from the viscera, joints, muscles, and cutaneous structures.

Collectively, there is an imprecise and diffuse organization of visceral primary inputs appearing consistent with an imprecise and diffuse localization by the CNS (*Table 13*).

Clinical implication: visceral pain may present as an imposter; where it is mistakenly interpreted as somatic pain. This can result in a totally erroneous diagnosis and treatment plan.

Visceral hypersensitization

The bladder is one of the few viscera that has recognized sensation when healthy and when diseased. As with irritable bowel syndrome (IBS), hypersensitivity to somatic stimuli is noted in people with interstitial cystitis (IC). Subjects with IC are significantly more sensitive to deep tissue measures of sensation related to pressure, ischemia, and bladder stretch than healthy subjects, showing an upward and left shift of reported discomfort with bladder filling (**Fig. 45**)[64].

TABLE 13: Differences between visceral and somatic pain processing

	Visceral pain	Superficial pain
Innervation	Spinal + vagal	Spinal
Injury	No	Yes
Noxious	Stretch Inflammation Ischemia	Damage Threat of damage
Localization	Poor	Excellent
Referred pain	The rule	The exception
Pathology	Not related to intensity	Related to intensity

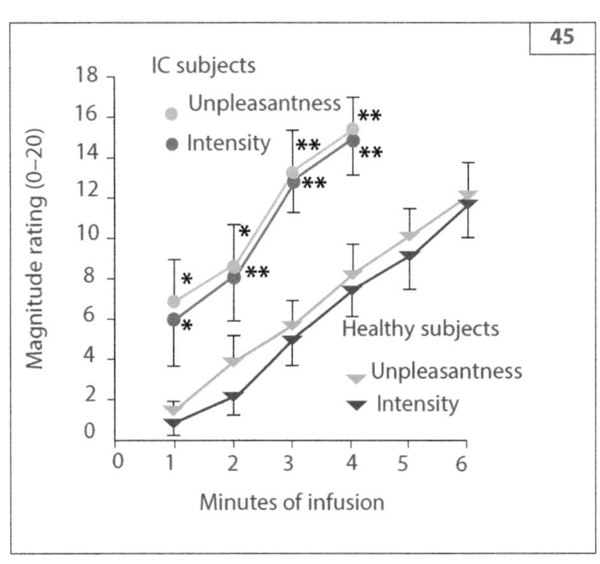

Fig. 45 Human subjects with interstitial cystitis (IC) show an upward and left shift of discomfort with bladder filling compared to normal, healthy subjects. Single asterisk indicates significantly different in subjects with IC *vs.* healthy subjects ($p<0.05$). Double asterisks indicate significantly different in subjects with IC *vs.* healthy subjects ($p<0.01$).

Cross-organ communication: visceral organs

As many as 40–60% of human patients diagnosed with IBS also exhibit symptoms and fulfill diagnostic criteria for IC; correspondingly, 38% of patients diagnosed with IC also have symptoms and fulfill diagnostic criteria for IBS[65,66]. Because neural cross-talk exists under normal conditions, alterations in neural pathways by disease or injury may play a role in development of overlapping chronic pelvic pain disorders and pelvic organ cross-sensitization (**Fig. 46**). Pezzone *et al.*[67] have developed a rodent model for studying pelvic organ reflexes, pelvic organ cross-talk, and associated striated sphincter activity that has shown: (1) colonic afferent sensitization occurs following the induction of acute cystitis; and (2) urinary bladder sensitization occurs following the induction of acute colitis. A possible explanation might be that the inflamed colon and urinary bladder have a common afferent axon that enters the spinal cord, resulting in the observed effect.

In the rat, approximately 14% of superficial and 29% deeper L6–S2 spinal neurons receive convergent inputs from both urinary bladder and colon[68]. In cats, approximately 30% of the sacral and thoracolumbar compound spinal interneurons have convergent inputs from both the urinary bladder and colon, and both of these visceral organs either excite or inhibit approximately 50% of the neurons[69]. These facts suggest that pelvic pain conditions and disorders might be a result of the interaction between pain-generating conditions of more than one visceral organ.

Clinical implication: animals presented for either urinary (bladder) or bowel (colon) problems should also have the other system evaluated.

Visceral pain and emotion

Human studies, as well as animal models, have demonstrated that visceral pain is strongly linked to emotion. The emotional state frequently alters function of the viscera[70], and the reverse is true – far more pronounced than with equal intensity of superficial pain. This tends to evoke an unending cycle of feedback between visceral pain and anxiety.

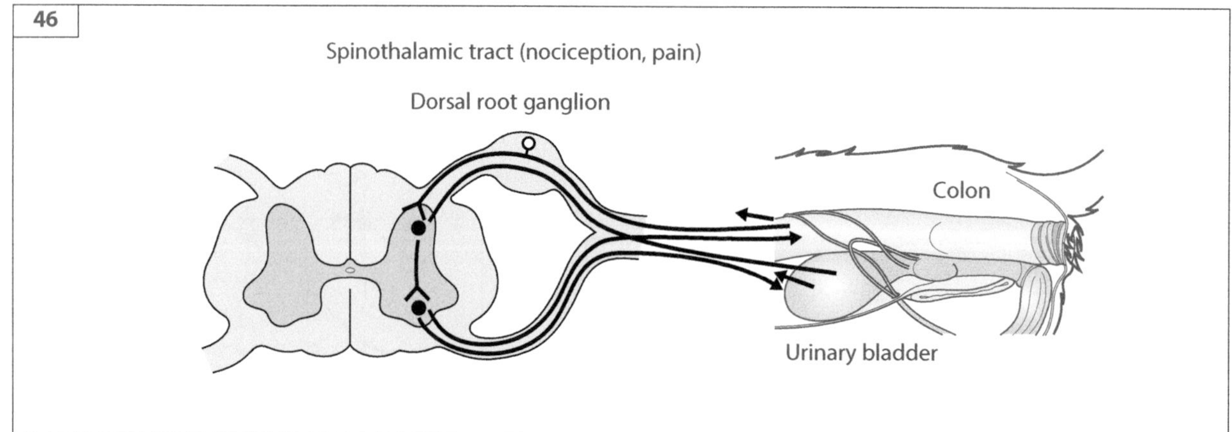

Fig. 46 Cross-organ convergence: convergence of colonic and urinary bladder afferent fibers onto a spinothalamic tract cell.

Clinical implication: it would appear appropriate to include an anxiolytic in a pharmacotherapeutic regimen targeting chronic visceral pain syndromes.

Visceral pain summary

Visceral pain is unique for several reasons:

- There is a poor correlation between the amount of tissue injury and visceral pain.
- Patterns of referred pain are a result of convergence of somatic and visceral afferents on the same dorsal horn neurons within the spinal cord.
- Clinical visceral pain is poorly localized (in humans), midline, and perceived as deep because, in part, of poor representation within the primary somatosensory cortex.
- More so than in somatic pain, visceral pain is accompanied by autonomic responses.
- Only a minority of visceral afferents are sensory: most relate to motor or reflex responses and few have specialized sensory terminals.
- Pain severity is transmitted by the sum of activity from nonspecific sensory receptors within mucosa, smooth muscle, and serosa.

Potentially useful agents in the management of visceral pain are presented in *Table 14*.

TABLE 14: Potentially useful agents in the management of visceral pain

Agent	Mode of action
κ opioid agonist	Peripheral kappa receptor agonists on visceral afferents reduce sP and CGRP
μ and δ opioids	Central μ and δ receptors reduce primary nociceptor activity and central hypersensitivity through PAG activity
NSAIDs	Block spinal cord and peripheral PG and central hypersensitivity
Ketamine, methadone, amantadine	Block dorsal horn NMDA receptors
Corticosteroids	Block expression of spinal cord NOS and reduces hypersensitivity
Gabapentin	Reduces central glutamate levels and NMDA binding for hypersensitivity
α_2-adrenoreceptor agonists	Facilitate descending inhibitory tracts through the PAG
Tricyclic antidepressants	Facilitate descending inhibitory tracts in PAG
Anticholinergics	Reduce colic and intestinal secretion
Somatostatin	Inhibits vasointestinal peptide and decreases colic and intestinal secretion. Reduces central hypersensitivity.

CGRP: calcitonin gene-related peptide; PAG: periaqueductal gray; PG: prostaglandin; sP: substance P; NMDA: N-methyl-D-aspartate; Nos: nitric oxide synthase; NSAID: nonsteroidal anti-inflammatory drug.

Classifying pain: mechanism-based

Some researchers[71] consider current methods of classifying pain as unsatisfactory, and for several reasons. Foremost is that pain syndromes are identified by parts of the body, duration and causative agents, rather than the mechanism involved. The argument holds that anatomical differences should be disregarded in favor of mechanisms that apply to either particular tissues or all parts of the body, rather than a particular part of the body (*Table 15*). For example, the term 'cancer pain' relates only to the disease from

TABLE 15: Summary of various pain states

Pain categories	Pain conditions	Pain mechanisms	Potential drug /targets	Animal models	Proof-of-concept
1. Transient stimulus-induced pains (nociceptive pain)	Procedural pain (injections/ minor injuries)	Nociceptor activation	VRs; Na^+-TTXs; MOR, nAChR	Thermosensitivity, mechanosensitivity, chemosensitivity	Minor surgical procedures
2. Tissue damage (inflammatory pain); spontaneous and provoked pain	Trauma/ postoperative pain; arthritis/ infection	Nociceptor activation; peripheral sensitization; central sensitization; phenotype switch	COX-2, EPR, 5-HTR, P_{2x}, BKR; IL-β TNR-α, TrkA, TrkB; Na^+-TTXr, ASIC, α^2, MOR, DOR, A1, $N\text{-}Ca^{++}$, NK1, nAChR, NMDA-R, GluR5, mGluR, PkCγ	Chemical irritants: capsaicin, mustard oil, formalin Experimental inflammation: carrageen, UVB, Freund's adjuvant, cytokines/growth factors	Dental postoperative pain; abdominal postoperative pain; thoracotomy; joint replacements; osteoarthritis
3. Injury: primary afferent (neuropathic pain); spontaneous and provoked pain	Peripheral nerve diabetic injury; neuropathy (human); toxic neuropathy; postherpetic neuralgia (human)	Extopic activity; phenotype switch; central sensitization; structural reorganization; disinhibition	Na^+-TTXr/ TTXs; α_2, NMDA-R, $N\text{-}Ca^{++}$, PKCγ; NGF/GDNF; GABA, AEAs, gabapentin; TCA, SNRIs	Peripheral nerve section; partial nerve section; loose ligatures; experimental diabetes, toxic neuropathies	Diabetic neuropathy (human); postherpetic neuropathy (human); radicular pain
4. Injury: central neuron (neuropathic pain); spontaneous and provoked pain	Spinal cord injury; stroke (humans)	Secondary ectopic activity; disinhibition; structural reorganization	GABA-R; Na^+-TTXs; AEAs; TCA, SNRIs	Spinal cord injury; ischemia; central disinhibition (e.g. strychnine/ bicuculline)	Spinal cord injury
5. Unknown mechanism	Irritable bowel syndrome; fibromyalgia (humans)	? Altered gain	COX-2, NMDA-R, Na^+ channels		Irritable bowel syndrome/ fibromyalgia

5-HTR: serotonin receptors; α_{2x}: adrenergic receptors; A_1: adenosine receptors; AEAs: antiepileptic agents, GABA-ergic compounds; ASIC: acid-sensing ion channel; BKR: bradykinin receptors; COX-2: cyclo-oxygenase 2; DOR: δ opiate receptors; EPR: prostaglandin receptors; GABA-R: γ-aminobutyric acid receptor; GluR5: kainate receptors; IL: interleukin; mGluR: metabotropic glutamate receptors; MOR: μ-opiate; nAChR: nicotinic acetylcholine receptor; $N\text{-}Ca^{++}$: voltage-gated calcium ion channels; NK1: neurokinin receptors; Na^+-TTXr: tetrodotoxin-resistant sodium ion channels; Na^+-TTXs: tetrodotoxin-sensitive sodium ion channels; NGF/GDNF: nerve growth factor/ glial-derived neurotrophic factor; NMDA-R: N-methyl-D aspartic acid receptors; P_{2x}: ligand-gated purino receptors/ion channels; PKCγ: protein kinase C gamma; SNRIs: serotonin and norepinephrine reuptake inhibitors. TCA: tricyclic antidepressants; TNR: tenascin R; TrkA, TrkB: high-affinity neurotrophin tyrosine kinase receptors; UVB: ultraviolet B; VR: vanilloid receptor.

which the patient suffers, not the mechanism of any pain the patient may experience. *A mechanism-based approach* is likely to lead to specific pharmacologic intervention measures for each identified mechanism within a syndrome. Advances in pain management are, then, contingent on first determining the symptoms that constitute a syndrome and then finding mechanisms for each of these. The clinical approach for a mechanism-based classification of pain is illustrated in **Fig. 47**.

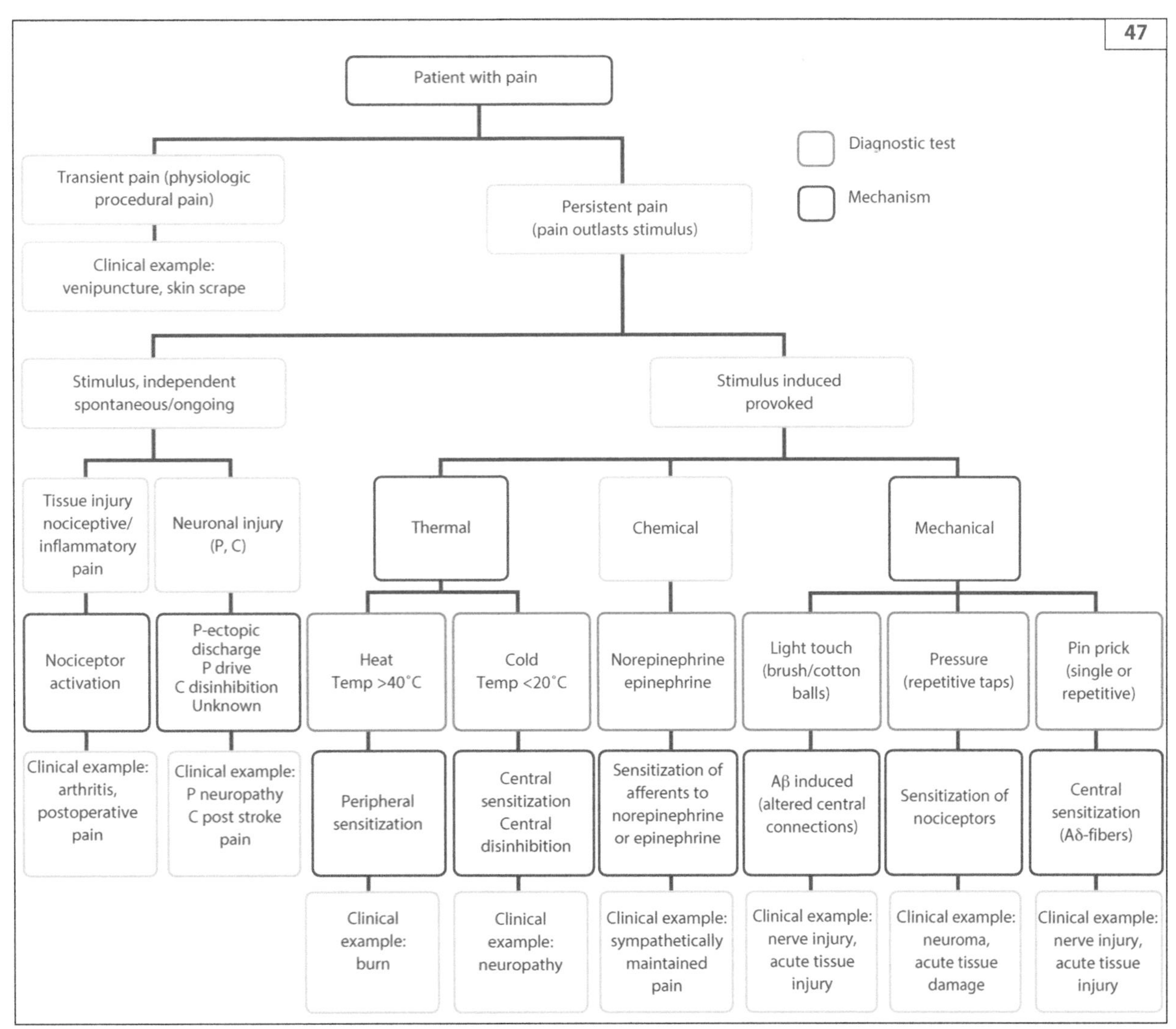

Fig. 47 Proposed scheme for a clinical approach to a mechanism-based classification of pain. C: central; P: peripheral.

Chapter 5

Pharmacologics (Various Drug Classes)

INTRODUCTION

Given a basic understanding of the neuroanatomy and neurochemistry of the pain generating process (**Fig. 48**), we can better understand how to alter this pathway with various drugs (*Table 16*).

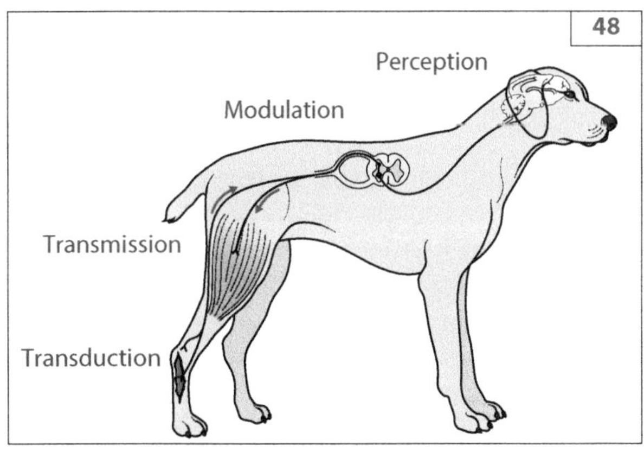

Fig. 48 The four physiologic processes of transduction, transmission, modulation, and perception offer specific targets for drug administration to alter the pain response.

TABLE 16: Classes of drugs which intervene in the physiologic processes of transduction, transmission, modulation, and perception

Perception	Modulation	Transmission	Transduction
Anesthetics	Local anesthetics	Local anesthetics	Local anesthetics
Opioids	Opioids	α_2 agonists	Opioids
α_2 agonists	α_2 agonists		NSAIDs
Benzodiazepines	Tricyclic antidepressants		Corticosteroids
Phenothiazines	Cholinesterase inhibitors		
	NMDA antagonists		
	NSAIDs		
	Anticonvulsants		

NMDA: N-methyl-D-aspartate; NSAID: nonsteroidal anti-inflammatory drug.

PHARMACOLOGIC PRINCIPLES

Several concepts need to be understood before discussing the various drug classes and their activities:

Pharmacokinetics is the study of what the body does to a drug.

Pharmacodynamics is the study of what a drug does to the body.

Hydrophilic is a term referring to a compound that has strong polar groups and therefore readily interacts with water.

Hydrophobic is a term referring to the repelling of water, or insolubility in water. Since biological membranes are rich in lipids (hydrophobic), hydrophilic drugs have difficulty crossing. Some membranes have mechanisms to transport specific molecules across the membrane.

Nonpolar substances can often diffuse straight through the lipid bilayer of cell membranes without requiring a membrane protein to assist in transport. Examples include oxygen, fatty acids, steroid hormones, and general anesthetics. Active transport denotes that specific binding of the transported substance occurs. Here, energy in the form of adenosine triphosphate (ATP) is required for a step in which the transporter is phosphorylated. Because energy is provided in this way, the transporter can move the substance to a higher concentration. Thus, these transporters always move the transported substance in one direction, regardless of the concentration gradient. The most widespread active transporter moves three Na^+ out of the cell while moving two K^+ into the cell to achieve a resting membrane potential (see Chapter 4; resting nerve membrane potential). In addition, there are active transporters both for Ca^{++} and for H^+. The latter, for example, are found in the stomach and participate in the secretion of acid into the stomach.

Phosphorylation is the addition of a phosphate (PO_4) group to a protein or organic molecule. Many enzymes are turned 'on' and 'off' by phosphorylation and dephosphorylation.

Drugs with low molecular weight, carrying no electrical charge, and highly **lipophilic** drugs can readily diffuse into various tissue compartments, such as the intra- and extracellular space or cerebrospinal fluid (CSF).

Clinical implication: highly lipid-soluble drugs such as fentanyl and oxymorphone rapidly diffuse out of the epidural space of cerebrospinal fluid into neighboring tissues, giving a relatively short analgesic effect. Since morphine is less lipid soluble, it yields a much longer duration of analgesia when administered by an epidural route.

Blood has a given **hydrostatic pressure**, which is often measured as one of the cardinal signs (together with temperature and respiration). It is this hydrostatic pressure that forces water and small molecules (molecular weight <30,000 Daltons) through certain membranes, such as the kidney's filtering device – the glomerulus.

It is the amount of free drug in blood that determines its availability for diffusion across membranes, and therefore its effect on a target tissue. However, many drugs bind to large molecules, such as plasma proteins (e.g. albumen). This **protein binding** restricts the drug's ability to diffuse across membranes or interact with target receptors. For example, the 'fraction bound' of the anticoagulant warfarin is 97%. This means that of the amount of warfarin in the blood, 97% is bound to plasma proteins. The remaining 3% (the fraction unbound) is the fraction that is actually active. The bound portion may act as a reservoir or depot from which the drug is slowly released as the unbound form. Drug binding is classified as extensive (>80%), moderate (50–80%), and low (<50%)[1]. Fortunately, there are not a great number of drugs that are extensively protein bound (*Tables 17–19*).

Clinical implication: if an animal is exceedingly hypoproteinemic, there is little available protein with which the drug can bind; therefore, a larger amount of the drug becomes 'free' or active. This can result in a greater clinical response to the drug than might be anticipated from the label dose.

TABLE 17: Commonly used drugs that are extensively (>80%) bound to plasma protein

Drug	Principal pharmacologic effect
Diazepam	Sedative, anticonvulsant
Digitoxin	Positive inotropic effect, heart rhythm stabilizer
Furosemide	Diuretic
Phenylbutazone	Anti-inflammatory
Phenytoin	Anticonvulsant, antiarrhythmic
Propanolol	β-adrenergic receptor blockade, antiarrhythmic
Quinidine	Antiarrhythmic, myocardial depressant
Valproate	Anticonvulsant
Warfarin	Anticoagulant

TABLE 18: Plasma protein binding of drugs at therapeutic concentrations in dogs

Drug	Concentration (μg/ml)	Binding (%)
Amphetamine	0.1	27
Chloramphenicol	20	39
Chlorpromazine		0.1 94
Digitoxin	0.05	89
Digoxin	0.01	27
Morphine	1	12
Propranolol	0.15–0.18	97
Sulfadiazine	100	17
Sulfadimethoxine	100	81
Sulfisoxazole	100	68
Thiopental	10	75

TABLE 19: Range of drug binding to plasma proteins in a variety of mammalian species

Drug	Binding range (%)
Amphetamine	20–40
Digitoxin	83–93
Digoxin	18–36
Morphine	12–34
Phenytoin	73–85
Propranolol	88–99
Sulfisoxazole	65–86

The liver and kidneys are the two major organs in the elimination of most drugs. When drugs are taken orally, they are absorbed through the gastrointestinal (GI) tract, and circulated directly to the liver via the portal vein. If the drug is rapidly and extensively metabolized by the liver, the substance undergoes extensive first-pass metabolism, with only a small amount of the dose reaching the systemic circulation (**Fig. 49**). If a drug is excreted by the liver into the bile from where it is then again absorbed by the intestine, it is said to undergo **entero-hepatic 'recycling'**.

Clinical implication: morphine (and most opioids), lidocaine, and propanolol are examples of drugs undergoing extensive first-pass metabolism and are therefore relatively ineffective.

Clinical implication: oral transmucosal administration of buprenorphine to cats and meloxicam to dogs has been shown to be very effective. This route has the advantage of avoiding hepatic first-pass elimination because venous drainage from the mouth is systemic.

The **elimination half-life** (t½) is the time required for the plasma concentration of a drug to decrease to 50% of an earlier value (*Table 20*). Note that this refers to *plasma concentration*, which may not reflect concentration in the target tissues, where the pH might be different due to inflammation.

Clinical implication: five half-lives is a convenient 'best guess' of how long it takes a drug to be 'washed out'. Keep in mind that this is just a rough estimate.

TABLE 20: Estimated time for drug elimination

1 half-life:	50% eliminated
2 half-lives:	75% eliminated
3 half-lives:	87.5% eliminated
3.3 half-lives:	90% eliminated
4 half-lives:	93.8% eliminated
5 half-lives:	97% eliminated

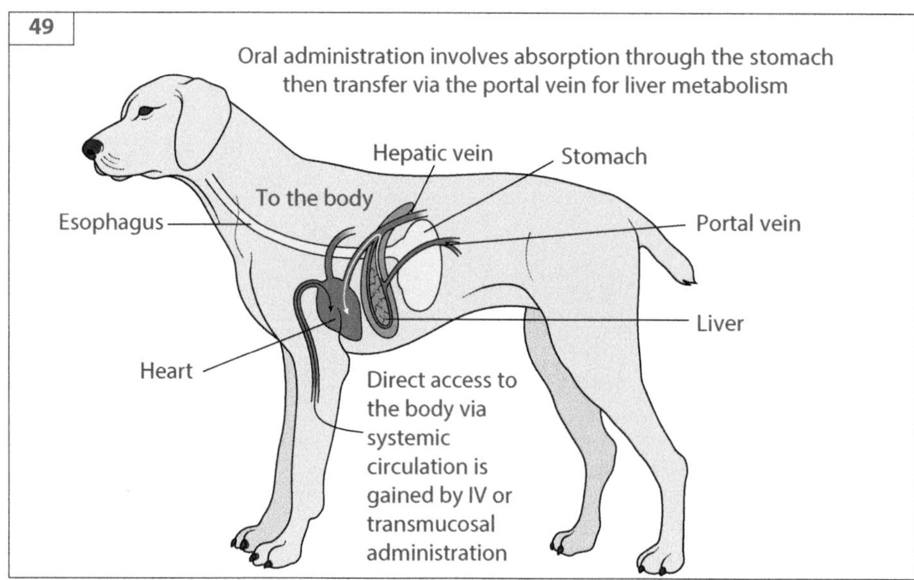

Fig. 49 First-pass metabolism is a consequence of oral drug administration and can markedly reduce its activity.

Antagonists can be classified as competitive or noncompetitive. **Competitive receptor antagonists** compete for the receptor site. Their effects are considered reversible, because they can be overcome by simply administering a higher dose of the agonist. **Noncompetitive receptor antagonists** produce an effect that cannot be overcome by increasing concentrations of the agonist; effects are irreversible until the drug is completely eliminated (approximately 5+ half-lives).

The term **receptor** refers to any large molecule (generally a protein) with which the drug combines to produce an effect.

The term **drug potency** has often been misrepresented by using opioids as examples (*Table 21*). That is, morphine is given a 'potency' of 1 and fentanyl is given a potency of 100. This does not mean that fentanyl will be much more effective as an analgesic. The analgesic effect at the opioid receptor is the same for both agents.

TABLE 21: Affinity* (often cited as potency) of different opioids for their receptor

	Receptor				
Drug	**Mu (μ)**	**Kappa-1 (κ_1)**	**Kappa-3 (κ_1)**	**Delta (δ)**	**Relative analgesic potency**
Full agonists					
Morphine	+++	+	+	++	1
Oxymorphone	+++	NA	NA	+	10
Hydromorphone	+++	?	?	?	10–15
Fentanyl	+++			+	80–150
Meperidine	+++	++	++	+	0.1
Methadone	+++			+	1.0–1.5
Codeine	++	+	+	+	?
Partial agonists					
Buprenorphine	P	–	–	?	25
Agonist–antagonists					
Butorphanol	P	+++	NA	NA	3–5
Pentazocine	P	++	+		0.25–0.5
Nalbuphine	– –	++	++		1
Antagonists					
Naloxone	– – –	– –	– –	–	
Nalmefene	– – –	– –	– –	– –	

*These affinities are based on different studies using many different assays, and it should be recognized that the relative affinity of the drug for a receptor may be dependent on the species, the cell type, and the specificity of the agonists or antagonists used in the study.
P = partial; + + + = high activity; + + = medium activity; + = low activity; – – – = greatest antagonism; – – = antagonism; – = least antagonism; ? = activity unknown or conflicting literature; NA = not available.

What it does mean is that fentanyl would rather bind to the μ-receptor with an attraction of 100× that of morphine. **The ranking is related to the drug's affinity for the receptor**, not its clinical response. For example, if equal concentrations of both morphine and fentanyl were offered to a restricted number of receptors, the fentanyl would preferentially replace any morphine molecules in the receptor sites because it has 100× the attraction for that receptor. Thus a lesser amount or dose of the fentanyl can be used relative to morphine; morphine is dosed in <u>milli</u>grams, whereas fentanyl is dosed in <u>micro</u>grams.

Clinical implication: if administration of a 'weak' opioid is followed by administration of a 'strong' opioid, the latter can displace the former, e.g. buprenorphine following butorphanol.

Many drugs have two or more three-dimensional structures, but the same chemical formula. These different configurations are termed **isomers**. This is analogous to your hands: they are the same, but they're not the same! They are mirror images of each other. When a drug exists as an equimolar mixture of these isomers, it is called a racemic mixture. The two components of this mixture may have similar or different receptor effects. An example is the drug medetomidine. Medetomidine is a racemic mixture of dexmedetomidine and levomedetomidine. Levomedetomidine is believed to be pharmacologically inactive, so its removal from the mixture leaves dexmedetomidine as a very potent drug at a much lower relative dose.

When the effects of one drug are additive to those of another drug, the drugs are considered to be **additive** or summative. For example, if two such drugs that produce analgesia are mixed together and administered, the analgesia produced is the sum of the individual analgesic activity of each drug (i.e. 1 +1 = 2). When the results of two drugs mixed together yields a result greater than the sum of their individual effects, they are considered **synergistic** (i.e. 1 + 1 = >2). An example of synergism is the mixing of drugs from two different drug classes, for example, acepromazine (a phenothiazine tranquilizer) and morphine or oxymorphone (opioids), or an opioid (morphine) and a α_2-agonist (medetomidine). Clinically, synergism is expected when drugs that act by different modes of action (multimodal) are combined.

Controlled substances

Quality emergency and critical care for animal patients cannot be accomplished without the use of controlled substances. Maintaining 'control' over controlled substances can be a confusing issue; however, being fully compliant with controlled drug regulations need not be a burden. Access to controlled substances varies by country, and one should be grateful for the right to use such powerful agents.

In the USA, the Drug Enforcement Administration (DEA) is empowered to enforce controlled substance laws and regulations. The DEA categorizes drugs of abuse into 'schedules' according to the likelihood for abuse. Substances are divided into five schedules, designated by the Roman numerals I-V:

Schedule I: have no currently accepted medical use and are those with the highest abuse potential, namely heroin, marijuana (currently under debate), and lysergic acid diethylamide (LSD).

Schedule II: are drugs with accepted medical value with high potential for abuse, such as pentobarbital, morphine, cocaine, and fentanyl.

Schedule III–V: have declining potential for abuse and include ketamine (III), diazepam (IV), and diphenoxylate and atropine (V).

All commercially available drugs used for euthanasia are controlled substances. Scheduling may vary by state/country and is frequently changing.

In the USA, all practitioners who prescribe controlled substances must be registered with the DEA, and only DEA registrants may actually prescribe controlled substance prescriptions to be filled at pharmacies. In some states, dual registry with both the state and federal DEA is required. In practices with multiple locations, there must be at least one DEA registrant for every location. Although the registrant may choose to issue power of attorney to facilitate controlled substance purchasing and accountability, the

DEA registrant retains ultimate responsibility for controlled substance disposition associated with his/her DEA registration and must still sign his/her name to medical records and written prescriptions for controlled substances. DEA registration is renewable every few years (check current local requirements).

Controlled substances are identified on the product container with a large capital C and corresponding Roman numeral inscribed within the C. Without access to the container, drug schedules can be obtained at http//www.dea.gov/pubs/scheduling.html (listed by generic name). Listings are also available in references such as the *Compendium for Veterinary Products* and the *Veterinary Drug Handbook*.

Schedule II drugs must be purchased on special drug order forms (DEA triplicate Form 222), and orders cannot be 'phoned in' to vendors. The order form limits order quantity to 10 Schedule II drugs. The drug invoice should be attached to the 222 form and stored in a readily retrievable file for a minimum of 2 years (location dependent). Drugs in Schedules III–V may be ordered by telephone or fax without any special order forms, yet the invoices must be signed by the registrant and filed separately from Schedule II invoices for a minimum of 2 years.

Controlled substances may not be ordered from a pharmacy or another practice for resale or for 'office use'. All controlled substance prescriptions to pharmacies must be for an individual patient and federal law prohibits transfer of that prescription to a patient other than for whom the original prescription was intended. Borrowing controlled substances from other practices is prohibited. Schedule II prescriptions are not refillable under any circumstances and a new, written prescription must be issued for every prescription of Schedule II drugs. Drugs in Schedules III–V may be refilled for five times or 6 months, whichever is sooner.

Controlled substances must be stored in a securely locked, substantially constructed cabinet or safe. Double locking of such safes is not required, but is considered good practice by most DEA inspectors. Any drug not used should be disposed of in the presence of a witness, with both persons noting the amount disposed of and method of disposal on the patient's medical record along with their full signatures. Records must easily trace the use of controlled substances from purchase to patient, and easily detect any discrepancies in controlled substance inventory.

The DEA requires that an initial controlled substance inventory be conducted on the first day of DEA registration as well as on the day of any change in DEA registrant information. An actual count inventory is also required every 2 years and is usually performed on May 1 or on the anniversary date of DEA registration. Subsequent biennial inventories must be conducted on the same date (or on as close a working day as possible).

A 'significant loss' of a controlled substance is undefined, although most practitioners consider a discrepancy of >10% to be significant. A DEA registrant's only obligation in the event of loss or theft is to report the loss to the DEA.

OPIOIDS

The analgesic effects of opium have been known for over 5,000 years, but unfortunately, abuse has limited the use of opioids. Society has attempted to find a balance between licit and illicit use, therapeutic versus adverse effects, and medical needs with legal issues. Regardless of the legal, administrative, and social obstacles, no other class of drugs has remained in use for the treatment of pain as long as opioids.

Opiate: any drug derived from opium, e.g. morphine.
Opioid: any synthetic narcotic with opiate-like activities, but is not derived from opium.

Opioid receptors

Knockout mice studies suggest that three opioid receptor types regulate distinct pain modalities (*Table 22*)[2]:

- Mu (μ) receptors (OP3) influence responses to mechanical, chemical, and supraspinal thermal nociception. Densities of receptor μ are not identical among individuals, as shown by binding studies in human postmortem brain samples[3].
- Kappa (κ) receptors (OP2) modify spinally-mediated nociception and chemical visceral pain.
- Delta (δ) receptors (OP1) increase mechanical nociception and inflammatory pain. To date there are no pure delta opiates commercially available.

Sigma receptors (σ) were once considered to be opioid receptors due to the antitussive actions of many opioid drugs being mediated via sigma receptors, and the first selective sigma agonists being derivatives of opioid drugs (e.g. allylnormetazocine). However, sigma receptors were found not to be activated by endogenous opioid peptides, and are quite different from the other opioid receptors in both function and gene sequence, so they are now uncommonly classified with the opioid receptors.

Opioid receptors are synthesized in the dorsal root ganglia (DRG) and transported from the cell body along intra-axonal microtubules into central and peripheral processes of the primary afferent neuron (**Fig. 50**). At the terminals, opioid receptors are incorporated into the neuronal membrane and become functional receptors. Upon activation by exogenous or endogenous opioids, opioid receptors couple to inhibitory G proteins, leading to direct or indirect suppression of cation currents and subsequent attenuation of substance P (sP) release. Inflammation enhances the peripherally directed axonal transport of opioid receptors, leading to an increase in their number (up-regulation) at peripheral nerve terminals. Further, pre-existing, but possibly inactive, neuronal opioid receptors may undergo changes in the inflammatory milieu (e.g. low pH), and become active. Ligands with a preference for μ receptors are generally most potent, but depending upon the circumstances, all three receptor types can be present and functionally active in subcutaneous tissue, viscera, or joints.

A **ligand** (Latin *ligare* = to bind) is a substance that is able to bind to, and form a complex with, a biomolecule to serve a biologic purpose. In a narrower sense, it is a signal triggering molecule, binding to a site on a target protein.

TABLE 22: Subtypes, location and function of the three major opioid receptors

Receptor	Subtypes	Location	Function
Mu (μ) OP_3	μ_1, μ_2, μ_3	Brain: cortex thalamus striosomes periaqueductal gray Spinal cord: substantia gelatinosa Intestinal tract	μ_1: supraspinal analgesia physical dependence μ_2: respiratory depression miosis euphoria reduced GI motility physical dependence μ_3: unknown
Kappa (κ) OP_2	$\kappa_1, \kappa_2, \kappa_3$	Brain: hypothalamus periaqueductal gray claustrum Spinal cord: substantia gelatinosa	spinal analgesia sedation miosis ADH release inhibition dysphoria
Delta (δ) OP_1	δ_1, δ_2	Brain: pontine nuclei amygdala olfactory bulbs deep cortex	analgesia antidepressant effects physical dependence

ADH: antidiuretic hormone; GI: gastrointestinal.

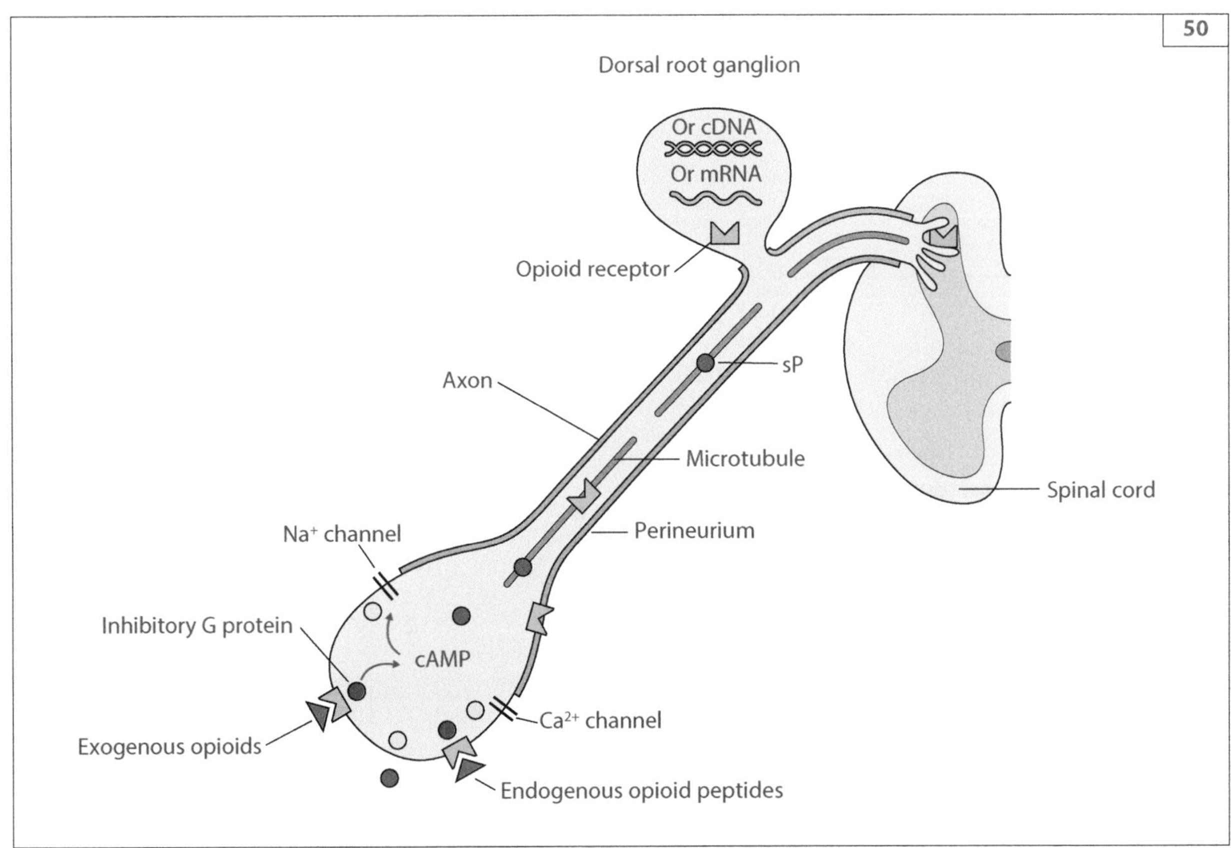

Fig. 50 Opioid receptor creation and transport. cAMP: cyclic adenosine monophosphate; cDNA: cyclic deoxyribonucleic acid; mRNA: messenger ribonucleic acid; sP: substance P.

Response to opioid receptor activation

In common with spinal and supraspinal opioid receptors, the binding of opioid agonists results in K^+ channel-mediated neuronal hyperpolarization, attenuation of Ca^{++} entry through voltage-gated Ca^{++} channels and reduced cyclic adenosine monophosphate availability, with resultant reduction in nociceptor activity (**Fig. 51**)[4]:

Cyclic adenosine monophosphate is a second messenger, used for intracellular signal transduction, e.g. transferring the effects of hormones, such as glucagon and epinephrine (adrenaline), which cannot pass through the cell membrane. It is involved in the activation of protein kinases and regulates the effects of epinephrine and glucagon. It also regulates the passage of calcium through ion channels.

- μ- and δ- (and to some degree κ-) agonists induce a membrane hyperpolarization through the activation of an inwardly flowing K^+ channel.
- Inhibition of the opening of voltage-sensitive Ca^{++} channels, that will subsequently depress the terminal release of neurotransmitters from the cell.
- Occupancy of the presynaptic μ and δ sites reduces the release of sP and/or calcitonin gene-related protein (CGRP), in part by an inhibition of the opening of voltage-gated calcium channels.

Substance P and calcitonin gene-related peptide are important neurotransmitters in the transmission of the pain response.

That said, research over the last decade suggests that morphine and other opioids do not have fixed actions, but operate on receptor mechanisms that are subject to alterations by other transmitters and receptors.

Supraspinal activity of opioids occurs at several locations within the brain and brainstem. The tenet that opioids are centrally acting (within the central nervous system [CNS]) is long standing. Yet, direct application of opioids at high concentrations to the peripheral nerve can produce a local anesthetic-like action, but this is not naloxone reversible. Models in which peripheral opioids appear to work are those that possess a significant degree of inflammation and are characterized by a hyperalgesic component.

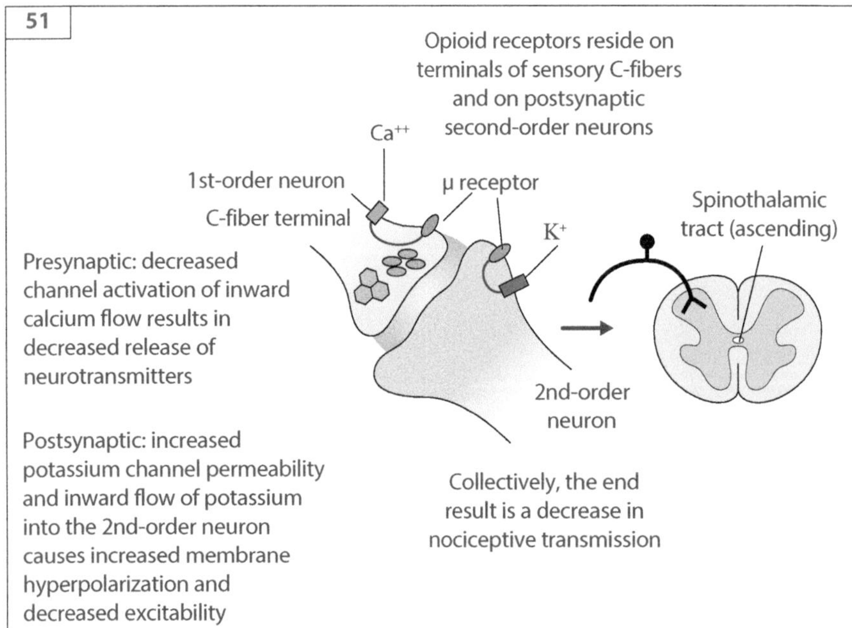

Fig. 51 Opioid-induced antinociception is mainly C-fiber mediated[5], where opioids act at both the pre- and postsynaptic sides of nerve junctions.

Mechanisms for this antihyperalgesic effect are presently unexplained, but injection of morphine into the knee joint of humans after surgery has shown a powerful sparing effect upon subsequent analgesic use.

Clinical implication: veterinary patients can benefit greatly from the addition of opioids injected into operated joints.

Although controversial, studies suggest that neuropathic pain secondary to peripheral nerve damage, more often than not, shows reduced sensitivity to opioids[6]. This is attributable to a reduction in spinal opioid receptors, nonopioid receptor-expressing Aβ-fiber-mediated allodynia, increased cholecystokinin (CCK) antagonism of opioid actions, and N-methyl-D-aspartate (NMDA)-mediated dorsal horn neuronal hyperexcitability, likely requiring a greater opioid inhibitory counter-effect.

Clinical implication: pain relief for neuropathic pain from peripheral nerve damage will be more pronounced when using drug combinations than from simply increasing the dose of an opioid.

Cholecystokinin and opioids

CCK is one of the most abundant of the neuropeptides present in brain and spinal cord small neurons. CCK and the opioids tend to have opposite effects, suggesting that the CCK system may represent an 'antiopioid' or 'antianalgesic' mechanism. CCK antagonists not only enhance opioid responses, they also reverse existing morphine tolerance[7]. Changes in the expression of the peptide CCK and its receptor (CCK-2) on primary afferent neurons may play a key role in the alterations of pain sensitivity and opioid responsiveness that occur in chronic pain conditions.

Opioid classifications

Opioids may be the best drugs available for pain control, and one might argue that 'serious pain control' cannot be implemented without them. Morphine, oxymorphone, fentanyl, hydromorphone, and meperidine are opioid agonists acting mainly at the μ receptor, for which they have a high affinity. The agonist–antagonists (butorphanol, nalbuphine, pentazocine) are able to reverse some effects of the pure agonists, but can produce analgesia. Buprenorphine is a κ antagonist, with high affinity for μ receptors, classified as a partial agonist, while butorphanol acts at the κ receptor and acts as a μ-antagonist. Opioid antagonists including naloxone, naltrexone, and nalmefene, reverse the actions of both μ- and κ-agonists (*Tables 23, and 24 overleaf*).

TABLE 23: Classification of opioids based upon binding activity

A pure opioid agonist binds to one or more types of receptor and causes certain effects, such as analgesia or respiratory depression (e.g. morphine)
A partial agonist binds at a given receptor causing an effect less pronounced than that of a pure agonist (e.g. buprenorphine is less effective than morphine). It is considered a partial agonist at the μ receptor and an antagonist at the κ receptor
An opioid antagonist binds to one or more types of receptor, but causes no effect at those receptors. By competitive displacement, an antagonist reverses the effect of an agonist (e.g. naloxone reverses morphine)
An agonist–antagonist binds to more than one type of effect receptor, causing an effect at one receptor, but no or a lesser effect at another receptor (e.g. butorphanol is considered a κ agonist and a μ antagonist, with minimal effect at the μ receptor)

TABLE 24: World Health Organization opioid classification

Strength	Functional
Weak opioids	***Full agonists***
Codeine	Morphine
Dihydrocodeine	Fentanyl
Dextropropoxyphene	Hydromorphone
Tramadol	Codeine
	Methadone
Strong opioids	Tramadol
Morphine	Meperidine (pethidine)
Methadone	
Fentanyl	***Partial agonists***
Hydromorphone	Buprenorphine
Meperidine (pethidine)	Pentazocine
Oxycodone	Butorphanol
Buprenorphine	
Levorphanol	***Agonists antagonists***
Dextromoramide	Nalbuphine
	Nalorphine
	Full antagonists
	Naloxone
	Naltrexone
	Alvimopan

Opioid side-effects

The most common side-effects seen with opioids include respiratory depression, nausea and vomiting, histamine release, constipation, and central excitement. In human medicine the common practice of coadministering antiemetics with opioids is being challenged due to the findings that the occurrence of vomiting associated with opioid administration for acute pain is low[8]. Urine production may be decreased for several hours following morphine administration; however, this does not appear to be related to arginine vasopressin (previously known as antidiuretic hormone or vasopressin) concentrations in the dog[9].

Opioid antagonists (naloxone, naltrexone, nalmefene) can be used to reverse the clinical side-effects (such as bradycardia) of opioids. However, if the patient is in pain, reversal of the opioid and its analgesic properties, may result in intense pain and related sympathetic stimulation which may be detrimental. In the case of bradycardia, administration of an anticholinergic (e.g. atropine or glycopyrrolate) would be more appropriate to restore the heart rate.

Opioid-induced hyperalgesia (OIH)

The chronic nature of cancer pain often requires prolonged opioid administration by various routes, and doses are often escalated over time, as the disease progresses. Clinical studies with humans report that opioids can unexpectedly produce hyperalgesia and allodynia, particularly during rapid opioid dose escalation[10,11]. Preclinical human studies have unexpectedly demonstrated that opioids can paradoxically enhance pain[12,13]. In a mouse model of bone cancer, King *et al.*[14] showed that in a dose-dependent manner, morphine enhanced, rather than diminished, spontaneous, and evoked pain. Additionally, morphine increased osteoclast activity and upregulated interleukin (IL)-1β within the femurs of sarcoma-treated mice, suggesting enhancement of sarcoma-induced breakdown of bone. The authors proposed that sustained morphine increases pain, osteolysis, bone loss, and spontaneous fracture, as well as markers of neuronal damage in DRG cells and expression of proinflammatory cytokines. Sustained opioid delivery through patches and controlled-release delivery systems has become more commonly used for pain management, and these data demonstrate that prolonged morphine treatment may have unexpected antianalgesic effects. Identifying the development of hyperalgesia is of clinical importance since patients receiving opioids to relieve pain may paradoxically experience more pain as a result of treatment. The precise mechanisms underlying OIH are poorly understood. The sensitization of pronociceptive pathways in response to opioid treatment appears to involve several pathways.

While there are many proposed mechanisms for OIH, five mechanisms involving the central glutaminergic system, spinal dynorphins, descending facilitation, genetic mechanisms, and decreased reuptake and enhanced nociceptive response have been described as the important mechanisms. Of these, the central glutaminergic system is considered the most common possibility. Yet another hypothesis is that OIH includes activation of the NMDA receptors, with inhibition of the glutamate transporter system and facilitation of calcium regulated intracellular protein kinase C, with cross-talk of neural mechanisms of pain and tolerance[15].

Clinicians should suspect OIH when the effect of opioid treatment seems to wane in the absence of disease progression, particularly if found in the context of unexplained pain behaviors or diffuse allodynia unassociated with the original pain, and increased levels of pain with increasing dosages. Treatment involves reducing the opioid dosage, tapering it off, or supplementation with NMDA receptor modulators.

Orally administered opioids

Oral administration yields low (<30% [morphine ~5%]) bioavailability[16,17] because opioids are metabolized in the liver. Codeine has the highest bioavailability, approaching 60%[18], and is often administered in combination with acetaminophen (**acetaminophen is lethal in cats**). Although morphine and hydromorphone are available as suppositories (*Table 25*), there appears to be little difference in efficacy or bioavailability (~20%) from oral administration[19]; however, this delivery form is an option if oral administration is unavailable.

TABLE 25: Oral/rectal preparations of morphine (for human use) in the USA

Duration of action	Preparation	Dosage formulation
Immediate release	Tablet/capsule	1.5 mg, 30 mg
	Soluble/sublingual	10 mg
	Solution	10 mg/5 ml; 10 mg/2.5 ml; 20 mg/5 ml; concentrate 20 mg/ml
	Suppository	5, 10, 20, 30 mg
Controlled/sustained release	MS Contin	15, 30, 60, 100, 200 mg
	Oramorph SR	15, 30, 60, 100 mg
	Kadian (food sprinkles)	20, 30, 50, 60, 100 mg
	Avinza (food sprinkles)	30, 60, 90, 120 mg

Opioid transdermal patch delivery system (TDPS)

The highly lipid-soluble opioid fentanyl lends itself to transdermal delivery and is available in a patch containing a drug reservoir (**Fig. 52**).
An ethylene-vinyl acetate copolymer membrane controls the rate of delivery to the skin. (A more recent development is the Matrix® adhesive delivery patch from Noven Pharmaceutical Inc.)

Due in part to the differences in dermal vascularization, drug uptake from the patch varies between the dog and cat. Studies suggest it takes 12–24 hours to reach peak effect in the dog[20,21], whereas peak values in the cat are reached sooner (2–18 hours)[22,23]. Fentanyl patches certainly have their place; however, they are not without concerns, which include: class II DEA accountability, expense, difficulty with maintaining placement, variable absorption, possible skin reaction, the need to shave the hair, and choosing an optimal location for placement. Following discharge home with a fentanyl patch, if a pet shows hyperexcitability the pet owner cannot differentiate if the behavior is due to uncontrolled pain or excessive opioid absorption. Arguably, fentanyl patches may have their optimal use in chronic conditions, such as terminal cancer. For postoperative pain, one might consider a patient requiring opioid administration as an in-house hospital patient wherein it can be closely monitored and treated with cost-efficient morphine; thereafter, discharging the patient only when appropriate pain management can be provided by oral medication, for example a nonsteroidal anti-inflammatory drug (NSAID) and/or tramadol.

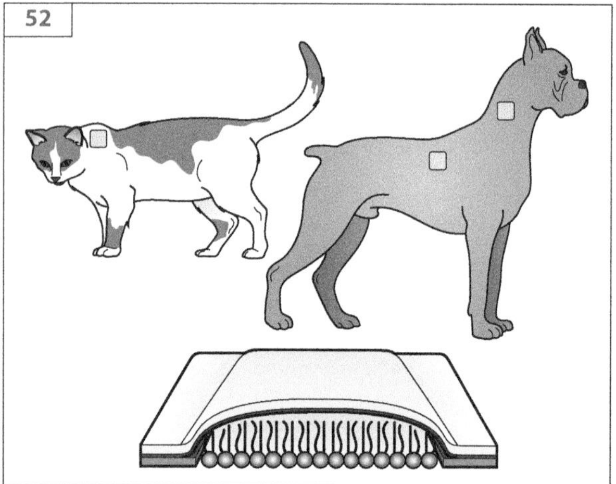

Fig. 52 Opioid (fentanyl) patch. Different sized patches deliver different doses. Crystal reservoir technology has allowed smaller patches with a more controlled drug release. Patches should be placed where the patient would have difficulty removing them.

The minimum analgesic plasma concentration of fentanyl required to achieve analgesia in humans and considered to apply also for dogs is 0.23 ng/ml[20]. This concentration has been reported with use of the fentanyl patch in dogs undergoing spinal surgery[24].

Buprenorphine TDPS has recently been developed for use in humans in three patch sizes: 35, 52.5, and 70 µg/h. Potential advantages of buprenorphine as an analgesic in dogs include its long duration of action, tendency not to induce vomiting, and negligible cardiovascular effects in healthy animals[25]. In humans, plasma concentration of buprenorphine gradually increases after the application of a 70 µg/h patch, and after 11 hours the minimum effective analgesic concentration (MEC) of 100 pg/ml is reached. Plateau levels of about 624 pg/ml are detected between 36 and 60 hours[26]. Although the MEC of buprenorphine for dogs has not been described, after IV administration of 0.02 mg/kg, plasma concentrations are found to be 0.26–2.36 ng/ml at 45–60 minutes postadministration[27] – similar to that obtained with a 70 µg/h patch[28]. Moll *et al.*[29] have reported that the clinical efficacy of a 70 µg/h patch was similar to that of SC administration of 20 µg/kg buprenorphine in dogs undergoing ovariohysterectomy. Plasma buprenorphine concentrations increased slowly during the first 36–48 hours and remained in a steady state for 108 hours. In humans, the minimum effective buprenorphine plasma concentration for analgesia is assumed to be 0.1 ng/ml[30], and a peak buprenorphine concentration of 0.3 ng/ml has been reported

70 hours after the application of a 52.5 μg/h patch[31]. Pieper *et al.*[32] has reported buprenorphine plasma levels greater than 1 ng/ml after application of the 52.5 μg/h patch. The delayed onset of antinociception after transdermal buprenorphine patch application may limit its perioperative use; however, it may prove useful for the management of chronic pain in dogs.

Intra-articular opioid delivery

Morphine is also used for intra-articular analgesia, and several investigators suggest that, in combination with bupivacaine, morphine works best from among the opioids[33].

Example: ~1 ml/10 kg of either 2.0% lidocaine or 0.5% bupivacaine, and 0.1–0.2 mg/kg morphine.

Spinal cord opioid delivery

Because opioid receptors are found in the spinal cord, opioids can be applied directly to these receptors by epidural or intrathecal administration. This takes advantage of smaller doses and central administration to minimize systemic uptake and possible side-effects associated with higher dose recommendations (*Table 26*).

Fentanyl transdermal solution; Elanco Animal Health Inc.

Arguably, little innovation in the opioid drug class has been made over the past several decades, particularly in veterinary medicine. Fentanyl is an exception. Fentanyl was first synthesized by Paul Janssen in 1959 under the label of his relatively newly formed Janssen Pharmaceutica. In the mid-1990s, Janssen developed and introduced into clinical trials the Duragesic patch, which is designed to deliver fentanyl over a period of 48–72 hours. Following the patch, a flavored lollipop of fentanyl citrate mixed with inert fillers was introduced under the brand name of Actiq, landmarking the first quick-acting formulation of fentanyl for use with chronic breakthrough pain in humans. More recently, fentanyl has been developed into an effervescent tablet for buccal absorption, much like the Actiq lollipop, followed by a buccal spray device for fast-acting relief. The USA Food and Drug Administration (FDA) has also approved a new fentanyl product, Onsolis® (Meda Pharmaceuticals Inc.), for breakthrough cancer pain. This delivery technology, a fentanyl buccal soluble film, is proposed to offer less abuse potential in its offering as a small disk.

TABLE 26: Opioid dosages for epidural analgesia in dogs and cats[34]

Drug class	Drug	Dose†	Onset (min)‡	Duration (h)‡
Opioid	Morphine§	Dog and cat: 0.1 mg/kg	20	20
	Hydromorphone§	Dog: 0.2 mg/kg: Cat: 0.1 mg/kg	15	
	Fentanyl	Dog: 0.006 mg/kg: Cat: 0.004 mg/kg	15	6
	Oxymorphone	Dog and cat: 0.05–0.1 mg/kg	15	10
	Buprenorphine	Dog: 0.005 mg/kg	30	18
	Butorphanol	Dog and cat: 0.25 mg/kg	10	2–4

†Decrease the dose by half for spinal administration of local anesthetics; decrease the epidural dose in geriatric, obese, and pregnant animals, and animals with space occupying lesions of the spinal cord or conditions in which venous engorgement is expected. Volume should be below 0.3ml/kg; do not exceed 6ml/dog or 1.5ml/cat (there are other volume recommendations: the author used these).
‡When specific onset and duration of action are not known for veterinary patients, they are extrapolated from human literature or from the onset and duration of parenterally administered drugs.
§Preservative-free morphine (for example: Duramorph) should be used for epidural or spinal administration of morphine.
Oxymorphone is variably available.
Avoid head-down positioning of the patient after epidurals; a block to T1 leads to intercostal paralysis, a block to C5–C7 leads to phrenic nerve paralysis.

The fentanyl transdermal patch was never 'approved' for use in veterinary medicine; however, the FDA and the EMA have recently approved a transdermal fentanyl solution for canine use – Recuvyra (Elanco Animal Health Inc.).

Recuvyra is licensed for preoperative administration to manage postoperative pain. A small volume of the liquid is applied with a special applicator onto the skin of the patient 2–4 hours prior to surgery. Within 5 minutes, the liquid evaporates, depositing fentanyl below the skin surface directly under the application site. Shortly following application and continuing over 4 days, fentanyl will diffuse from the skin into the dog's blood stream providing analgesia. As a precaution, it is recommended that the solution be administered with protective clothing, including gloves, and contact with the application site is to be avoided for 72 hours.

This transdermal fentanyl solution is a clear, colorless to light yellow solution containing 5% w/v (50 mg/ml) fentanyl as the active pharmaceutical ingredient. It is indicated for the control of pain associated with orthopedic and soft tissue surgery in dogs, with opioid effects lasting up to 7 days. The recommended dose is 1.2 mg/lb (2.7 mg/kg) applied topically to the dorsal scapular area 2–4 hours prior to surgery.

The solution is drawn up through a special needleless adaptor applied to the vial. Special syringes are used because of the interaction between the carrier solution and 'rubber' plungers of most plastic syringes. An applicator tip is then attached to the syringe for administration to the site, where the haircoat need not be clipped. Application to a single spot is restricted to 0.5 ml, with repeat repositioning and application at sites no closer than 1 inch (2 cm) apart until the entire calculated volume has been applied. (Absorption characteristics may vary by administration site. Safety and efficacy in cats, horses, or other species and administration at different sites have not been evaluated.)

Side-effects and precautions associated with this transdermal fentanyl solution are consistent with other delivery forms of the potent opioid fentanyl. The concomitant use of Recuvyra with other opioids or other CNS depressants (sedatives, hypnotics, general anesthetics, phenothiazines, and skeletal muscle relaxants) has not been extensively explored; nor has the drug been evaluated in dogs in the presence of cytochrome P450 3A4 inhibitors.

Once applied to the skin, solvent evaporation results in super-saturation of both a penetration enhancer and the active fentanyl (**Fig. 53**). The fentanyl is absorbed and sequestrated into the stratum corneum layer of the skin from which it is absorbed into the bloodstream. Unlike parenteral injections of fentanyl citrate in dogs where the terminal half-life of fentanyl is determined by the elimination rate, fentanyl from transdermal solution exhibits absorption-dependent (flip-flop) pharmacokinetics (*Table 27*). The absorption rate of fentanyl from skin is much slower than the elimination rate from blood and therefore the primary factor responsible for prolonged fentanyl blood concentrations is extended absorption (**Fig. 54**).

TABLE 27: Pharmacokinetic parameters in a typical (n = 215) Recuvyra canine patient

Terminal half-life	Time to 0.5 ng/ml	Time to 1.0 ng/ml	C_{max}	t_{max}	t_{lag}
74.0 h	1.6 h	3.08 h	1.83 ng/ml	13.6 h	0.552 h

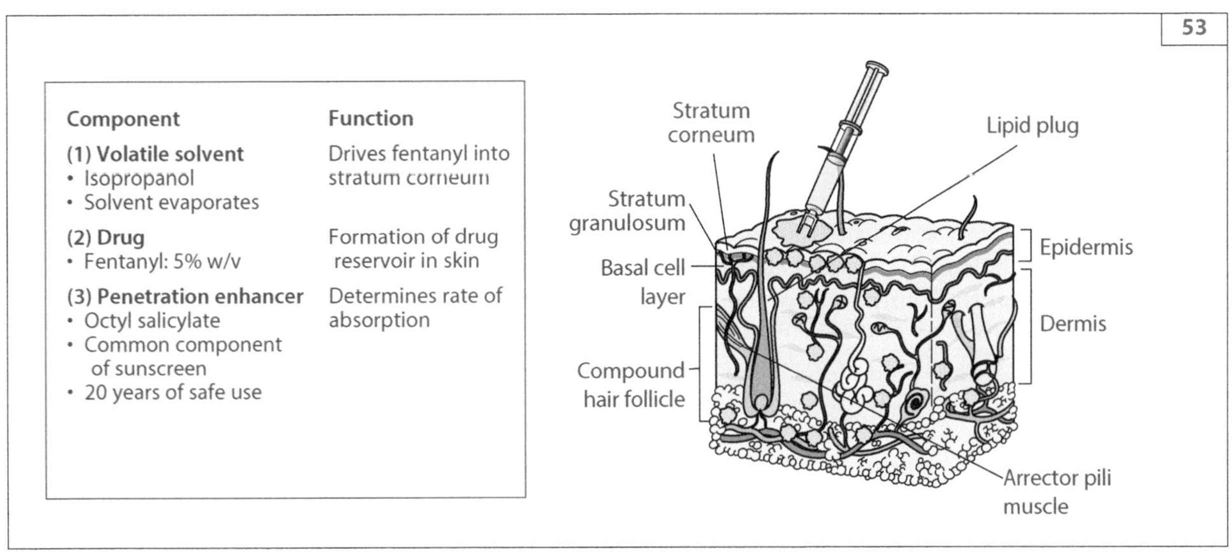

Component	Function
(1) Volatile solvent • Isopropanol • Solvent evaporates	Drives fentanyl into stratum corneum
(2) Drug • Fentanyl: 5% w/v	Formation of drug reservoir in skin
(3) Penetration enhancer • Octyl salicylate • Common component of sunscreen • 20 years of safe use	Determines rate of absorption

Fig. 53 The Medistend ™ volatile liquid transdermal drug delivery system consists of three principle components: (1) volatile solvent, (2) active drug, and (3) penetration enhancer.

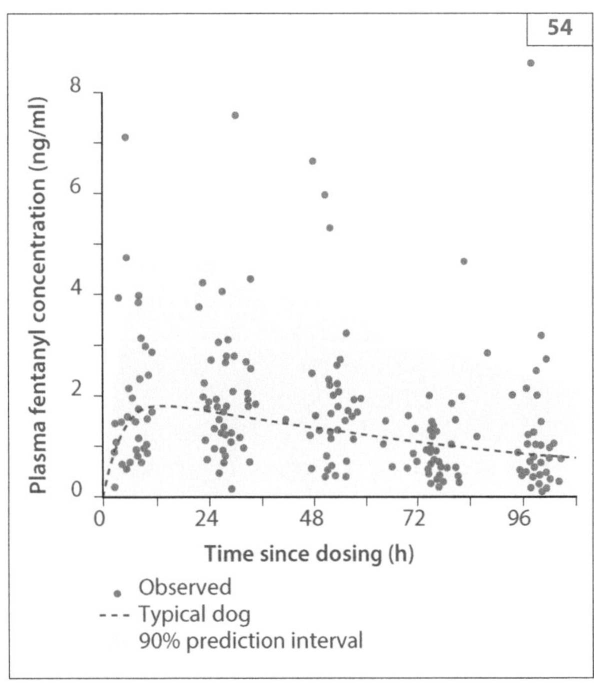

Fig. 54 Plasma fentanyl concentrations over approximately 4 days following a single administration 2–4 hours prior to orthopedic or soft tissue surgery (n = 215 dogs). The shaded area is the range of expected plasma fentanyl concentrations in 90% of dogs.

In two randomized multi-centered, double-masked, active-controlled field studies across 25 investigative sites, the transdermal fentanyl solution (n = 249 dogs) group showed non-inferior efficacy compared to the control (oxymorphone hydrochloride; n = 253 dogs) group. In canine safety studies administering 1×, 2× and 3× the labeled doses every 4 days for a total of 3 doses on the ventral abdomen (which results in approximately 30% greater exposure with similar peak exposure, compared to dorsal scapular application), critical adverse events were not seen at the labeled dose. Two dogs died on days 4 and 7 in the 2× group. Death was due to endotoxic shock as a result of severe GI stasis complicated by continued hypothermia and sedation, conditions considered unrelated to the active agent. Heart rate and respiration rate in individual treated dogs began decreasing within 4 hours of dosing. The largest drop in mean body temperatures occurred within 12–24 hours after dosing. Decreased food consumption was a consistent finding and was dose dependent. Dogs in the 1× group returned to pretreatment food consumption by day 12.

In a 16 week laboratory animal safety study topical fentanyl solution was administered at doses corresponding to 1× (n = 8 dogs), 2× (n = 4 dogs), and 3× (n = 4 dogs) the label dose, every 7 days for 16 weeks:

- Sedation lasted from 2 to 4 days after each dose.
- Maximal sedative effect (moderate sedation) was seen in the 1× group on days 2 and 3.
- Subjects appeared to show 'tolerance' of sedation with subsequent dosing.
- The day after dosing showed the greatest overall decrease in body temperature.
- The lowest body temperature in the 1× group on days 2 and 3 after the first dose was 99°F (37.2°C).
- Dogs showed bradycardia (<70 bpm) on the second and/or third days after dosing.
- Heart rate decreases did not require treatment and were not severe in the 1× group.
- The lowest respiratory rate in the groups was 12 bpm.
- Inappetence and weight loss were seen frequently in all groups.
- Abnormalities associated with increased white blood cells (WBC), decreased hemoglobin, and decreases in mean corpuscular hemaglobin concentration were mild, occurring in all groups.
- Gross necropsy findings for all groups did not reveal any treatment-related findings and no histopathologic findings were reported in the 1× group.

This topical fentanyl solution is available in 10 ml, amber-colored glass vials, and it is suggested that broached vials be discarded after 30 days.

This innovative delivery form of the popular opioid fentanyl has potential for changing the way clinicians address perioperative pain management.

Tramadol

Tramadol has become a very popular analgesic adjunct over the past decade, having gained a worldwide reputation as an effective, safe, and well-tolerated drug for inhibition of moderate pain in human patients (*Table 28*). It has come to fill the gap on the World Health Organization (WHO) analgesic ladder between the 'weak analgesics' (NSAIDs) and the strong opioids of the morphine-type. In veterinary medicine, arguably, tramadol has become the most embraced drug with the least supportive, evidence-based data in current times. The original compound comprised S- and R-enantiomers that could easily be separated by solubility differences. Pharmacologic testing of the individual enantiomers showed the R-enantiomer to be the stronger analgesic and erroneously this was further presumed to come from the trans-configuration, therefore the compound was named tramadol. Both enantiomers are required for full analgesic activity. The (+)-enantiomer inhibits serotonin (SE) reuptake and has weak affinity for opioid receptors (**Fig. 55**), while the (-)-enantiomer inhibits norepinephrine (NE) (noradrenaline) reuptake. Each enantiomer independently produces centrally mediated analgesia and the combination of enantiomers produces a greater than the additive effect of each enantiomer alone (they are synergistic).

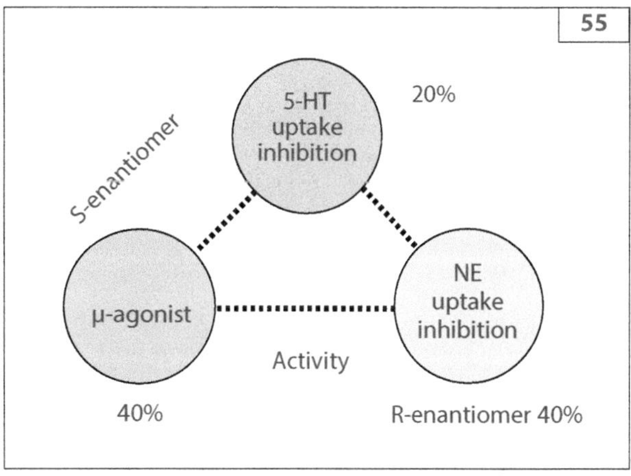

Fig. 55 Most (60%) of the activity associated with tramadol is as a tricyclic antidepressant/serotonin (5-HT) reuptake inhibitor. Less than half of its activity is as an opioid. NE: norepinephrine.

TABLE 28: Trade names for tramadol in different countries

Grünenthal GmbH, which still owns the patent on Tramadol, has cross-licensed the drug to pharmaceutical companies internationally. Thus, Tramadol is marketed under many trade names around the world, including:

- **Acugesic** (Malaysia, Singapore)
- **Adolonta** (Spain)
- **Algifeno** (Bolivia)
- **Algesia** (Philippines)
- **Anadol** (Bangladesh, Thailand)
- **Boldol** (Bosnia, Herzegovina)
- **Calmador** (Argentina)
- **Campex** (Pakistan)
- **Contramal** (Belgium, France, India, Italy, Turkey, Sudan, Hungary)
- **Crispin** (USA)
- **Dolcet** (combined with paracetamol)
- **Dolol** (Denmark)
- **Dolzam** (Belgium, Luxembourg)
- **Dromadol** (United Kingdom)
- **Exopen** (South Korea)
- **Ixprim** (France, Ireland)
- **Lumidol** (Bosnia, Herzegowina, Croatia)
- **Mabron** (Bahrain, Bangladesh, Bulgaria, Czech Republic, Estonia, Iraq, Jordan, Latvia, Lithuania, Malaysia, Oman, Romania, Singapore, Slovakia, Sri Lanka, Sudan, Yemen)
- **Mandolgin** (Denmark)
- **Mandolgine** (Denmark)
- **Mosepan** (USA)
- **Matrix** (combined with paracetamol) (Honduras, Guatemala)
- **Nobligan** (Argentina, Denmark, Iceland, Mexico, Norway, Portugal, Sweden)
- **Osteodol** (India)
- **Oxxalgan PR** (Greece)
- **Palitex** (India)
- **Poltram** (Poland)
- **Pyredol** (combined with paracetamol) (Vietnam, Bolivia)
- **Ralivia** (Canada)
- **Ryzolt** (USA)
- **Sinergix** (combined with ketorolac) (Mexico)
- **Sintradon** (Serbia)
- **Siverol** (Philippines)
- **Tandol** (South Korea)
- **Tiparol** (Sweden)
- **Tonoflex** (Pakistan)
- **Topalgic** (France)
- **Tradol** (Bangladesh, Ireland, Mexico, Singapore, Venezuela)
- **Tradolan** (Austria, Denmark, Finland, Iceland, Romania, Sweden)
- **Tradolgesic** (Thailand)
- **Tradonal** (Belgium, Indonesia, Italy, Luxembourg, Netherlands, Philippines, Spain, Switzerland)
- **Tralglt** (Czech Republic, Georgia, Romania, Slovakia)
- **Tralodle** (Italy)
- **Tramacet** (combined with paracetamol) (Canada, Mexico, Costa Rica, South Africa)
- **Tramacip** (India)
- **Tramadex** (Israel)
- **Tramadin** (Finland)
- **Tramadol HEXAL** (Denmark, Finland, Germany, Hungary)
- **Trexol** (Mexico)
- **Trumen** (Bangladesh)
- **Tramadol** (Australia, Belgium, Canada, Chile, Estonia, France, Netherlands, Romania, New Zealand, Norway, Spain, United Kingdom, USA)

continued

TABLE 28: Trade names for tramadol in different countries (continued)

- **Tramadol Stada** (Sweden)
- **Tramadol-Sandoz** (Hungary)
- **Tramadol-Ratiopharm** (Hungary, many European countries)
- **Tramadolor** (Austria, Estonia, Germany, Hungary, Latvia, Lithuania, Luxembourg, Romania)
- **Tramadolor ID** (Hungary)
- **Tramaigic** (Hungary, Czech Republic, Slovakia)
- **Tramagit** (Romania)
- **Tramahexal** (Australia)
- **Tramake** (United Kingdom)
- **Trama-Klosidol** (Argentina)
- **Tramal** (Bulgaria, Colombia, Pakistan, Netherlands, Finland, Croatia, Morocco, Slovenia, Austria, Poland, Croatia, Morocco, Slovenia, Austria, Poland, Brazil, Chile, Romania, Australia, New Zealand, Germany, Switzerland, Lebanon, Israel, Philippines, Egypt, Thailand)
- **Tramalgic** (Hungary)
- **Tramal Gotas** (Ecuador)
- **Tramazac** (India, Myanmar, Sri Lanka)
- **Tramed** (USA)
- **Tramedo** (Australia)
- **Tramoda** (Thailand)
- **Tramol** (Iceland)
- **Tramundal** (Austria)
- **Tridol** (South Korea)
- **Tridural** (Canada)
- **Trodon** (Serbia)
- **Ultracet** (combined with paracetamol) (Brazil, USA)
- **Ultradol** (Bangladesh)
- **Ultram and Ultram ER** (USA)
- **Ultramed** (combined with paracetamol) (India)
- **Veldrol** (Mexico)
- **VAMADOL PLUS** (India)
- **Volcidol** (Thailand)
- **Zafin** (combined with paracetamol) (Chile)
- **Zaldlar** (combined with paracetamol) (Belgium, Chile, Croatia, Czech Republic, Mexico, Poland, Portugal, Slovenia, Spain, Russia)
- **Zaledor** (combined with paracetamol) (Chile)
- **Zamadol** (United Kingdom)
- **Zamudol** (France)
- **Zodol** (Chile, Ecuador, Peru)
- **Zydol** (United Kingdom, Ireland, Australia)
- **Zytram** (Canada, Iceland, New Zealand, Spain)
- **Zytrim** (Spain)

Only preparations for oral administration to humans are available in the USA. Metabolism of tramadol through hepatic demethylation to (the M1-metabolite) O-desmethyl-tramadol is reported in several species (including dog and cat), and O-desmethyl-tramadol has been shown to bind to the μ-opioid receptor with a much higher affinity than the parent drug, likely providing its analgesic effect. Metabolic clearance is proposed to be through hepatic metabolism and renal excretion of unchanged drug. The lower clearance in cats compared to dogs may reflect the lower capacity of the liver to biotransform tramadol in cats (*Table 29*).

The unique characteristics of tramadol were identified by incomplete inhibition of IP tramadol-induced antinociception with SC naloxone, compared with the complete inhibition of antinociception induced by codeine and morphine in the mouse abdominal constriction test (**Fig. 56**)[35].

Tramadol possesses weak agonist actions at the μ-opioid receptor, releases SE, and inhibits the reuptake of NE. While its action is not like that of other opioids, tramadol is a synthetic analog of the phenanthrene alkaloid codeine. Tramadol does not inhibit cyclo-oxygenase activity (NSAID mode of action). Seizure risk is cautioned in human patients receiving CNS drugs that reduce seizure threshold, such as tricyclic antidepressants (TCAs), selective SE-reuptake inhibitors (SSRIs), monoamine oxidase inhibitors, or neuroleptics. Tramadol may also be associated with GI bleeding, exacerbated by concurrent use with a NSAID (Author's personal observation[36])[37,38]. In May 2009, the USA FDA issued a Warning Letter[39] to Johnson & Johnson, alleging that a promotional website commissioned by the manufacturer had 'overstated the efficacy' of the drug, and 'minimized the serious risks'.

One study[40] in human patients demonstrated that both tramadol and its M1 demethylated

TABLE 29: Pharmacokinetic parameters for orally administered tramadol

	Tramadol		O-desmethyl-tramadol	
	Dog	**Cat**	**Dog**	**Cat**
Availability	65±38%	93±7%		
T½			2.18±0.55 h	4.82±0.32 h
Elimination half-life	1.71 h	3.4 h		
C_{max}	1402.75±696 ng/ml	914±232 ng/ml		
T_{max}	1.04±0.51 h	0.42 h		

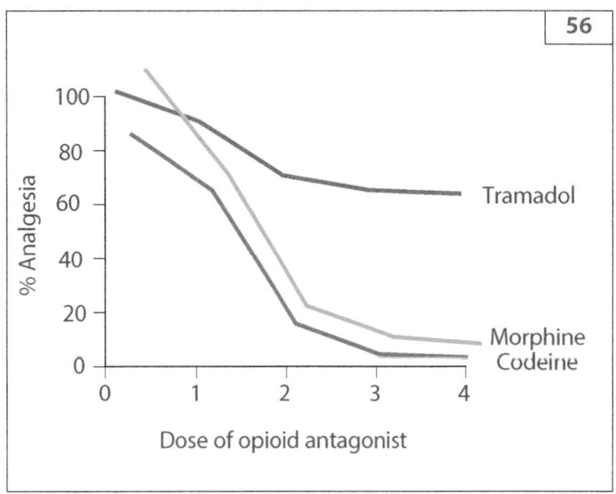

Fig. 56 Comparison of antagonist reversal of opioid analgesia. While the traditional μ-receptor agonists (morphine and codeine) show pronounced analgesic reversal with the opioid antagonist naloxone, tramadol does not, confirming that it is not a 'pure' opioid.

metabolite penetrate into synovial fluid, significantly reducing synovial fluid concentrations of sP. IL-6 synovial fluid concentrations were not significantly decreased. In dogs, the systemic clearance of orally administered tramadol is almost five times faster than in humans, with at least 32 metabolites identified[41]. In a different study[42], simulated oral dosing regimens at 5 mg/kg every 6 hours and 2.5 mg/kg every 4 hours were predicted to produce tramadol and M1 levels consistent with analgesia in humans, noting that pharmacodynamic studies are lacking to confirm the plasma concentrations needed to provide analgesia in dogs. The fraction of tramadol metabolized to M1 calculated for study dogs was 15.65±4.1%, indicating that demethylation of tramadol to M1 in dogs is a relatively minor pathway. The short elimination half-life of M1 following oral tramadol administration (2.18±0.55 h (with T_{max} of 0.50±0.20 h)) illustrates the need for frequent dosing to maintain effective plasma concentrations. MEC (plasma) for tramadol and M1 have been reported to be 298±410 and 39.6±34 ng/ml, respectively, in postoperative humans. McMillan *et al.*[44] (2008) reported that the levels of M1 following IV tramadol administration were low and near the lower limits of assay quantification (9.8–19.7 ng/ml). With support from the afore mentioned findings, Giorgi *et al.*[45] reported that the sustained release formulation of tramadol may not have suitable pharmacokinetic characteristics to be administered once-a-day as an effective and safe treatment for pain in the dog. The bioavailability of tramadol is apparently similar to that in humans (65±35%). In cats, tramadol is rapidly absorbed after oral administration and eliminated relatively slowly[46].

Tramadol has rivaled morphine for postoperative analgesia in bitches undergoing ovariohysterectomy[47]. In a study involving 42 dogs with oral neoplasms, investigators concluded that an opioid–NSAID combination was the best option for pain control; however, if the use of an NSAID is contraindicated, then administration of tramadol alone may be a good alternative[48].

Most analgesic combination products currently marketed for moderate-to-severe pain are mixtures of codeine, hydrocodone, oxycodone, or propoxyphene with aspirin (acety salicyclic acid), acetaminophen, or ibuprofen (examples: Ultracet: tramadol + acetaminophen; Tylenol 1–4: acetaminophen + codeine).

Opioid overview

Opioids are relatively safe. Subcutaneous administration of opioids (particularly in cats) is the least desirable route of administration. Potential side-effects include:

- Sedation or CNS depression.
- Excitement or dysphoria.
- Bradycardia.
- Respiratory depression.
- Panting.
- Laryngeal reflex depression.
- Histamine release (particularly with IV administration).
- Vomition and defecation (nausea).
- Constipation (longer-term use).
- Urinary retention (more common with epidural administration).
- Hyperthermia (especially in cats [with hydromorphone]).

Mechanistic summary of opioids

- Act at μ, δ, and κ opioid receptors.
- Hyperpolarize by increased K^+ conductance; block transmitter release by blocking calcium conductance. Act in brain, spinal cord, and at peripheral afferent terminals.
- Brainstem – periaqueductal gray (PAG): activates several mechanisms, including increased activity in descending/ascending pathways.
- Spinal cord: act in the substantia gelatinosa to block C-fiber release and hyperpolarizes dorsal horn nociceptive neurons.
- Periphery: act to alter the excitability in terminals located in an inflammatory milieu; only block hyperalgesia.
- Central: raise nociceptive thresholds.

Opioids at-a-glance

Meperidine (pethidine)

- Less sedation than morphine.
- More likely to cause histamine release; IV can cause excitement in animals. NOT to be given IV.
- Anticholinergic effects associated with structural similarity to atropine.
- In humans, the metabolite normeperidine is a neurotoxic CNS stimulant associated with adverse reactions[49].
- Very short acting (<2 hours in cats).

Oxymorphone

- Does not cause histamine release.
- May induce panting.

Methadone

- Does not cause histamine release.
- NMDA and SSRI activity.

Hydromorphone

- More sedation than oxymorphone, but shorter duration.
- No histamine release with IV administration.
- Hyperthermia in cats.

Fentanyl

- Rapid onset of action (2–3 minutes).
- Short duration of action (thermal threshold testing revealed that 10 μg/kg IV lasts approximately 2 hours in cats).

Butorphanol

- Agonist (κ)–antagonist (μ).
- Weak analgesic, with analgesic ceiling effect.
- Short duration of analgesia (~ 40 minutes in the dog; approximately 90 minutes after IV dosing in cats).

Buprenorphine

- Agonist (strong for μ-receptor)–antagonist (κ -receptor).
- Slow onset (30–60 minutes), long acting (8–12 hours).
- Affinity for μ-receptor makes reversal more difficult.

- Most popular opioid used in small animal practice in the UK, Australia, New Zealand, and South Africa.
- Oral transmucosal administration very effective in the cat.
- Considered by some to be the best opioid investigated in the cat[50].

Codeine
- 'International standard' weak opioid.
- Substantially improves analgesia of nonopioids (e.g. NSAIDs).

Tramadol
- 40% activity at the μ-receptor, 60% as SE and NE neuronal reuptake inhibitor (monoaminergic).
- Reduces synovial fluid concentrations of sP and IL-6 in human patients with knee osteoarthritis[40].
- Augments analgesia of opioids[51] and NSAIDs[52].
- Bioavailability is about 65%, with a short half-life (<1.7 hours) in dogs; bioavailability is 93% with a half life of 3.4 hours in the cat.
- Simulated oral dosing regimens at 5 mg/kg Q6h and 2.5 mg/kg Q4h in the dog are predicted to produce tramadol and M1 levels consistent with analgesia in humans[40].
- Effective in neuropathic pain[53].
- Low abuse potential.
- Possible potentiation of bleeding, especially when combined with a NSAID.
- Lack of evidence-base for dosing, efficacy, and safety in dogs and cats.

Preoperative and acute pain management opioid doses are presented in *Tables 30* and *31 overleaf*.

TABLE 30: Opioid preoperative doses

Drug	Dose	Species	Route	Duration
Morphine	0.5–1.0 mg/kg	Canine	IM, SC	3–4 h
	0.5 mg/kg + 0.1–1.0 mg/kg/h	Canine	IV	As long as infusion lasts
	0.1 mg/kg preservative-free morphine	Canine/feline	Epidural	12–24 h
	0.05–0.1 mg/kg	Feline	IM, SC	3–4 h
	1–5 mg in 5–10 ml	Canine	Intra-articular	
Meperidine	3–5 mg/kg	Canine/feline	IM, SC	1–2 h
Methadone	0.1–0.5 mg/kg	Canine/feline	IM, SC	2–4 h
Oxymorphone	0.05–0.1 mg/kg	Canine	IM, IV, SC	3–4 h
	0.03–0.05 mg/kg	Feline	IM, SC	3–4 h
Hydromorphone	0.1–0.2 mg/kg	Canine	IM, IV, SC	2–4 h
Fentanyl	5 μg/kg + 3–6 μg/kg/h	Canine	IV	Infusion
	2–3 μg/kg + 2–3 μg/kg/h	Feline	IV	Infusion
	2.7 mg/kg	Canine only	Transdermal	4–7 days
Butorphanol	0.1–0.2 mg/kg	Canine/feline	IM, IV, SC	3–4 h
Pentazocine	1–3 mg/kg	Canine/feline	IM, IV, SC	2–4 h
Nalbuphine	0.03–0.1 mg/kg	Canine/feline	IM, IV, SC	2–4 h
Buprenorphine	5–20 μg/kg	Canine/feline	IM, IV, SC	8–12 h

TABLE 31: Opioids for acute pain management[34]

Drug	Route	Dose (dog)	Dose (cat)	Notes
μ-Agonists				
Morphine	SC, IM, slow IV	0.5–1 mg/kg	0.2–05 mg/kg	Lasts 2–4 h
	CRI	0.1–0.3 mg/kg/h	0.1–0.2 mg/kg/h	
	Epidural	0.1 mg/kg	0.1 mg/kg	Use preservative-free morphine
	Oral	2–5 mg/kg		Sustained-release tablets. Dose *bid*
Hydromorphone	SC, IM, IV	0.05–0.2 mg/kg	0.05–0.1 mg/kg	Lasts 2–6 h
	CRI	0.015–0.03 mg/kg/h	0.015–0.03 mg/kg/h	
Oxymorphone	SC, IM, IV	0.05–0.4 mg/kg	0.02–0.1 mg/kg	Lasts 2–4 h
Methadone	SC, IM, IV	1–1.5 mg/kg		Lasts 2–4 h
Fentanyl	IV	2–5 μg/kg	1–3 μg/kg	Lasts 15–20 min
	CRI	2–5 μg/kg/h	1–4 μg/kg/h	
	Transdermal patch	2–4 μg/kg/h	2–4 μg/kg/h	Apply 12–24 h preoperatively Lasts 3–4 days
Partial μ-agonist				
Buprenorphine	SC, IM, IV	0.005–0.02 mg/kg	0.005–0.02 mg/kg	Lasts 8–12 h Will antagonize α-agonists
	Transmucosal		0.01–0.02 mg/kg	Lasts 6–8 h
Agonist–antagonist				
Butorphanol	SC, IM, IV	0.1–0.4 mg/kg	0.1–0.4 mg/kg	Lasts 1–4 h
	Oral	0.5–2 mg/kg	0.5–1 mg/kg	Lasts 8–12 h
	CRI	0.1–0.5 mg/kg/h	0.1–0.3 mg/kg/h	

CRI: constant rate infusion.

TABLE 32: MLK (morphine/lidocanine/ketamine) formulae and constant rate infusion (CRI) administration[34]

Drug	Amount added to 1 l of crystalloid given at 10 ml/kg/h	Amount added to 1 l of crystalloid given at 5 ml/kg/h	Drug CRI
Morphine	24 mg	48 mg	0.24 mg/kg/h
Hydromorphone* (replaces morphine)	2 mg	4 mg	0.02 mg/kg/h
Lidocaine	300 mg	600 mg	3 mg/kg/h
Ketamine	60 mg	120 mg	0.6 mg/kg/h
±Medetomidine	100 μg	200 μg	1 μg/kg/h

*Fentanyl may also be substituted for morphine.

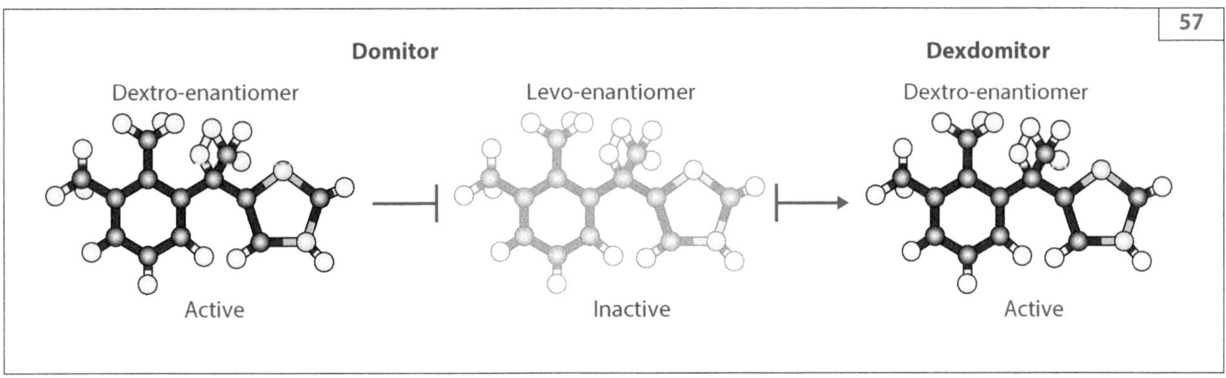

Fig. 57 Dexmedetomidone provides sedation and analgesia using only the active enantiomer of medetomidine.

A multimodal technique with the implementation of morphine has been described[54] and has been widely used. This combination reduces the amount of inhalant anesthetic agent required for maintenance of anesthesia (45% minimum alveolar concentration [MAC] reduction), although there appears to be little advantage over the morphine dose alone (*Table 32*).

α_2-AGONISTS

The prototypical α_2-adrenergic agonist used in veterinary medicine has been xylazine. Since its introduction in 1962, xylazine has been used, mostly in horses and ruminants, as a sedative-analgesic or anesthetic adjuvant (it is NOT an anesthetic). The newer α_2-adrenergic agonists, medetomidine and dexmedetomidine, have gained acceptance in companion animal practice where they demonstrate lower anesthetic mortality than xylazine. Medetomidine is an equal mixture of two optical enantiomers, of which dexmedetomidine is a potent α_2-agonist, while levomedetomidine is pharmacologically inactive. Medetomidine has a high affinity for the α_2-receptor, with an α_2/α_1 binding ratio of 1620, compared with ratios of 260, 220, and 160 for detomidine, clonidine, and xylazine, respectively[55]. Currently, it is uncommon practice (in the USA) to administer large doses of an α_2-agonist as a single agent, but it is commonly accepted that low doses are very useful when used as adjuncts in a balanced analgesic protocol.

Since its USA launch in 2007, medetomidine has been phased out (in the USA) and replaced by dexmedetomidine. Dexmedetomidine is the dextrorotary enantiomer of the racemic mixture medetomidine (**Fig. 57**). It is approximately twice as potent as medetomidine in terms of its ability to produce sedation and analgesia. Dexmedetomidine is supplied as a 0.5 mg/ml solution, which allows clinicians to use the same injection volume as medetomidine because the dexmedetomidine dilution has the same potency as medetomidine.

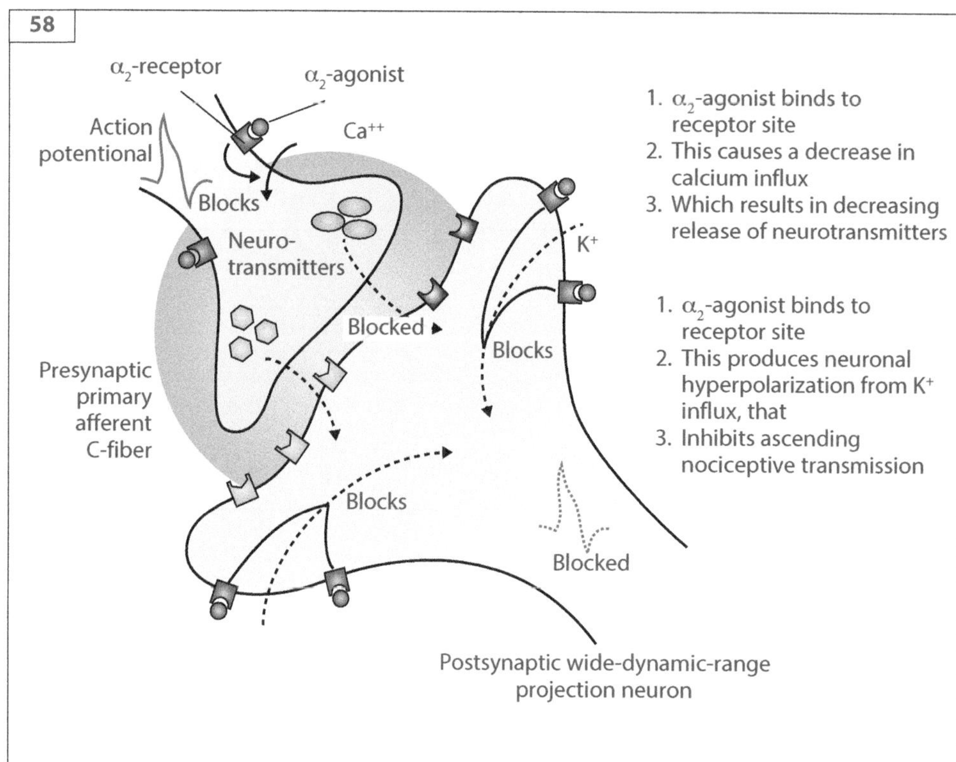

Fig. 58 At the level of the dorsal horn, activation by norepinephrine or an α_2-agonist has both a pre- and a postsynaptic activity that leads to analgesia.

Presynaptic α_2-adrenoceptors secrete NE, which binds with postsynaptic adrenoceptors to stimulate target cell response governing autonomic functions. Dexmedetomidine produces rapid sedation by selectively binding to α_2-adrenoceptors in the neuron, inhibiting release of NE necessary for neurotransmission.

Bulbospinal noradrenergic pathways can regulate dorsal horn nociceptive processing by the release of NE and the subsequent activation of α_2-adrenergic receptors. Epidural delivery of α_2-agonists can produce potent analgesia in humans and animals[56]. Although the receptor is distinct, spinal action of an α_2-agonist is mediated by a mechanism similar to that of spinal opioids: 1) α_2 binding is presynaptic on C-fibers and postsynaptic on dorsal horn neurons; 2) α_2-receptors can depress the release of C-fiber transmitters; and 3) α_2-agonists can hyperpolarize dorsal horn neurons through a Gi-coupled K^+ channel (**Fig. 58**).

Dense populations of α_2-adrenoceptors are concentrated in the mammalian spinal cord dorsal horn, both pre- and postsynaptically, and on non-noradrenergic nociceptive neurons. On presynaptic α_2-adrenoceptors, when G_0 proteins are activated, a decrease in calcium influx is mediated, leading to decreased release of neurotransmitters and/or neuropeptides, including glutamate, vasoactive intestinal peptide, CGRP, sP, and neurotensin. At postsynaptic α_2-adrenoceptors, Gi protein-coupled potassium channels produce neuronal hyperpolarization that dampens ascending nociceptive transmission, thereby producing postsynaptically-mediated spinal analgesia. The sedative–hypnotic effects are apparently mediated by activation of supraspinal α_2-adrenoceptors located in the brainstem, where there is a relatively high density of α_2-agonist binding sites.

α_2-mediated analgesia (in neuropathic pain) involves spinal muscarinic and cholinergic receptor activation with nitric oxide (NO) mechanisms, supporting that α_2 receptors may be primarily located on spinal cholinergic interneurons[57]. Spinal α_2 receptors, in conjunction with PAG opioid receptors, mediate the analgesic actions of NO. Sedative effects are presumed to be mediated at the level of the brainstem. It is generally accepted that effects of spinal α_2-adrenoceptor agonists are not naloxone reversible and show no cross-tolerance to opioids.

Potential α_2-agonists features include (*Table 33*):

- Sedation, muscle relaxation, and anxiolysis.
- Short-duration hypertension accompanied by a compensatory baroreceptor-mediated reflex bradycardia.
- Decreased respiratory rate, but with pH, PaO_2, and $PaCo_2$ maintained within normal limits.
- Both cats and dogs may vomit: cats (~90%) > dogs (~20%).
- GI atony with possible gas accumulation.
- Increased urinary output.
- Transient hypoinsulinemia and hyperglycemia have been reported in dogs.

The hemodynamic effects of α_2-agonists in the dog have typically been described as a biphasic blood pressure response with decreased heart rate and cardiac index, and increased systemic vascular resistance index and central venous pressure[58].

TABLE 33: Data taken from an educational demonstration in a live dog, demonstrating the physiologic responses to an α_2-agonist (medetomidine); anticholinergic (atropine); and reversal agent (antipamezol)

Parameters (normal)	Heart rate (bpm) (70–110)	Mean BP (mmHg) (60–100)	Cardiac output (L/min) (2.5–6)	O_2 saturation (%) (95–100)	Mucous membrane color (pink,1–3 s)	PaO_2 (mmHg) (500–600)	$PaCO_2$ (mmHg) (40–55)	Respiration rate (breaths/min) (6–20)
Baseline (1.1 % isoflurane)	91	76	2.95	98	pink, fast	575	52	20
(10 µg/kg; IM) medetomine admin								
+ 5 min	49	96	1.33	93	pale, slow	630	55	24
+ 15 min	50	90	1.36	95	pinker, slow	563	54	18
(0.04 mg/kg, IV) anticholinergic admin								
+ 3 min	77	125	1.45	100	pink, faster	602	59	13
(50 µg/kg; IM) antipamezol admin								
+ 1 min	86	147	1.56	99	pink, fast	X	X	15
+ 5 min	89	96	2.3	98	pink, fast	597	54	12

(Drs. WJ Tranquilli and KA Grimm; University of Illinois, to Pfizer Animal Health Veterinarians.)

BP: blood pressure; bpm: beats per minute; X: not measured.

The initial increase in blood pressure results from peripheral vasoconstriction caused by activation of postsynaptic α_2-receptors in peripheral vascular smooth muscle (seen clinically as peripheral blanching and 'muddy' oral mucous membranes). This is associated with increased vagal tone and decreased heart rate (phase 1). Blood pressure then falls as vasoconstriction wanes and a central hypotensive effect predominates (phase 2). Sympathetic nervous tone is decreased, and this phase is associated with a prolonged decrease in heart rate (**Fig. 59**). The exact location and the specific receptors responsible for the central hypotensive effect are not known.

Dexmedetomidine contains only the active enantiomer without levomedetomidine; therefore, differences in drug metabolism between dexmedetomidine and medetomidine can be expected, such as a lesser inhibitory effect on concomitantly used ketamine. One study[59] showed a greater analgesic duration for dexmedetomidine than medetomidine at equivalent doses in dogs. In cats, McKusick *et al.*[60] showed that premedication with dexmedetomidine before ketamine anesthesia resulted in a quicker recovery than if premedicated with the racemic medetomidine. Also in cats, Granholm *et al.*[61] showed that the percentage of subjects with normal heart rate and normal pulse character after drug administration was higher with dexmedetomidine than medetomidine.

Dexmedetomidine dosing is based on a given canine body weight considering the level of sedation/analgesia desired and the route of administration. The available concentration of dexmedetomidine (0.5 mg/ml) provides clinicians a simple volume-for-volume substitution of dexmedetomidine for medetomidine. In dogs there are two FDA-approved doses for sedation and analgesia (500 μg/m² IM and 375 μg/m² IV), and two approved doses for premedication (125 μg/m² IM and 375 μg/m² IM). There is only a single FDA-approved dose for sedation and analgesia in cats (40 μg/kg). This cat dose is based on the body surface area (BSA) of a 4.5 kg cat. Dexmedetomidine dosing is based on an animal's BSA rather than body weight to minimize variations in sedative and analgesic effects. BSA is defined as the measured or calculated surface of an animal's body and is a better indicator of metabolic mass than body weight because it is less affected by abnormal adipose (fat) tissue mass. This is relevant in small animals because the specific (mass-related) metabolic rate of animals decreases with increasing body size. Accordingly, the μg/kg dose increases as an animal's body weight decreases (*Tables 34,* and *35* [62].

Because medetomidine is so widely used, and because medetomidine has traditionally been positioned for best use in combination with other agents, the manufacturer has provided guidance for the use of dexmedetomidine with other sedatives, analgesics, and anesthetic agents (*Tables 36–40 overleaf*)[62]. The TKX (tiletamine–zolazepam, ketamine, and xylazine) combination has been widely used in cats, particularly in trap-and-neuter and shelter operations. Its drawbacks include limited analgesia and erratic recovery. These limitations prompted replacement of the xylazine with medetomidine and replacement of the ketamine with butorphanol, creating the TTD protocol (tiletamine–zolazepam, butorphanol, and medetomidine).

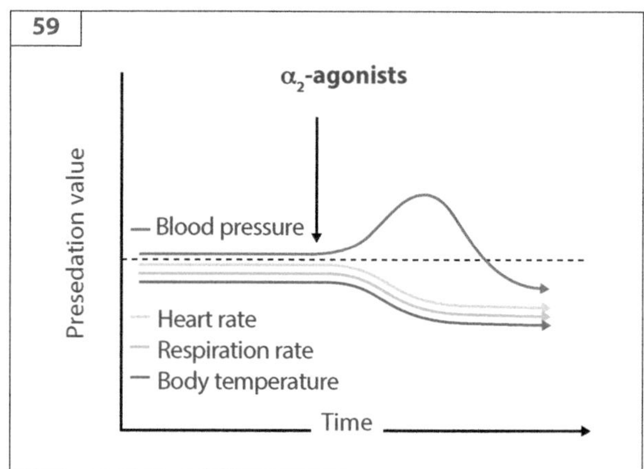

Fig. 59 In the periphery, α_2-agonists cause vasoconstriction. This causes an increase in systemic vascular resistance, resulting in increased blood pressure. To maintain cardiac output, the heart rate decreases to compensate for the increased blood pressure.

TABLES 34 and 35: Guides to determine dose requirements of dexmedetomidine (500 µg/ml) in dogs (*Table 34*) and cats (*Table 35*), using body surface area

34	Dexmedetomidine dose for cooperative sedation/ preanesthesia in dogs (125 µg/m² IM)*			Dexmedetomidine dose for moderate sedation/ preanesthesia in dogs (375 µg/m² IM or IV)			Dexmedetomidine dose for profound sedation in dogs (500 µg/m² IM)		
Weight (kg)	**Total dose in ml†**	**Dose in ml/kg†**	**Dose in µg/kg**	**Total dose in ml†**	**Dose in ml/kg†**	**Dose in µg/kg**	**Total dose in ml†**	**Dose in ml/kg†**	**Dose in µg/kg**
2	0.04	0.02	10.02	0.12	0.060	30.06	0.16	0.080	40.08
2.5	0.05	0.02	9.30	0.14	0.056	27.90	0.19	0.076	37.21
5	0.08	0.015	7.38	0.22	0.044	22.15	0.30	0.060	29.53
7.5	0.10	0.013	6.45	0.29	0.039	19.35	0.39	0.052	25.80
10	0.12	0.012	5.86	0.35	0.035	17.58	0.47	0.047	23.44
12.5	0.14	0.011	5.44	0.41	0.033	16.32	0.55	0.044	21.80
15	0.15	0.010	5.12	0.46	0.031	15.36	0.62	0.041	20.48
20	0.19	0.009	4.65	0.56	0.028	13.95	0.74	0.037	18.60
25	0.22	0.009	4.31	0.65	0.026	12.95	0.86	0.035	17.27
30	0.24	0.008	4.06	0.73	0.024	12.19	0.98	0.033	16.25
35	0.27	0.008	3.86	0.81	0.023	11.58	1.08	0.031	15.44
40	0.30	0.007	3.69	0.89	0.022	11.07	1.18	0.030	14.77

*The preanesthetic dose (125 µg/m² IM, cooperative sedation/preanesthesia) can be used IM with an opioid (morphine, 0.25 mg/kg hydromorphone, 0.05 mg/kg or butorphanol, 0.2 mg/kg) to produce a moderate degree of sedation similar to that induced by 375 µg/m² IM of dexmedetomidine.

†The total doses in ml and doses in ml/kg in this table have been derived from the µg/kg BSA dose and have been rounded up or down, as appropriate, to accommodate practical dosing. As a result, a perfect match in values based on calculation conversions between columns will not necessarily occur.

TABLE 35 **BSA specific dexmedetomidine dose (IM) for sedation/analgesia in cats**

Weight (kg)	Total dose in ml	Dose in ml/kg	Dose in µg/kg
2	0.21	0.105	52.4
2.5	0.24	0.097	48.7
3	0.28	0.092	45.8
3.5	0.30	0.087	43.5
4	0.33	0.083	41.6
4.5	0.36	0.080	40
5	0.39	0.077	38.6
5.5	0.41	0.075	37.4
6	0.44	0.073	36.4

BSA: body surface area.

TABLE 36: Dexmedetomidine–opioid combinations in dogs and cats for profound sedation

	Drug dose				
Species	Dexmedetomidine (μg/kg)	Butorphanol (mg/kg)	Hydromorphone (mg/kg)	Morphine (mg/kg)	Buprenorphine† (mg/kg)
Dogs	5–10 IV	0.1–0.2 IV	0.03–0.05 IV	0.25–0.5 IV	–
	15–20 IM	0.3–0.4 IM	0.05–0.1 IM	0.5–1 IM	–
Cats	15–25 IV	0.2–0.3 IV	0.03–0.05 IV	–	0.01–0.02 IV
	20–40 IM	0.3–0.4 IM	0.05–0.1 IM	–	0.02–0.04 IM

*Note that buprenorphine has a slower onset than other opioids.

TABLE 37: Dexmedetomidine–butorphanol–midazolam and dexmedetomidine–butorphanol–diazepam combinations for profound sedation and immobilization of healthy dogs and cats

	Drug dose		
Species	Dexmedetomidine (μg/kg)	Butorphanol (mg/kg)	Midazolam or diazepam (mg/kg)
Dogs	2.5–5 IV	0.2 IV	0.2 IV
	5–10 IM	0.3 IM	0.4 IM
Cats	10–15 IV	0.2 IV	0.2 IV
	20–25 IM	0.3 IM	0.4 IM

TABLE 38: Dexmedetomidine–ketamine combinations in dogs and cats*

	Drug dose	
Species	Dexmedetomidine (μg/kg)	Ketamine (mg/kg)
Dogs	5–10 IV	1–2 IV
	15–20 IM	3–4 IM
Cats	15–25 IV	2–3 IV
	20–40 IM	3–5 IM

*The combinations induce a surgical plane of anesthesia that lasts 20 min (low doses) to 40 min (high doses).

The TTD protocol has proved safe for use in **both** dogs and cats, replacing the TKX combination. To incorporate dexmedetomidine into this protocol, the medetomidine component is substituted with an equal volume of dexmedetomidine, yielding the TTDex combination (*Table 40*).

Mechanistic summary of α_2-agonists

- Act at α_2-adrenergic receptor.
- Hyperpolarize by increased K^+ conductance; block transmitter release by blocking calcium conductance.
- Act in the brain to produce sedation and depress arousal.

TABLE 39: Dexmedetomidine–butorphanol–ketamine ('kitty magic') combination in cats*

	Drug dose			
Level of sedation/procedure	**Dexmedetomidine (0.5 mg/ml)**	**Butorphanol (10 mg/ml)**	**Ketamine (100 mg/ml)**	**Atipamezole† (5 mg/ml)**
Profound sedation-analgesia	0.1 ml (11.1 μg/kg)	0.1 ml (0.22 mg/kg)	0.1 ml (2.2 mg/kg)	0.1 ml (111.1 μg/kg)
Castration or laceration repair	0.2 ml (22.2 μg/kg)	0.2 ml (0.44 mg/kg)	0.2 ml (4.4 mg/kg)	0.2 ml (222.2 μg/kg)
Ovariohysterectomy, onychectomy, abdominal procedures	0.3 ml (33.3 μg/kg)	0.3 ml (0.66 mg/kg)	0.3 ml (6.6 mg/kg)	0.3 ml (333.3 μg/kg)

*Based on a 4.5 kg (10 lb) cat. All drugs (except atipamezole) can be mixed in one syringe and administered as a single IM injection. If given IV, the drug doses in this combination should be halved; however, if a deeper plane of anesthesia is desired, the full IM dose can be given IV.
†If reversal is necessary for safe recovery.

TABLE 40: Tiletamine–zolazepam–butorphanol–dexmedetomidine (TTDex) combination in dogs and cats

Desired purpose	**IM dosages of individual components***	**Volume (ml/kg IM) of reconstituted TTDex†**
Premedication (mild to moderate sedation)	Tiletamine–zolazepam, 1 mg/kg Butorphanol, 0.05 mg/kg Dexmedetomidine, 2.5 μg/kg	0.01
Chemical restraint (profound sedation)	Tiletamine–zolazepam, 2 mg/kg Butorphanol, 0.1 mg/kg Dexmedetomidine, 5 μg/kg	0.02
Surgical plane of anesthesia	Tiletamine–zolazepam, 3 mg/kg Butorphanol, 0.15 mg/kg Dexmedetomidine, 7.5 μg/kg	0.03

*Each agent (tiletamine–zolazepam, butorphanol, and dexmedetomidine) may be drawn up separately according to the dosage listed in this table. If given IV, drug doses in this combination should be halved; however, if a deeper plane of anesthesia is desired, the full IM dose can be given IV.
†Alternately, tiletamine–zolazepam powder can be reconstituted using 2.5 ml of butorphanol (10 mg/ml) and 2.5 ml of dexmedetomidine (0.5 mg/ml) as diluents. If given IV, drug doses in this combination should be halved; however, if a deeper plane of anesthesia is desired, the full IM dose can be given IV.

- In the spinal cord, produce analgesia and depress sympathetic outflow.
- In the spinal cord, act in the substantia gelatinosa to block C-fiber release and hyperpolarize dorsal horn nociceptive neurons, producing analgesia.
- Effects on neuropathic pain may reflect mild sympatholytic action.

α_2-agonists at-a-glance

- Not first-line analgesic agents, but excellent analgesic adjuncts.
- At low doses, both sedation and analgesia are dose-dependent.
- Ceiling effect at higher dosages.
- Co-administration with anticholinergics to alleviate bradycardia is controversial.
- A volume of atipamezole equal to that of the α_2-agonist can be used for reversal after the procedure has been completed if indicated by patient management.
- Atipamezole reverses not only the α_2-agonist-induced bradycardia but also the drug's sedative and analgesic effects.
- The recommended route of administration for atipamezole is IM; however, a single IV bolus can be given in an emergency situation.
- Atipamezole is frequently used to reverse sedation in cats, but it is not FDA approved for use in cats.
- Inclusion in a premedication protocol markedly reduces the required dose of induction and maintenance anesthetic agents.
- Up to 20% of dogs and 90% of cats will vomit after administration.
- Increased urine output is reported in both dogs and cats.
- Transient hypoinsulinemia and hyperglycemia is reported in dogs.
- α_2-agonists are sedative-analgesics, NOT anesthetics. Therefore, under their influence, the animal is still arousable and may still bite in response to a noxious stimulus.
- Reflex bradycardia and bradyarrhythmias are common. Heart rates may decrease by 50%[63].
- Blood pressure may fall by one-quarter to one-third and cardiac output may decrease by one-third to one-half of baseline values.
- Should be avoided in animals with severe cardiovascular disease, respiratory disorders, liver or kidney disease, diabetes, or in conditions of shock, severe debilitation, or stress due to extreme heat, cold, or fatigue.
- General rule is to halve the IM dose if the IV route is used.

MEMBRANE STABILIZERS

Neuropathic pain is often a result of many underlying mechanisms, yet, there may be a dominant mechanism that, when treated, reduces pain to a tolerable level. For example, if ectopic impulse generators, due to abnormal sodium channel activity located in injured or abnormally functioning primary afferent fibers, are generating increased traffic entering CNS pathways, treatment with a sodium channel-blocking agent that reduces ectopic firing may dramatically reduce pain. With such recognition, mechanism-based pain management is an area of intense research[64]. This includes reducing transmitter release from pronociceptive neurons by opioids or α_2 calcium channel-binding drugs, by inhibiting postsynaptic excitatory receptors, such as the NMDA or alpha-amino-3-hydroxy-5-methyl-isoxazole-4-propionic-acid (AMPA)–kainate receptors, by potentiating inhibitory transmitters through reduced transmitter uptake or by agonist administration, and by use-dependent sodium channel blockers.

Trafficking, up- and down-regulation, and even functional modulation of Na^+ channels, are the primary players in neuropathic membrane remodeling and hyperexcitability, with K^+ channels playing an important role. Many drugs that block Na^+ channels are available for clinical use. Local anesthetics are the most widely used: lidocaine and bupivacaine. When applied at high concentrations to a nerve, impulse conduction and pain stop when the impulse originates distal to the application site. This is effective for both adaptive and maladaptive pain. Low concentrations of lidocaine, two to three orders of magnitude lower than those required to block normal impulse propagation, selectively suppress subthreshold oscillations, as well as ectopic neuroma and DRG discharge, yielding a similar CNS response. Such sensitivity to sodium channel blockage is the basis for these drugs being given systemically without serious toxicity from failure of normal neuronal conduction within the cardiovascular and nervous systems. However, Pypendop[65] has recommended that lidocaine NOT be administered IV to cats for reducing isoflurane requirements because of cardiovascular depression.

In the normal resting state, the nerve has a negative membrane potential of -70 mV. This resting potential is determined by the concentration gradients of two major ions, Na^+ and K^+, and the relative membrane permeability to these ions (also known as leak currents). The concentration gradients are maintained by the sodium/potassium ATP pump (in an energy-dependent process) that transports sodium ions out of the cell and potassium ions into the cell. This active transport creates a concentration gradient that favors the extracellular diffusion of potassium ions. In addition, because the nerve membrane is permeable to potassium ions and impermeable to sodium ions, 95% of the ionic leak in excitable cells is caused by K^+ ions in the form of an outward flux, accounting for the negative resting potential. The recently identified 2-pore domain potassium (K2P) channels are believed to be responsible for leak K^+ currents.

When a nerve is stimulated, depolarization of the nerve occurs, and impulse propagation progresses. Initially, sodium ions gradually enter the cell through the nerve cell membrane. The entry of sodium ions causes the transmembrane electric potential to increase from the resting potential. Once the potential reaches a threshold level of approximately -55 mV, a rapid influx of sodium ions ensues. Sodium channels in the membrane become activated, and sodium ion permeability increases; the nerve membrane is depolarized to a level of +35 mV or more.

Once membrane depolarization is complete, the membrane becomes impermeable to sodium ions again, and the conductance of potassium ions into the cell increases. The process restores the excess of intracellular potassium and extracellular sodium and reinstates the negative resting membrane potential. Alterations in the nerve cell membrane potential are termed the **action potential**. Leak currents are present through all the phases of the action potential, including setting of the resting membrane potential and repolarization. It is proposed that local anesthetics enter the lipoprotein cell membrane and bind to a receptor site in the sodium channel to prevent sodium ion movement, thereby blocking propagation of the action potential over a critical length of the nerve.

Vasodilation is often associated with administration of local anesthetics, and with vasodilation comes a more rapid diffusion of active drug and shorter duration of action. Addition of a vasoconstrictor to the local anesthetic solution decreases local perfusion, delays the rate of vascular absorption of local anesthetic, and therefore prolongs anesthetic action. Epinephrine (5 mg/ml or 1:200,000) is most commonly added to the local anesthetic for its vasoconstrictive effect.

Clinical implication: do not administer epinephrine together with a local anesthetic in areas of compromised vascularization, e.g. frostbite.

Cocaine was isolated in 1860 and first used as a local anesthetic in 1884. The search for a less toxic and less addictive substitute led to the development of the aminoester local anesthetic procaine in 1904. Since then, several synthetic local anesthetic drugs have been developed and put into clinical use, notably lidocaine in 1943, bupivacaine in 1957, and prilocaine in 1959.

Systemic local anesthetics have long been used for analgesia, particularly in humans, for neuropathic pain. The primary mode of action of IV lidocaine is a dose-dependent blockade of spontaneous ectopic activity in peripheral nerves and DRG cells[66]. Importantly, these effects occur at plasma concentrations that are lower than those required to produce a frank block of nerve conduction (5–10 μg/ml); for lidocaine, effective concentrations may be on the order of 1–3 μg/ml. Neuropathic pain relief could be explained, in part, by the actions on the CNS, such as postsynaptic modification of NMDA-receptor activity[67].

Long-term use of systemic (parenteral) local anesthetics (e.g, lidocaine) in humans is often precluded by tachyphylaxis and dose-related toxic effects. Orally administered lidocaine-like antiarrhythmics, such as mexilitene, have been used as an alternative with favorable results (in humans)[68]. The topical application of lidocaine (e.g. lidocaine patch) is reported to be effective for some forms of nerve injury pain (e.g. postherpetic neuralgia [PHN]), offering the advantage of fewer side-effects because plasma concentrations are well below toxic levels (*Table 41*).

Tachyphylaxis is a rapid decrease in the response to a drug after repeated doses over a short period of time. Increasing the dose of the drug will not increase the pharmacologic response. Tachyphylaxis may develop with an initial dose.

TABLE 41: IV lidocaine clinical efficacy in humans

Clinical state	Efficacy	Reference
Postoperative		
Abdominal – opiate sparing	–	69
Cardiac – opiate sparing	–	70
Abdominal hysterectomy	–	71
Cholecystectomy	+	72
Cancer		
Bony metastases	+	73
Neuropathy	–	74
	+	75, 76
Nerve injury		
Nerve injury – VAS	+	77, 78
Nerve injury – allodynia	+	79
Stroke – stroke pain	+	80
Postherpetic neuralgia	+	75, 81
Fibromyalgia	+	82
Diabetic neuropathy	+	83, 84

VAS: Visual Analog Scale.

Mechanistic summary of IV lidocaine

- IV lidocaine is NOT recommended for cats due to cardiovascular depression.
- Lidocaine is a sodium channel blocker.
- Sodium channels appear to be responsible for spontaneous activity in nerve terminals after local tissue and nerve injury.
- IV sodium channel blockers at concentrations that do not block enough sodium channels to suppress conduction will block the ectopic generators.
- Low dose IV sodium channel block is antihyperalgesic and antiallodynic, and may have little effect upon high intensity stimulus-induced acute nociceptor-mediated pain.
- Mixing local anesthetics (e.g. lidocaine for its quick onset together with bupivacaine for its long duration of action) is a popular clinical practice; however, compromising actions of one agent on the other has not been explored.

A problem with systemic lidocaine is its short duration of action and the need to administer IV. This first issue is solved by administration of an anticonvulsant, whose mode of action is Na^+ channel blockade (e.g. phenytoin, lamotrigine, carbamazepine, oxcarbazepine, and zonisamide)[85]. TCAs circumvent the requirement for IV administration.

LOCAL ANESTHETICS

Local anesthetics act by blocking voltage-gated sodium channels, which are responsible for the transient increase in the permeability of excitable membranes to Na^+ that is normally produced by depolarization of the membrane. This anesthetic effect elevates the threshold and slows the rate of rise of the action potential; at lower concentrations it slows conduction velocity. Aδ and C-fibers are more susceptible to local anesthetics than large fibers; they are blocked earlier and to a greater degree, apparently related to the shorter internodal distances of smaller nerve fibers.

The functional blockade density and duration of action of a local anesthetic for a peripheral nerve block are dependent on both the concentration of local anesthetic used (sufficient to inhibit sodium channels) and the use of a critical drug volume to achieve a sustained critical exposure length. Raymond *et al.*[86] interpreted three nodes of Ranvier as the minimal nerve length exposure necessary to block effective nerve transmission (corresponding to a nerve length of approximately 3.4 mm) (**Fig. 60**). Campoy *et al.*[87] reported that in the dog, lidocaine volumes of 0.3 and 0.05 ml/kg produced sufficient distribution for performing brachial plexus, and sciatic nerve blocks, respectively.

Topical local anesthetics for neuropathic pain could depend on peripheral factors, such as ectopic discharges from sensitized cutaneous nerves bombarding the dorsal horn of the spinal cord. Damaged or regenerating sensitized fibers undergo changes in the number and location of sodium channels, and ectopic impulses from injured peripheral nerves may be sensitive to lower concentrations of local anesthetics than are required for blocking normal impulse conduction[88]. A topical lidocaine patch holds promise for treatment of neuropathic pain conditions, as it has shown benefit for several human neuropathic pain states, including incisional neuralgia, painful diabetic neuropathy, complex regional pain syndrome, and postamputation stump pain[89].

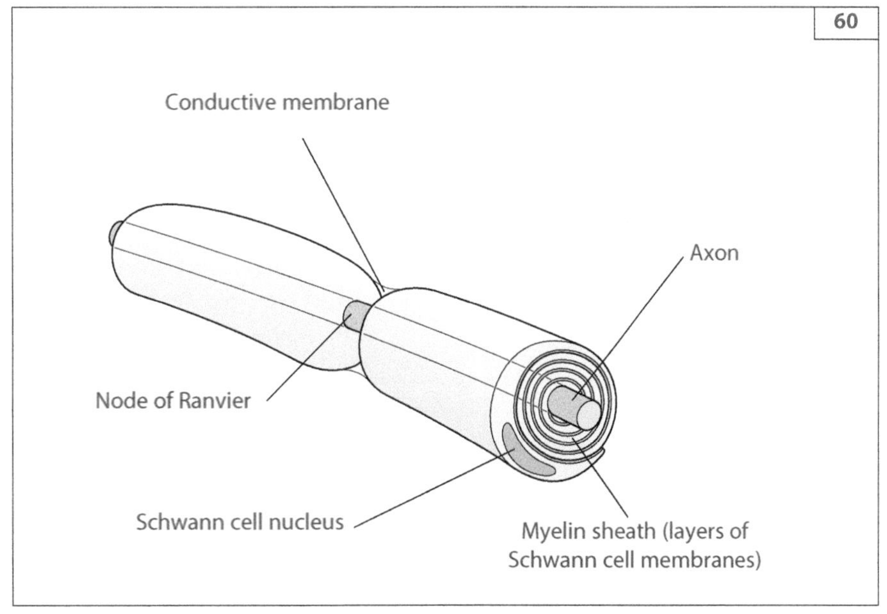

Fig. 60 Node of Ranvier. Local anesthetic must cover approximately three nodes (3 mm) to yield an effective nerve block.

Local anesthetics are typically under-utilized to block specific nerve trunks or instilled into a body cavity; however, epidural and spinal administration is increasingly more widely used (**Fig. 61**). Lidocaine spray (10%), producing mucosal anesthesia for up to 2 mm depth, 1–2 minutes after application, for a duration of 15–20 minutes is used for oral, nasal, and pharyngeal mucous membranes. Sterile lidocaine jelly (2%) is also available for use in association with catheter placement.

A 1:1 mixture of lidocaine and prilocaine is commercially available for transcutaneous application as EMLA cream. Each gram (milliliter) of the cream contains 25 mg of lidocaine and 25 mg of prilocaine. Reported biovailability is 3% for lidocaine and 5% for prilocaine[90]. Although this transcutaneous agent is used for various procedures in veterinary medicine, it is questionable whether it is more effective than local infiltration of either agent alone[91].

61

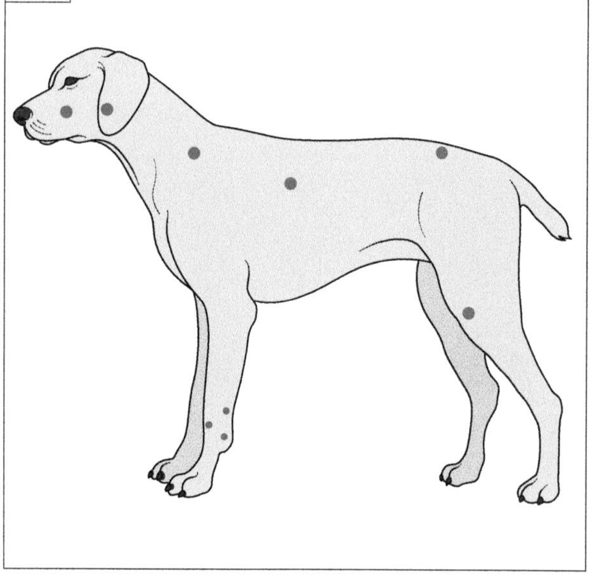

Fig. 61 Local anesthetics can be used in a variety of anatomic locations: maxilla, mandible, axilla, thorax, epidurum, and distal joints.

Local anesthetics at-a-glance

- The amide link (lidocaine, bupivacaine) or ester link (procaine, benzocaine) for the different local anesthetics determine the drug disposition within the body.
  - Metabolism of ester-linked local anesthetics is primarily by nonspecific pseudocholinesterase enzymatic hydrolysis in the plasma.
  - Amide local anesthetics are metabolized primarily in the liver.
- Local anesthetics are weak bases, and the predominant form of the compound in solution at physiologic pH is the ionized or cationic form.
- At clinical doses vasodilation is present, whereas at low concentrations, local anesthetics tend to cause vasoconstriction.
- Adding a vasoconstrictor to the local anesthetic decreases local perfusion, delays the rate of vascular absorption and prolongs anesthetic action. Epinephrine (5 µg/ml or 1:200,000) is commonly used for such a response.
- There are presently no data on the concept of mixing local anesthetics, for example, a short onset and duration agent with a different agent of long onset and duration.
- Harmful side-effects are usually associated with accidental IV administration or administration of large amounts of anesthetic following aggressive regional administration. Always aspirate before injecting. Bupivacaine can cause cardiac dysrhythmias and ventricular fibrillation if injected IV.
- Clinical applications (*Table 42*):
  - Local infiltration:
    - Soaker catheters.
  - Topical anesthesia.
  - IV administration NOT recommended for cats.
  - Epidural block.
  - Spinal (supra-arachnoid) block.
  - Peripheral nerve block.
  - Intra-articular administration (**Fig. 62**).

TABLE 42: Specific nerve blocks and indications

Nerve block	Indication	Area blocked
Antebrachial nerves (radial/ulnar/median)	Distal forelimb and paw	Antebrachium and paw
Intercostal nerves	Thoracotomy	Chest wall
Brachial plexus	Forelimb and elbow	Forelimb, especially distal to the elbow
Auriculotemporal and great auricular nerves	Total ear canal ablation and bulla osteotomy	External and middle ear
Inferior alveolar nerve	Mandibular (dental) surgery	Mandible
Infraorbital nerve	Maxillary (dental) surgery	Maxilla
Articular branches of main peripheral nerves	Joint surgery	Joint capsule

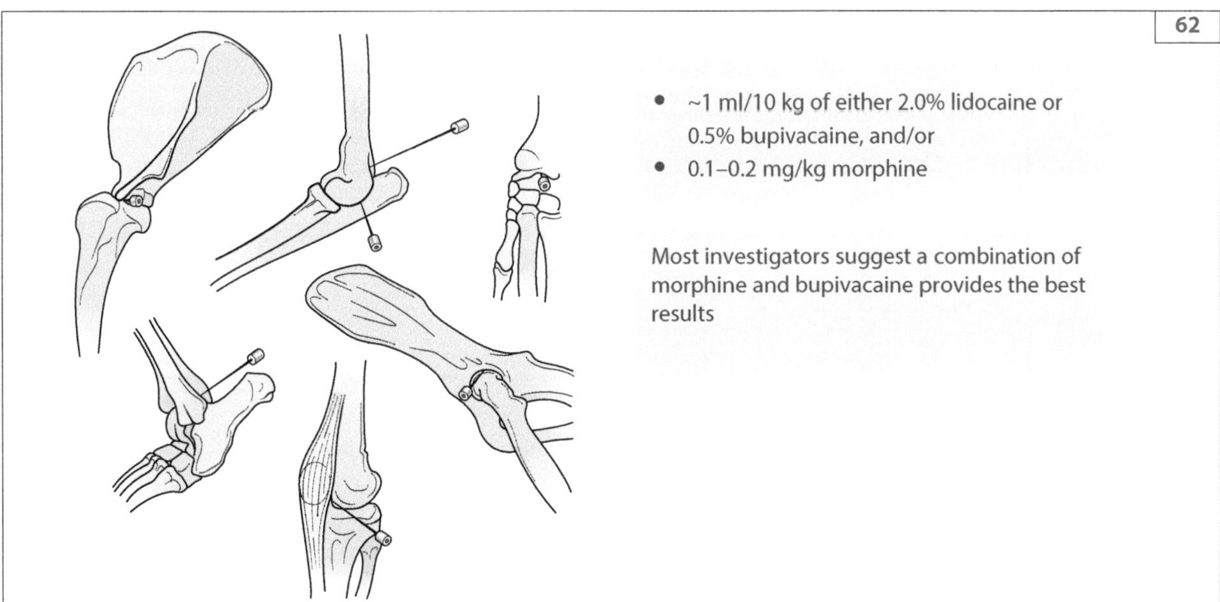

Fig. 62 Intra-articular analgesia is often achieved with a local anesthetic agent, augmented with an opioid.

In October 2011, the FDA approved the extended-release liposome injection formulation of bupivacaine (Exparel, Pacira Pharmaceuticals) for human use. This new product is designed to extend the duration of analgesia provided by bupivacaine. Based on human clinical trial data, this product provides continuous and extended postsurgical analgesia for up to 72 hours compared with bupivacaine's analgesic time of 7 hours or less. To date there are no data available for the use of this product in veterinary practice.

TRICYCLIC ANTIDEPRESSANTS

For many years drugs with a characteristic tricyclic structure have been used to treat depression in humans. Imipramine was one of the first drugs in this class, and only a few years after its introduction in 1958, its analgesic properties were identified[92] (**Fig. 63**). For a number of years, TCAs were the mainstay for treatment of neuropathic pain in humans (having been replaced by the gabapentanoids, gabapentin and pregabalin). Although treatment of neuropathic pain with TCAs in humans is evidence-based, it is not clear how these drugs actually relieve pain. Most research is based on their ability to inhibit presynaptic reuptake of NE and SE, but these drugs also act as NMDA-receptor antagonists and apparently block ion channels (*Table 43*).

TCA mode of action

TCAs are characterized by their multiple modes of action, with a particular ability to inhibit reuptake of monoamines (SE and NE) from presynaptic terminals. Additionally, TCAs block several receptors (cholinergic, adrenergic, histaminergic) and ion channels, including Na+ channels. Mechanism of TCA action might best be identified as five drugs in one:

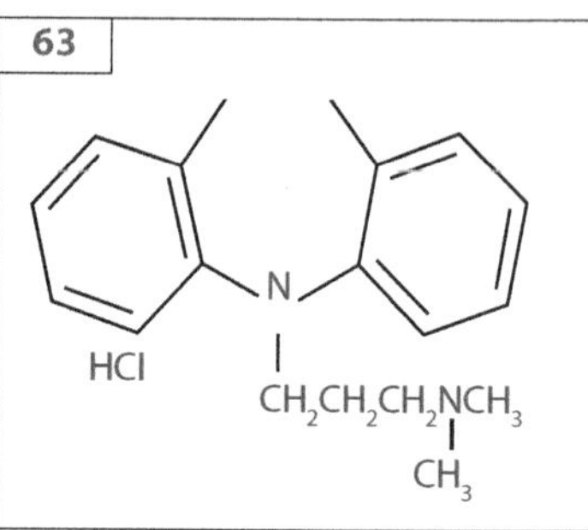

Fig. 63 Imipramine: one of the first tricyclic antidepressants.

1 SSRI.
2 NE reuptake inhibitor.
3 Anticholinergic-antimuscarinic drug.
4 Alpha-1 adrenergic antagonist.
5 Antihistamine.

NE is an inhibitory transmitter that activates descending inhibitory pathways and has been associated with hyperalgesia in patients. SE can activate the primary afferent nerve fibers via 5-HT_3 receptors. In addition, SE can cause mechanical hyperalgesia, most likely by effects on the 5-HT_{1A}-receptor subtype. Opioids can be

TABLE 43: Tricyclic antidepressant exploration for human use over the decades

Clinical development	Pharmacologic discoveries
1958: Report of antidepressant effect	
1960: First suggestion of analgesic effect	1960–1980: Presynaptic reuptake inhibition (norepinephrine and serotonin)
	Postsynaptic receptor blockage (α-adrenergic, cholinergic, histaminergic)
1970–1980: Observations of analgesic effect in painful diabetic neuropathy	
1980: First controlled trial in painful diabetic neuropathy	1980: μ-opioid receptor interaction
1984-to date: Numerous controlled trials in neuropathic pain	
	1988: NMDA-antagonist-like effect
1990–to date: Systematic reviews	
	1992: Calcium channel blockade
	1998: Sodium channel blockade

Hansson PT, *et al.* (2001). *Neuropathic Pain: Pathophysiology and Treatment.* IASP Press **21**:169–183.

NMDA: N-methyl-D-aspartate.

displaced from their binding sites with initial administration of antidepressants. With chronic administration, antidepressants can lead to modifications in opioid receptor densities, leading to increased endogenous opioid levels. It has been observed that TCAs given in the preoperative period may be useful in preventing nerve injury-induced sensory changes that contribute to the development of chronic postsurgical neuropathic pain[93]. However, chronic administration of amitriptyline was required for preventive analgesic effect because amitriptyline given only at the time of surgery did not have any effect on the development of chemogenic hypersensitivity. Additionally, antidepressant medications can bind to the NMDA receptor complex, which acutely reduces intracellular calcium accumulation. Longer-term administration alters the receptor binding of NMDA. Additionally, antidepressants can inhibit potassium, calcium, and sodium channel activity.

Opioid activity of TCAs may have the same effect as inhibition of NE and SE reuptake, enhancing activity of neurons in the network comprising diffuse noxious inhibitory controls, although TCAs have low affinity for the μ-opioid receptor[94]. Therefore, their opioid effect is likely to be minimal. Tricyclic NMDA activity is likely analgesic by way of its inhibition of neuronal hyperexcitability[95]. α-adrenergic receptor blockade in peripheral neuropathy may be relieving pain generated or maintained by noradrenergic stimulation of highly sensitive receptors, such as those identified on sprouts from diseased peripheral nerves[96]. Antihistamines have been shown to relieve pain, and TCAs may play a role in analgesia through their antihistaminergic action. TCAs may actually stabilize both diseased peripheral nerves and hyperexcitable neurons of the CNS by blocking sodium channels[97]. Only a few studies have shown calcium channel blockade with tricyclics. SSRIs, lacking NE reuptake, having weaker ion-channel blocking effects, and having no postsynaptic effects are rendered less effective than the TCAs.

TCAs express many modes of action, which could contribute to pain relief. Because of their multimodal mechanisms of action, their efficacy may be greater than other agents that demonstrate a more selective pharmacologic effect. The number-needed-to-treat (NNT) for TCAs is quite similar across different human neuropathic pain conditions, with values of 2–3, meaning that every second or third patient with neuropathic pain that is treated with a TCA will experience more than 50% pain relief[98]. Genetic polymorphism of different drug metabolizing enzymes likely explains the pharmacokinetic variability of these drugs[99].

TCAs were the first evidence-based neuropathic pain treatments to be studied, and it is now understood that pain relief and relief of depression are independent effects[100–102]. Duloxetine (human medicine) is a selective, relatively balanced SE and NE reuptake inhibitor (SNRI), recently shown to provide centrally acting analgesia to human patients with osteoarthritic knee pain, yet showing a different adverse-event profile from that of NSAIDs[103]. Amitriptyline is best known as an inhibitor of catecholamine reuptake, although it is also a strong local anesthetic[104], and is likely to relieve neuropathic pain by suppressing ectopic discharge. The newer non-TCAs, such as selective SSRIs, antidepressants that alter both serotonergic and noradrenergic neurotransmission, and NE selective antidepressants, have preferential use in human medicine because of better tolerability; however, their efficacy for neuropathic pain relief is not yet as convincing (*Table 44 overleaf*).

Mechanistic summary of antidepressants

TCAs (amitriptyline, imipramine):

- Block the reuptake of SE and NE in the CNS. They also have antihistamine effects.
- TCAs are used for the treatment of chronic and neuropathic pain in humans at lower doses than required for treatment of depression.

Antidepressants at-a-glance

- May be 5HT selective or NE/5HT selective.
- Most reliable efficacy is noted with mixed inhibitors, but possibly NE alone.
- Hypothesized to augment tone in bulbospinal monamine pathways and in ascending pathways to the forebrain.
- Some antidepressants also have NMDA and sodium channel blocking properties, which may account for some side-effects.

TABLE 44: Antidepressants and mechanisms of action in producing analgesic effects

	Reuptake inhibition			Receptor blockade			
	Serotonin	Norepinephrine	α-adrenergic	H1-histaminergic	Muscarinic cholinergic	Opioid receptor interaction	Quinidine-like effect
Classic TCAs							
Imipramine	+	+	+	+	+	+	+
Clomipramine	+	+	+	+	+	+	+
Amitriptyline	+	+	+	+	+	+	+
Deslpramine	–	+	+	+	+	+	+
Nortriptyline	–	+	+	+	+	+	+
SSRIs							
Paroxetine	+	–	–	–	–	?	–
Citalopram	+	–	–	–	–	?	–
Fluoxetine	+	–	–	–	–	+	–
SNRIs							
Venlafaxine	+	+	–	–	–	?	–
Tetracyclines							
Mianserin	–	+	+	+	–	+	–

Hansson PT, *et.al.* (2001). *Neuropathic Pain: Pathophysiology and Treatment.* IASP Press **21**:169–183.
SNRI: serotonin and norepinephrine reuptake inhibitor; SSRI: selective serotonin reuptake inhibitor; TCA: tricyclic antidepressant.

Drugs similar to antidepressants

Tramadol is a synthetic analog of the phenanthrene alkaloid codeine, and is typically classified as an 'atypical' opioid; however, based upon its greater (60%) activity involving the monoamine pathway, this author prefers to consider it more akin to a TCA. Accordingly, those clinicians enamoured with tramadol might find a renewed interest in TCAs for pain management protocols. A new molecular entity, structurally similar to tramadol is tapentadol (Nucynta, Grunenthal Pharma). Tapentadol is a centrally acting analgesic with a dual mode of action as both an agonist at the μ-opioid receptor and as a NE reuptake inhibitor[105–107]. Its general potency is somewhere between tramadol and morphine. Tapentadol is similar in structure to the M1 metabolite of tramadol, is approved for the treatment of moderate to severe acute pain in humans, but has potential for off-label use in chronic pain, and has Schedule II classification in the USA (Class A in the UK).

Tapentadol will likely not find a role in veterinary practice due to its low bioavailability (~3%), short half-life (~3.7 h), and an efficacious dose in the dog generally 2–3× greater than morphine, on a 1 mg dose per body weight basis.

Bicifidine represents yet another class of drug similar to the TCAs. While the drug is purported to be a SE transporter (SERT) and NE transporter (NET) inhibitor, it also has effects at the dopamine transporter (DAT), effectively making it a broad-spectrum monoamine transporter inhibitor or 'triple reuptake inhibitor'. While its efficacy at the DAT is lower than its efficacy at either the SERT or the NET, it is still capable of increasing the perisynaptic concentration of all three monoamines. Preliminary results suggest that bicifadine has an analgesic efficacy slightly stronger than codeine and approximately equivalent to tramadol[108].

SEROTONIN

The idea that combined blockade of SE, otherwise known as 5-hydroxytryptamine (5-HT) and NE uptake might be useful in the treatment of pain has gained recognition from recent data on antidepressants and utilization of tramadol. There are at least seven major subtypes of SE receptor, several of which have been identified in the spinal cord[109]. The SERT is best recognized as the site of action of the SSRIs, which increase availability of SE at the synaptic junction for receptor binding.

Neurotransmitters such as SE (and NE) are recognized by receptors on the surface of the recipient (postsynaptic) cell, which upon this stimulation, in turn, relays the signal. About 10% of the neurotransmitters are lost in this process; the other 90% are released from the receptors and taken up again by monoamine transporters into the sending (presynaptic) cell: a process called reuptake. SSRIs inhibit the reuptake of SE in the presynaptic cell. As a result, the SE stays in the synaptic gap longer than it normally would, and may be recognized again (and again) by the receptors of the postsynaptic cell, thereby stimulating it more (**Fig. 64**).

Although metabolism occurs very rapidly, storage protects SE against metabolism. It is synthesized and stored in presynaptic neurons (serotonergic neurons, pineal gland, and catecholaminergic neurons). Outside the CNS, SE synthesis is limited to enterochromaffin cells of the GI tract, and platelets, where 90–95% of the body's SE is stored. Platelets are unable to synthesize SE, yet they avidly take up the amine from plasma, using the same transporter used by neurons[110]. Although SE is a relatively weak platelet activator, in the presence of proaggregatory factors, such as adenosine diphosphate, epinephrine and collagen, SE significantly potentiates aggregation[111].

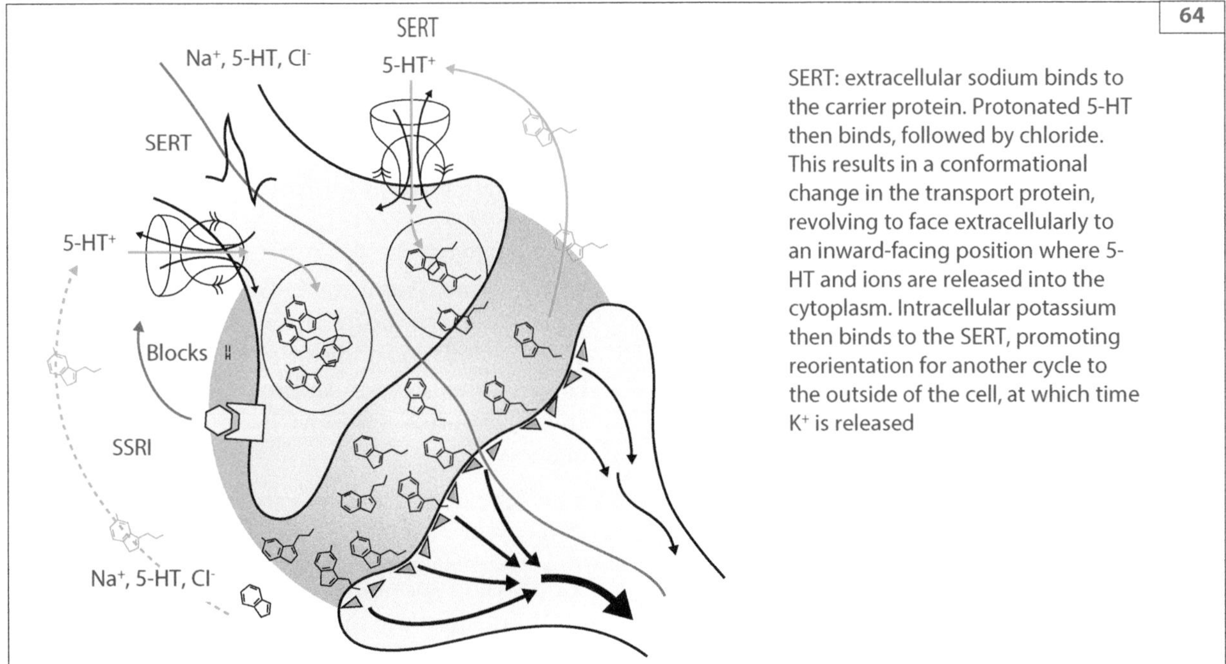

Fig. 64 Selective serotonin reuptake inhibitors (SSRIs) increase the extracellular level of the neurotransmitter serotonin by inhibiting its reuptake into the presynaptic cell, increasing the level of serotonin available to bind to the postsynaptic receptor. Left side of figure illustrates the effect of a SSRI, whereas the right side depicts the normal reuptake of serotonin. 5-HT: 5-hydroxytryptamine; SERT: serotonin transporter.

Accordingly, any intervention that affects platelet SE content or its release from dense granules may theoretically have an impact on haemostasis and thrombosis.

In studies performed in humans, all SSRIs have consistently caused a drastic decrease in platelet SE content after several weeks of treatment, reaching levels around or below 10% of the pretreatment SE levels[112]. A similar effect has been shown with clomipramine[113]. This potential for GI bleeding associated with the administration of antidepressants is particularly noteworthy in recognition of the increased veterinary use of tramadol with NSAIDs. Sixty percent of the activity of tramadol is associated with the monoamine pathway, and De Abajo *et al.*[112] have documented the synergistic effect of NSAIDs together with SSRIs for causing upper GI bleeding in the human population.

Excess SE can give rise to the 'SE syndrome', characterized by: 1) autonomic hyperactivity (diarrhea, mydriasis, tachycardia, tachypnea, hypertension, diaphoresis, fever); 2) neuromuscular signs (hyper-reflexia, myoclonus and secondary hyperthermia, tremors, rigidity, seizures; pyramidal rigidity [advanced stage]); and 3) altered mental status (confusion, agitation, and excitement).

Substances that can contribute to SE syndrome[114] include:

- Food or medication that facilitates SE synthesis:
  - L-Tryptophan.
  - Cheese.
- Medications that increase presynaptic release of SE:
  - Amphetamine.
  - Methylphenidare.
  - 3,4-methylenedioxymethanamphetamine (MDMA, Ecstasy).
- Medications that inhibit SE reuptake into the presynaptic neuron (including all SSRIs and TCAs):
  - Amitriptyline.
  - Bupropion.
  - Chlorpheniramine.
  - Clomipramine (Clomicalm).
  - Duloxetine.
  - Fentanyl.
  - Fluoxetine (Reconcile).
  - Paroxetine.
  - Pethidine.
  - Sertraline.
  - Tramadol.
  - Trazodone.
  - Venlafaxine.
- Medications that inhibit the metabolism of SE:
  - Amtrak (preventic collar).
  - Linezolid.
  - Selegiline.
- Medications that act as SE agonists at the postsynaptic membrane:
  - Buspirone.
  - Lithium.
  - LSD.

SE antagonists include: cyproheptadine, chlorpromazine, and methysergide.

ANTICONVULSANTS

Even before peripheral and central sensitization had been defined in detail, the first controlled clinical trials in humans with the anticonvulsant carbamazepine established its efficacy in relieving the pain of trigeminal neuralgia and diabetic neuropathy. Only carbamazepine, phenytoin, gabapentin, and lamotrigine have been studied in randomized human clinical trials for relief of pain in neuropathic pain disorders. Currently, only carbamazepine and gabapentin (pregabalin) have proved effective in humans.

Lamotrigine (Lamicital®, GlaxoSmithKline) is an anticonvulsant drug used in humans to treat epilepsy and bipolar disorder. It is the only Food and Drug Administration approved drug as a mood stabilizer since lithium. Its mode of action is unknown.

Carbamazepine blocks ionic conductance by suppressing spontaneous Aδ- and C-fiber activity without affecting normal nerve conduction[115]. However, carbamazepine has not been widely embraced in human medicine because of side-effects, interaction with other drugs metabolized in the liver, and erratic pain relief.

Anticonvulsants are a category of medications grouped together based only on their ability to suppress epileptic seizures. Anticonvulsants together with antiarrhythmic drugs can be looked at as sodium channel or other channel neuronal activity regulators. Evidence firmly supports that anticonvulsants and local anesthetic drugs relieve neuropathic pain[116,117]. Based on NNT calculations, gabapentin is comparable with TCAs for efficacy on neuropathic pain, and is presently used more frequently than any anticonvulsant for human chronic pain.

Gabapentin was developed as an analog of the neurotransmitter γ-aminobutyric acid (GABA), but it has since been shown not to interact with either $GABA_A$ or $GABA_B$ receptors. Gabapentin does not interact with any known antiepileptic drug receptor site. It does not exhibit affinity for common CNS receptors, including adrenergic (α_1, α_2, β), cholinergic (muscarinic, nicotinic), dopaminergic (D_1, D_2), histamine, SE (S_1, S_2), nor opiate (μ, δ, κ) receptors[118].

Although not a Na^+ channel blocker, gabapentin depresses ectopic discharge by suppression of Ca^{++} conductance. Its mode of action is associated with binding to a highly specific [^{3}H] gabapentin-binding site in the brain, the α2δ site, on voltage-gated calcium channels (VGCC). Its mechanism of action is, therefore, likely associated with modulation of certain types of Ca^{++} currents (**Fig. 65**)[119]. Gabapentin is unlike other antiepileptic drugs in that it does not affect voltage-dependent Na^+-channels[120]. Gabapentin (and pregabalin) reduces the stimulated synaptic influx of calcium, thereby reducing transmitter release within 10–30 minutes of application. As a result, the stimulated release of transmitters such as glutamate, NE, GABA, sP, CGRP, and acetylcholine at the neuromuscular junction, and spinal inhibitory glycine, are all reduced.

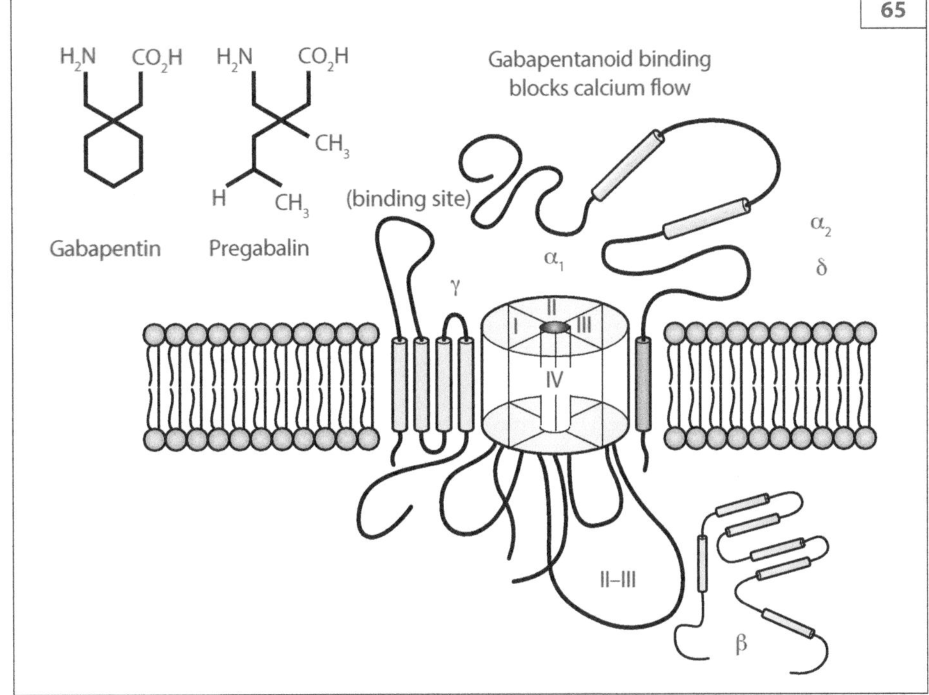

Fig. 65 Gabapentin's mechanism of action is unclear; however, its use is associated with the modulation of calcium flow.

Administered alone, gabapentin does not produce analgesia. It is, however, effective at the level of the dorsal horn on inflammation-induced pain. Its most popular use is as an adjunct to other drugs (e.g. NSAIDs for osteoarthritis and cancer pain as part of a multimodal treatment protocol), and for prophylaxis prior to procedures anticipated to be quite painful.

Gabapentin was originally synthesized to treat human spasticity; however, it has been found to be effective in chronic pain and anxiety disorders. Gabapentin has no effect on the nocifensive behaviors observed during the acute phase of the formalin test, but does block the development of the late phase, demonstrating a selective antihyperalgesic action[121,122]. It is an effective antihyperalgesic agent in a knee joint model of acute arthritis induced by administration of kaolin and carrageenan[123,124]. Gabapentin has demonstrated analgesic efficacy for human patients with painful diabetic neuropathy and postherpetic neuralgia (NNT of 3.8 and 3.2, respectively).

Gabapentin has also been observed to possess pre-emptive analgesic activity[125,126]. A single pre-emptive administration of the drug dose-dependently blocked the development of both static allodynia and thermal hyperalgesia for over 48 hours. Functional disruption of the α2δ subunit by gabapentin may result in an inhibition of excitatory neurotransmitter release. This leads to a decrease in mechanosensitivity during mechanical manipulation of a joint[127]. Such activity adds supports to efficacy of gabapentin's peripheral effect[128], in addition to its central effect. Gabapentin has been shown to modulate the effect of sP by inhibiting its facilitation mechanism in the rat[129], while Boileau *et al.*[130] showed that a compound chemically related to pregabalin and gabapentin (PD-0200347), reduced the production of several catabolic factors, including matrix metalloproteinases (MMPs) and inducible NO synthase (iNOS) in a canine anterior cruciate ligament sectioning model.

In a limited number of client-owned dog study[131], perioperative administration of gabapentin as part of a multimodal analgesic protocol for forelimb amputation did not show a benefit. The investigators suggested a number of reasons why gabapentin might not have made a difference, principal to which is support of earlier studies determining that gabapentin has antihyperalgesic effects, not antinociceptive effects. This proposes that gabapentin would not be of use until there is hyperalgesia, and that its analgesic efficacy might be time-dependent.

Gabapentin at-a-glance

- Originally introduced as an antiepileptic drug.
- Apparently, has no analgesic effect at GABA receptors.
- Well suited for neuropathic pain.
- Gabapentin is highly bioavailable in dogs (~80%).
- Gabapentin is metabolized by the liver and excreted almost exclusively by the kidneys. $T_{1/2}$ is approximately 3–4 hours.
- Gabapentin does not alter nociceptive thresholds; therefore, does not produce analgesia, but assists other drugs' analgesic response.
- Appears effective only against hypersensitivity induced by tissue damage or neuropathy, and may well be referred to as an antihypersensitive agent.
- Gabapentin does not interact with any known antiepileptic drug receptor sites.
- It does not exhibit affinity for common CNS receptors, including adrenergic (α_1 α_2, β), cholinergic (muscarinic, nicotinic), dopaminergic (D_1, D_2), histamine, SE (S_1, S_2), or opiate (μ, δ, κ) receptors[118].

Apparently, anticonvulsants that act synaptically, such as barbiturates, are nonanalgesic, while membrane stabilizing anticonvulsants are analgesic. Corticosteroids also have membrane-stabilizing properties, which may be a major mechanism of pain control when depot-form corticosteroids are injected. Topical forms of the TCA doxepin, gabapentin, lidocaine[132], and bupivacaine, as well as ketamine, are now available for use in humans.

NMDA ANTAGONISTS

A single brief noxious stimulus results first in a pricking pain sensation by the afferent myelinated Aδ-fibers. A moment later, afferent long-latency unmyelinated C-fibers convey a burning, throbbing, aching pain. Both of these impulses are received in sequence by the same second-order neuron. Repetition of the brief noxious stimulus at less than 3-second intervals will result in magnification of the secondary burning component conveyed by the C-fibers, termed temporal summation or 'wind-up'. NMDA-receptor antagonists block prolonged depolarization and temporal summation of electrically stimulated C-afferent fibers, without abolishing Aδ activation.

The channel associated with the NMDA receptor is blocked by normal resting physiologic levels of magnesium, and no change in excitability of the neurons possessing NMDA receptors can occur until this is removed. The magnesium block is removed only by a shift in the membrane voltage towards depolarization. Binding of glutamate to the receptor alone is insufficient to activate the channel. Further, glycine is a required co-agonist with glutamate for activation of the receptor: the release and binding of glycine and glutamate are needed together with a non-NMDA-induced depolarization to remove the magnesium block (**Fig. 66**).

Importantly, NMDA antagonists are not only effective in preventing the development of pronociceptive changes, but may also reduce hyperalgesia, even when the changes have already developed[133]. Some preclinical studies report a synergistic interaction between opioids and NMDA antagonists. This synergism is found in acute pain models, in which NMDA antagonists are normally rather inactive[134].

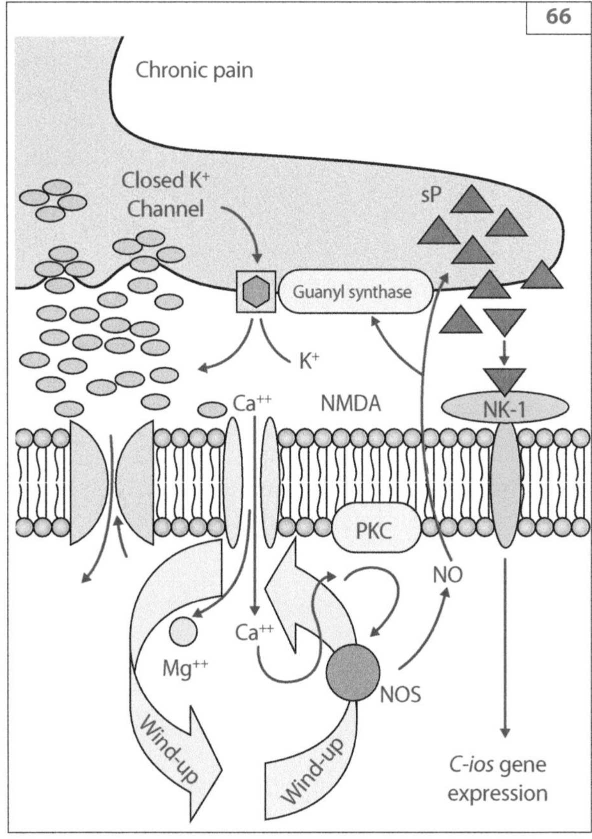

Fig. 66 Central nervous system wind-up involves the N-methyl-D-aspartate (NMDA) receptor which, when activated, allows the conduction of calcium into the neuronal axon through a channel previously blocked by a magnesium 'plug'. NK-1: neurokinin-1; NO: nitric oxide; NOS: nitric oxide synthase; PKC: protein kinase C; sP: substance P.

Ketamine

Ketamine was synthesized in 1963, deriving its name from being a 'keto' derivative of an amine. It has a chiral center in the cyclohexanone ring, thereby existing as optical isomers. The S(+) isomer has a fourfold greater affinity for the NMDA receptor compared to the R(−) isomer, has twice the analgesic potency, and presents fewer psychomimetic effects[135]. (S-ketamine is now available commercially.) Ketamine binds to many sites in the central and peripheral nervous systems, including nicotinic, muscarinic, opioid, AMPA, kainite, and $GABA_A$ receptors[136]. Ketamine also inhibits SE and dopamine reuptake and down-regulates voltage-gated Na^+ and K^+ channel function[137]. It preserves sympathetic reflexes that help support blood pressure. In human clinical studies, low-dose ketamine given before surgical incision in combination with opioids produced a 60% reduction in patient-controlled analgesia morphine use postoperatively[138]. In a study of dogs undergoing ovariohysterectomy, Slingsby and Waterman-Pearson[139] demonstrated that ketamine was effective, but short-acting.

At high doses, ketamine causes dissociative anesthesia, whereby subjects are awake but dissociated from the environment. Dorsal horn wind-up is inhibited by low-dose ketamine, whereas it is enhanced by low-dose morphine, differentiating the analgesic role of NMDA blockade versus opiate agonism[140]. Additionally, NMDA blockade does not alter tactile or thermal sensory thresholds.

An important field of ketamine application is for neuropathic pain in humans. Studies report relief from both spontaneous and evoked pain by prolonged treatment with ketamine for neuropathic pain syndromes of either peripheral or central origin[141]. Some report effectiveness of ketamine in neuropathic pain after chronic SC infusion[142] or oral administration[143]. Dysphoric and psychotomimetic effects are the major limiting problems with the clinical use of ketamine (and dextromethorphan) in the treatment of (human) pain.

The analgesic action of low, subanesthetic doses of ketamine acts predominantly from blockade of the NMDA receptor. In its resting state, the NMDA receptor is inactive and does not participate in synaptic modulation because its ion channel is plugged by magnesium. The magnesium plug is dislodged by postsynaptic depolarization or when serine residues on the channel protein are phosphorylated following activation of calcium-dependent intracellular protein kinases. The NMDA receptor's ion channel must be open or 'active' before ketamine can bind to, or dissociate from, its binding site within the channel. Binding of ketamine to phencyclidine sites within the ion channel decreases the channel's opening time and frequency, thus reducing calcium ion influx and dampening secondary intracellular signaling cascades.

The NMDA–receptor–channel complex is activated only by intense synaptic transmission across the second-order neuron and not by routine physiologic transmission. Accordingly, meta-analyses of human clinical trials indicate that ketamine supplementation of opioids for acute postoperative pain does not significantly improve analgesia; however, ketamine does benefit 'pathologic' pain as a 'central sensitization modulator' (antiallodynic, antihyperalgesic, and opioid tolerance-reversing) in pain states of neuropathic or cancer pain.

Amantadine

Amantadine is an orally available NMDA-antagonist, first recognized as an antiviral agent and later found to be useful in the treatment of Parkinson's disease. Administered IV, amantadine abolished or reduced pathologic pain in humans with chronic neuropathic pain[144] and surgical neuropathic pain in cancer patients[145]. Amantadine PO reduced experimental sensitization and pain in human patients with chronic back pain[146]. Lascelles *et al.*[147,148] have reported that the administration of amantadine might be a useful adjunct therapy for clinical management of osteoarthritic and cancer pain in dogs refractory to a NSAID.

Topical NSAIDs, such as diclofenac, are employed to treat musculoskeletal pain on the premise that their analgesic effect is mediated by a local action on nociceptive afferent fibers (nociceptors), namely to suppress prostaglandin E_2. However, topical application of diclofenac results in local tissue concentrations greatly exceeding those achieved by systemic administration and diclofenac appears to be able to act as a sodium channel blocker to mediate local anesthetic-like effects[149,150]. It is postulated that this action occurs through the NMDA receptor. It is reported that *in vivo* diclofenac can exert a selective, competitive inhibition of peripheral NMDA receptors at muscle concentrations achievable after topical administration of diclofenac-containing preparations[151].

NMDA antagonists at-a-glance

(Ketamine, tiletamine, amantadine, methadone, dextromethorphan [possibly gabapentin])

- Ketamine acts both centrally and peripherally at multiple receptor sites, including NMDA, opioid, AMPA, kainate, and $GABA_A$ receptors.
- Oral administration of ketamine produces few adverse effects and may be more effective than SC administration[152].
- Microdoses of ketamine have little, if any, side-effects, and the best use of the drug is with an analgesic, such as an opioid.
- Amantadine was originally developed as an antiviral drug for use in humans, and is available as an oral preparation. It is well absorbed in the GI tract and excreted relatively unchanged in urine.
- The pharmacology of amantadine in dogs and cats has not been well established; however, the pharmacokinetics of amantadine in cats has been described[153].
- In humans, amantadine has been used for neuropathic pain.
- Amantadine is used in veterinary patients for allodynia and opioid tolerance, allowing lower opioid doses and complementing opioid analgesia.
- Amantadine is available in 100 mg capsules and as a 10 mg/ml elixir.
- The feline toxic dose of amantidine is 30 mg/kg[154].
- Behavioral side-effects from amantadine in dogs and cats begin at 15 mg/kg PO[146].
- Methadone and dextromethorphan (the active ingredient in many over-the-counter cough syrups) are opioid derivatives. Both are weak, noncompetitive NMDA-antagonists.
- Methadone also functions as a NE-reuptake inhibitor.
- Methadone is commonly used for cancer pain in human patients because of its high oral bioavailability, rapid onset, and time to peak analgesic effect as well as the relatively long duration of activity.
- In contrast to its pharmacokinetics in humans, methadone has a short elimination half-life, rapid clearance, and low bioavailability in dogs[14], accounting for its infrequent use.
- Erratic absorption, short elimination half-life, rapid clearance, and adverse effects limit the usefulness of dextromethorphan for therapeutic purposes in dogs[155].
- Parenteral formulations of dextromethorphan are currently unavailable.

EVIDENCE FOR PHARMACOLOGIC TREATMENT OF NEUROPATHIC PAIN

Damage to the somatosensory system represents a potential risk for the development of neuropathic pain, and such damage to the nervous system can be caused by a variety of disorders ranging from simple nerve cuts to complex genetic disorders compromising axonal transport. Several human disease conditions giving rise to neuropathic pain have been studied (namely diabetic polyneuropathy, postherpetic neuralgia, peripheral nerve injury, human immunodeficiency virus [HIV] neuropathy, and trigeminal neuralgia); however, neuropathic pain has not been well studied in companion animal diseases. Since animals suffer many diseases in common with humans (e.g. diabetes), and the nervous system of companion animals is very similar to that of humans, it is tempting to presume that many of our pets suffer from neuropathic pain, even though we might be inadequately trained to recognize it.

Pharmacologic management is presently the most important therapeutic option for chronic neuropathic pain in both humans and animals. Treatment recommendations in humans usually depend on the simple assessments of the patients' pain intensity and functionality without taking the possible underlying mechanisms into account. As a result, the possibility to target mechanisms of pain optimally with specific therapies may be obscured; this 'treatment targeting' is even more complex in the nonverbal veterinary patient.

However, there is a need to find the best possible evidence for symptom control. Without head-to-head comparisons between different compounds, NNT and numbers-needed-to-harm (NNH) collected either retrospectively or prospectively are alternative methods for determining efficacy across both compounds and conditions, and can serve as guidance for treating veterinary patients.

Finnerup *et al.*[156] have reviewed the human literature for treatment of neuropathic pain, noting that 69 new randomized controlled trials have been published in the past 5 years compared with 105 published trials in the preceding 39 years. Obviously, this is an area of considerable interest. **Fig. 67–69** show their findings.

Although these data summarize human trials, the authors point out that the NNT has not decreased over the past several decades. One reason for this is likely due to the fact that the primary outcome measure in most pain trials is based on a one-dimensional recording of pain intensity. In veterinary practice, this is usually the only outcome measure considered. In consequence, these human data may give guidance to management considerations of neuropathic pain in pets, especially in disease states considered to be similar to those in humans.

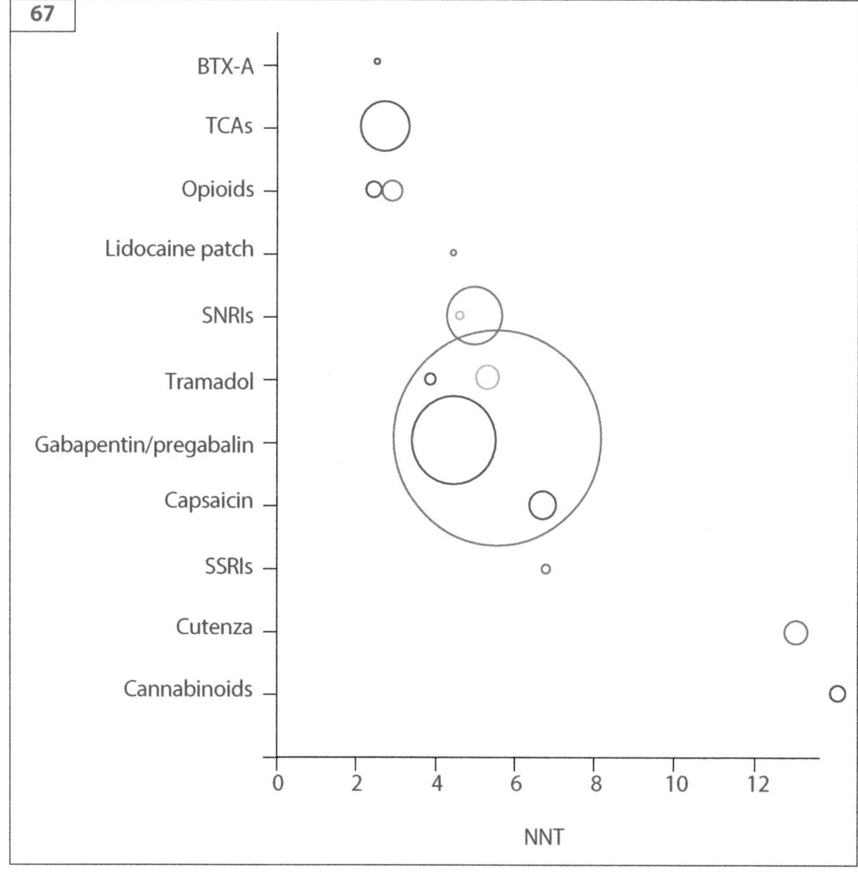

Fig. 67 Combined number-needed-to-treat (NNT) values for various drug classes in all central and peripheral neuropathic pain conditions (not including trigeminal neuralgia). Circle sizes indicate the relative number of patients who received active treatment drugs. Differences in study design and the patient population preclude a direct comparison of NNT values across drug classes. (After Reference 156.) BTX-A: botulinum toxin type A; SNRI: serotonin and norepinephrine reuptake inhibitor; SSRI: selective serotonin reuptake inhibitor; TCA: tricyclic antidepressant.

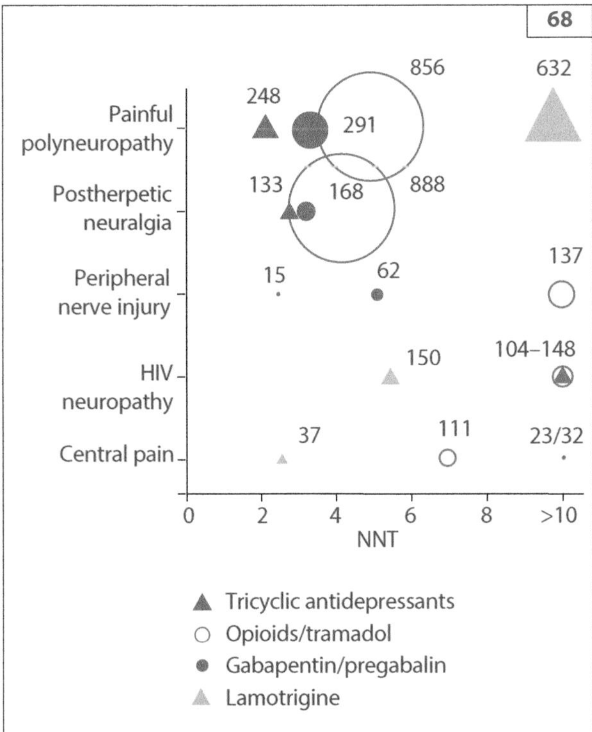

Fig. 68 Combined number-needed-to-treat (NNT) values for different drug classes against specific disease etiologies. Symbol sizes indicate the relative number of patients who received active treatment drugs in the trials. (After Reference 156.) HIV: human immunodeficiency virus.

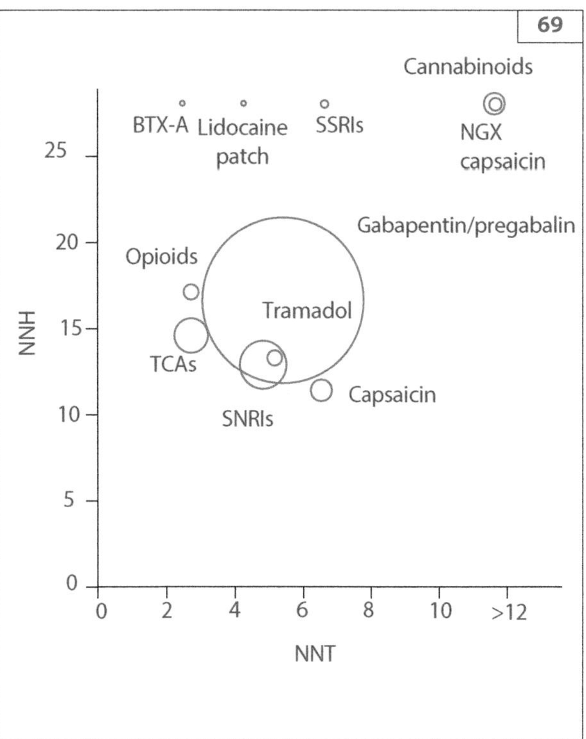

Fig. 69 Relationship between number-needed-to-treat (NNT) values for 50% pain relief and number-needed-to-harm (NNH) values for the number of patients to drop out of the study due to side-effects. It is noted that differences in study design and placebo response may influence NNH and NNT values. Circle sizes and the related numbers indicate the number of patients who received active treatment drugs in trials for which data were available. (After Reference 156.) BTX-A: botulinum toxin type A; NGX: Neuroges X (capsaicin dermal patch); SNRI: serotonin and norepinephrine reuptake inhibitor; SSRI: selective serotonin reuptake inhibitor; TCA: tricyclic antidepressant.

BISPHOSPHONATES

Bisphosphonates (also called diphosphonates) are a class of drugs that prevent the loss of bone mass, and are used to treat osteoporosis and bone cancer. Bone has constant turnover, and is kept in balance (homeostasis) by osteoblasts that create bone and osteoclasts that digest bone. Bisphosphonates inhibit the digestion of bone by osteoclasts. Osteoclasts also have constant turnover and normally destroy themselves by apoptosis, a form of cell suicide. Bisphosphonates encourage osteoclasts to undergo apoptosis[157].

Bisphosphonates were developed in the 19th century, but were first investigated in the 1960s for use in disorders of bone metabolism. The initial rationale for their use in humans was their potential in preventing the dissolution of hydroxylapatite, the principal bone mineral, thus arresting bone loss. In the 1990s, the actual mechanism of their action was demonstrated with the initial launch of alendronate by Merck Pharmaceutical.

All bisphosphonate drugs share a common P-C-P 'backbone'. The two phosphonate (P) groups covalently linked to carbon (C) determine both the name 'bisphosphonate' and the function of the drug. The long side-chain (R_2) determines the chemical properties, the mode of action, and the strength of bisphosphonate drugs. The short side-chain (R_1), often called the 'hook', mainly influences chemical properties and pharmacokinetics (**Fig. 70**, *Table 45*).

About 50% of administered bisphosphonate is excreted unchanged by the kidney. The remainder has a very high affinity for bone tissue, and is rapidly adsorbed onto the bone surface.

Mechanistic summary of bisphosphonates

Bisphosphonates' mechanisms of action all stem from their structures' similarity to pyrophosphate. A bisphosphonate group mimics pyrophosphate's structure, thereby inhibiting activation of enzymes that utilize pyrophosphate.

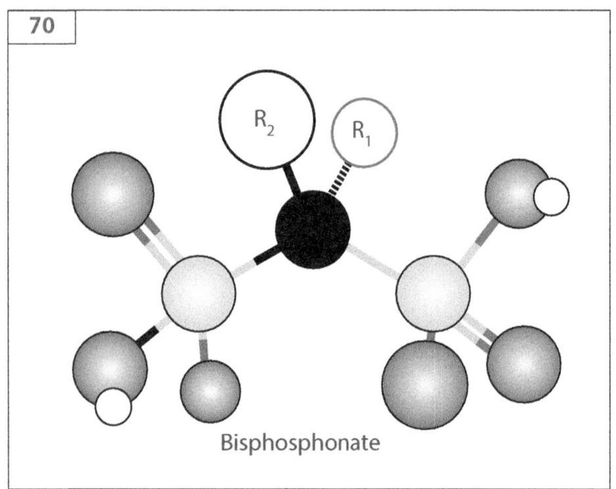

Fig. 70 All bisphosphonate drugs share a common P-C-P 'backbone'. The two phosphonate (P) groups covalently linked to carbon (C) determine both the name 'bisphosphonate' and the function of the drug. The long side-chain (R_2) determines the chemical properties, the mode of action, and the strength of bisphosphonate drugs. The short side-chain (R_1), often called the 'hook', mainly influences chemical properties and pharmacokinetics.

Bisphosphonate-based drug specificity comes from the two phosphonate groups (and possibly a hydroxyl at R_1) that work together to co-ordinate calcium ions. Bisphosphonate molecules preferentially 'stick' to calcium and bind to it. The largest store of calcium in the body is in bones, so bisphosphonates accumulate to a high concentration only in bones. Bisphosphonates, when attached to bone tissue, are 'ingested' by osteoclasts, the bone cells that breaks down bone tissue.

Drugs such as the bisphosphonates that block osteoclast activity, can markedly reduce bone pain[158,159]. There is little information on their use in dogs for palliation of bone pain, but drugs such as pamidronate and zoledronate are increasingly being used, and early information suggests a decrease in pain for about 40% of cases[160]. Bisphosphonates are typically administered at relatively high doses IV; however, oral administration of low-dose bisphosphonate has been reported to improve severe pain and regional osteoporotic changes in human patients with complex regional pain syndrome type I[161].

TABLE 45: 'R' side-chains associated with the various bisphosphonates

Agent	R_1 side chain	R_2 side chain
Etidronate	-OH	$-CH_3$
Clodronate	-Cl	-Cl
Tiludronate	-H	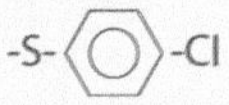 -S-(phenyl)-Cl
Pamidronate	-OH	$-CH_2-CH_2-NH_2$
Neridronate	-OH	$-(CH_2)_5-NH_2$
Olpadronate	-OH	$-(CH_2)_2N(CH_3)_2$
Alendronate	-OH	$-(CH_2)_3-NH_2$
Ibandronate	-OH	$-CH_2-CH_2N(CH_3)(CH_2)_4-CH_3$
Risedronate	-OH	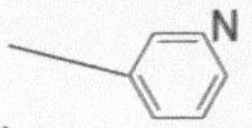 (pyridinyl ring, N)
Zoledronate	-OH	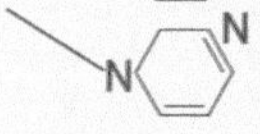 (imidazolyl ring, N, N)

CAPSAICIN

Creams, lotions, and patches containing capsaicin, generally in the range of 0.025–0.1% by weight, are sold in many countries, often without the requirement of a prescription, for the managemet of neuropathic and musculoskeletal pain (e.g. osteoarthritis). Capsaicin treatment typically involves the application of a topical anesthetic until the area is numb. Then the capsaicin is applied by a therapist wearing rubber gloves and a face mask. The capsaicin remains on the skin until the patient starts to feel the 'heat', at which point it is promptly removed. A high-concentration capsaicin 8% patch is now approved for use in the European Union and USA.

Capsaicin is the active component of chilli peppers. It is an irritant, producing a sensation of burning in any mammalian tissue with which it comes into contact, and was first reported to have analgesic properties in 1850. It is the active ingredient in riot control pepper spray chemical agents.

Capsaicin is an agonist for the TRPV1 receptor, a transmembrane, mixed Na^+/Ca^{++} ion channel complex which provides integrated responses to temperature, pH, and endogenous lipids. Temperatures of 43°C (109.4°F) or higher, or acidity of pH of <6.0 can directly activate the channel, but combinations of these two stimuli can activate the channel at substantially lower temperatures or pH values.

In contrast to transient activation, which follows normal environmental stimuli or inflammatory responses to tissue injury, activation of transient receptor potential (TRP) V1-expressing nerve fibers by exposure to a chemically stable exogenous agonist, such as capsaicin, can generate a biochemical signal with a persistent effect. The TRPV1 channel is highly calcium permeable, allowing considerable amounts of calcium to flow into nerve fibers. Additionally, TRPV1 is expressed on intracellular organelles, so capsaicin application can cause release of calcium from the endoplasmic reticulum and induces additional intracellular calcium release from internal stores via calcium-dependent calcium release.

These responses, as well as osmotic swelling and inhibition of mitochondrial respiration lead to impaired local nociceptor function for extended periods, 'defunctionalization' (**Fig.** 71)[162].

Resiniferatoxin is a potent capsaicin analog. Intrathecal resiniferatoxin administration leads to selective targeting and permanent deletion of the TRPV1-expressing C-fiber neuronal cell bodies in the DRG[163,164]. Loss of these C-fiber neurons interrupts the transmission of pain information from the body to second-order spinal cord neurons, which in turn convey the information to the brain. Yet, noxious and non-noxious mechanosensation, proprioception, and locomotor capability are retained. Intrathecal resiniferatoxin (1.2 mg/kg, 100 mg/ml solution) has been reported to produce a prolonged antinociceptive response in dogs with bone cancer[165].

SUMMARY

Opioid analgesics have provided the most consistent and effective analgesia for many years and are still the best drugs available for both acute and severe pain control in small animals. It is frequently said that one cannot implement 'serious' pain management without the availability of opioids. Opioids are the cornerstone of perioperative pain management, where they are commonly supplemented with other classes of drugs, such as α_2-agonists, NSAIDs, and local anesthetics. The actual agents

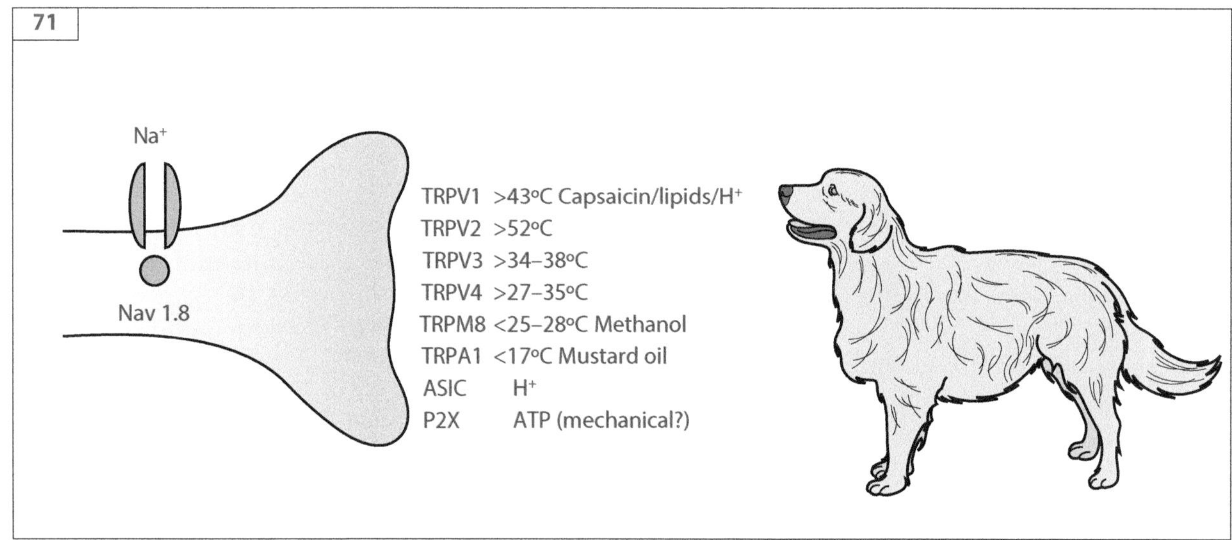

Fig. 71 With chronic exposure to capsaicin, neurons are depleted of neurotransmitters, leading to reduction in sensation of pain and blockade of neurogenic inflammation. ASIC: acid-sensing ion channel; ATP: adenosine triphosphate; P2X: subtype of ATP receptor; Nav 1.8: tetrodotoxin [TTX]-resistant voltage-gated sodium channel; TRP: transient receptor potential.

administered within these classes of drugs are patient-dependent, and include selection criteria of: the patient's physiologic status, pain syndrome treated, concurrent drug administration, delivery form, duration of effect, potential for side-effects, drug familiarity of the prescriber, and cost.

Whereas opioids are the cornerstone treatment for 'severe' and perioperative pain, NSAIDs are the cornerstone for 'lesser' pain states treated longer term. This is because of the NSAID characteristics as anti-inflammatories, analgesics, and antipyretics. Further, administration is easier and side-effects of NSAIDs are fewer than with extended-use opioids. Accordingly, the WHO suggests the management of pain by implementing the WHO analgesic ladder (**Fig**. 72).

As veterinary medicine becomes more sophisticated in delivering pain therapy, drug profiles from human medicine are being considered (and often implemented) for veterinary application. Consequently, a number of drugs administered in human medicine are being used in veterinary medicine based on an anthropomorphic approach and empirical or anecdotal support. However, considering that veterinary clinical trials with many of these drugs (such as tramadol, amantadine, and gabapentin) are presently nonexistent, the use of such drugs may have their role in veterinary medicine, provided: 1) the drug's mode of action is understood; 2) that the pharmacokinetics have been studied in the target species; and 3) that physiology as well as pathophysiology between human and the veterinary target species is similar.

Neuropathic pain can be thought of as the 'maladaptive pain state', potentially resultant from any significant noxious insult. It is much easier to identify in man than in nonverbal animals. Although not evidence-based, **Fig**. 73 suggests a logical approach to managing the progressive pain state, wherein pain management utilizes a multimodal scheme, and drug classes are added rather than substituted. The doses are empirical, and one could debate the order of implementation from bottom to top. The merit of this approach is the addition of agents from different drug classes, attempting to block as many of the pain pathway segments (transduction, transmission, modulation, and perception) as possible.

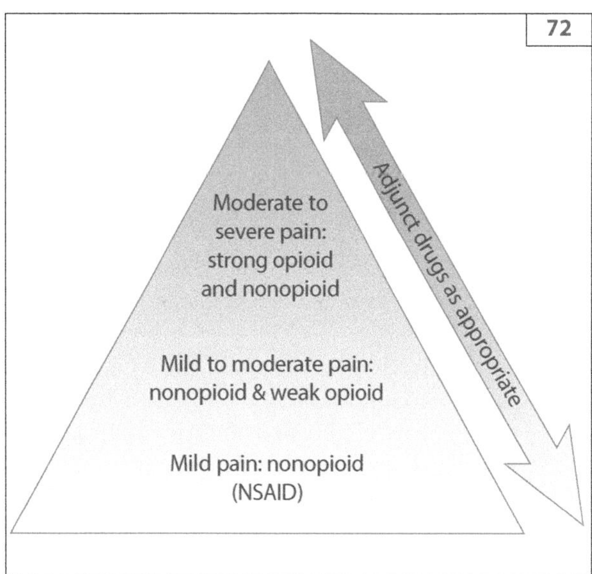

Fig. 72 World Health Organization analgesic ladder was developed to give guidance for treating cancer pain in humans; however, it has been adapted for treating various pain states in both human and veterinary patients.

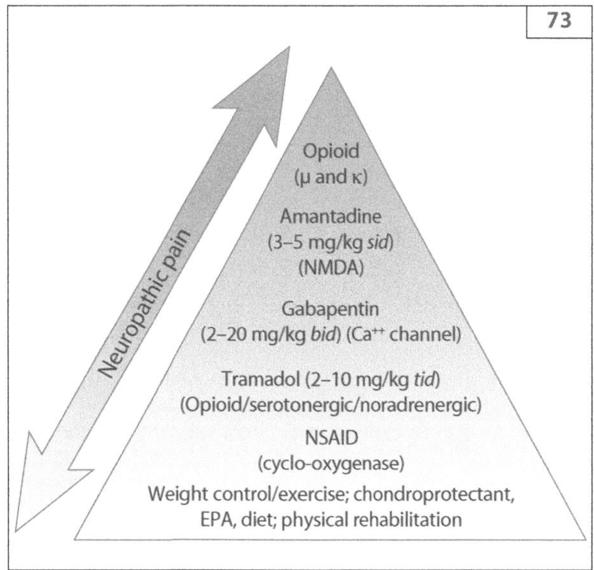

Fig. 73 A multimodal drug scheme would be a logical approach to managing progressive neuropathic pain. Logic resides in each drug's independent efficacy, and each drug's different mode of action/site of action. EPA: eicosapentaenoic acid; NMDA: N-methyl-D-aspartate; NSAID: nonsteroidal anti-inflammatory drug.

There exist a plethora of potential sites of analgesic action that may be exploited with the development of agents directed toward both peripheral and spinal targets (*Tables 46* and *47*).

Idealized criteria for new analgesic therapy in chronic pain:

- Analgesic properties:
  - Moderate-strong analgesic activity.
  - Delayed onset of action is acceptable for treating chronic pain; fast onset of action is required for treating acute or breakthrough pain.
  - No or low analgesic tolerance profile.
  - Not cross-tolerant to morphine.
- Side-effect profile compatible with chronic use:
  - Nonsedating.
  - No, or minimal, respiratory depression.
  - Minimal GI, cardiovascular, renal effects.
  - No or minimal physical drug dependence.
  - Minimal mood-altering activity.
  - Not immunosuppressant.
- Pharmaceutical considerations:
  - Acceptable bioavailability for oral use preferred; alternatives = nasal, rectal, oral transmucosal, transdermal, or injectable use.
  - Half-life and duration of action consistent with chronic use; 1× a day (*sid*) dosing.
  - No drug accumulation with chronic use.
  - Nontoxic metabolite(s).
  - Known and acceptable drug interactions; compatible use with opioids, NSAIDs.
  - Acceptable for use in senior populations.
- Mechanism of action considerations:
  - Nonopioid mechanisms of action preferred.
  - Agonists at non-μ opioid receptors may have advantages.
  - Indirect opioid agonists/peptide releasers, opioid potentiators, and opioid tolerance inhibitors may be useful.
  - Drugs with novel or 'unknown' mechanisms of action are good.

TABLE 46: Various drug classes, mechanism of action and effective application.

Drug class	Mechanism	Acute	Tissue injury	Nerve injury
Opioid (morphine)	Opioid receptors on high threshold C-fibers	X	X	X
NMDA antagonist (ketamine)	Blocks glutamate-spinal facilitation	O	X	X
NSAID	Inhibits PG synthesis at injury site and spinal cord	O	X	O
IV lidocaine	Blocks sodium channels	O	O	X
Anticonvulsant (gabapentin)	Reduces spontaneously active neurons	O	O	X
TCA (amitryptyline)	Increases catecholamine levels	O	O	X

NMDA: N-methyl-D-aspartate; NSAID: nonsteroidal anti-inflammatory drug; PG: prostaglandin; TCA: tricyclic antidepressant; X: effective; O: ineffective.

- Analgesics that also treat the emotive aspects of chronic pain, stress, or depression are useful.

Major themes in analgesic product development

- Opioid combination products:
  - Increased analgesic potency, and/or
  - Increased analgesic efficacy, and/or
  - Reduced side-effects, and/or
  - Reduced tolerance/dependency potential.
- Central opioid receptor analgesics:
  - Opioid-active partial μ-agonist.
  - Morphine metabolite (M6G).
  - μ–δ opioid analgesic.
  - κ-agonist analgesic.
  - Controlled-release drug delivery systems.
- Peripheral opioid receptor analgesics:
  - Peripheral μ-agonist.
  - Peripheral κ-agonist.
- Anti-inflammatory analgesics:
  - COX-2 inhibitors.
  - COX–LOX inhibitors.
  - COX–NO-releasing compounds.
  - Disease-modifying compounds.
- Novel mechanism of action:
  - Ion channel blocking drugs.
  - Cannabinoid analgesics.
  - Muscarinic/nicotinic/α_2-agonist drugs.
  - Special-use products (e.g. unique efficacy for one disease condition or one species, such as osteoarthritis in cats).

TABLE 47: Summary of peripheral pain mechanisms and potential targets for new analgesics

Peripheral mechanism	Peripheral target	Type of drug
Nociceptor activation	Sodium channels	TTX-s channel blocker
Ectopic activity (neuroma, DRG)		TTX-r channel blocker
Nociceptor sensitization	Calcium channels	N-channel blocker
		L-channel blocker
	Acid-sensitive ion channel	Channel blocker
	P2X 3 receptor	Receptor antagonist
	VR1 receptor	Receptor agonist or antagonist
	Opioid receptors	μ, δ, and κ receptor agonists
	Cannabinoid receptors	CBI and CB2 agonists
	Nicotinic receptors	Receptor agonist
	Adrenergic receptors	α_2 agonist
		α_1 antagonist
	Prostanoid receptors	EP antagonist
	Prostanoid production	COX I/II inhibitors
	Serotonin receptors	5-HT$_1$D agonist
		5-HT$_2$ antagonist
	Kinin receptors	B1 antagonist
		B2 antagonists
	Glutamate receptors	NMDA antagonists
	Nerve growth factor	Trk A receptor antagonist
	Cytokines	IL-1β receptor antagonist
		Interleukin-converting enzyme inhibitor
	Protein knase	TNF-α receptor antagonist
		Kinase isotype inhibitor

5-HT: 5-hydroxytryptamine; COX: cyclo-oxygenase; DRG: dorsal root ganglion; EP: prostaglandin E$_2$ receptor; IL: interleukin; NMDA: N-methyl-D-aspartate; TNF: tumor necrosis factor; TTX-r: tetrodotoxin-resistant ion channel; TTX-s: tetrodotoxin-sensitive ion channel; VR: vanillioid receptor.

Table 48 presents data on optimizing premedications.

Example protocols are presented in *Table 49 overleaf*. **Fig. 74** shows an algorithm for treating postoperative maladaptive pain.

Patients given 'follow-up' opioids should not be given antagonists to a previously administered opioid agonist, e.g. butorphanol should not follow morphine.

Obviously, the administration of postoperative opioids takes time to show effect (30–60 minutes IM). During this time, diazepam (0.2 mg/kg IV) can be administered to deepen the plane of sedation, providing time for the opioid to take effect. Low doses of acepromazine (0.01–0.02 mg/kg IV (dog); 0.02–0.05 mg/kg (cat)) can be administered for mild discomfort/dysphoria. If opioid overdosing is suspected as the origin of postoperative excitation, a slow titration of naloxone can be given to effect (4 μg/kg diluted to 10 ml and given at 1 ml increments Q1min).

Various analgesic drugs and premedicants commonly used in the dog and cat are presented in Appendix 1 *Tables 1* and *2*. These drugs are often used together in multimodal protocols, where they are administered at lower doses.

TABLE 48: Optimizing premedications: synergism of multimodal analgesia

Premedication	Induction agent	Gaseous anesthetic
μ-agonist opioid • Efficacious • Inexpensive (morphine) • Relatively safe • MOA: opioid receptors	Lower end of dose range should be used when premedications give heavy sedation and analgesia	Patients often will require much lower inhalant concentrations (0.5–1.5%) to maintain anesthesia when sedatives and analgesics are administered pre-emptively
α_2-agonist[166] • Synergistic to opioids • At lower doses	Induction agents should be given slowly and to effect, as their need may be reduced by as much as 50–70%	
NSAID[167] • Sensitizes opioids to receptors		

MOA: mode of action; NSAID: nonsteroidal anti-inflammatory drug.

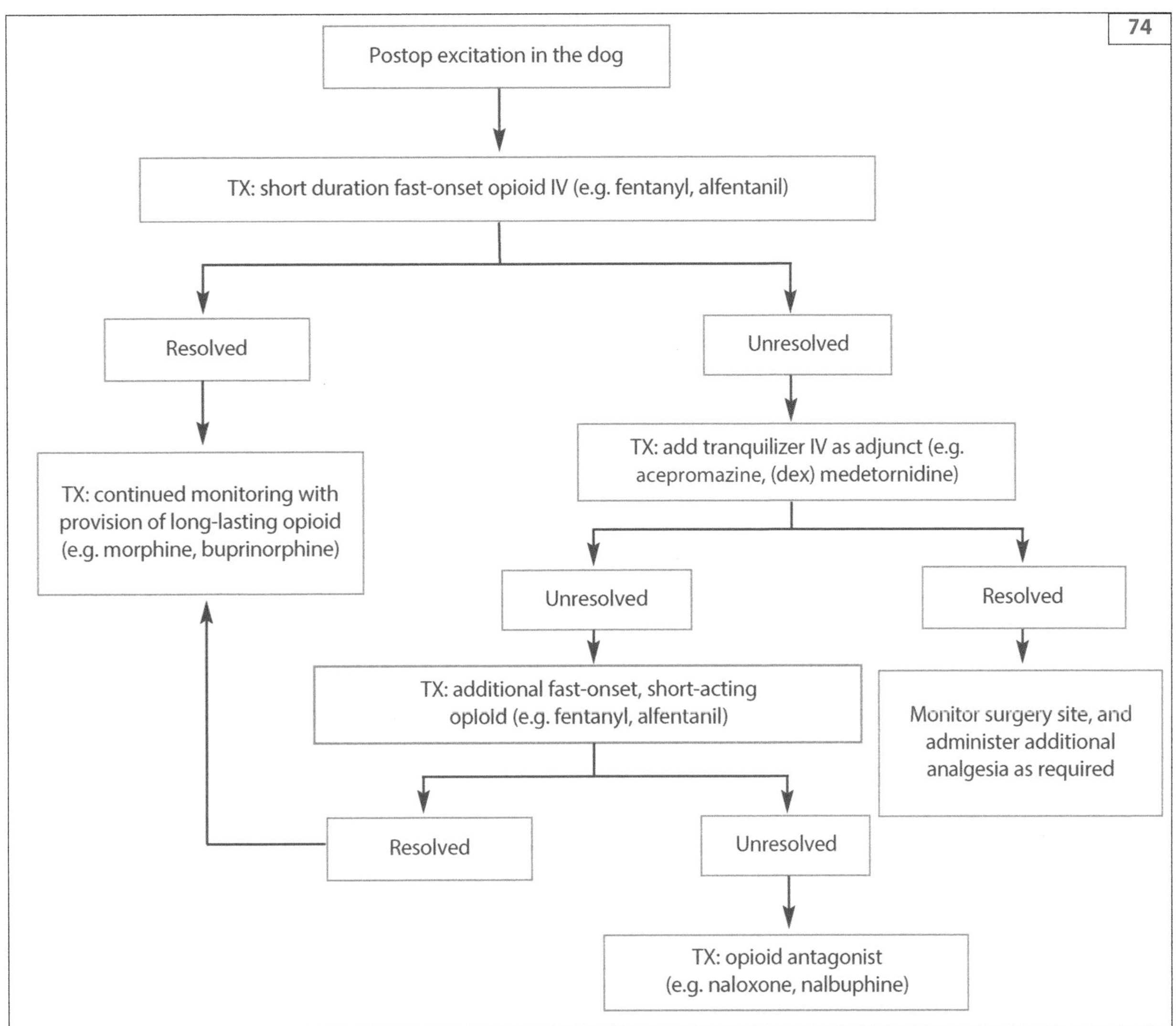

Fig. 74 Algorithm for treating (TX) postoperative maladaptive pain*.
*Patients recovering from surgery must be carefully assessed to determine if excitement, whining, or agitation is resultant from pain, dysphoria, or disorientation. When in doubt, treat with an analgesic, with response to treatment serving as confirmation of pain. Response to the administration of acepromazine suggests dysphoria or disorientation which plays a role in excitation. Adapted from Pascoe (2000)[25].

TABLE 49: Example protocols

Procedure	Anticipated degree of pain	Example Protocol A	Example Protocol B
Canine OHE and castration	Mild to moderate	**Premedication** Acepromazine#, 0.05 – 0.2 mg/kg SC, IM +Buprenorphine*, 0.01–0.03 mg/kg SC, IM ± Atropine, 0.0–0.04 mg/kg SC, IM or Glycopyrrolate, 0.005–0.01 mg/kg SC, IM** + COX-1-sparing NSAID **Intraoperative analgesia** Incisional block: Bupivacaine, 1.5 mg/kg (with 1:200,000 epinephrine) **Postoperative analgesia** Repeat dose of opioid 4–6 h following the initial dose, or sooner if needed NSAID PO *sid* ×7 days starting 24 h after initial dose	**Premedication** Medetomidine, 0.005–0.020 mg/kg IM + Morphine*, 0.5–1.0 mg/kg IM or Hydromorphone*, 0.2 mg/kg IM ± Atropine, 0.01–0.04 mg/kg SC, IM or Glycopyrrolate, 0.005–0.01 mg/kg SC, IM** + COX-1-sparing NSAID **Postoperative analgesia** Repeat dose of opioid 4–6 h following the initial dose, or sooner if needed NSAID PO *sid* × 7 days starting 24 h after initial dose
Feline OHE	Moderate	**Premedication** Acepromazine#, 0.05–0.2 mg/kg SC, IM + Hydromorphone*, 0.05–0.1 mg/kg SC, IM ± Atropine, 0.01–0.04 mg/kg SC, IM or Glycopyrrolate, 0.005–0.01 mg/kg SC, IM** **Intraoperative analgesia** *Incisional block*: Bupivacaine (with 1:200,000 epinephrine), 1.5 mg/kg **Postoperative analgesia** Repeat dose of opioid 4–6 h following the initial dose, or sooner if needed	**Premedication** Medetomidine, 0.02 mg/kg IM + Buprenorphine, 0.01–0.02 mg/kg IM + Ketamine, 2–4 mg/kg IM **Postoperative analgesia** Repeat buprenorphine 6–8 hrs after initial dose Buprenorphine, 0.01–0.02 mg/kg buccal every 8–12 h for 2–4 days beginning 4–6 h after last IM dose ± NSAID for 5–7 days
Feline castration	Mild to moderate	**Premedication** Acepromazine#, 0.05–0.2 mg/kg SC, IM + Hydromorphone*, 0.05 mg/kg SC, IM ± Atropine, 0.01–0.04 mg/kg SC, IM or Glycopyrrolate, 0.005–0.01 mg/kg SC, IM**	Same as for OHE, but may omit the postoperative opioid
Feline onychectomy	Moderate to severe	**Premedication** Acepromazine#, 0.05–0.2 mg/kg SC, IM + Hydromorphone*, 0.05–0.1 mg/kg SC, IM ± Atropine, 0.01–0.04 mg/kg SC, IM or Glycopyrrolate, 0.005–0.01 mg/kg SC, IM** **Intraoperative analgesia** *Declaw block*: Bupivicaine, 1.5 mg/kg maximum dose or Lidocaine 2.0 mg/kg +	**Premedication** Apply 25 µg/h fentanyl patch 6–12 h before surgery or at time of surgical prep (may cover half of the absorptive surface of the patch in cats <5 kg) Medetomidine, 0.02 mg/kg IM + Morphine*, 0.2–0.5 mg/kg IM ± Atropine, 0.01–0.04

Procedure	Anticipated degree of pain	Example Protocol A	Example Protocol B
		Bupivacaine 0.75 mg/kg (without epinephrine) **Postoperative analgesia** *In hospital*: Hydromorphone*, 0.05 mg/kg IM or SC, 4–6 h after initial doses and repeat as needed *At home:* Buprenorphine, 0.01–0.02 mg/kg buccal every 8–12 h for 2–4 days beginning 4-6 h after last hydromorphone dose ± NSAID for 5-7 days	mg/kg SC, IM or Glycopyrrolate, 0.005–0.01 mg/kg SC, IM** **Intraoperative analgesia** *Declaw block:* Bupivacaine, 1.5 mg/kg maximum dose (without epinephrine) **Postoperative analgesia** May need to repeat opioid dose 1–2 times to cover immediate postoperative pain or until fentanyl patch becomes effective. Remove fentanyl patch in 3–5 days ± NSAID for 5–7 days
Canine routine dentistry	Mild to moderate	**Premedication** Acepromazine#, 0.05–0.2 mg/kg SC, IM + Buprenorphine*, 0.01–0.02 mg/kg SC, IM ± Atropine, 0.01–0.04 mg/kg SC, IM or Glycopyrrolate, 0.005–0.01 mg/kg SC, IM** + COX-1-sparing NSAID **Postoperative analgesia** ± Deracoxib, 1–2 mg/kg PO *sid* × 7 days starting 24 h after initial NSAID dose Should be strongly considered with moderate to severe gingivitis	**Premedication** Medetomidine, 0.005–0.010 mg/kg IM + Morphine*, 0.5–1.0 mg/kg IM or Hydromorphone*, 0.2 mg/kg IM ± Atropine, 0.01–0.04 mg/kg SC, IM or Glycopyrrolate, 0.005–0.01 mg/kg SC, IM** + COX-1-sparing NSAID **Postoperative analgesia** ± Deracoxib, 1–2 mg/kg PO *sid* × 7 days starting 24 h after initial NSAID dose Should be strongly considered with moderate to severe gingivitis
Canine dentistry with extractions	Moderate to severe	**Premedication** Acepromazine#, 0.05–0.2 mg/kg SC, IM + Buprenorphine*, 0.01– 0.02 mg/kg SC, IM ± Atropine, 0.01–0.04 mg/kg SC, IM or Glycopyrrolate, 0.005–0.01 mg/kg SC, IM** + COX-1-sparing NSAID *Infraorbital, mandibular, or other regional nerve blocks*: Bupivacaine, 1.5 mg/kg maximum dose (± 1:200,000 epinephrine) **Postoperative analgesia** Deracoxib, 1–2 mg/kg PO *sid* × 7 days starting 24 h after initial NSAID dose	**Premedication** Medetomidine, 0.005–0.010 mg/kg IM + Morphine*, 0.5–1.0 mg/kg IM or Hydromorphone*, 0.2 mg/kg IM ± Atropine, 0.01–0.04 mg/kg SC, IM or Glycopyrrolate, 0.005–0.01 mg/kg SC, IM** + COX-1-sparing NSAID **Intraoperative analgesia** *Infraorbital, mandibular, or other regional nerve blocks*: Bupivacaine, 1.5 mg/kg maximum dose (± 1:200,000 epinephrine) **Postoperative analgesia** Deracoxib, 1–2 mg/kg PO *sid* × 7 days starting 24 h after initial NSAID dose

(continued)

TABLE 49: Example protocols (continued)

Procedure	Anticipated degree of pain	Example Protocol A	Example Protocol B
Feline routine dentistry	Mild to moderate	**Premedication** Acepromazine#, 0.05– 0.2 mg/kg SC, IM + Hydromorphone*, 0.05 mg/kg SC, IM ± Atropine, 0.01–0.04 mg/kg SC, IM or Glycopyrrolate, 0.005–0.01 mg/kg SC, IM** ± NSAID for 5–7 days	**Premedication** Medetomidine, 0.02 mg/kg IM + Buprenorphine*, 0.01–0.02 mg/kg IM + Ketamine, 2–4 mg/kg IM **Postoperative analgesia** Repeat buprenorphine (IM or buccal) 6–8 h after initial dose or as needed if gingivitis is moderate to severe ± NSAID for 5–7 days
Feline dentistry with extractions	Moderate to severe	**Premedication** Acepromazine#, 0.05–0.2 mg/kg SC, IM + Hydromorphone*, 0.05–0.1 mg/kg SC, IM ± Atropine, 0.01–0.04 mg/kg SC, IM or Glycopyrrolate, 0.005–0.01 mg/kg SC, IM** **Intraoperative analgesia** *Infraorbital, mandibular, or other regional nerve blocks*: Bupivacaine, 1.5 mg/kg maximum dose (± 1:200,000 epinephrine) **Postoperative analgesia** ± NSAID for 5–7 days	**Premedication** Medetomidine, 0.02 mg/kg IM + Buprenorphine*, 0.02 mg/kg IM + Ketamine, 2–4 mg/kg IM **Intraoperative analgesia** *Infraorbital, mandibular, or other regional nerve blocks*: Bupivacaine, 1.5 mg/kg maximum dose (±1:200,000 epinephrine) **Postoperative analgesia** Repeat buprenorphine 6–8 h after initial dose Buprenorphine, 0.01–0.02 mg/kg buccal every 8–12 h for 2–4 days beginning 4–6 h after last IM dose ± NSAID for 5–7 days
Canine laparotomy	Moderate to severe	**Premedication** Morphine*, 0.5–1.0 mg/kg SC, IM ± Atropine, 0.01–0.04 mg/kg SC, IM or Glycopyrrolate, 0.005–0.01 mg/kg SC, IM** **Intraoperative analgesia** *Incisional block*: Bupivacaine (with 1:200,000 epinephrine), 1.5 mg/kg maximum dose *Constant rate infusions*: Morphine* (0.05–0.2 mg/kg/h) (or other opioid CRI options) **Postoperative analgesia** Oral morphine, 0.5–1.0 mg/kg following discontinuation of CRI ± NSAID therapy for 7–10 days after discharge (if appropriate for gastrointestinal condition)	**Premedication** Hydromorphone*, 0.2 mg/kg SC, IM + Fentanyl patch placed 12–24 h prior to surgery or at time of surgical prep ± Atropine, 0.01–0.04 mg/kg SC, IM or Glycopyrrolate, 0.005–0.01 mg/kg SC, IM** **Intraoperative analgesia** Lidocaine CRI (0.025–0.050 mg/kg/min) **Postoperative analgesia** May need to repeat opioid dose 1–2 times to cover immediate postoperative pain or until fentanyl patch becomes effective; remove fentanyl patch in 3–5 days

Procedure	Anticipated degree of pain	Example Protocol A	Example Protocol B
Feline laparotomy	Moderate to severe	**Premedication** Hydromorphone*, 0.05– 0.1 mg/kg SC, IM ± Medetomidine, 0.02 mg/kg IM ± Atropine, 0.01–0.04 mg/kg SC, IM or Glycopyrrolate, 0.005–0.01 mg/kg SC, IM** **Intraoperative analgesia** *Incisional block*: Bupivacaine, 1.5 mg/kg maximum dose *Constant rate infusions*: Hydromorphone (0.03–0.05 mg/kg/h) (or other CRI options) **Postoperative analgesia** Buprenorphine, 0.01–0.02 mg/kg buccal every 8–12 h for 2–4 days beginning 4–6 h after discontinuing CRI ± NSAID for 5–7 days	**Premedication** Morphine*, 0.25 mg/kg SC, IM ± Acepromazine#, 0.05–0.1 mg/kg SC, IM ± Atropine, 0.01–0.04 mg/kg SC, IM or Glycopyrrolate, 0.005–0.01 mg/kg SC, IM** + Apply 25 µg/h fentanyl patch 6–12 h prior to surgery or at time of surgical prep **Postoperative analgesia** May need to repeat opioid dose 1–2 times to cover immediate postoperative pain or until fentanyl patch becomes effective; remove fentanyl patch within 3–5 days ± NSAID for 5–7 days
Canine cruciate repair or rear limb orthopedic procedure	Moderate to severe to excruciating	**Premedication** Acepromazine#, 0.05–0.2 mg/kg SC, IM + Morphine*, 1.0 mg/kg SC, IM ± Atropine, 0.01–0.04 mg/kg SC, IM or Glycopyrrolate, 0.005–0.01 mg/kg SC, IM** + COX-1-sparing NSAID PO **Intraoperative analgesia** *Epidural*: Morphine, 0.1 mg/kg (not to exceed 6–7 ml total volume) ± Bupivacaine, 1.0 mg/kg *Intra-articular*: Bupivacaine, 1.0–2.0 mg/kg ± Morphine (1.0 mg in 5 ml saline) **Postoperative analgesia** May need to repeat dose of morphine (oral or parenteral) every 4–6 h as needed after epidural analgesia is no longer effective NSAID PO *sid* starting 24 h after surgery for 7 days	**Premedication** Medetomidine, 0.005–0.010 mg/kg IM + Hydromorphone*, 0.2 mg/kg SC, IM ± Atropine, 0.01–0.04 mg/kg SC, IM or Glycopyrrolate, 0.005–0.01mg/kg SC, IM** + COX-1-sparing NSAID PO + apply appropriate size fentanyl patch 12–24 h preoperatively or at time of surgical prep **Intraoperative analgesia** *Intra-articular*: Bupivacaine, 1.0–2.0 mg/kg ± Morphine (1.0 mg in 5 ml saline) (for surgeries involving the joint) **Postoperative analgesia** Hydromorphone*, 0.2 mg/kg IM, SC 4 h after initial dose May repeat as needed until fentanyl patch is effective NSAID PO *sid* starting 24 h after surgery for 7 days
Canine forelimb orthopedic procedure	Moderate to severe to excruciating	**Premedication** Acepromazine#, 0.05–0.2 mg/kg SC, IM + Morphine*, 1.0 mg/kg SC, IM ± Atropine, 0.01–0.04 mg/kg SC, IM or Glycopyrrolate, 0.005–0.01 mg/kg SC, IM** +COX-1-sparing NSAID	**Premedication** Medetomidine, 0.005–0.010 mg/kg IM + Hydromorphone*, 0.2 mg/kg SC, IM ± Atropine, 0.01–0.04 mg/kg SC, IM or Glycopyrrolate, 0.005–0.01

(continued)

TABLE 49: Example protocols (continued)

Procedure	Anticipated degree of pain	Example Protocol A	Example Protocol B
		Intraoperative analgesia *Brachial plexus block*: Bupivacaine, 1.0–2.0 mg/kg (for procedures distal to the elbow) Consider Ketamine CRI (0.5 mg/kg IV followed by 10 µg/kg/min during surgery and 2 µg/kg/min for 24 h following surgery) **Postoperative analgesia** Morphine*, 1.0 mg/kg SC, IM 4 h after initial dose and repeat as needed NSAID PO *sid* starting 24 h after surgery for 7 days	mg/kg SC, IM** + COX-1-sparing NSAID + apply appropriate size fentanyl patch 12–24 h preoperatively or at time of surgical prep **Intraoperative analgesia** *Intra-articular*: Bupivacaine, 1.0–2.0 mg/kg (for surgeries involving the joint) **Postoperative analgesia** May need to repeat opioid dose 1–2 times to cover immediate postoperative pain or until fentanyl patch becomes effective; remove fentanyl patch in 3–5 days NSAID PO *sid* starting 24 h after surgery for 7 days
Feline forelimb orthopedic procedure	Moderate to severe to excruciating	**Premedication** Acepromazine#, 0.05–0.2 mg/kg SC, IM + Morphine*, 0.25 mg/kg SC, IM ± Atropine, 0.01–0.04 mg/kg SC, IM or Glycopyrrolate, 0.005–0.01 mg/kg SC, IM** **Intraoperative analgesia** *Brachial plexus block*: Bupivicaine, 1.5 mg/kg (for procedures distal to the elbow) **Postoperative analgesia** Buprenorphine, 0.01–0.02 mg/kg buccal every 8–12 h for 2–4 days beginning 4–6 h after initial dose of opioid ± NSAID for 5–7 days	**Premedication** Medetomidine, 0.02 mg/kg IM + Hydromorphone*, 0.05–0.1 mg/kg IM ± Atropine, 0.01–0.04 mg/kg SC, IM or Glycopyrrolate, 0.005–0.01 mg/kg SC, IM** + Apply 25 µg/h fentanyl patch 8–12 h prior to surgery or at time of surgical prep **Intraoperative analgesia** Consider Ketamine CRI (0.5 mg/kg IV followed by 10 µg/kg/min during surgery and 2 µg/kg/min for 24 h following surgery) **Postoperative analgesia** May need to repeat opioid dose 1–2 times to cover immediate postoperative pain or until fentanyl patch becomes effective, ± NSAID for 5–7 days
Feline rear limp orthopedic procedure	Moderate to severe to excruciating	**Premedication** Acepromazine#, 0.05–0.2 mg/kg SC, IM + Morphine*, 0.25 mg/kg SC, IM ± Atropine, 0.01–0.04 mg/kg SC, IM or Glycopyrrolate, 0.005–0.01 mg/kg SC, IM** **Intraoperative analgesia** Consider epidural morphine, 0.1 mg/kg	**Premedication** Medetomidine, 0.02 mg/kg IM + Hydromorphone*, 0.05–0.1 mg/kg IM ± Atropine, 0.01–0.04 mg/kg SC, IM or Glycopyrrolate, 0.005–0.01 mg/kg SC, IM** + Apply 25 µg/h fentanyl patch placed 8–12 h prior to surgery or at time of surgical prep

Procedure	Anticipated degree of pain	Example Protocol A	Example Protocol B
		Postoperative analgesia Buprenorphine, 0.01–0.02 mg/kg buccal every 8–12 h for 2–4 days beginning 4–6 h after initial dose of opioid ± NSAID for 5–7 days	**Intraoperative analgesia** Ketamine CRI (0.5 mg/kg IV followed by 10 µg/kg/min during surgery and 2 µg/kg/min for 24 h following surgery) **Postoperative analgesia** May need to repeat opioid dose 1–2 times to cover immediate postoperative pain or until fentanyl patch becomes effective ± NSAID for 5–7 days
Canine pancreatitis	Moderate to severe to excruciating	Interpleural lidocaine, 1.5 mg/kg followed by interpleural bupivacaine (no epinephrine), 1.5 mg/kg every 3–6 h Parenteral opioids	*Constant rate infusions*: Lidocaine, 0.025–0.050 mg/kg/min ± Morphine, 0.1mg/kg/hr or Ketamine 0.5 mg/kg IV loading dose followed by 2 µg/kg/min + parenteral opioid or Fentanyl 2–5 µg/kg IV loading dose followed by 2–5 µg/kg/h Consider microdoses of Medetomidine, 0.001–0.002 mg/kg IM or IV
Canine osteoarthritis	Mild to severe	Weight management + controlled exercise NSAID PO *sid*	Weight management + controlled exercise NSAID PO *sid* ± Polysulfated glycosaminoglycan, 2 mg/lb (4.4 mg/kg), IM twice weekly for 4 weeks If refractory to standard NSAID therapy or if progressed to severe stages, consider adding nontraditional pharmaceuticals (e.g. acetaminophen+codeine, amantadine, gabapentin) and/or alternative therapies (e.g. acupuncture, physical therapy)

*Consult other references for dosages of other drugs from the same class.

**Anticholinergics (e.g. atropine and glycopyrrolate) have been listed as an option in a number of protocols. Use of anticholinergics should always be based on evaluation of the patient, the anesthetic protocol, and the experiences of the veterinarian. These agents should fit into the protocol on an individual patient basis and should not necessarily be a routine component of every premedicant protocol. Further, the lower end of the atropine dose may not always be effective in alleviating bradycardia.

#Maximum dosage of acepromazine in cats is 1 mg total dose and is 3–4 mg total dose in dogs. Acepromazine dosages as low as 0.01 mg/kg may be effective in dogs, but higher dosages are generally required for adequate sedation in cats.

Dexmedetomidine may be substituted for medetomidine.

Although deracoxib has been cited as the example postoperative NSAID, various NSAIDs can be substituted.

When selecting a perioperative NSAID, it should be COX-1-sparing, i.e. deracoxib, meloxicam, or firocoxib. The new topical fentanyl, Recuvyra™, can be substituted as the preoperative opioid.

COX: cyclo-oxygenase; CRI: constant rate infusion; NSAID: nonsteroidal anti-inflammatory drug; OHE: ovariohysterectomy.

The FDA has not approved some of these drugs or the listed routes of administration for use as canine or feline analgesics; these constitute extra-label indications under the Animal Medicinal Drug Use Clarification Act (AMDUCA). It is the veterinarian's responsibility to comply with the rules and regulations required by this Act. Refer to the FDA/CVM website (www.fda.cvm.org) and the publication, 'FDA and the Veterinarian' (http://www.fda.gov/cvm/index/fdavet/cov12.htm) for more information.

Chapter 6

Nonsteroidal Anti-inflammatory Drugs

INTRODUCTION

Nonsteroidal anti-inflammatory drugs (NSAIDs) are the fastest growing class of drugs in both human and veterinary medicine. This reflects their broad use as anti-inflammatories, analgesics, and antipyretics (**Fig. 75**). Perhaps this supports devoting a separate chapter to the subject.

As with antibiotics, NSAIDs can be considered to have been introduced in successive generations to date: 1) first generation: aspirin (ASA), phenylbutazone, meclofenamic acid; 2) second generation: carprofen, etodolac, meloxicam; and 3) third generation: tepoxalin, deracoxib, firocoxib, mavacoxib, and robenacoxib. However, unlike the logic of 'saving the big gun antibiotic' for last, so as to avoid microbial suprainfections, logic would dictate using the optimal NSAID at the earliest opportunity, so as to avoid the physiologic complication of 'wind-up'.

Currently, several NSAIDs (ASA, carprofen, cinchophen, deracoxib, etodolac, firocoxib, robenacoxib, mavacoxib, flunixin, ketoprofen, meloxicam, phenylbutazone, tepoxalin, tolfenamic acid, and vedaprofen) have approval in various countries for the control of canine perioperative and/or chronic pain. NSAIDs approved for feline use are far more limited (meloxicam, tolfenamic acid, ketoprofen, carprofen, robenacoxib, and ASA are generally approved in various countries for short-term administration). (See Appendix 1 *Tables 3* and *4*.)

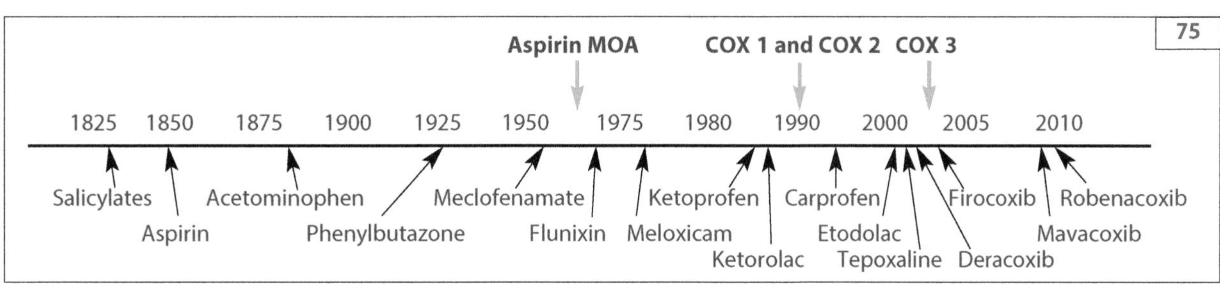

Fig. 75 Evolution of nonsteroidal anti-inflammatory drugs (NSAIDs). Following discovery of aspirin's mode of action and the discovery of cyclo-oxygenase (COX) 1 and 2, a number of NSAIDs have been approved for use in the dog and cat. MOA: mode of action.

ARACHIDONIC ACID PATHWAY

In most respects NSAIDs can be characterized as a class, although there are molecule-specific characteristics among individual drugs. NSAIDs manifest their mode of action in the arachidonic acid (AA) cascade (**Fig. 76**).

AA is an ubiquitous substrate derived from the continual degradation of cell membranes. Corticosteroids express their activity in the early stages of this course. AA is thereafter metabolized to various eicosanoids via the cyclo-oxygenase (COX) pathway to prostaglandins (PGs) or via the lipoxygenase (LOX) pathway to leukotrienes (LTs). Under the influence of local tissues, these end-product prostanoids can be proinflammatory and enhance disease processes and pain.

There are four families of **eicosanoids:** prostaglandins, prostacyclins, the thromboxanes, and the leukotrienes. For each there are two or three separate series, derived either from an omega (ω)-3 or omega-6 essential fatty acid.

Clinical implication: since corticosteroids act earlier in the pathway than do nonsteroidal anti-inflammatory drugs, administering both groups of drugs together is somewhat redundant.

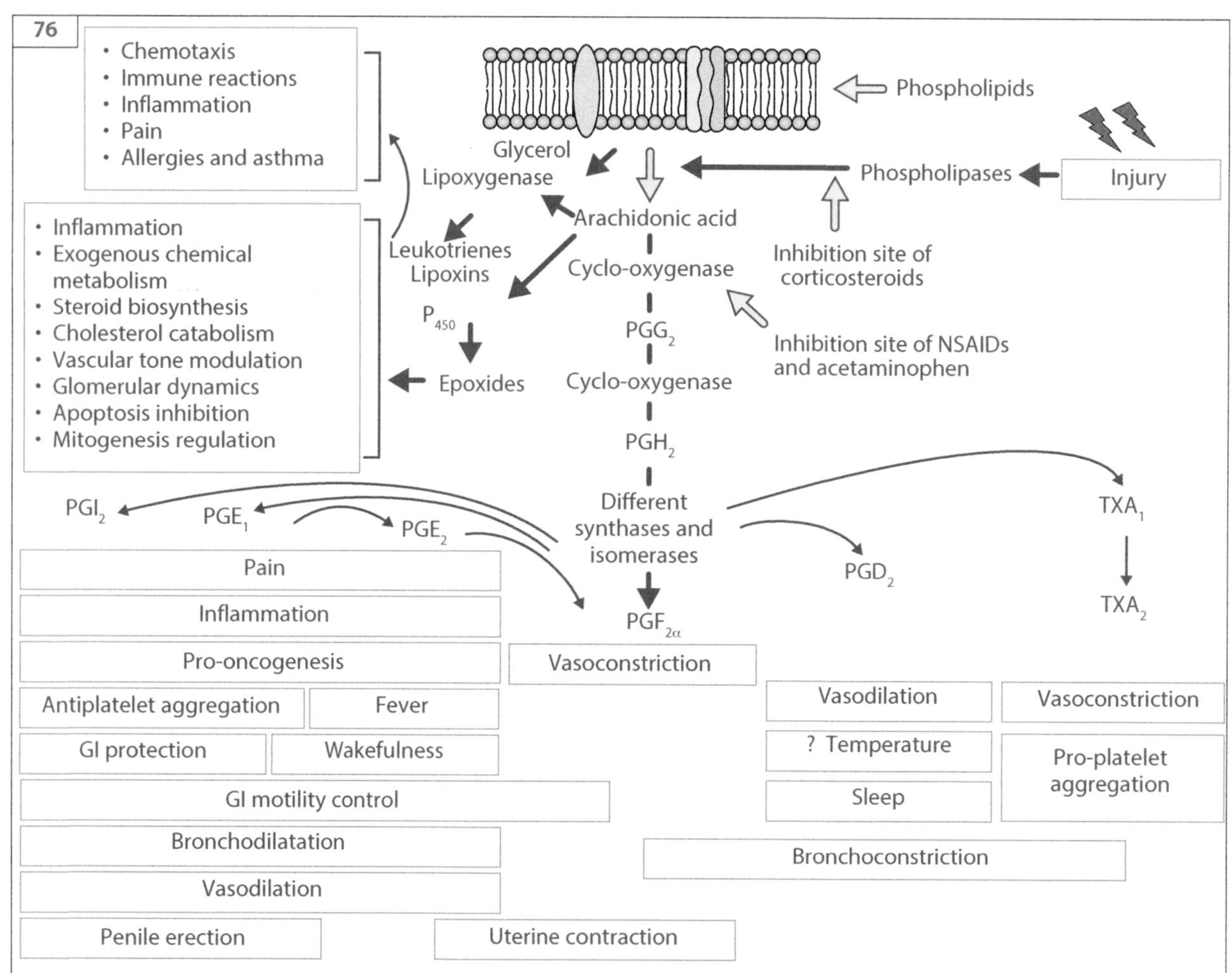

Fig. 76 The arachidonic acid pathway generates a variety of eicosanoids which play various roles in different physiologic functions. GI: gastrointestinal; NSAID: nonsteroidal anti-inflammatory drug; PG: prostaglandin; TXA: thromboxane A.

It is important to note that the function of many prostanoids is tissue-dependent, for example PGs may contribute to pain and inflammation in the arthritic joint, while they enhance normal homeostatic functions of vascularization, and bicarbonate and mucous secretion in the gastrointestinal (GI) tract (*Table 50*).

At one time it was believed that blocking the COX pathway led to a build up of the substrate AA, which would then lead to increased production of LTs. This idea has been challenged by some authors[1].

Because corticosteroids have their mode of action at a location higher in the AA cascade than do NSAIDs, it is inappropriate to use the drugs concurrently, and doing so markedly increases the risk for adverse reactions[2–4]. Data from humans show that the risk of NSAID-induced GI complications is doubled when a NSAID is used concurrently with a corticosteroid[5].

COX ISOZYMES

Approximately 20 years following the discovery of the AA pathway as the mode of action for the NSAID ASA, it was discovered that the COX enzyme exists as at least two isoenzymes: COX-1 and COX-2[6,7]. These two distinct COX isoforms have been identified as products of two separate genes[8]. Early thinking was that COX-1-mediated PGs were constitutive physiologically (accounting for normal platelet, renal, and GI functions), and should be retained, while COX-2-mediated PGs were pathologic and should be eliminated for the control of inflammation and pain (**Fig.** 77).

TABLE 50: Major prostanoids and their functions

Prostanoid	Primarily found in	Major biologic action
TXA_2	Platelets Monocytes	Platelet aggregation Vasoconstriction Bronchoconstriction Cellular proliferation
PGI_2 (prostacyclin)	Vascular endothelium	Inhibition of inappropriate platelet aggregation Vasodilation Bronchodilation
	Vascular sub-endothelium	Vascular permeability Bronchodilation Inflammation Cholesterol efflux from arteries
PGE_2	Renal medulla Gastric lining Platelets	Vasodilation Inflammation Na^+–K^+ excretion/ reabsorption
	Microvascular endothelium	Bronchodilation Presynaptic adrenergic activity Cardio-protection
$PGF_{2\alpha}$	Brain Uterus	Vasoconstriction Bronchoconstriction Uterine constriction
PGD_2	Mast cells Brain	Sleep regulation Bronchoconstriction Temperature control Vasodilation

PG: prostaglandin; TXA: thromboxane A.

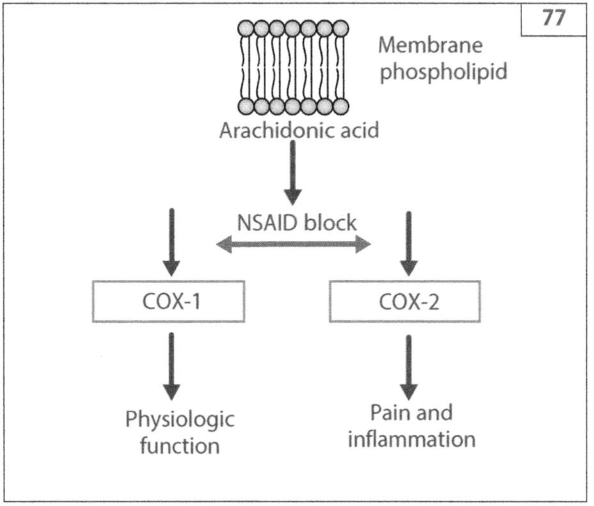

Fig. 77 Cyclo-oxygenase (COX)-1-mediated prostaglandins (PGs) tend to be more associated with constitutive physiologic functions, while COX-2-mediated PGs tend to be more associated with pain and inflammation. NSAID: nonsteroidal anti-inflammatory drug.

COX-2-selective NSAIDs were designed for this purpose: the selective suppression of COX-2-mediated PGs (**Fig. 78–80**).

In contrast to COX-1, COX-2 is not widely expressed under normal physiologic conditions, but is up-regulated in cells, such as synoviocytes, fibroblasts, monocytes, and macrophages, under the influence of proinflammatory mediators. The overall amino acid sequence of COX-1 and COX-2 is similar, the only difference in humans between the two isoforms being in the active site region that occurs at residue 523, where the isoleucine residue in COX-1 is replaced by a valine residue in COX-2. This single difference has been shown to have a marked effect on the overall size and shape of the binding site, apparently the basis for COX-2 inhibitor selectivity (**Fig. 81**).

The IC_{50} is defined as the concentration of drug (NSAID) needed to inhibit the activity of the enzyme (COX) by 50%. In keeping with the above rationale, one would like to have a high concentration of NSAID before causing 50% inhibition of COX-1 ('good guy') and a low concentration of NSAID to reach the IC_{50} for COX-2 ('bad guy'):

$$\frac{IC_{50}\text{ of COX-1 (good)} \quad \text{HIGH}}{IC_{50}\text{ of COX-2 (bad)} \quad \text{LOW}}$$

The higher the numerator and lower the denominator, the higher the absolute value. Therefore, a greater COX-1/COX-2 ratio suggests (theoretically) the more optimal performing NSAID. With this in mind, pharmaceutical companies began designing NSAIDs for which it takes a low concentration to inhibit COX-2, but a high concentration to inhibit COX-1. Many factors, such as species, incubation time, and enzyme source, can influence the data obtained from enzyme preparations. Additionally, particularly when measuring COX-2 potency, the kinetics of inhibition are very complex and time dependent.

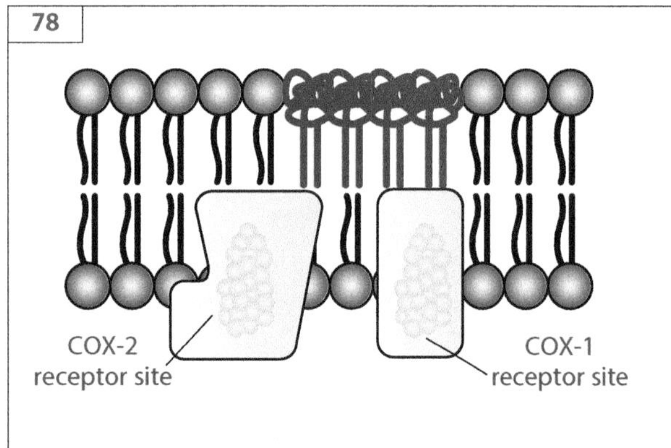

Fig. 78 The cyclo-oxygenase (COX)-1 receptor site differs from the COX-2 receptor site by only a single amino acid; however, the COX-2 site has a larger entry port and characteristic side pocket. Small, traditional nonsteroidal anti-inflammatory drugs (NSAIDs) fit into both sites, blocking both COX-1 and COX-2-mediated prostaglandin production from arachidonic acid, hence the term *nonselective NSAID.*

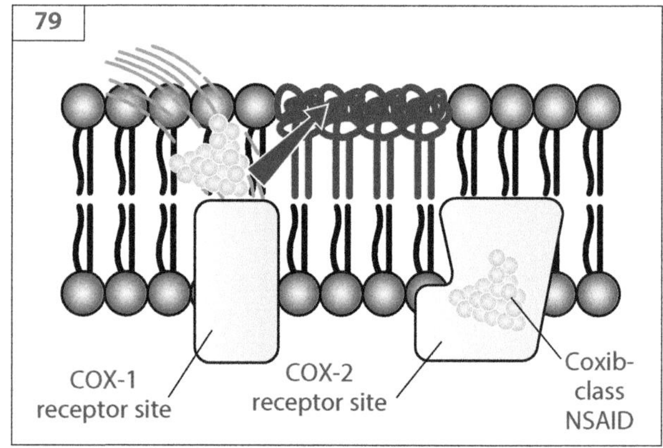

Fig. 79 Coxib-class nonsteroidal anti-inflammatory drugs (NSAIDs) were designed to be too large for the cyclo-oxygenase (COX)-1 receptor site (at labeled dose); however, they fit hand-in-glove within the COX-2 receptor site. These drugs spare COX-1-mediated prostaglandin (PG) production, and block COX-2-mediated PG production, that is they are COX-1 *sparing* and COX-2 *selective.*

80

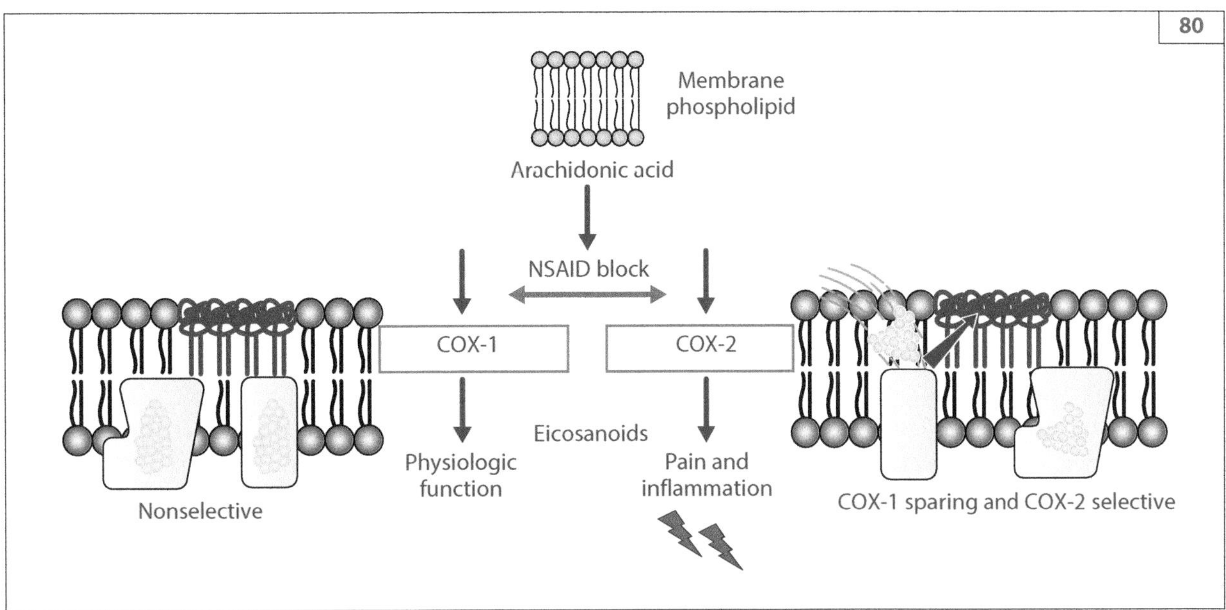

Fig. 80 Overview of cyclo-oxygenase (COX)-1 and COX-2 nomenclature and clinical relevance. NSAID: nonsteroidal anti-inflammatory drug.

81

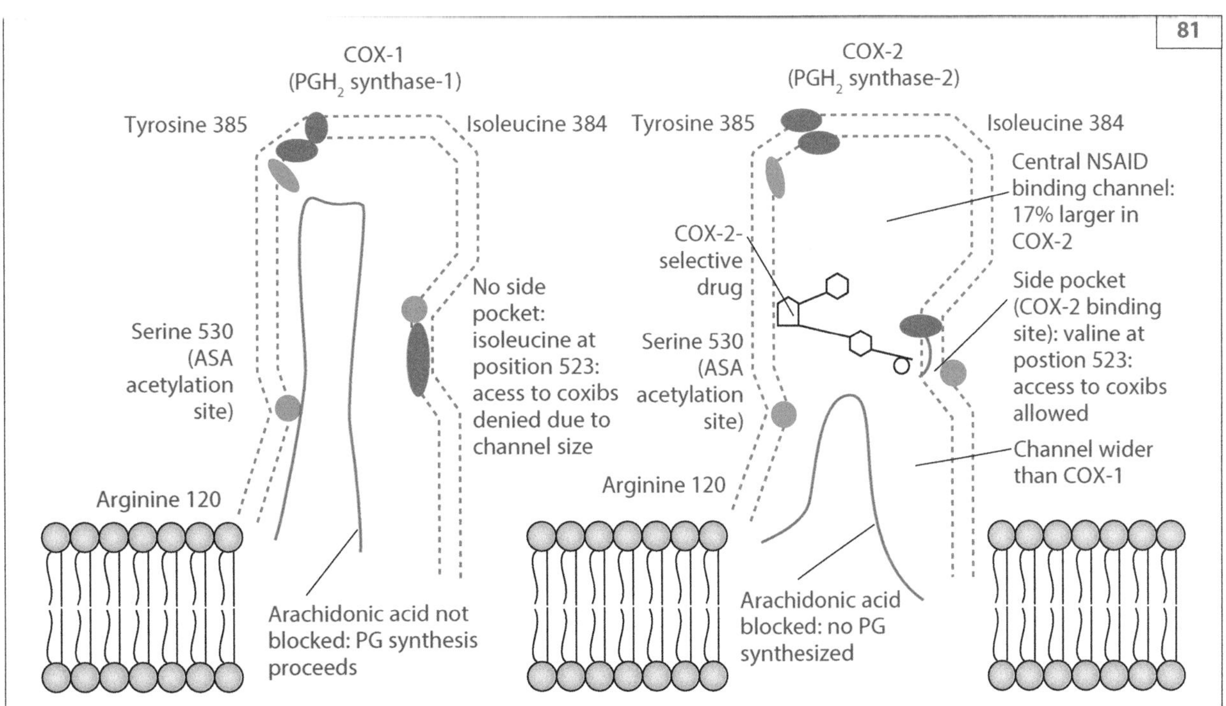

Fig. 81 In humans, the two cyclo-oxygenase (COX) isoforms differ by a single amino acid; this single difference, however, influences COX-2 inhibitor selectivity. ASA: acetyl salicylic acid; NSAID; nonsteroidal anti-inflammatory drug; PG: prostaglandin.

Consequently, different values have been reported for the same drug. Although COX-1:COX-2 ratios vary by investigator, relative ratio standings provide insight as to a drug's expected species-specific COX activity (*Table 51*). Complicating this issue, some report ratios of COX-2/COX-1 rather than the more conventional COX-1/COX-2.

It has been suggested that a COX-1/COX-2 ratio of <1 would be considered COX-1 *selective*, a ratio >1 as COX-2 *preferential*, a ratio >100 as COX-2 *selective* and a ratio >1,000 as COX-2 *specific*. Selectivity nomenclature is used loosely and such comparative ranking has not been associated with clinical correlation. Hence, almost all discussions of COX data presented by pharmaceutical manufacturers include the disclaimer, 'clinical relevance undetermined', because the data are sourced *in vitro*.

In vitro refers to a procedure performed not in a living organism, but in a controlled environment, such as in a test tube or Petri dish.

In vivo is experimentation using a whole, living organism as opposed to a partial or dead organism, or in an *in vitro* controlled environment.

We now know that the 'good-guy-COX-1', 'bad-guy-COX-2' approach is naive, recognizing that COX-2 is needed constitutively for reproduction, central nervous system (CNS) nociception, renal function, and GI lesion repair. In fact, the physiologic functions associated with COX activity overlap (**Fig. 82**). Accordingly, there is likely a limit as to how COX-2 selective a NSAID can be without causing problems, for example inhibiting endogenous repair of a gastric lesion, which requires COX-2; this limit is not known. More important than how COX-2 selective an NSAID might be, is whether or not the NSAID is COX-1 sparing (does it preserve homeostatic physiology, e.g. maintain normal GI protection)? Further, it is logical to avoid a COX-1-selective NSAID (COX-1:COX-2 ratio <1) perioperatively, so as not to enhance bleeding. The coxib-class, third generation NSAIDs, with their high COX 1:2 ratio and COX-1-sparing feature, have been shown to be associated with less risk for GI complications in human studies[14].

At the time of writing, only the following nonsteroidal anti-inflammatory drugs are documented as **cyclo-oxygenase-1 sparing:** firocoxib, deracoxib, meloxicam, ± carprofen.

COXIB-CLASS NSAIDs

Human coxib-class NSAIDs were designed to be more safe for the GI tract, although any NSAID can cause adverse reactions (adverse drug event, ADE). Analogous safety profiles have not been extensively investigated in the canine. Coxib-class NSAIDs were not designed to be more safe for renal or hepatic function and they have been associated with potential cardiovascular risks in humans (but not dogs or cats). Fortunately, companion animals are not at risk for coxib-class NSAID cardiovascular problems (atherosclerosis)[15] as are humans, and it may well be that the canine is an optimal target species for this class of drugs.

TABLE 51: Canine COX-1:COX-2 ratios of contemporary veterinary nonsteroidal anti-inflammatory drugs reported by different investigators

Investigator	Drug	Ratio of IC_{50} COX-1:COX-2
Kay-Mungerford *et al.*[9]	Meloxicam	12.2
	Carprofen	1.8
	Ketoprofen	0.4
Brideau *et al.*[10]	Meloxicam	10
	Carprofen	9
	Ketoprofen	6.5
Streppa *et al.*[11]	Meloxicam	2.7
	Carprofen	16.8
	Ketoprofen	0.2
	Aspirin	0.4
Li *et al.*[12]	Carprofen	5
	Celecoxib	6.2
	Deracoxib	36.5
	Firocoxib	155

COX: cyclo-oxygenase.

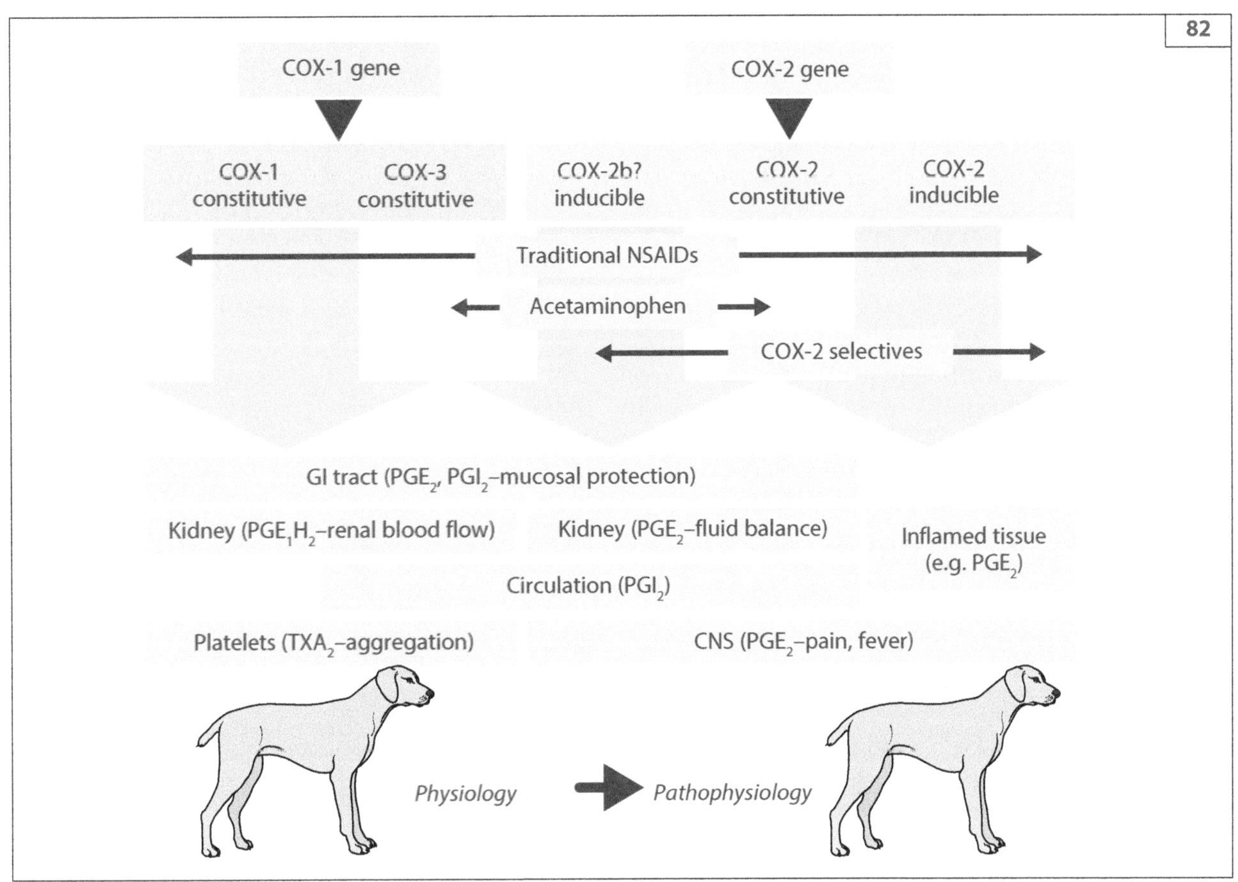

Fig. 82 Clinical relevance of cyclo-oxygenase (COX) activity overlap, as influenced by the patient's general health, fitness, age, and other medications. Based on these variables, the nonsteroidal anti-inflammatory drug (NSAID) may have a large influence on pain and inflammation but little influence on constitutive physiology (dog on the right). In contrast, based on these variables, the NSAID may have a large influence on constitutive physiology (dog on the left). (After Reference 13.) CNS: central nervous system; GI: gastrointestinal; PG: prostaglandin; TXA: thromboxane A.

The label precaution regarding potential sulfonamide hypersensitivity is likely theoretical. Trepanier[16] reported that 'sulfur drugs' other than the antimicrobial sulfonamides do not produce a similar pathogenesis for the same hypersensitivity.

Clinical implication: problems associated with the drug Vioxx being withdrawn from the human market are not seen in the dog.

DUAL PATHWAY INHIBITORS

NSAIDs are a mainstay in the treatment of inflammatory disease and are among the most widely used drugs worldwide. They are anti-inflammatory, antipyretic, and analgesic and are prescribed as first choice for the treatment of rheumatic disorders and, in general, inflammation. The main limitation in using NSAIDs resides in their side-effects, including GI ulcerogenic activity and bronchospasm. The mechanism of action of these drugs is attributed to the inhibition of COX, and, consequently, the conversion of AA into PGs. It is hypothesized that the undesirable side-effects of NSAIDs are due to the inhibition of COX-1 (constitutive isoform), whereas the beneficial effects are related to the inhibition of COX-2 (inducible isoform). AA can also be converted to LTs by the action of 5-lipoxygenase (5-LOX). LTC_4, LTD_4, and LTE_4 are potent bronchoconstrictors, whereas LTB_4 is chemotactic for leukocytes and plays an important role in the development of GI ulcers by contributing to the inflammatory process. Thus, developing dual inhibitor compounds that will simultaneously inhibit COX and 5-LOX could enhance their individual anti-inflammatory effects and reduce the undesirable side-effects associated with NSAIDs, especially of the GI tract.

The first commercialized dual pathway inhibitor, analgesic and anti-inflammatory agent was (human use) licofelone. Merckle's licofelone differs from both conventional NSAIDs and COX-2 specific inhibitors in that it inhibits not only COX but also 5-LOX, an enzyme associated with the production of proinflammatory and gastrotoxic LTs. Some evidence suggests that NSAID-induced GI toxicity may involve shunting AA metabolism to the 5-LOX pathway, thereby increasing the production of gastrotoxic LTs. Inhibition of 5-LOX may therefore offer a new approach to reducing the GI toxicity associated with NSAID use, while retaining the analgesic and anti-inflammatory properties of NSAIDs and COX-2 specific inhibitors.

The veterinary dual pathway inhibitor tepoxalin has demonstrated *in vivo* inhibitory activity against COX-1, COX-2, and 5-LOX in dogs at the approved recommended dosage[17], yet there are no data to suggest it is more safe than traditional, or COX-2-selective NSAIDs. Tepoxalin actually inhibits COX-1 more than COX-2. In the dog, tepoxalin is a dual inhibitor for a short period of time only; but, in the cat tepoxalin pharmacokinetics indicate it is potentially a balanced COX and LOX inhibitor throughout its kinetic profile[18].

ASPIRIN

ASA presents unique risk factors to the canine patient. ASA is both topically and systemically toxic (even at low doses of 5–10 mg/kg *sid*), chondro-destructive, causes irreversible platelet acetylation, and is associated with GI bleeding of approximately 3 ml/day[19,20]. The American Medical Association reports that 16,500 people die each year associated with NSAID toxicity[21], with an over-representation of ASA. Pet owners often consider ASA benign because it is available over-the-counter (OTC) and the media suggest it is safe. Even low-dose ASA has consistently been associated with GI petechiation and hemorrhage. ASA does not have a USA Food and Drug Administration (FDA) license for use in the dog, and the plasma concentrations regarded as being therapeutic are relatively close to the toxic levels[22]. In theory, since ASA causes GI lesions, it would be inappropriate to progress sequentially from ASA to a strongly COX-2-selective NSAID (which might restrict the COX-2 necessary for repair of GI petechiation or erosion), without an adequate washout period following the ASA. It is also perilous to use ASA together with another NSAID or together with a corticosteroid.

Since **aspirin** (acetyl salicylic acid) is not a controlled agent, can be bought in large quantities, and is extensively advertised on television, most pet owners believe it is without potential danger.

Clinical implication: arguably, it would be most appropriate to start a nonsteroidal anti-inflammatory drug (NSAID) protocol with a coxib-class NSAID for patients at low risk, rather than start with a traditional NSAID and switch to a coxib-class NSAID.

Development of gastric mucosal hemorrhage, erosion, and ulceration associated with administration of NSAIDs is largely attributed to reduction of PGE synthesis in the gastric mucosa. PGs play a key role in protection of the GI mucosal barrier by: 1) increasing mucus and bicarbonate secretion; 2) enhancing mucosal blood flow; 3) stimulating epithelial cell growth; and 4) suppressing acid secretion.

ASA can cause direct cellular toxicosis, independent of the inhibition of PG synthesis. ASA may cause gastric mucosal injury via two mechanisms: 1) direct damage to the gastric epithelial cell; and 2) indirect damage caused by its anti-PG effects[23]. The erosive effects of ASA on the canine stomach have been known since 1909, when Christoni and Lapressa administered 150–200 mg of ASA to dogs and noted gastric lesions[24]. Interestingly, the discovery of ASA's ulcerogenic properties resulted in its use to induce gastroduodenal ulcer disease in animal models[25,26]. Topical irritation and physical damage to the gastric mucosal barrier may result from a pH-mediated effect of mucosal hydrophobicity, and from direct contact between ASA and gastric epithelium. In the highly acidic gastric lumen, ASA is mostly nonionized and lipid-soluble. In this form, it can freely diffuse into mucosal cells where, at neutral pH, ASA becomes ionized and water-soluble. The water-soluble form cannot penetrate lipid cell membranes and consequently becomes trapped in mucosal cells. The presence of intracellular ASA causes increased membrane permeability, leading to an influx of hydrogen ions (H^+) from the gastric lumen or an increased 'back-diffusion' of acid across the gastric mucosal barrier. This increased acid back-diffusion is crucial in initiating and perpetuating mucosal injury. The result is edema, inflammation, hemorrhage, erosions and ulceration, as well as submucosal capillary damage (**Fig. 83**).

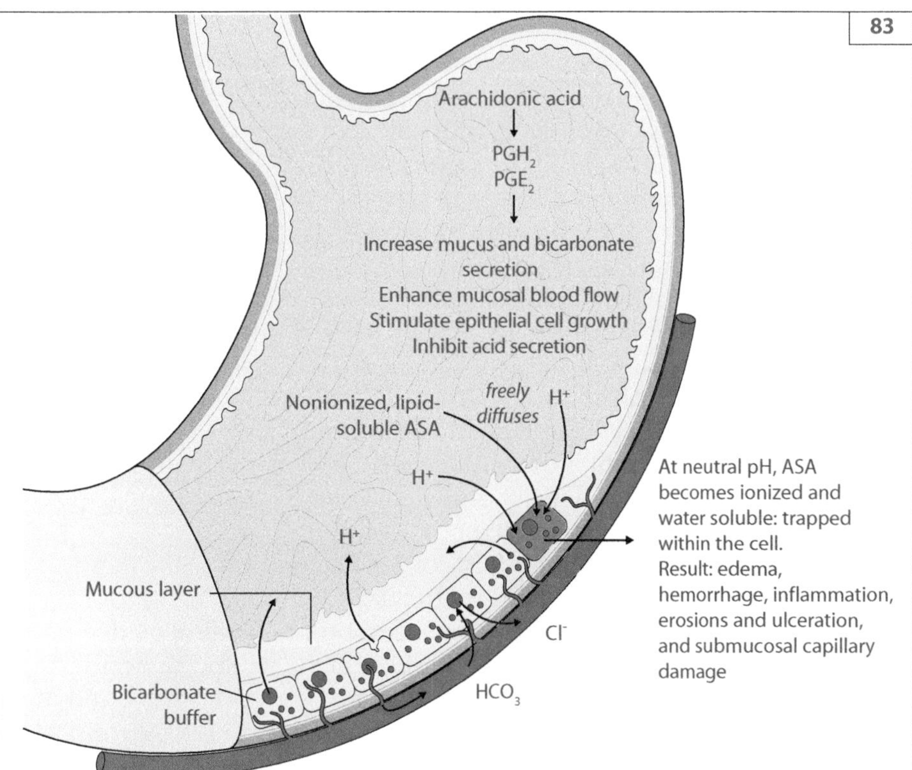

Fig. 83 Prostaglandin (PG)-dependent mechanisms of gastric mucosal protection and influence of aspirin (ASA) on gastric mucosa.

Risk factors for NSAID-induced GI complications (human) are shown in *Table 52* (**Fig. 84**).

Standard formulations of buffered ASA have been shown **not** to provide sufficient buffering to neutralize gastric acid or to prevent mucosal injury[27]. Enteric-coated ASA causes less gastric injury in humans, compared with that from administration of nonbuffered or buffered ASA, but absorption is quite variable[28,29], with coated tablets having been observed to pass in the feces.

Acute inflammation is normally a localized protective response where leukocytes (polymorphonuclear leukocytes [neutrophils; PMNs]) play a pivotal role, not only to destroy invading microbes, but also to wall off injured tissues[31]. ASA causes increased leukocyte adherence within the gastric and mesenteric microcirculation, which has been shown to contribute significantly to the creation of lesions in the stomach lining[32]. As an adaptive protective mechanism, both man and dog up-regulate expression of COX-2 by the gastric mucosa and increase generation of 15(R)-epi-lipoxin A4, so-called 'aspirin-triggered lipoxin' (ATL). Lipoxin A4 and its carbon-15 epimer ATL have potent inhibitory effects on neutrophil chemotaxis, adherence, transmigration, and superoxide anion production[33]. ASA administration results in inhibition of gastric PG synthesis, which contributes to the generation of hemorrhagic lesions in the mucosa. However, ASA-induced acetylation of COX-2 results in the generation of ATL, which counteracts the detrimental effects of depletion of mucosal PGs, thereby reducing the severity of gastric damage[34] (**Fig. 85**).

Data from animal and human studies have shown that the combination of ASA and a selective COX-2 inhibitor results in greater gastric injury than that observed following the administration of either drug alone[35]. This is a result of COX-2 inhibitors (selective or nonselective) blocking the activity of the enzyme 15(R)-HETE (hydroxyeicosatetraenoic acid). Blocking either of the enzymes 5-LOX or 15(R)-HETE results in blockade of ATL synthesis and blockade of the inhibitory effects of ASA on neutrophil adherence to endothelial cells. Herein, the AA substrate now follows a different pathway, leading to the generation of LTB_4. Endogenous chemical mediators generated by the host govern leukocyte trafficking from the vasculature to active sites[36], and in this context LTB_4 is among the most potent PMN chemoattractant known[37].

TABLE 52: Risk factors for NSAID-induced GI complications (human)[2]

	Risk factor	Estimated increased risk
Established	Prior clinical GI event (ulcer/complication)	2.4–4×
	Advanced age (65+ years)	2–3.5×
	Concurrent anticoagulation therapy	3×
	Concurrent corticosteroid use	2×
	High-dose NSAID or multiple NSAID use	2–4×
	Major comorbidity (e.g. heart disease)	Variable
Probable	Long-term NSAID use	
	Coexisting *H. pylori* infection	
	Dyspepsia caused by an NSAID	

GI: gastrointestinal; NSAID: nonsteroidal anti-inflammatory drug.

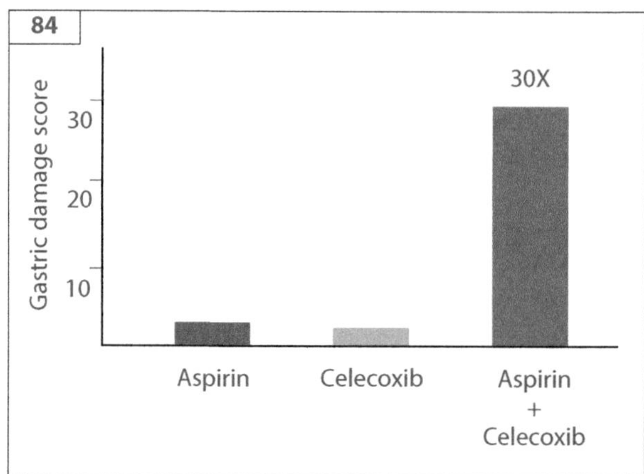

Fig. 84 Some human patients take high-dose aspirin (ASA) for their cardiac condition and a 'third generation' nonsteroidal anti-inflammatory drug for their musculoskeletal discomfort, thereby increasing their potential for gastric damage. This has been shown to increase the risk for gastric damage significantly[31].

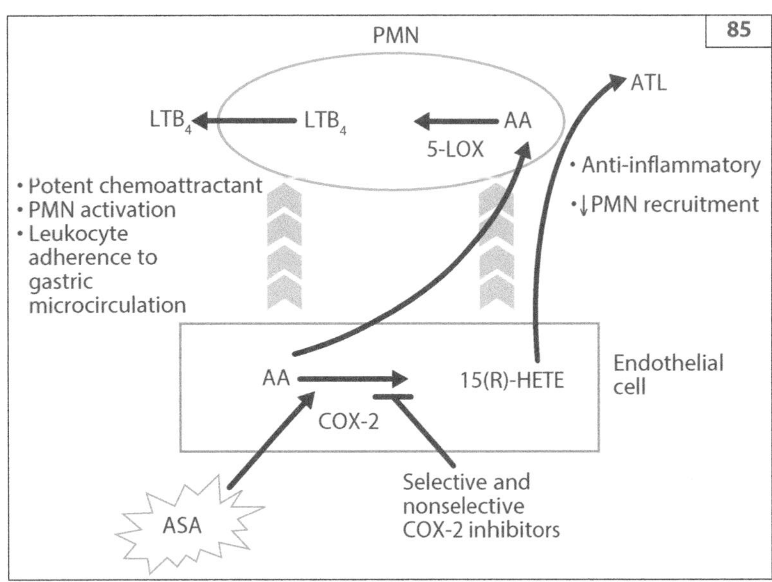

Fig. 85 Potential for increased gastrointestinal damage from the concurrent use of aspirin (ASA) with another nonsteroidal anti-inflammatory drug (NSAID) resides with the aspirin-triggered lipoxin (ATL) pathway. ATL is a protective mechanism with ASA consumption, which is blocked with the concurrent administration of another NSAID, giving rise to an alternative pathway for arachidonic acid (AA) that actually enhances the potential for ASA toxicity[34]. COX: cyclo-oxygenase; HETE: hydroxyeicosatetraenoic acid; LOX: lipoxygenase; LT: leukotriene; PMN: polymorphonuclear leukocyte.

The end result of administering ASA together with another NSAID is that: 1) production of the protective protein ATL is blocked; and 2) the risk of gastric damage is amplified by the strong recruitment of leukocytes by LTB_4.

ACETAMINOPHEN (PARACETAMOL)

Acetaminophen is a popular OTC analgesic included in many headache, influenza, cold, and pain relief medications. It is a relatively safe and effective drug in humans, but it can be associated with serious problems in companion animals. Acetaminophen is considered a moderate analgesic and antipyretic, but with no anti-inflammatory attributes. For this reason, it is not a 'true' NSAID.

Toxicity in dogs commonly causes liver damage, while methemoglobinemia is the primary toxic manifestation in cats. The toxic dose of acetaminophen is 100–200 mg/kg in dogs and as low as 60 mg/kg in cats[38]. Oxidation of acetaminophen by cytochrome P450 results in the formation of the reactive metabolite N-acetyl-para-benzoquinoneimine (NAPQI), which is responsible for the toxic effects of acetaminophen ingestion. In the cat, glucuronidation is limited because of reduced activity of the UDP-glucuronosyltransferase enzyme, and therefore the drug is slow to be eliminated and increased shunting to P450 occurs with subsequent toxic metabolite formation.

Clinical implication: just one regular-strength acetaminophen (e.g. Tylenol 325 mg) can be toxic in a 4 kg cat, causing cyanosis, methemoglobinemia, Heinz body anemia, facial swelling, icterus, and death. Further, 95% of reported toxicities are from deliberate administration by the owner, because they did not know acetaminophen could be toxic in the cat.

Acetaminophen has been used for mild to moderate pain in humans. It provides enhanced analgesia when combined with NSAIDs or codeine[39]. In osteoarthritis, most human studies show that acetaminophen provides effective pain relief, although it seems less effective than NSAIDs[40]. Yet, it is recommended in first-line therapy to relieve pain in several clinical guidelines, such as those of the American College of Rheumatology or the European League of Associations of Rheumatology, based on its high safety profile. Acetaminophen has shown some efficacy in animal models of neuropathic pain[41].

Its passage through the blood–brain barrier is quite fast, and the concentrations found in the cerebrospinal fluid are similar to plasma concentrations[42].

One hypothesis for the molecular mechanism of acetaminophen action is inhibition of COX (specifically COX-3). However, 1 year after COX-3 discovery, its existence was questioned. Currently, the published data suggest there is no convincing evidence about the contribution of COX to the analgesic action of acetaminophen. Although the definitive mode of action of acetaminophen remains unknown, it is known that it strengthens the serotonin bulbospinal pathway and mobilizes spinal 5-HT (serotonin) to exert its analgesic effect[43]. The endocannabinoid system, suppression of inducible nitric oxide synthase, the adrenergic system, and the cholinergic system have all been proposed to play a role in the analgesic action of acetaminophen[44]. It is commonly accepted that the antipyretic effect of acetaminophen involves the inhibition of COX[45]. At normal doses acetaminophen has good digestive tolerance, does not alter hemostasis, and does not induce nephrotoxicity.

Some clinicians use acetaminophen as the first line of analgesic therapy in dogs with renal compromise where NSAIDs cannot be used or in dogs that appear to be otherwise intolerant to NSAIDs (e.g. vomiting or GI ulceration)[46]. Acetaminophen can be used on its own or in a preparation combined with codeine and is initially dosed at approximately 10–15 mg/kg *bid*.

Combination acetaminophen and opioids

Codeine

Tylenol #3: 30 mg codeine + 300 mg acetaminophen.
Tylenol #4: 60 mg codeine + 300 mg acetaminophen.

Oxycodone

2.5 mg oxycodone HCl + 325 mg acetaminophen.
5 mg oxycodone HCl + 325 mg acetaminophen.
7.5 mg oxycodone HCl + 325 mg acetaminophen.
7.5 mg oxycodone HCl + 500 mg acetaminophen.
10 mg oxycodone HCl + 325 mg acetaminophen.
10 mg oxycodone HCl + 650 mg acetaminophen.

Hydrocodone

Vicodin contains 500 mg paracetamol and 5 mg hydrocodone.
Vicodin ES contains 750 mg paracetamol and 7.5 mg hydrocodone.
Vicodin HP contains 660 mg paracetamol and 10 mg hydrocodone.

Ketoprofen

Ketoprofen is a COX-1-selective NSAID, and is purported to provide some 5-LOX inhibition. Ketoprofen is not registered for use in cats or dogs in the USA. It is licensed for short-term use in the cat and dog and medium to long-term use in the dog at a reduced dose rate in the UK.

Tolfenamic acid

Tolfenamic acid injection is licensed in the UK for use in cats with upper respiratory disease in conjunction with antibiotics as an antipyretic; and in dogs for postoperative pain and inflammation. A 3-day treatment regimen is to be followed by 4 days of no medication. (Author's comment: this often leads to poor pet owner compliance.)

Cinchophen

Cinchopen was introduced in 1910 as a treatment for gout. It is used in experimental animals to cause gastric ulcers and is associated with liver toxicity. Cinchophen is chemically related to salicylate, and is associated with poor safety.

Phenylbutazone

Phenylbutazone is registered for use in dogs in the USA (and cats in Europe); however, its use in small animals is not common because of its toxicity profile (GI ulceration, renal failure, and bone marrow depression). The major use of phenylbutazone is in horses.

Among the 'contemporary' NSAIDs available in companion animal practice, four compounds tend to lead the market: carprofen, deracoxib, meloxicam, and firocoxib.

Carprofen

Carprofen is approved in oral and injectable formulations to treat pain and inflammation associated with osteoarthritis and postoperative pain associated with surgery in dogs. The injectable formulation has a different pharmacokinetic profile than the tablet: C_{max} of 8.0 µg/ml at 1.5–8 hours *vs.* C_{max} of 16.9 µg/ml at 0.5–3 hours, respectively[47]. Carprofen is a member of the arylpropionic acid class of NSAIDs and is COX-2 selective. Its classification as a COX-1-sparing NSAID is controversial. Carprofen has been associated with idiosyncratic hepatotoxicosis (as differentiated from hepatopathy, an increase in liver enzymes). The manufacturer reports the incidence of hepatic adverse events in dogs treated with carprofen is less than 0.06%[48]. In some countries a single injectable dose of carprofen is approved for pain relief in cats. Some suggest carprofen's COX activity is insufficient to explain its clinical efficacy, proposing that it may act through inhibition of the activation of nuclear factor kappa-B (NF-κB)[49].

Deracoxib

Deracoxib was the first coxib-class NSAID approved for veterinary use. It has been shown to be both COX-1 sparing and COX-2 selective both *in vitro* and *in vivo*[50,51]. Deracoxib has demonstrated effective analgesia for acute postoperative pain following cruciate ligament stabilization[52] as well as pain relief in canine clinical trials of osteoarthritis and dental pain[53,54]. More recently, deracoxib was shown to have similar activity to piroxicam in controlling canine transitional cell carcinoma[55]. COX inhibition is thought to play a major role in the antitumor effects of COX inhibitors, although effects independent of COX have been reported. Lascelles *et al.*[2] reported on a series of deracoxib ADEs focusing on GI complications. The investigators' conclusion was that most cases were associated with inappropriate NSAID use (overdosing and/or concurrent use with a different NSAID or corticosteroid). Originally, the drug was launched with two dosing recommendations: 3–4 mg for perioperative use, and 1–2 mg/kg for long-term use. Unfortunately, the former dose was approved and propagated before the latter. As a consequence, the higher dose was used by many clinicians for an extended period. Lascelles' paper strongly suggested that the lower dose be used for all scenarios. This paper (and others) gave recognition that for most NSAIDs, ADEs were approximately 64% GI, 21% renal, and 14% hepatic. Due to the limited data on pharmacokinetics in cats, deracoxib use is discouraged in this species.

Firocoxib

Firocoxib is a COX-1-sparing, COX-2-selective NSAID approved for the management of pain and inflammation associated with canine osteoarthritis. Its clinical efficacy and ADE profile has not been demonstrated to be different from other coxib-class NSAIDs. Firocoxib has a relatively low safety margin and overdoses of 3-, 5- or 10-times the recommended therapeutic dose were associated with adverse side-effects in registration trials, some of them serious or fatal. It is not tolerated as well in puppies as in older dogs, and palatability is relatively low at 68.5%. Based on registration trials, efficacy of firocoxib appears not to be inferior to meloxicam, etodolac, and carprofen.

Meloxicam

Meloxicam is a member of the oxicam family of NSAIDS, and is both COX-1 sparing and COX-2 selective. The elixir presentation is a highly palatable, honey-based presentation. Since 2003, the oral (liquid) formulations of meloxicam have been licensed in the USA for use in dogs only, with the January 2005 product insert specifically warning in bold-face type: '**Do not use in cats**'. An injectable formulation for use in dogs was approved by the FDA in November 2003, with a formulation for cats, for surgical use only, approved in October, 2004.

In the USA, per the manufacturer's clinical instructions as of July 2010, injectable meloxicam is indicated in operative use with felines as a single, one-time dose only, with specific and repeated warnings not to administer a second dose. In June 2007, a new oral version of meloxicam was licensed in Europe for the long-term relief of pain in cats. As of June 2008, meloxicam is registered for long-term use in cats in Australia, New Zealand, and throughout Europe.

The liquid oral formulation is available as both 1.5 mg/ml and 0.5 mg/ml; while the SC injectable solution is available as 5 mg/ml.

Along with the introduction of new pain management drugs over the past several years, has also come the development of new delivery forms. Meloxicam trasmucosal oral spray (OroCAM/RevitaCAM: Abbott Laboratories, North Chicago, IL) is such an example. This product is bioequivalent to the oral suspension[56], but is sprayed onto the buccal and/or gingival mucosal surfaces. Dosage for the control of pain and inflammation associated with osteoarthritis in dogs is 0.1 mg/kg, *sid*. The product is supplied in three vial sizes containing 6 ml, 11 ml, and 33 ml of meloxicam solution. Each vial has a different metered dose pump delivering a dose of 0.25 mg, 0.5 mg, or 1.075 mg meloxicam per spray, respectively.

In pharmacokinetic studies, maximum concentration (C_{max}) was achieved 2 hours after dosing, with a secondary peak or shoulder seen at 8 hours. Many characteristics of the product are similar to the oral solution; however, the T_{max} is 31% less. It is purported that the IC_{50} for plasma would be exceeded within 15 minutes after administration, contrasting with 30–60 minutes for oral dosing with the oral suspension[56]. This product feature demonstrates how first-pass metabolism by the liver can be avoided by mucosal mist application.

Given the innovative delivery form of this popular NSAID, with its COX-2 selectivity, COX-1-sparing features, and short time to plasma C_{max}, the transmucosal oral spray will find its place in clinical practice. Dog owner acceptance of the oral spray will dictate commercial success.

More recent NSAIDs

Mavacoxib, a triangular shaped, chewable tablet was introduced to the European Union (EU) market in late 2009. The approved indication is 'for the treatment of pain and inflammation associated with degenerative joint disease in dogs, in cases where continuous treatment exceeding 1 month is indicated'. This NSAID has focused on the concept of 'stronger-longer'. Mavacoxib is a monthly treatment (2 mg/kg), where the initial dose is given, repeated 14 days later, and then monthly dosed for up to a maximum of seven consecutive doses (6.5 months). The most common side-effects noted in the European Medicines Agency submission dossier were loss of appetite, diarrhea, and vomiting (consistent with the NSAID class of drugs).

In dogs, mavacoxib is intermediately specific to COX-2, with a COX-2/COX-1 ratio of 21.2. Mavacoxib tablets are COX sparing at recommended doses in dogs. The majority of the product is excreted in the feces. The tablet contains an artificial beef flavor (soybean origin) with desiccated pork liver powder. Investigating population pharmacokinetics of mavacoxib in osteoarthritic dogs, Cox *et al.*[57] reported that their model predicts a typical $T_{½}$ of 21 days in 1-year-old, 10 kg laboratory dogs. The model also predicts that young adult laboratory Beagle dogs (1–2 years of age) will have a $T_{½}$ that is typically 29–39% shorter than that of an identically sized, 10-year-old osteoarthritic patient.

Robenacoxib is a NSAID of the coxib class, which selectively inhibits COX-2. The active substance, robenacoxib, is a structural analog to diclofenac (**Fig. 86**). Robenacoxib is approved in the EU for both cats and dogs, while it is approved only for the cat (as of 2011) in the USA. Within the EU, robenacoxib is available as tablets and as a solution for injection, while in the USA it is available only as tablets for cats.

The approved EU indications are:

Tablets

Cats: Treatment of acute pain and inflammation associated with musculoskeletal disorders at a once daily dose of 1 mg/kg body weight for up to 6 days.

Dogs: Treatment of pain and inflammation associated with chronic osteoarthritis at a once daily dose of 1 mg/kg body weight as long as required (as directed by the veterinarian).

Solution for injection (single SC dose of 2 mg/kg, both dog and cat)

Cats: Treatment of pain and inflammation associated with soft tissue surgery.

Dogs: Treatment of pain and inflammation associated with orthopaedic or soft tissue surgery.

The approved USA indication:

Tablets

Cats: Treatment for the control of postoperative pain and inflammation associated with orthopedic surgery, ovariohysterectomy, and castration in cats ≥5.5 lbs (2.5 kg) and ≥6 months of age; 1mg/kg once daily for up to a maximum of 3 days.

Preoperatively: administer approximately 30 minutes prior to surgery.

Postoperatively: tablets may be given with or without food.

Dogs: Not approved in USA.

Solution for injection: not approved in USA.

No antimicrobial preservative is added to the injectable multidose preparation. Ethanol is present to enhance the preservative efficacy. The artificial beef flavor is only contained in the dog formulation and is sourced from desiccated pork liver powder and not of ruminant origin, associated with a risk of spongiform encephalopathy. T_{max} for the cat is 1 hour and 0.5 hours for SC injection and oral administration. The same is true for the dog. The systemic bioavailability of robenacoxib tablets is 49% in cats without food. In dogs, the average systemic bioavailability of robenacoxib tablets is 62% with food and 84% without food. Bioavailability was 88% after SC injection. The drug is rapidly metabolized by the liver in both cats and dogs. Robenacoxib is excreted predominately via the biliary route (65–70%) in both dogs and cats, with the remainder via the kidneys.

86

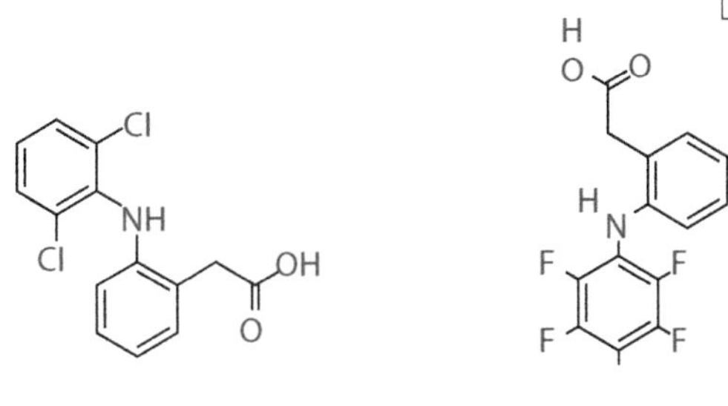

Cl NH Cl OH O

H O O H N F F F F

Fig. 86 Molecular structure of diclofenac (left); robenacoxib (right).

Clinical implication: some nonsteroidal anti-inflammatory drugs (NSAIDs) are more palatable than others, and tablet acceptance is often a challenge in the cat. NSAID acceptance can often be enhanced by 'top-dressing' with an extremely palatable agent, such as Viyo Recuperation™.

A number of publications have accompanied the introduction of robenacoxib to the market[58–65]. Consistently, robenacoxib has shown no inferiority to meloxicam, with a suggestion of improved safety based on inhibition of COX-1 (**Fig. 87**).

NSAID SAFETY

Comparative safety of different NSAIDs in dogs is difficult to determine. Such a query compares the incidence of problems with one NSAID to that of a second NSAID. Incidence would then be a ratio consisting of the number of dogs with problems (numerator) over the number of dogs treated with that drug over a period in time (denominator). Not all ADEs are reported and not all reported ADEs are directly causal, therefore the numerator is unknown. The denominator is also unknown, because it is impossible to determine the number of dogs on a drug at any given time. For these reasons, accurate comparative data are unobtainable.

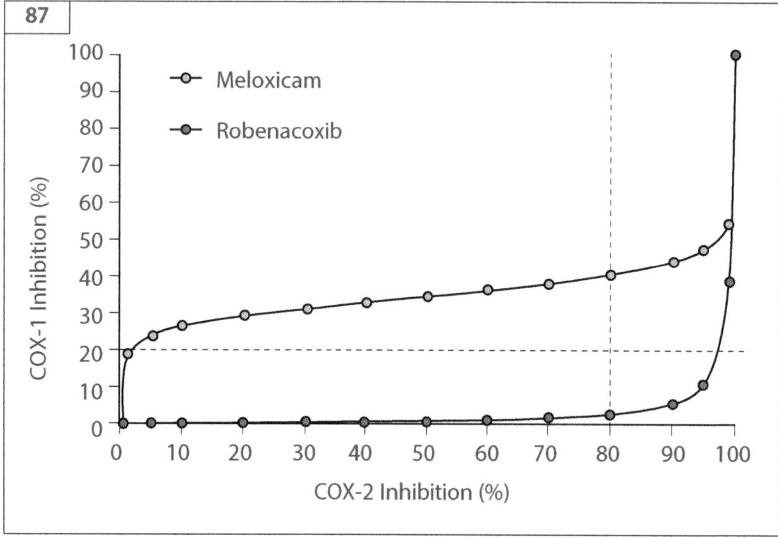

Fig. 87 Inhibition percentages of COX-2 and corresponding inhibition percentages of COX-1 for a range of concentrations of robenacoxib in the cat. Dotted lines indicate cut-off values for inhibition of COX-1 (20% inhibition COX-1 = percentage above which a risk of side-effects is assumed) and COX-2 (80% inhibition for COX-2 = percentage above which a good therapeutic effect is expected). Data for meloxicam, generated in a previous investigation, are included for comparison. (After Reference 61.)

Accordingly, most NSAID manufacturers can state with credibility, 'no NSAID has been proved safer than (XX)'. Nevertheless, all ADEs should be reported to the FDA and drug manufacturer so that general trends can be tracked and documented.

Clinical implication: currently, there is no process by which it can be proved that a given nonsteroidal anti-inflammatory drug (NSAID) is more safe than a different NSAID.

ADE reports at the USA FDA Center for Veterinary Medicine provide some insights as to why ADEs from NSAID use might be so high[66]:

- 23% of pet owners state that veterinarians never discuss adverse effects of the medication.
- 22% of pet owners state they are not given client information sheets about the prescribed drugs which are provided by pharmaceutical companies for the purpose of pet owner education.
- 14% of prescribed NSAIDs are dispensed in other than original packaging, thereby denying pet owners drug information provided on the label.
- only 4% of pet patients prescribed drugs are given preadministration blood analyses.

As a class of drug, NSAIDs are most commonly associated with adverse reactions to the GI tract (64%), renal system (21%), and liver (14%), respectively[66]. There is no published information relating to similar feline ADEs with NSAIDs. GI problems associated with NSAIDs can be as benign as regurgitation or as serious as gastric ulceration and perforation. Vomiting has been identified as the most frequent clinical sign associated with gastric perforation[66]. Pet owners should be informed that while taking an NSAID, if their pet experiences vomiting, the drug should be stopped and the patient should promptly be examined. This is a conservative approach since dogs are considered a 'vomiting species' and some NSAIDs are associated with more vomiting than others (*Table 53*).

TABLE 53: Gastrointestinal adverse events reported in USA clinical trials

Drug	Vomiting	Diarrhea
Carprofen	3.1% (3.8)	3.1% (3.8)
Etodolac	4.3% (1.7)	2.6% (1.7)
Deracoxib	2.9% (3.8)	2.9% (1.9)
Tepoxalin	2.0% (4.8) at 7 days 19.6% at 28 days	4.0% (0) at 7 days 21.5% at 28 days
Meloxicam	25.5% (15.4)	12.1% (7.4)
Firocoxib	3.9% (6.6)	0.8% (8.3)

Values represent mean of test article (placebo)
Data sourced from drug inserts. Caution should be used in comparing adverse events among different drugs because of differences in study populations, data collection methods, and reporting methods

NSAID-associated GI ulceration

Gastric perforations are most frequently found near the pyloric antrum of the stomach and have a poor prognosis if not discovered early and treated aggressively[2,26]. Risk factors identified with NSAID-associated gastric ulceration are most commonly seen with inappropriate use: 1) overdosing; 2) concurrent use of multiple NSAIDs; and 3) concurrent use of NSAIDs with corticosteroids. For nearly 50 years 'steroid ulceration' has been recognized with the sole use of corticosteroids, attributed to a steroid-induced gastric hypersecretion of acid together with a decreased rate of mucus secretion[67].

Lascelles *et al.*[2] observed that 23/29 GI perforations in a NSAID retrospective review occurred in the area of the pyloric antrum (**Fig. 88**). Reasons for this anatomical focus being at higher risk include speculation that it is subject to recurrent bathing by irritable bile reflux through the pylorus. Apart from a few studies that have examined the effect of NSAIDs on gastric mucosal production of prostanoids[17,68,69], COX selectivity has largely been determined using *in vitro* assays, and assumptions have been made about GI effects based on these *in vitro* data. Given the variability in results from *in vitro* assays, and the lack of understanding of COX physiology in the canine proximal GI tract, making assumptions about the clinical effects of various NSAIDs based on *in vitro* data may lead to erroneous conclusions.

Wooten *et al.*[70] reported an assessment of the *in vivo* action of NSAIDs in the region of the GI tract which appears to be at greatest risk for ulceration in the dog. Purpose-bred mongrel dogs were given a COX-1-selective NSAID (ASA 10 mg/kg *bid* PO), a COX-2-preferential NSAID (carprofen 4.4 mg/kg *sid* PO), and a COX-2-selective NSAID (deracoxib 2 mg/kg *sid* PO), or placebo for 3 days, with a 4-week washout period between treatments. Endoscopic mucosal biopsies were obtained from the pyloric and duodenal mucosa, and evaluated histologically, measuring COX-1 and COX-2 protein expression with Western blotting and prostanoids via enzyme-linked immunosorbent assay (ELISA) (**Fig. 89**). This investigation can be considered clinically relevant as it reflects the effect of a drug treatment on the actual tissue levels of prostanoids, not the drug effect on the total possible production of prostanoids by a tissue, as has previously been inferred from *in vitro*-sourced COX ratios.

Remember: *in vivo* refers to data obtained in the live animal, whereas *in vitro* refers to data obtained in the laboratory.

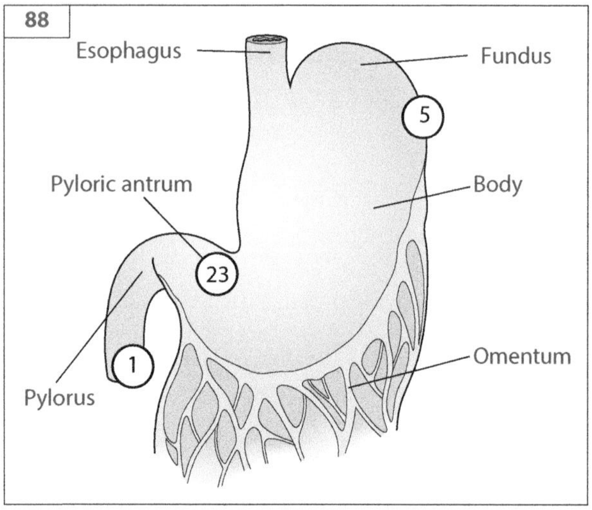

Fig. 88 In a retrospective nonsteroidal anti-inflammatory drug-associated gastrointestinal perforations study, 23/29 perforations were identified in the pyloric antrum[2].

PG levels were found to be significantly higher in the pylorus than in the duodenum, which may be explained by differences in COX expression in the pylorus *vs.* the duodenum, where the need for protection from refluxed bile is high. The 'more traditional' NSAIDs (ASA and carprofen) decreased the total concentration of PGs in the gastric mucosa, while PG levels were not altered by the coxib-class NSAID (deracoxib).

Thromboxane (TX) has been shown to be indicative of COX-1 activity in the GI tract of several species[71]; however, TXB_2 linkage to COX-1 activity in the canine GI tract is speculated, but not confirmed. Carprofen administration also significantly reduced TXB_2 concentrations compared to deracoxib, suggesting that carprofen inhibits COX-1 in the gastric mucosa, whereas deracoxib had no effect on TXB_2 (COX-1) concentrations.

Other investigators have reported *in vivo* findings for commonly used NSAIDs. Sessions *et al.*[68] reported that carprofen and deracoxib were both COX-1 sparing, while Punke *et al.*[72] reported that firocoxib and meloxicam were COX-1 sparing, and tepoxalin was not.

Findings from these studies demonstrate that different NSAIDs reduce prostanoid production

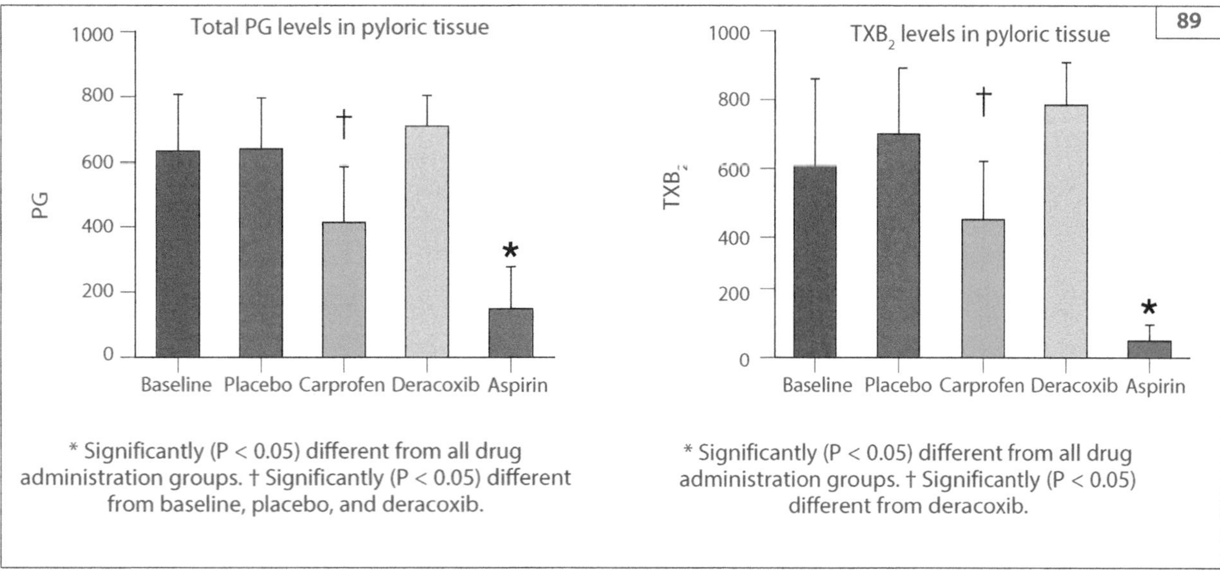

Fig. 89 Total prostaglandin (PG) and thromboxane B_2 (TXB_2) pyloric tissue levels in an *in vivo* study of traditional *vs*. coxib-class nonsteroidal anti-inflammatory drug[70].

by a different degree in the canine pylorus and duodenum, and this appears to be related to their COX selectivity. This begs the question, why NSAIDs that appear to be highly selective for COX-2 have been shown to be apparently associated with perforating ulcers in the pylorus and duodenum of the dog. To date, the only study assessing the association between a selective COX-2 inhibitor (deracoxib) and gastroduodenal perforation revealed that in almost all cases (26/29) of ulceration in dogs receiving the coxib-class NSAID, an inappropriately high dose, or concurrent administration with other NSAIDs or corticosteroid, or rapid switching (<24 hours) from one NSAID to another was identified[70]. This suggests that when GI perforation occurs following administration of a selective COX-2 inhibitor, other factors, such as over-dosing, concurrent administration of drugs inhibiting prostanoid production, rapid change from one NSAID to another, or hitherto unrecognized factors, play a major role in the production of ulceration. This is corroborated by documentation that 75–80% of all ADE reports with deracoxib use are associated with inappropriate use[73].

Clinical implication: it is imperative that pet owners be well-informed regarding appropriate drug dose, dosing interval, and the potential risk associated with concurrent use of multiple medications.

NSAIDs and renal function

Through regulation of vascular tone, blood flow, ion and water balance, and renin, PGs are important for normal renal function[74]. In situations of decreased systemic blood pressure or circulating blood volume, PGs assist to regulate and maintain renal blood flow to maintain a mean arterial pressure ranging from 60 to 150 mmHg[75]. Both the COX-1 and the COX-2 isoforms are expressed in the kidney of dogs, rats, monkeys, and humans where they both play constitutive roles (**Fig. 90**).

NSAID complications associated with hypovolemia and hypotension have led to acute renal failure and death in both dogs and cats[76]. Information regarding COX-1 and COX-2 distribution or expression under varying conditions of the feline kidney is unknown. Meloxicam is, perhaps, the most frequently administered NSAID in cats, and repeated (off label) use has been associated with acute renal failure in cats. (In 2010 the Metacam® USA label was changed to read: 'Warning. Repeated use of meloxicam in cats has been associated with acute renal failure and death. Do not administer additional injectable or oral meloxicam to cats. See contraindications warnings and precautions for detailed information'.)

Clinical implication: at recommended dosing, no one nonsteroidal anti-inflammatory drug is safer than another on renal function in dogs and cats.

Blood urea nitrogen and creatinine elevations occur relatively late in renal disease, therefore screening urine for protein has been suggested for early disease detection. Any positive screening result should be followed by measurement of urine protein:creatinine ratio for a more complete assessment. Any patient with compromised renal function is at risk with any NSAID administration.

NSAIDs and hepatic function

Serious liver injury can occur from acetaminophen (paracetamol) overdose in humans and dogs (>10 mg/kg, *bid*). Technically, acetaminophen is not a true NSAID since it is considered analgesic but not anti-inflammatory. Acetaminophen toxicity in cats presents primarily as methemoglobinemia and Heinz body anemia, likely from enhanced susceptibility of feline erythrocytes to oxidative injury[77]. Acetaminophen should not be administered to cats.

Clinical implication: since acetaminophen is not a 'true' nonsteroidal anti-inflammatory drug (NSAID), it can be used together with traditional or coxib-class NSAIDs in the dog.

Drug-induced hepatopathy (defined as an elevation of liver enzyme values) is a rare, but potentially serious adverse consequence of several drug classes, including NSAIDs, volatile anesthetics, antibiotics, antihypertensives, and anticonvulsants. This can occur with all NSAIDs. In comparison, idiosyncratic hepatotoxicosis has become associated with the rare (estimated 0.02% incidence[78]) lethal liver toxicity of carprofen. All dogs with hepatotoxicosis have a hepatopathy (increase of liver enzyme values) (*Table 54*, **Fig. 91**); however, not all cases of hepatopathy are lethal. This hepatotoxicosis does not appear to be associated with dose or duration of administration, and no epidemiologic study has shown the hepatotoxicosis to be breed-related. A hypothesis for carprofen-related hepatotoxicosis is that reactive acyl glucuronide metabolites are generated that can covalently bind and heptenize hepatocyte proteins, thereby promoting a toxic immunologic response in the liver[79–81].

TABLE 54: Approximate plasma half-life of hepatic enzymes in the dog and cat

Enzyme	Dog	Cat
Alanine aminotransferase	40–61 h	3.5 h
Aspartate aminotransferase	12 h	1.5 h
Glutamate dehydrogenase	18 h	–
Alkaline phosphatase		
Hepatobiliary isoenzyme	66 h	6 h
Corticosteroid isoenzyme	74 h	–
Intestinal isoenzyme	6 min	2 min

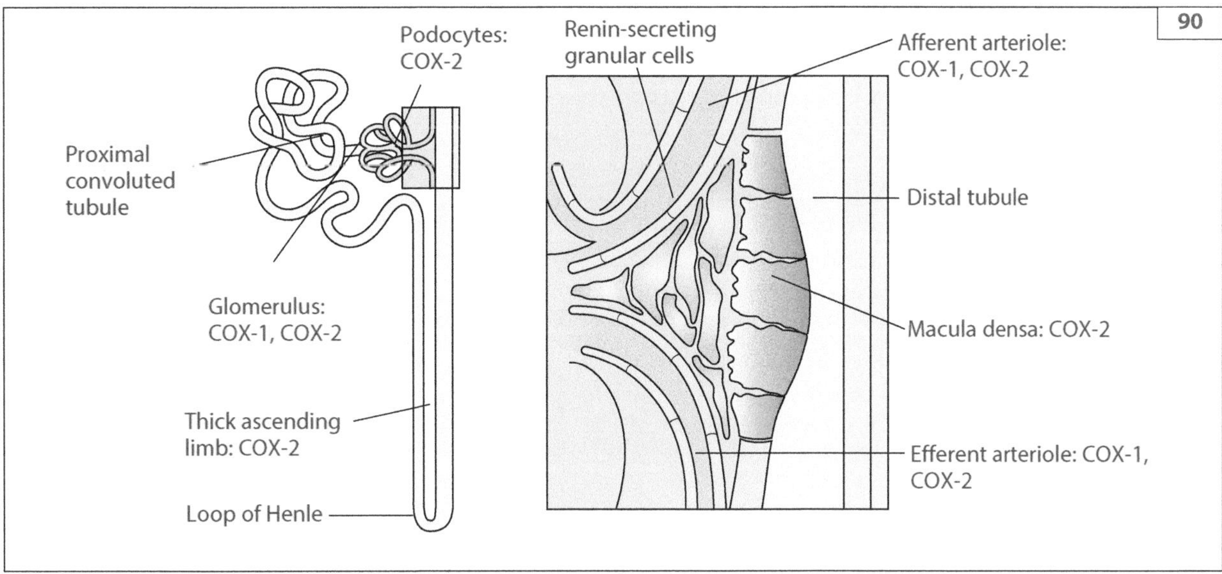

Fig. 90 Cyclo-oxygenase (COX) presence in the kidney.

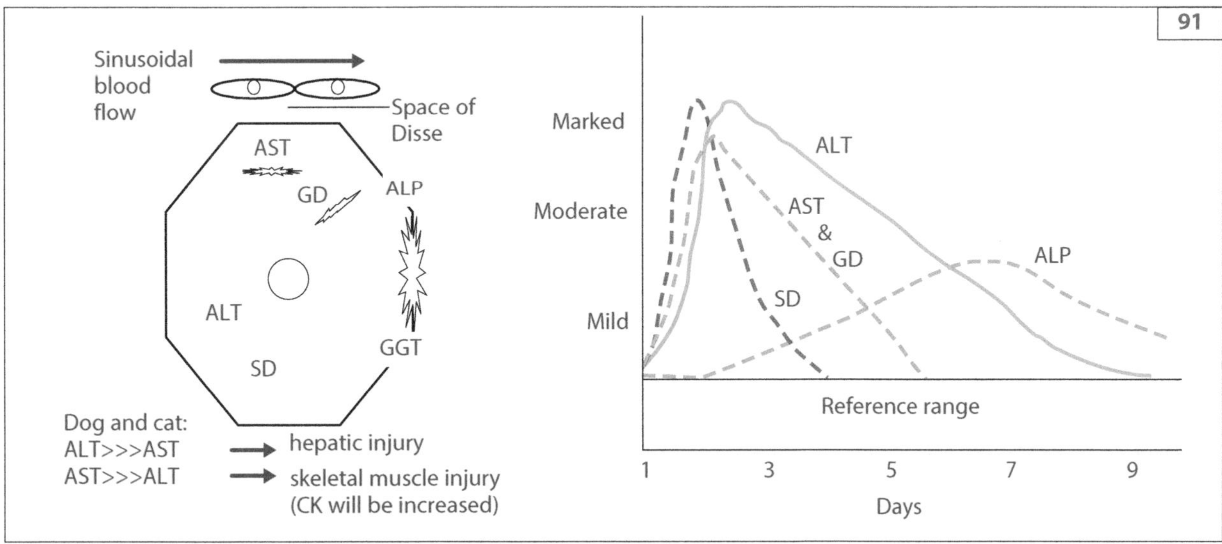

Fig. 91 Subcellular location of hepatobiliary enzymes and relative magnitude and duration of increase of plasma activities following acute, severe, diffuse injury to the liver. ALP: alkaline phosphatase; ALT: alanine aminotransferase; AST: aspartate aminotransferase; CK: creatine kinase ; GD: glutamine dehydrogenase; GGT: γ -glutamyltransferase; SD: sorbitol dehydrogenase.

It is well advised to characterize liver enzymes before and during NSAID administration, especially when an NSAID is being administered long-term. However, an increase in liver enzymes is difficult to interpret, as any chronic drug administration can cause an elevation, and liver enzymes are not a good measure of hepatic function. When liver enzymes are elevated and concern for liver function is present, liver function tests should be performed (**Fig. 92**). Mere elevation of liver enzymes may not be cause for discontinuing an NSAID.

Commonly used OTC NSAIDs are presented in *Table 55*.

Akaline phosphatase (ALP) has a high **sensitivity** for the detection of liver disease (86%), but poor **specificity** for liver disease (49%). 39% of all dogs and 51% of dogs over 8 years have increased ALP activity.

TABLE 55: Commonly used over-the-counter (OTC) nonsteroidal anti-inflammatory drugs

OTC brand	Generic name
Actron®	Ketoprofen
Advil®	Ibuprofen
Aleve®	Naproxen sodium
Bayer®	Aspirin
Ecotrin®	Aspirin
Excedrin®	Aspirin, acetaminophen, and caffeine
Motrin IB®	Ibuprofen
Nuprin®	Ibuprofen
Orudis KT®	Ketoprofen

Antiulcer agents

One goal of antiulcer treatment is to lower intragastric acidity so as to prevent further destruction of the GI tract mucosa. Cimetidine, a histamine H_2-receptor blocker, is commonly used. Cimetidine requires dosing 3- to 4-times daily; however it is not effective in preventing NSAID-induced gastric ulceration. Omeprazole is a substituted benzimidazole that acts by inhibiting the hydrogen-potassium adenosine triphosphate (ATP)ase (proton pump inhibitor) that is responsible for production of hydrogen ions in the parietal cell. It is 5- to10-times more potent than cimetidine for inhibiting gastric acid secretion and has a long duration of action, requiring once-a-day administration (*Table 56*). Omeprazole may be useful in decreasing gastric hyperacidity, but has minimal effect on ulcer healing. Misoprostol is a synthetic PGE_1 analog used to prevent gastric ulceration. It decreases gastric acid secretion, increases bicarbonate and mucus secretion, increases epithelial cell turnover, and increases mucosal blood flow. Both cimetidine and misoprostol require dosing 3- to 4-times daily and adverse reactions mimic those of gastritis and ulcerations.

Washout

Washout between NSAIDs is poorly researched. However, one survey report suggests that failure to implement a washout between different NSAIDs may put the patient at risk for GI pathology[2]. One must consider the reason for changing NSAIDs when considering a washout period. If the reason for change is efficacy, in the healthy dog 'washout' is a lesser issue than if the reason for change is intolerance. With intolerance, a minimal washout time should be no less than the time required to recover from adverse clinical signs. Most agree that washout following ASA is a unique scenario, due in part to the phenomena of ATL[34]. Five to 10 days washout following ASA is probably adequate.

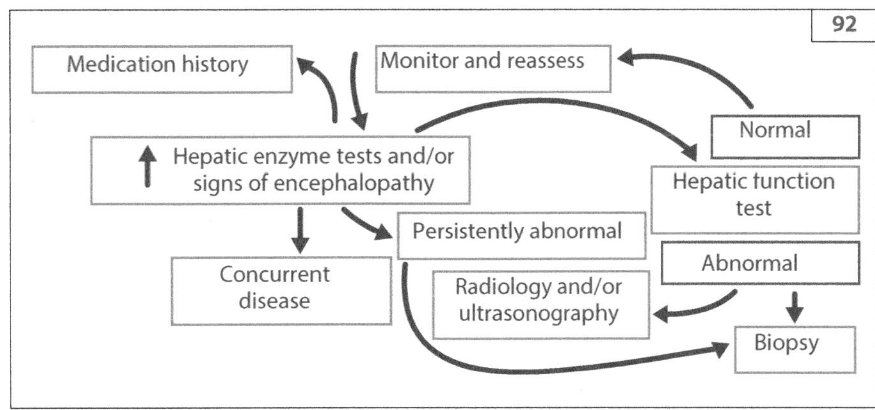

Fig. 92 Simplified algorithm for investigation of abnormal hepatic tests in an animal without severe anemia. Concurrent extrahepatic diseases, such as lymphocytic–plasmacytic enteritis, pancreatitis, heart failure, and endocrinopathies, can cause hepatic tests to be abnormal.

TABLE 56: Pharmacologic agents for nonsteroidal anti-inflammatory drug gastrointestinal prophylaxis and treatment

Group	Generic name	Brand name	Dose
Proton pump inhibitor	Omeprazole	Prilosec	Canine: 0.7 mg/kg, PO
	Lansoprazole	PrevAcid	
	Rabeprazole	AcipHex	
	Pantoprazole	Protonix	
	Esomeprazole	Nexium	
Prostaglandin analog	Misoprostol	Cytotec	Canine: 2-5 g/kg, *tid*, PO
H_2 blocker	Cimetidine	Tagament	Canine/Feline: 10 mg/kg,*tid*, PO, IV, IM Feline: 3.5 mg/kg, *bid*, PO or 2.5 mg/kg, *bid*, IV
	Ranitidine	Zantac	Canine: 2 mg/kg, *tid*, PO, IV
	Famotidine	Pepcid	Canine/Feline: 0.5 mg/kg, *sid*, PO, IV, IM, SC or 0.25 mg/kg, *bid*, PO, IV, IM, SC
	Nizatidine	Axid	Canine: 2.5-5 mg/kg, *sid* PO
Mucosal sealant	Sucralfate	Carafate	Canine: 0.5-1 g, *tid-bid*, PO Feline: 0.25 g, *tid-bid*, PO

One study has been conducted where injectable carprofen was followed at the next *sid* dosing with deracoxib[82]. In this study of a limited number of healthy dogs, no difference was noted in following injectable carprofen with either oral carprofen or oral deracoxib. Pain relief during a washout period can be obtained by the use of other class drugs, for example acetaminophen, tramadol, amantadine, gabapentin, or opioids.

Clinical implication: there is no evidence base for a specific 'washout period' between different nonsteroidal anti-inflammatory drugs (NSAIDs) or NSAIDs and a corticosteroid.

Enhancing responsible NSAID use

Every pet who is discharged with medication, including NSAIDs, should have the following questions addressed:

- What is the medication supposed to do?
- What is the proper dose and dosing interval?
- What potential adverse response(s) are possible?
- What should the owner do if an adverse response is observed?

Both verbal and written instructions should be given to the owner. Preadministrative urinalysis and blood chemistries are well advised prior to dispensing NSAIDs for two primary reasons. Firstly, the pet may be a poor candidate for any NSAID, that is it may be azotemic or have decreased liver function. (These physiologic compromises may not preclude the use of NSAIDs, but such a determination must be justified.) Secondly, a baseline status should be established for subsequent comparison, should the patient show clinical signs suggestive of drug intolerance. For the patient on a long-term NSAID protocol, the frequency of laboratory profiling should be determined by clinical signs and age. Minimal effective dose (MED) should always be the therapeutic objective, and routine examinations of the animal constitutes the practice of good medicine. Since alanine aminotransferase (ALT) is more specific than serum alkaline phosphatase (SAP) as a blood chemistry for liver status, an elevation 3–4-times laboratory normal should prompt a subsequent liver function test. Because the kidney expresses both COX isozymes constitutively, no one NSAID can be presumed safer than another for renal function, and any patient that is hypotensive or insufficiently hydrated is at risk for NSAID administration.

NSAIDs play a major role in a perioperative protocol for healthy animals, due to their features as anti-inflammatories, analgesics, and antipyretics. NSAID inclusion helps prevent CNS 'wind-up' and provides synergism with opioids[83]. Surgery cannot be performed without resultant iatrogenic inflammation, and the best time to administer the anti-inflammatory drug is pre-emptively (before the surgery). It is imperative that surgical patients be sufficiently hydrated if NSAIDs are used perioperatively. Under the influence of gaseous anesthesia, renal tissue may suffer from under-perfusion, at which point PGs are recruited to assist with this perfusion, and if the patient is under the influence of an anti-PG (NSAID), renal function may be at risk. In human medicine, some suggest that NSAIDs should not be withheld from adults with normal preoperative renal function because of concerns about postoperative renal impairment[84].

NSAIDs and bone healing

Among their many uses, COX inhibitors (NSAIDs) are widely administered for musculoskeletal conditions, including post-surgical orthopedic analgesia. It has been hypothesized that these agents may modulate bone, ligament, or tendon healing by inhibiting PG production. Results from animal models do suggest that NSAIDs and COX-2 inhibition may have a minimal effect on bone, tendon, and ligament healing, especially at earlier stages, but bear no significant impact on the ultimate long-term outcome. In a review on the subject[85], the authors proposed that despite the contribution of PGs in the dynamic process of normal bone healing and pathophysiology, alternative mechanisms may maintain normal bone function in the absence of COX-2 activity. Direct comparison studies suggest that retardation of bone healing from selective COX-2 inhibitors is lesser in magnitude than that from nonselective NSAIDs[78].

A tenet of support for internal fracture fixation is **early ambulation** and therefore increased vascularization to the healing bone. Analgesia also allows for early ambulation, thereby encouraging fracture repair through increased circulation.

COMPARATIVE NSAID EFFICACY

There are few objective pain assessment models for soft tissue, from which to compare NSAID efficacy. It is difficult to differentiate NSAID efficacy in the perioperative setting because most clinicians administer NSAIDs as part of a multimodal (balanced) analgesic protocol. Perioperative analgesia from an NSAID alone is rarely sufficient. Injectable carprofen was designed for perioperative use; yet for labeled IM administration, the injectable product has a different pharmacokinetic profile than the oral product, due to its mixed-micelle formulation. Given IM, the maximum concentration (C_{max}) of the injectable (C_{max}: 8.0 µg/ml at 1.5–8 hr) is half that of the oral formulation (C_{max}: 16.9 µg/ml at 0.5–3 hr), and is reached later[47]; suggesting that it be given several hours prior to surgery for maximal pain-preventive effect.

In contrast, force plate gait analysis in an orthopedic model has become the standard for ranking NSAID efficacy in canids on an objective basis[86]. Although several NSAID manufacturers have made public their studies comparing one or two products, none have compared the large group of NSAIDs most commonly used in clinical practice. Dr. Darryl Millis[87] and colleagues at the University of Tennessee reported such a study (**Fig. 93**), conducted independent of commercial support, using the force plate gait analysis model, which is considered to be the gold standard for objective assessment.

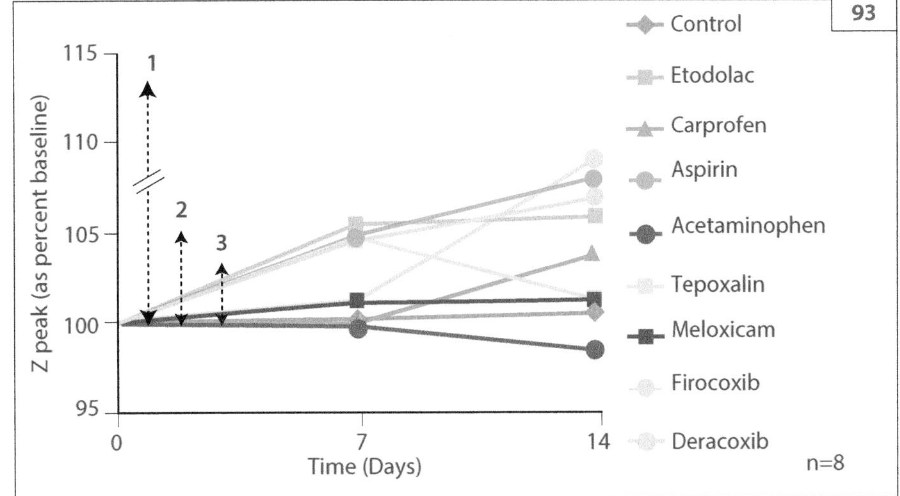

Fig. 93 Comparative efficacy of contemporary nonsteroidal anti-inflammatory drugs (NSAIDs) used in dogs. Responses from modalities other than NSAIDs are shown as double-ended arrows[86,116,117]. 1: approximate change seen with weight loss; 2: approximate change seen with high eicosapentaenoic acid diet; 3: approximate change seen with Dasuquin.

Measuring ground reaction forces is the most common way to assess weight bearing in dogs objectively. Using a force plate platform, investigators can compare, with certainty, the degree of lameness over a period of time. In its simplest terms, force plate gait analysis measures ground reaction forces that result when a dog places its limb during a specific gait. The three orthogonal ground reaction forces generated – vertical, craniocaudal, and mediolateral – represent the total forces transmitted through one limb to the ground. Typically, peak force in the vertical axis is used to measure limb function objectively. When comparing NSAID efficacy, lame dogs (often with long-standing anterior cruciate ligament compromise) are walked over a force plate during a given treatment regimen. Comparing the relative amount of weight placed by the compromised limb on the force plate under different NSAID regimens generates a relative rank of NSAID efficacy, or pain relief (**Fig. 94**, *Table 57*).

Kinematic gait analysis, or motion analysis, is used less frequently than force platform analysis, but its use is increasing, mostly in research laboratories. Kinematic evaluation measures changes in joint angles with gait, the velocity and acceleration of changes in joint angles, stride length, as well as gait swing and stance times. Kinematic evaluation is often combined with force platform gait analysis, providing a powerful method of detecting abnormalities and response to therapy.

TABLE 57: Comparison of nonsteroidal anti-inflammatory drug efficacy studies used for USA Food and Drug Adminstration approval

Drug	Primary assessment method	Ground reaction force assessment
Carprofen	Subjective owner and veterinary assessment indicated improvement more likely in treated dogs	No significant difference between placebo dogs and treated dogs
Etodolac	Ground reaction forces	Peak vertical force improved 0.4%, 2.3%, and 1.6% with placebo, low-dose, and high-dose treatments, respectively Vertical impulse improved 0.4%, 0.13%, and 0.22%, respectively
Deracoxib	Ground reaction forces	Peak vertical force improved 7.4% with treatment *vs.* placebo Vertical impulse improved 4.9% with treatment compared with placebo
Tepoxalin	Subjective changes compared with carprofen, no placebo comparison Subjective improvement similar to carprofen	Not measured
Meloxicam	Subjective assessment of lameness, weight bearing, pain on palpation, and overall improvement compared with placebo Significant improvement noted on Day 14 of one 14-day study Significant improvement noted in the parameter of overall assessment on Day 7 by veterinary assessors and on Day 14 by owners in a second study	Not measured
Firocoxib	Subjective comparison to etodolac No comparison to placebo Subjective efficacy comparable to etodolac	Ground reaction forces were determined in a subset of patients Results were comparable between firocoxib and etodolac

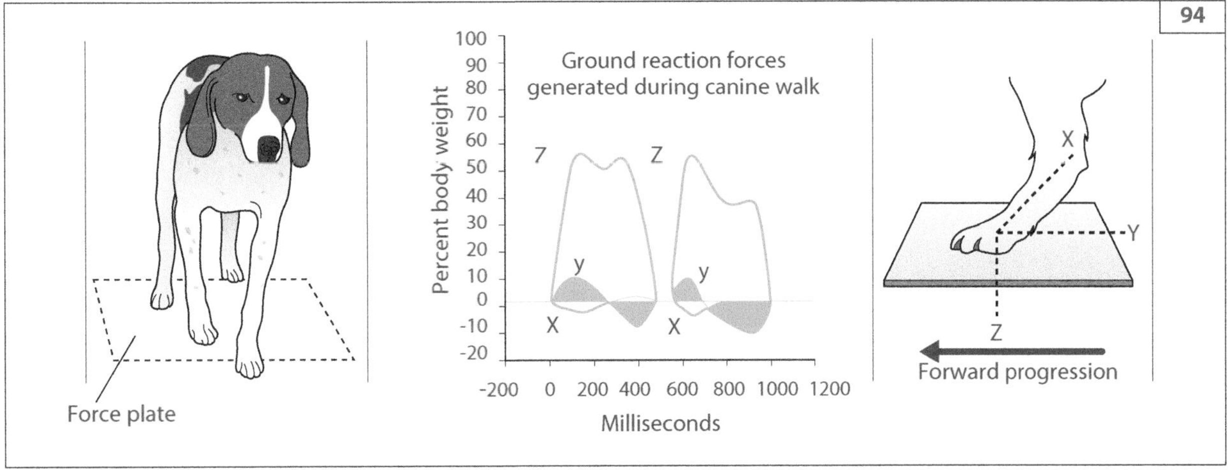

Fig. 94 Each gait generates a specific pattern of ground reaction forces. The first peak in vertical forces (Z) of the m-shaped pattern of the walk represents the peak vertical forces associated with initial paw strike. Y and X represent the craniocaudal and mediolateral forces, respectively. Breaking and propulsion impulses are indicated by the shaded areas of the craniocaudal graphs.

Objective measurement of lameness severity in cats is quite difficult, as cats do not comply with force plate protocols. However, pressure mats have been used to reveal the distribution of pressures associated with paw contact[88] so that pressures on each digital pad and on the metacarpal pad can be measured quantitatively following onychectomies. Use of the pressure mat to evaluate lameness in cats will likely see further development. The use of acceleration-based activity monitors may also allow for future objective measurement of improved mobility following treatment for degenerative joint disease (DJD) in the cat[89].

NSAID ADMINISTRATION

Time of administration (chronotherapy)

Time of administration is a common question arising from NSAIDs labeled for dosing once daily, that is should the drug be administered in the morning or in the evening? Some argue that morning administration is most logical, taking advantage of C_{max} during that time of the day when the dog might be most active. Others suggest the NSAID should be dosed so that C_{max} is reached to ensure maximal rest for the animal; proposing that the animal performs best following a good night's rest. There is no consensus.

With or without food

Many of the contemporary NSAIDs are labeled for use either with or without food. Administration with food takes advantage of the increased production of gastric bicarbonate and associated buffering. Feeding an NSAID together with food may enhance acceptability in some dogs.

NSAID compatibility with other agents

NSAIDs are highly protein bound and may compete with binding of other highly protein bound drugs, particularly in the hypoproteinimic animal, resulting in altered drug concentrations. Fortunately, the number of other highly protein bound drugs is minimal. Drugs and agents that may be influenced by the concurrent administration of NSAIDs are shown in *Table 58 p.183*.

Because pet owners tend to be using more and more 'natural' products, some of which can potentially influence the concurrent use of a NSAID, it is well advised to ask owners for a complete listing of everything they are giving their pet PO (*Table 59*).

NSAIDs and cancer

Human studies have shown that patients receiving long-term NSAID therapy have a reduced risk of colorectal cancer[90]. Such observations have led to researching the role of NSAIDs as a preventative measure against cancer development and as adjunctive antineoplastic therapy. Published data also suggest that control of oncologic pain can impact the course of cancer progression[91].

PGs play a major role in cancer development, including inhibition of immune surveillance, promotion of angiogenesis, and inhibition of apoptosis[92,93]. High levels of PGs are found in tumors of many types that may exert effects in an autocrine or paracrine fashion, and up-regulation of COX-2 has been directly associated with tumor aggression[94].

In addition to decreasing PG production via inhibition of COX-2, NSAIDs also have COX-independent anticancer mechanisms, including activation or inhibition of cellular signaling pathways via up-regulation or inhibition of oncogenes. Preliminary results of a study involving deracoxib, a COX-2-selective inhibitor, as therapy for transitional cell carcinoma, have demonstrated stable disease in nine of nine dogs[95]. Many oncologists are now prescribing COX-2 inhibitors in conjunction with traditional modalities of surgery, radiation therapy, and chemotherapy for a variety of tumors.

CATS AND NSAIDS

There are approximately 69 million cats in the USA[96] and approximately 10 million in the UK[97]. Radiographically detectable DJD is apparently as high as 90% in cats over 12 years of age[98]. Efficacy of NSAIDs for relief of chronic pain in the cat is difficult to demonstrate, but empirically embraced. Probable reasons for the relative void of evidence base for NSAIDs in cats include:

- Assumption by pharmaceutical manufacturers that the market for cat analgesics is not financially rewarding.
- Difficulty of identifying pain in cats, and therefore indications for administration.
- Scarcity of information about NSAIDs in cats.
- Potential risk of NSAID toxicity in cats.

Salicylate toxicity in cats is well established. Cats present a unique susceptibility for NSAID toxicity because of slow clearance and dose-dependent elimination (**Fig. 95**). Cats have a low capacity for hepatic glucuronidation of NSAIDs[99], which is the major mechanism of metabolism and excretion for this class of drug. Meloxicam and piroxicam are metabolized by oxidation, and therefore less affected by this constraint[100], as is robenacoxib. **Cats are particularly susceptible to acetaminophen toxicity** due, in part, to defective conjugation of the drug and conversion to a reactive electrolytic metabolite. Acetaminophen toxicity in cats results in methemaglobinemia, liver failure, and death.

Because of its delivery form as an elixir, meloxicam is sometimes used preferentially in small dogs and cats. Only carprofen injectable, meloxicam injectable, and robenacoxib are approved for use in the cat (country dependent). There are only limited data to support the safe chronic use of NSAIDs in cats[101]. The manufacturer of meloxicam has recommended reducing the original approval dose from 0.3 to 0.1 mg/kg because of some initial GI problems, and recent label warnings (USA) of acute renal failure have discouraged repeated use. In many regions of the world, meloxicam has been licensed for long-term use in cats. This suggests particular attention be given to accurate dosing of small dogs and cats. The NSAID robenacoxib, has been licensed for up to 6 days therapy in cats. As with all NSAIDs in dogs or cats, potentially causal gastric ulcerations have been observed. For most of the NSAIDs used in cats, it is not known if repeated long-term dosing alters the pharmacokinetics or pharmacodynamics of the drug. Further, considerable variability of NSAID pharmacokinetics between cats is noted and there is no practical way to differentiate 'fast' metabolizers from those that are slower. It is, therefore, unlikely that a set mg/kg dose and dosing schedule will work equally well for all cats in all pain states.

TABLE 58: Nonsteroidal anti-inflammatory drug (NSAID) potential drug interactions

Drug	May increase the toxicity of	May decrease the efficacy of	Toxicity may be increased by
Classical NSAIDs (clinically significant COX-1 inhibition)	Warfarin, methotrexate, valproic acid, midazolam, furosemide, spironolactone, sulfonylureas, heparin	Furosemide, thiazide, ACE inhibitors, β-blockers	Aminoglycosides, furosemide, cyclosporine (renal), glucocorticoids (GI), heparin, gingko, garlic, ginger, ginseng (hemorrhage)
Coxibs and relatively COX-2-selective agents	Warfarin, methotrexate, valproic acid, midazolam, furosemide, spironolactone, sulfonylureas	Furosemide, thiazides, ACE inhibitors, β-blockers	Aminoglycosides, furosemide, cyclosporine (renal), glucocorticoids (GI)
Phenylbutazone, acetaminophen	Warfarin, sulfonylureas		Phenobartital, alcohol, rifampin, metoclopramide

Trepanier LA (2005). Potential interactions between nonsteroidal anti-inflammatory drugs and other drugs. *J Vet Emergency and Critical Care* **15**(4):248–253.
ACE: angiotensin-converting enzyme; COX: cyclo-oxygenase; GI: gastrointestinal.

TABLE 59: Potential herb–drug interactions

Herb	Interacting drugs	Results
St. John's wort	Cyclosporine, fexofenadine, midazolam, digoxin, tacrolimus, amitriptyline, warfarin, theophylline	Decreased plasma drug concentrations
Ginkgo	Warfarin, heparin, NSAIDs, omeprazole	Bleeding Decreased plasma concentrations
Ginseng	Warfarin, heparin, NSAIDs opioids	Bleeding Falsely elevated serum digoxin levels (laboratory test interaction with ginseng) Decreased analgesic effect (laboratory test interaction with ginseng)
Garlic Chamomile Ginger	Warfarin Heparin NSAIDs	Bleeding

Goodman L, Trepanier L (2005). Potential drug interactions with dietary supplements. *Compendium* (SAP) October:780–789.
NSAID: nonsteroidal anti-inflammatory drug.

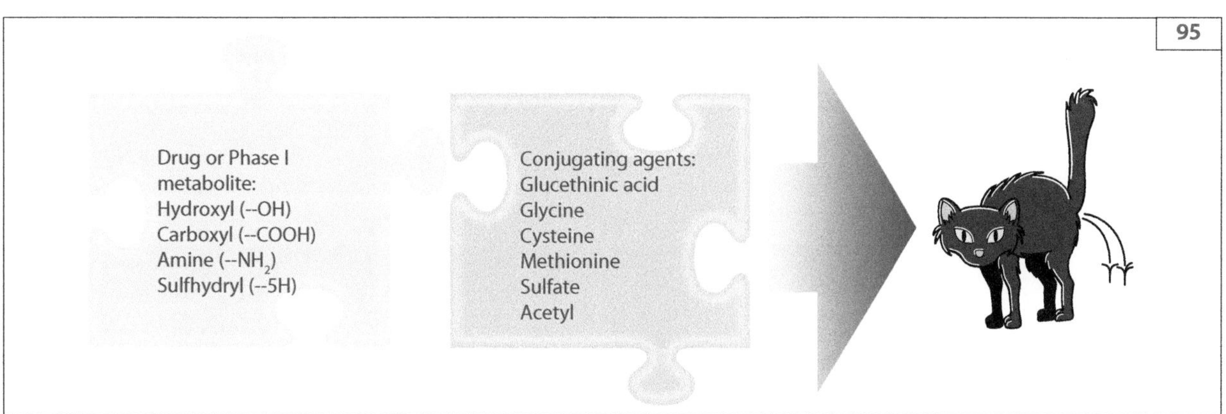

Fig. 95 Cats are deficient in the transferring enzyme glucuronly transferase, therefore the process of eliminating many drugs is slow, with enhanced potential for drug toxicity.

The most common cause of chronic feline pain (as in the dog) is thought to be DJD, affecting 60–90% of cats[102–111]. Dramatic responses have been reported from NSAID administration, indicating that there is a large opportunity for safe, effective long-term NSAID therapy within the population of aged cats with DJD. Control of protracted inflammation and pain is important in many other feline diseases. These include various cancers, particularly where definitive treatment is not possible, or in some cases for the antineoplastic effect an NSAID might offer[112–115].

LOOKING TO THE FUTURE

NSAIDs are the fastest growing class of drugs in both human and veterinary medicine because of their relatively safe resolution of a wide range of pathologic conditions. Based upon current understanding of their mode of action, future NSAIDs will likely **not** be developed to be 'stronger-longer' (i.e. supremely COX-2 selective, with a very long half-life). Instead, NSAID development may well offer species- and/or disease-specific molecules, increased safety profiles, and augmenting benefits, such as nitric oxide inhibition. At present this class of drug offers immense benefits, constrained most often only by issues of safe, responsible use.

Improving safety

The following guidelines can be used to minimize risk factors for NSAID ADEs:

- Proper dosing.
- Administer MED.
- Dispense in approved packaging together with owner information sheets.
- Avoid concurrent use of multiple NSAIDs and NSAIDs with corticosteroids.
- Refrain from the use of ASA.
- Provide pet owners with both oral and written instructions for responsible NSAID use.
- Conduct appropriate patient chemistry/urine profiling. Do not use in patients with reduced cardiac output or in patients with overt renal disease.
- Conduct routine check-ups and chemistry profiles for patients on chronic NSAID regimens. Do not fill NSAID prescriptions without conducting patient examinations.
- Caution pet owners regarding supplementation with OTC NSAIDs.
- Administer GI protectants for high at-risk patients on NSAIDs.
- Avoid NSAID administration in puppies and pregnant animals.
- NSAIDs may decrease the action of angiotensin-converting enzyme inhibitors and furosemide, a consideration for patients being treated for cardiovascular disease.
- Geriatric animals are more likely to be treated with NSAIDs on a chronic schedule, therefore their 'polypharmacy' protocols and potentially compromised drug clearance should be considered.
- Provide sufficient hydration to surgery patients administered NSAIDs.
- Report ADEs to the product manufacturers.

SUMMARY

NSAIDs are a magnificent class of agents that have changed the practice of both human and veterinary medicine. Their utilization will likely continue for decades to come as we learn more specific applications and features of these molecules. Additionally, NSAIDs are market leaders for pharmaceutical companies, and public awareness is a tenet in the overall marketing strategy for these agents. Consequently, this class of drugs is not only a fundamental cornerstone of medical practice, but also an area of public scrutiny. As with all medications, adverse reactions from NSAIDs are possible, however the benefits far out-weigh problems associated with their use. With responsible use of NSAIDs, we must always strive for the MED, within established dosing ranges, and assess the benefit:risk ratio for each individual patient.

Chapter 7

Nutraceutical Mechanisms and Therapy

INTRODUCTION

The widespread interest in nutraceuticals began in 1997 with publication of the book entitled, '*The Arthritis Cure*', by Dr. Jason Theodosakis[1]. Three years later, USA sales of nutraceuticals topped $640 million[2]. The world market for pet nutraceuticals was worth $960 million in 2004; about 60% of this was for dogs, 25% for cats, and 10% for horses[3]. Joint health products for pets accounted for nearly half of the market, followed by vitamins, minerals, amino acids, and antioxidants.

NUTRIGENOMICS

In 2004 the canine genome was mapped. In addition to insights into genetic disease, this breakthrough has enabled scientists to investigate how biochemical processes work at the level of gene expression. This has led to the science of nutrigenomics. In both humans and dogs, progression from a healthy phenotype to a chronic disease phenotype occurs by changes in gene expression or by differences in activities of proteins and enzymes. Since dietary factors participate in the regulation of gene expression, it is intuitive that a subset of genes regulated by diet must be involved in disease initiation, progression, and severity.

Genomics: the study of function, interactions and dynamics of all genes in the genome, including their interactions with environmental factors.

Nutrigenomics (nutritional genomics): the study of nutritional effects on gene expression.

A goal of nutrigenomics is to maintain and improve individual health and manage individuals with disease via personalized nutrition. This science involves studying how diet influences gene transcription, protein expression, and metabolism. Comparing the amount and type of specific gene transcripts between health states and between exposure to different nutritional regimens, the biologic routes that tissues take in terms of protein expression and metabolism can be identified. Such transcripts can then be used as markers to evaluate the effects of nutritional intervention on the animal as a whole. Use of such information allows nutrient strategies to be developed, with the potential to create 'functional foods' that might affect the clinical course of diseases, such as cancer, diabetes, osteoarthritis

(OA), and others. An example of nutrigenomic application is the popular utilization of high-eicosapentaenoic acid (EPA) diets for the management of canine osteoarthritis. When dietary EPA (20:5n-3) is substituted for arachidonic acid (AA; 20:4n-6) in the production of eicosanoids, a different and less inflammatory set of compounds results.

Nutrigenomics may reveal:

- The effects of nutrition on development, prevention, and treatment of canine diseases.
- The optimal concentration of nutrients appropriate for all life and development stages.
- The effects of nutritional factors on gene expression.
- The efficacy of nutraceuticals[4].

BACKGROUND

Nutraceutical, a term combining the words 'nutrition' and 'pharmaceutical', is a food or food product that provides health and medical benefits, including the prevention and treatment of disease. Nutraceuticals are natural, bioactive chemical compounds that have health promoting, disease preventing, or medicinal properties. They are prescribed drugs in a limited number of countries, but are primarily provided as dietary supplements delivered over-the-counter (OTC). A dietary supplement is a product that contains nutrients derived from food products that are concentrated in liquid or capsule form. **A supplement that can be administered orally to promote good health and is not a drug is considered a nutraceutical.** Functional foods, as differentiated, have components or ingredients added to give a specific medical or physiologic benefit, other than a purely nutritional effect. In Japan, functional foods must meet three requirements: 1) be presented in their naturally occurring form, rather than a capsule, tablet, or powder; 2) be consumed in the diet as often as daily; and 3) should regulate a biologic process in the hope of preventing or controlling disease[5]. Functional food is characterized (from traditional food) 'if it is satisfactorily demonstrated to affect beneficially one or more target functions in the body, beyond adequate nutritional effects in a way which is relevant to either the state of well-being and health or the reduction of the risk of a disease[6].

Dietary supplements are regulated in the USA by the Food and Drug Administration (FDA) in a different manner from either OTC or prescription drugs. As laid out in the USA Dietary Supplement Health and Education Act of 1994, the manufacturer is responsible for determining that the supplement is safe and that any representations or claims made about it are adequately substantiated. Dietary supplements do not need to be approved by the FDA before they are marketed, and subsequently do not carry consumer confidence of FDA-endorsement. There are literally hundreds-to-thousands of nutraceutical products in the marketplace, each with varying levels of evidence for safety or efficacy and great variability in compliance with labeled content claims.

Since the focus of these works is pain management, attention herein is given to the role of nutraceuticals as chondroprotectants, where they are purported to influence the commonly painful disease of OA.

Clinical implication: Buyer beware!

Degenerative joint disease (DJD) or OA poses major therapeutic problems in pets as well as humans. Treatment with nonsteroidal anti-inflammatory drugs (NSAIDs) is designed to reduce pain and inflammation, the hallmarks of the disease. Yet long-term use of NSAIDs, notably with complications of inappropriate use[7], has been associated with adverse effects, including gastrointestinal (GI) ulceration, hepatic toxicity, renal failure and, in some cases, negative effects on chondrocytes and cartilage[8]. Such issues have led researchers to seek alternatives/adjuncts to NSAIDs for managing OA (*Table 60*). Originally, these compounds were considered to serve as building blocks for cartilage and exogenous sources of cartilage matrix components. The long-standing rationale for using nutraceuticals is that provision of precursors of cartilage matrix in excess quantities may favor matrix synthesis and repair of articular cartilage. More recent findings (mostly *in vitro*) have shown that some nutraceuticals may play a major role in the development and progression of the 'total joint disease' OA process.

Chondrocytes are the only active cells in cartilage, responsible for the creation and maintenance of the cartilage matrix.

TABLE 60: Nutraceuticals used for osteoarthritis

Ascorbic acid	Hyaluronic acid
Avocado/soybean unsaponifiables	Hydrolysate collagen
Boswellia serrata	Methylsulfonylmethane
Bromelain	Milk and hyperimmune milk
Cat's claw	n3-PUFAs
Chondroitin sulfate	Phycocyanin
Cetyl myristoleic oil	*Ribes nigrum*
Collagen hydrolysate	*Rosa canina*
Curumin	SAMe
Chitosan	Selenium
Devil's claw	Strontium
Flavonoids	Silicium
Glucosamine SO4/ Acetyl/HCl	Turmeric Vitamin D
Green lipped mussel	Vitamin E
Ginger	Willow

PUFA: polyunsaturated fatty acid; SAMe: S-adenosylmethionine.

According to the North American Veterinary Nutraceutical Association (NAVNA), a nutraceutical is 'a non-drug substance that is produced in a purified form and administered orally to provide compounds required for normal body structure and function with the intent of improving health and well-being'. Further, the NAVNA defined a **chondroprotective** as an agent that intends to 'stimulate cartilage matrix production by chondrocytes, inhibit matrix degradation, and potentially inhibit periarticular microvascular thrombosis'. The two most popular nutraceuticals for OA are glucosamine and chondroitin sulfate.

Understanding the concepts

OA involves cartilage damage from enzymatic degradation of the extracellular matrix. This results in loss of proteoglycans and the cleavage of type II collagen[9]. Matrix metalloproteinases (MMPs) and aggrecanases play a major role among the degradative enzymes. MMPs are similar in structure but differ somewhat in their preferred substrates. Collagenases (MMP-1, -8, and -13) cleave the intact triple helix of collagen[10]. Thereafter, the collagen fragments are susceptible to further proteolysis by gelatinases (MMP-2 and -9), enzymes that can also cleave aggrecan[11]. Stromelysins (MMP-3, -10, and -11) are capable of degrading aggrecan, denatured type II collagen, and small proteoglycans of the extracellular matrix[12]. Aggrecanases are principal mediators of aggrecan degradation, releasing core protein and glycosaminoglycan (GAG) constituents of aggrecan into the synovial fluid[13]. A number of cytokines, most importantly interleukin (IL)-1, are considered central to the induction of degradative enzyme and inflammatory mediator synthesis. Cytokines appear to be first produced by cells of the synovial membrane[14] and later by activated chondrocytes[15]. Generally, IL-1 is presumed to enhance cartilage degeneration and inhibit efforts at repair.

The body does a poor job of repairing hyaline cartilage. Destruction goes either unresolved, or is replaced by fibrocartilage, an inferior form of cartilage. Appreciating the tight correlation between structure and function of cartilage, replacement of hyaline cartilage brings with it the inferior performance of fibrocartilage.

Therefore, it is imperative to retain hyaline cartilage as best as is possible (structure = function) (**Fig. 96, Fig. 97**).

To understand the supposition behind the use of nutraceuticals, and particularly chondroprotectives, several tenets must be understood. GAGs (**96**) are long chains of disaccharides. There are three major types in cartilage: chondroitin sulfate-4 and -6, keratin sulfate, and dermatin sulfate. Chondroitin is the prevalent form in cartilage. GAGs are vital in the hydration of cartilage, as they are the primary (negatively charged) water-binding constituents within the cartilage matrix.

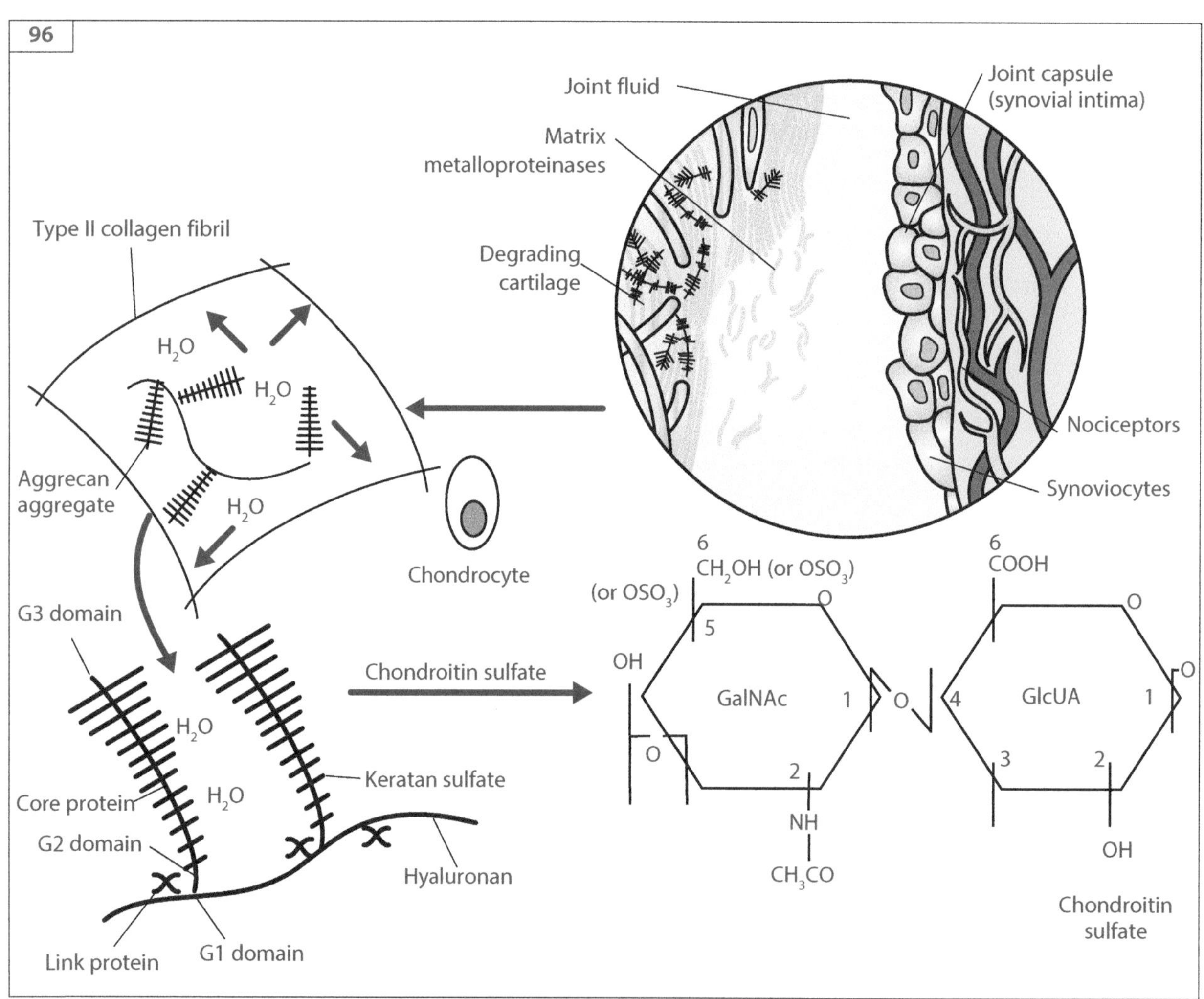

Fig. 96 Graphic illustrating the composition of normal hyaline (articular) cartilage. This cartilage manifests a strong correlation between structure and function.

CHONDROITIN SULFATE

Chondroitin sulfate is a long-chain polymer of galactosemine sulfate and gluceronic acid constituting the majority of GAGs. It is one of two primary GAGs responsible for binding of water in cartilage. The other primary GAG is keratin sulfate. Loss of GAGs, particularly chondroitin sulfate, occurs early in OA. This loss contributes to alterations in water binding in cartilage and subsequently to impaired cartilage mechanics and accelerated cartilage breakdown. Chondroitin sulfate appears to inhibit degradative enzymes, such as metallease, associated with OA. These degradative enzymes break down both cartilage matrix and hyaluronan in synovial fluid.

Hyaluronan is a component of both the cartilage matrix and synovial fluid.

Exogenous chondroitin-4 has been derived primarily from mammalian tissues, whereas chondroitin-6 is derived primarily from aquatic species, including shark, cartilage. The proposed mechanisms of action for chondroitin sulfate are somewhat similar to glucosamine (*Table 61*): stimulation of GAG synthesis, and inhibition of degradative enzyme synthesis, including MMPs. In contrast to glucosamine, chondroitin sulfate is known to inhibit IL-1-induced type II collagen degeneration[16], and improves synovial fluid viscosity by increasing hyaluronic acid concentration[17].

The molecular weight of chondroitin sulfate directly influences its absorption after oral administration, where higher GI permeability is achieved for low-molecular weight chondroitin sulfate[34]. The form and source of chondroitin sulfate also apparently influence its pharmacokinetic profile; in humans, chondroitin sulfate of bovine origin is superior to that obtained from shark cartilage, due to differences in molecular mass, degree of sulfation, and relative amounts of iduronate and glucuronate[35,36]. Due to size (range from 6 to 50 kDa), the form of chondroitin sulfate that is ultimately available after oral administration may be affected by intestinal degradation and metabolism within the liver[37]. The gastric mucosa contains several GAG-degrading enzymes, such as exoglycosidases, sulfatases, and hyaluronidase-like enzymes, capable of digesting chondroitin sulfate. This recognition, as well as the observation that charged molecules with a molecular mass exceeding about 180 kDa are unlikely to be absorbed without an active carrier system, suggest that perhaps the parent chondroitin sulfate is unlikely to be absorbed intact.

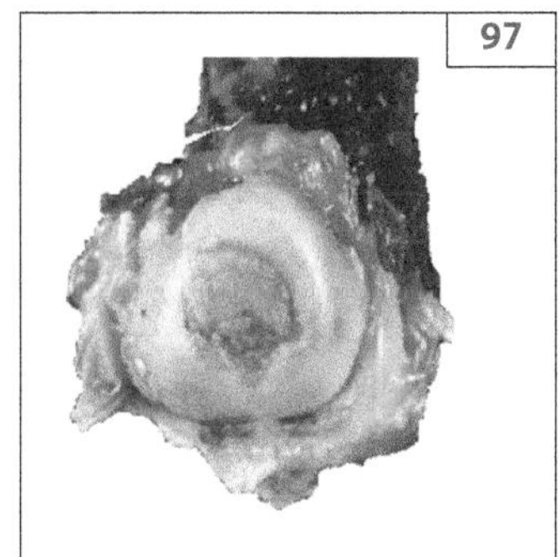

Fig. 97 Damaged sections of hyaline cartilage are often replaced with the inferior performing fibrocartilage.

TABLE 61: Proposed mechanisms of action for glucosamine and chondroitin sulfate. Each agent has been reported to have both proanabolic and anticatabolic or anti-inflammatory activities

Glucosamine
Stimulation of GAG synthesis[16,117]
Inhibition of COX-independent anti-inflammatory properties[19,20]
Inhibition of IL-1-stimulated gene expression or protease expression[21–27]
Chondroitin sulfate
Stimulation of synthesis of PG[28–31]
Inhibition of degradative enzymes and inhibition of IL-1-stimulated gene expression[17,32,33]
Inhibition of production from proinflammatory genes, including MMPs[24,25,27]

COX: cyclo-oxygenase; GAG: glycosaminoglycan; IL: interleukin; MMP: matrix metalloproteinase; PG: prostaglandin.

The monosaccharide building blocks of chondroitin sulfate (glucuronic acid and N-acetylglucosamine) created by its digestive hydrolysis might be absorbed, yet these hydrosylates might show different biologic and biochemical properties than those of the parent structure, upon which beneficial attributes have been proposed .

Clinical implication: it is debatable whether these large molecules are actually absorbed following oral administration, and if so, whether the 'biproducts' of these absorbed agents perform the same in the body as do their parent structures, from which data for efficacy have been identified.

Clearly, all chondroitin sulfate is not the same. Chondroitin sulfate is expensive, and it is possible that some suppliers may dilute it with compounds that include sugars, such as maltose, or other GAGs, such as dermatan sulfate, keratin sulfate, heparin, or hyaluronic acid that can cause analytical methods to overestimate the content. Therefore, despite language like 'quality tested' appearing on labels, there is no basis to compare one product against another or to judge the quality of different products. Consumerlab.com (an independent testing group that tests, and publishes data, on human and veterinary supplements for labeling accuracy and product purity[38]). reported in 2007 that 73% of 'joint formulas' tested, failed to meet their own label claim for chondroitin content[38]. It is incumbent on the consumer to be knowledgeable about the product and the manufacturer. Consumers should buy from manufacturers that use USP grade materials. They should stay away from products that are backed only by testimonials and not supported by scientific research. 'We believe what's happening with chondroitin is economic adulteration. Some manufacturers substitute with cheaper materials that look like the more expensive, real ingredients' says Dr. Tod Cooperman, MD, president of Consumerlab.com.

In a placebo-controlled double-blind study in dogs with OA, owners and veterinarians were unable to distinguish between chondroitin sulphate or placebo supplemented dogs after 12 weeks of follow-up[39].

GLUCOSAMINE

Glucosamine action *in vitro* includes a reduction in proteoglycan degradation and inhibition of the synthesis and activity of degradative enzymes and inflammatory mediators, such as aggrecanases, MMPs, nitric oxide (NO), and prostaglandin (PG)E_2, with anabolic effects of GAG stimulation and proteoglycan production, including aggrecan, but no effect on type II collagen[26]. Glucosamine also appears to inhibit nuclear factor kappa-B (NF-κB) activity[23].

Nuclear factor-κB plays a major role in inflammation and regulation of the immune response.

Glucosamine is a hexosamine sugar proposed to act as a precursor for the disaccharide units of GAGs. Nutritional glucosamine is suggested to provide the body with extra 'building blocks' for the creation of the cartilage matrix. Most glucosamine in the body is in the form of glucosamine-6-phosphate[40], while glucosamine is commercially available in three forms: glucosamine hydrochloride, glucosamine sulfate, and N-acetyl-D-glucosamine. The form of glucosamine apparently influences its activity. Glucosamine hydrochloride and glucosamine sulfate appear to inhibit equine cartilage degeneration more consistently than N-acetylglucosamine *in vitro*[41]. In addition, there is a suggestion that GAG synthesis may be through promoting incorporation of sulfur into cartilage[42].

Investigators have reported that in human patients, glucosamine sulfate increases the expression of cartilage aggrecan core protein and down regulates, in a dose-dependent manner, MMP-1 and -3 expression[43]. Such transcriptional effects are supported by reports that glucosamine sulfate increases proteoglycan synthesis with no effect on their physiochemical form, on type II collagen production, or on cell proliferation in a model of human osteoarthritic chondrocytes[16].

In trials assessing improvement in long-term symptomatic evaluation of human knee OA, it was observed that glucosamine hydrochloride does not induce symptomatic relief in knee OA to the same extent as glucosamine sulfate[44,45].

This raises the question of the importance of sulfate and its contribution to the overall effects of glucosamine.

Glucosamine sulfate is very hygroscopic and unstable. Consequently, during manufacturing, varying amounts of potassium or sodium chloride are added to improve stability. Due to concerns over valid labeling, commercially available capsules or tablets of glucosamine sulfate were analyzed. The amount of free-base varied from 41% to 108% of the milligram content stated on the label; the amount of glucosamine varied from 59% to 138%, even when expressed as sulfate[46]. Therefore, the results obtained with one single preparation of glucosamine sulfate, even when registered as a drug in Europe, cannot be extrapolated to the vast majority of OTC preparations sold without the appropriate quality controls.

Persiani *et al.*[47] reported that glucosamine is bioavailable both systemically and in the joint after oral administration of crystalline glucosamine sulphate in human osteoarthritic patients. 'The formulation used is the original crystalline glucosamine sulphate 1500 mg once-a-day soluble powder preparation which is a prescription drug in most European and extra-European countries, and differs from glucosamine formulations available in the USA and other countries. In fact, the USA Dietary Supplements Health and Education Act of 1994 documented the appearance of several poorly characterized dietary supplements containing either inadequate active ingredient quantity, or other glucosamine salts (e.g. hydrochloride), derivatives (e.g. N-acetyl-glucosamine), or dosage forms and regimens. This might also provide an explanation for the finding that when other salts, formulations and/or daily regimens have been used in clinical trials, the results have not been favorable. In particular, the 2006 National Institutes of Health-sponsored Glucosamine/Chondroitin Arthritis Intervention Trial (GAIT) trial in knee OA, indicated that the symptomatic effect of glucosamine hydrochloride at the dose of 500 mg *tid* did not differ significantly from placebo. This confirmed the skepticism concerning the several confounders and problematic study design of some trials, and the possible suboptimal exposure of the patients to the active molecule that might also come from the adopted dose and dosing interval.

It is interesting to note that the only clinically relevant results in the GAIT study were observed in the subgroup of more severe patients when glucosamine hydrochloride was combined with chondroitin sulphate, supporting the hypothesis that increasing the sulphate concentrations may have therapeutic effects[48].

Some suggest it is unlikely that the clinical effects of glucosamine (sulphate) are linked to a mere stimulation of GAG synthesis, but support the theory that glucosamine sulphate inhibits IL-1-induced gene expression, possibly via the suppression of the cytokine intracellular signaling pathway and NFκB activation, thus reversing the proinflammatory and joint degenerating effects of IL-1[47]. Crystalline glucosamine sulphate reportedly inhibits IL-1-stimulated gene expression of cyclo-oxygenase (COX)-2, inducible nitric oxide synthase, tumor necrosis factor-α (TNF-α), IL-6, IL-1, MMP-3, and aggrecanase 2[49]. Largo *et al.*[23], found that glucosamine sulfate inhibits NF-κB activation and PGE_2 synthesis induced by IL-1β in human chondrocytes, where NF-κB is considered a key regulator of tissue inflammation, since it controls the transcription of a number of proinflammatory genes that regulate the synthesis of cytokines, chemokines, and adhesion molecules. NF-κB activity has been shown essential for MMP-1 and MMP-3 up-regulation[50]. Glucosamine sulfate also inhibited the gene expression and the protein synthesis of COX-2 induced by IL-1β , while no effect on COX-1 synthesis was seen.

Kuroki *et al.*[51] have shown that within a canine articular cartilage and synovium explant co-culture system, glucosamine or chondroitin sulfate alone retards increased expression of proteinases and inflammatory mediators associated with IL-1, while the combination of glucosamine + chondroitin sulfate primarily retarded detrimental effects on matrix molecules. This corroborates findings of the first reported study showing the synergism of chondroitin sulfate plus glucosamine in chondrocyte GAG synthesis[30].

Some have questioned the potential for biologic activity of glucosamine, pointing out that the bioavailability from a single or multiple dose of glucosamine HCl is only 10–12% in dogs[52,53].

It is questionable whether substantial amounts of glucosamine reach the circulation following oral ingestion[54], and it is proposed that glucosamine is not essential for the biosynthesis of cartilage – glucosamine is only one of many substrates from which other metabolites are derived for the synthesis of cartilage matrix[55].

Despite challenges of efficacy, significant clinical improvement has been reported in dogs with DJD after 70 days of treatment with glucosamine–chondroitin sulfate[56], and glucosamine–chondroitin sulfate treatment has also resulted in clinical improvement in humans[57] and horses[58] with DJD. Studies have demonstrated that glucosamine is a safe, nontoxic product with rare adverse effects. There are no known contraindications or drug interactions[59]. Lenox *et al.*[60] have reported that in healthy dogs, short-term (21 days) oral glucosamine–chondroitin sulfate administration does not affect glycemic control or cause diabetes mellitus.

Glucosamine and chondroitin sulfate in combination

Orally administered glucosamine hydrochloride and chondroitin sulfate in combination has become a popular nutraceutical offering. A multicenter, double-blind, placebo- and celecoxib controlled study (GAIT study) of 1,583 human patients with stifle joint OA receiving 1500 mg glucosamine, 1200 mg chondroitin sulphate, or both, revealed the supplementations not to reduce stifle joint pain better than placebo[61]. In a subgroup of that same study, in patients with moderate-to-severe pain, the response of the combination glucosamine plus chondroitin sulfate was significantly better. In this same subgroup, the positive control, celecoxib, showed no response. Worthy of note is that the study was conducted under pharmaceutical rather than dietary-supplement regulations, therefore agents identical to the ones used may not be commercially available. Nevertheless, 'analysis of the primary outcome measure did not show that either supplement, alone or in combination, was efficacious'[62]. In contrast, some nutraceutical manufacturers cite the GAIT study results as testimonial that where an evidence-based efficacious drug (celecoxib) does not work, glucosamine plus chondroitin sulfate does!

Results from the GAIT study are not conclusive: some suggest it shows glucosamine and chondroitin sulfate combination is not effective, while others interpret the data to suggest it is. 'Rabbit or duck' (**Fig. 98**)?

Subsequent to the GAIT study, in an editorial appearing in the *New England Journal of Medicine*, Dr. Marc Hochberg, MD, states 'If patients choose to take dietary supplements to control their symptoms, they should be advised to take glucosamine sulfate rather than glucosamine hydrochloride and, for those with severe pain, that taking chondroitin sulfate with glucosamine sulfate may have an additive effect'[55].

Studies of *in vivo* or *in vitro* efficacy of veterinary products are limited, and efficacy claims are frequently made from subjective assessments, which include owner testimonials or clinical trials lacking peer review. A literature review suggests the bioavailability of these products in dogs after oral intake is limited and questions the availability of sufficient amounts to prevent or treat OA, whereas parenteral application (either IM or intra-articular) seems to approach the *in vitro* effect. Further, clinical efficacy is confused by reference to *in vitro* research data, studies in other than target species, or reports void of objective, placebo-controlled, double-blinded studies or any studies at all[62,63]. The Arthritis Foundation recommends that when a supplement has been studied with good results, the brand used in the study should be determined, and that product bought[64]!

Despite the scarcity of *in vivo* data, Chan *et al.*[65] have revealed the marked effects glucosamine + chondroitin sulfate + manganese has on the expression of genes encoding putative mediators of OA. Studying the effects on bovine cartilage explants, this combination was shown to: 1) decrease NO production by 50–66%, noting that NO is associated with cartilage degradation, inhibition of cartilage matrix inhibition, and chondrocyte apoptosis; 2) repress PGE_2 by 70%, noting that PGE_2 is associated with pain and inflammation; 3) decrease both MMP-3 and MMP-13, associated with cleavage of extracellular matrix proteins, and type II collagen, respectively; and 4) up-regulate tissue inhibiting metalloproteinase (TIMP)-3 transcription (approximately 300%) while also up-regulating genes encoding both type II collagen and aggrecan.

AVOCADO/SOYBEAN UNSAPONIFIABLES

Avocado/soybean unsaponifiables (ASUs) have become a nutraceutical compound of recent investigative interest (**Fig.** 99). The unsaponifiable portions of avocado and soybean oils are extracted via hydrolysis, and the extracts have been shown to treat several connective tissue diseases effectively66. Synergism between the avocado and soya components, and their relative ratios, appear to be important67. In vitro studies show that ASU extracts reduce proinflammatory mediators, including: IL-1 , IL-6, IL-8, macrophage inflammatory protein-1 , NO, MMP-13, TNF- , and PGE268–71. Such findings are important because they suggest that excessive production of PGE2 due to overexpression of COX-2 may be achieved with or without limited use of NSAIDs and their associated adverse effects.

It has been observed that osteoblasts isolated from subchondral OA bone demonstrate an altered phenotype[72]. They produce increased amounts of alkaline phosphatase, osteocalcin, transforming growth factor-β1(TGF-β1), insulin-like growth factor-1, and urokinase plasminogen activator. OA osteoblasts are also resistant to parathyroid hormone stimulation, possibly contributing to abnormal bone remodeling and bone sclerosis in OA[73]. Henrotin *et al.*[74] showed that ASU prevents the OA osteoblast-induced inhibition of matrix molecule production, suggesting promotion of OA cartilage repair.

Osteoblasts (from the Greek words for 'bone' and 'germ' or embryonic) are mononucleate cells that are responsible for bone formation.

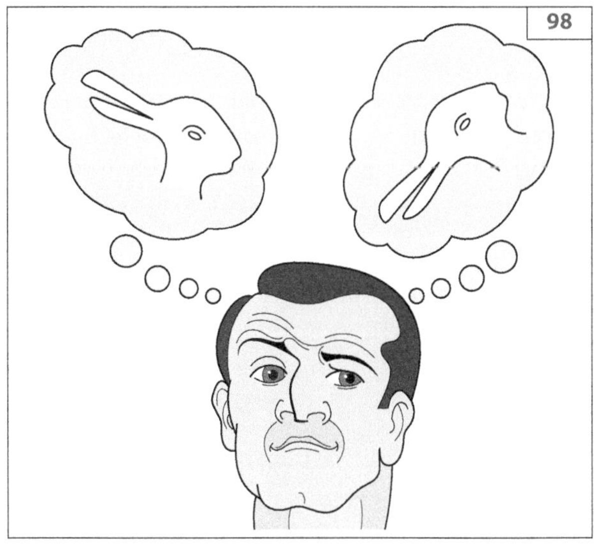

Fig. 98 Duck or rabbit? Glucosamine and chondroitin sulfate combination efficacy.

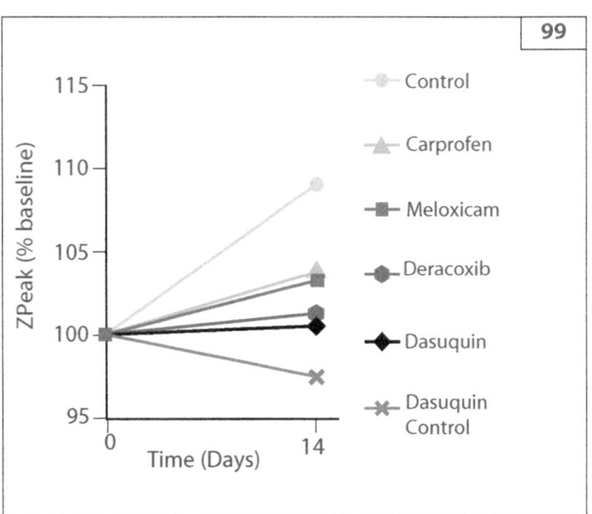

Fig. 99 Force plate gait analysis, showing that the avocado/soybean unsaponifiable product (Dasuquin) yields an efficacy similar to contemporary nonsteroidal anti-inflammatory drugs on peak vertical force measured in dogs treated for stifle osteoarthritis (N=8). (After Reference 79.)

OA is a total joint disease, which includes the involvement of subchondral bone (**Fig. 100**). Abnormal remodeling of the subchondral bone plate exposed to excessive nonphysiologic mechanical loads causes it to become stiffer, no longer effective as a shock absorber, thus increasing mechanical strain on overlying cartilage. It is proposed that intervention that reduces bone sclerosis might slow progressive cartilage degradation. In addition, because microcracks, vascular channels, and neovascularization provide a link between subchondral bone and cartilage, IL-6, TGF-β, and perhaps other factors produced by osteoblasts may contribute to the abnormal remodeling of OA cartilage[75].

Transforming growth factor-β is a protein that controls proliferation, cell differentiation, and other functions in most cells.

Since tidemark microcracks appear early in OA cartilage, it is speculated that soluble mediators produced by sclerotic subchondral osteoblasts may modulate chondrocyte metabolism and contribute to cartilage degradation. Aligning this theory together with ASU prevention of inhibitory effects of osteoarthritic subchondral osteoblasts on aggrecan, and type II collagen synthesis by chondrocytes, investigators propose that ASU may act via a new mechanism of action at the subchondral bone level in protecting cartilage[74]. Among study horses, ASU failed to ameliorate increasing lameness, response to joint flexion, or synovial effusion; however, GAG synthesis in the articular cartilage was increased compared with placebo-treated, OA-affected joints[76]. Investigators concluded that ASU extracts may have an anabolic effect directly on chondrocytes to increase GAG synthesis and, hence, help prevent articular cartilage damage by enhancing the articular cartilage matrix structure.

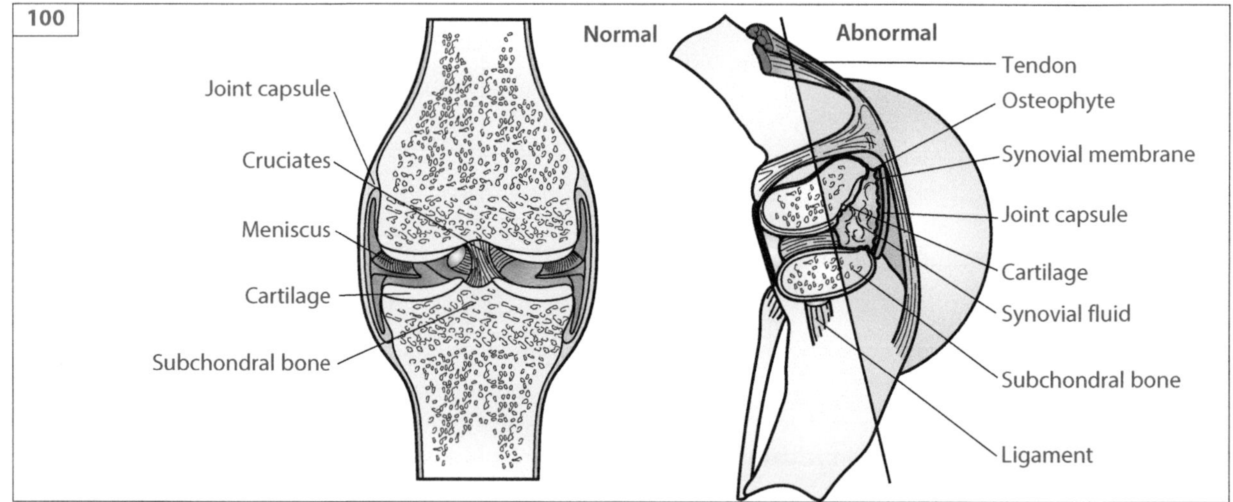

Fig. 100 Anatomy of the femoral–tibial joint. The arthritic joint is analogous to a totally diseased 'organ', with loss of cartilage, sclerosis of subchondral bone, inflammation of the synovial membrane, osteophyte formation, and pain.

In a canine study[77], ASU (4 mg/kg every 3 days or daily) increased both TGF-β_1 and TGF-β_2 levels in the stifle synovial fluid. TGF-β_1 levels reached maximum values at the end of the second month and then decreased after the third month, while TGF-β_2 levels marginally increased during the first 2 months, followed by a marked increase at the end of the third month. TGF-β is a stimulator of extracellular matrix production, like collagen type II and proteoglycan, in chondrocytes[78].

ASU has been demonstrated to alter the translocation of NF-κB from the cytoplasm to the nucleus with subsequent transcription of multiple proinflammatory mediators[71]. Finally, Millis[79] has shown with force plate gait analysis, that the combination ASU + glucosamine + chondroitin sulfate + manganese may have an efficacy in dogs similar to that of NSAIDs.

Clinical implication: some consider nuclear factor-κB to be the 'supreme commander' in controlling the generation of proinflammatory mediators.

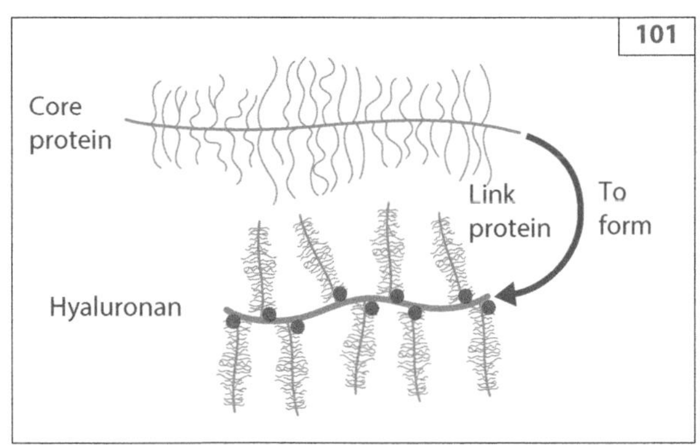

Fig. 101 The aggrecan aggregate is the 'functional unit' of cartilage, containing over 100 aggrecan monomers.

HYALURONIC ACID

The proteoglycan aggrecan molecule of articular cartilage is attached via a link protein to hyaluronic acid. The entire complex is referred to as a proteoglycan or aggrecan aggregate (**Fig. 101**). Hyaluronic acid acts as an aggregating factor between the collagen, PG aggregate, and cartilage structural network as a whole. Synovial fluid contains high concentrations of hyaluronic acid, derived from Type B synoviocytes embedded within the intimal lining of the joint capsule. The viscoelastic properties of synovial fluid are determined by hyaluronic acid, and with the progression of OA, hyaluronic acid concentrations decrease with a resultant decrease in the viscoelastic properties of the synovial fluid. Intra-articular injection of hyaluronic acid, called 'viscosupplementation', has demonstrated significant improvement of symptoms in patients with OA[80].

By definition, injectable hyaluronic acid (e.g. Legend®) is not a nutraceutical. However, it can be considered a chondroprotective agent and there are several commercially available forms of hyaluronic acid, differing by treatment regimens, total dosing, and average molecular weights. Support for use of hyaluronic acid resides in the improvement of OA symptoms with few side-effects. It is unlikely that sustained beneficial effects of hyaluronic acid therapy result from temporary restoration of the synovial fluid lubrication and viscoelasticity[81]. Perhaps hyaluronic acid therapy has disease-modifying biologic activity and an impact on OA progression. Four potential mechanisms have been proposed for the beneficial clinical effects noted from hyaluronic acid therapy:

1. Restoration of elastic and viscous properties of the synovial fluid.
2. Biosynthetic-chondroprotective effect on cells (hyaluronans can induce endogenous synthesis of hyaluronic acid by synovial cells, stimulate chondrocyte proliferation, and inhibit cartilage degradation)[80,82–84].
3. Anti-inflammatory effects[85,86]; analgesic effect[87,88].
4. Pozo *et al.*[89] reported that intra-articular hyaluronic acid reduced nerve impulse activity in nociceptive afferent fibers in a cat model of acute arthritis.

PHYCOCYANIN

Phycocyanin, composed of two protein subunits with covalently bound phycobilins that are the light-capturing part of the blue pigment in blue-green algae, is considered the active agent in PhyCox®, commercialized as PhyCox-JS®. There are some data suggesting that C-phycocyanin is a selective COX-2 inhibitor[90]. Phycocyanin has been shown to have antioxidant and anti-inflammatory properties *in vitro* and *in vivo* (rodents)[91,92]. Other ingredients in PhyCox-JS, which may contribute to product efficacy, include glucosamine, flaxseed oil, tumeric, EPA, and docosahexaenoic acid (DHA). PhyCox-JS is not a drug, but positioned as an animal nutraceutical of natural botanical origin (PhyCox). There are no pharmacokinetic studies for phycocyanin in the dog. The observational study performed by the manufacturer was based on owner observations of dogs on the ingredient PhyCox and not the commercial product PhyCox-JS, and study design was weak. Further, PhyCox-JS has not been studied in use together with a NSAID.

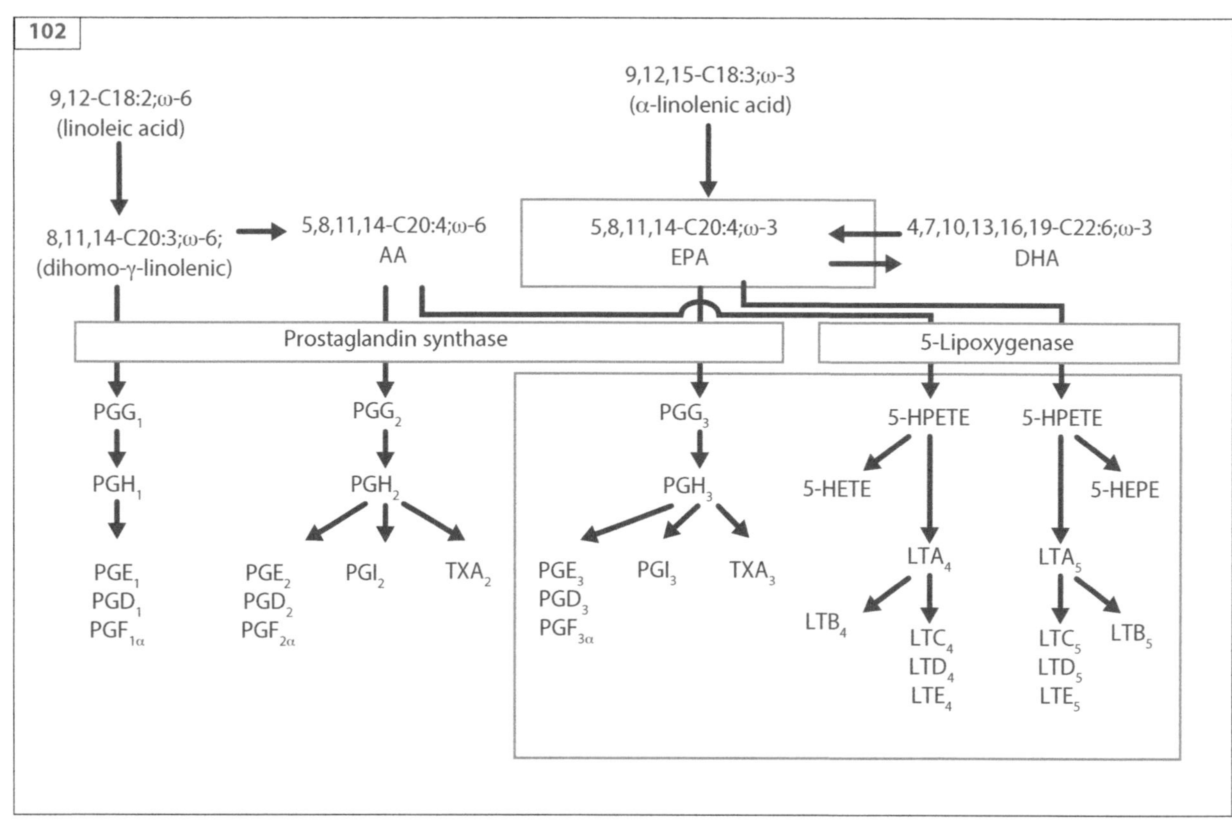

Fig. 102 Eicosapentaenoic acid (EPA) is the substrate for synthesis of many eicosanoids which act as mediators of inflammation. AA: archidonic acid; DHA: docosahexaenoic acid; HEPE: hydroxyeicosapentaenoic acid; HETE: hydroxyeicosatetraenoic acid; HPETE: hydroperoxyeicosatetraenoic acid; LT: leukotriene; PG: prostaglandin; TX: thromboxane.

EICOSAPENTAENOIC ACID

Both AA and EPA act as precursors for the synthesis of eicosanoids, important molecules functioning as hormones and mediators of inflammation (**Fig. 102**). The amounts and types of eicosanoids synthesized are determined by the availability of the polysulfated fatty acid precursor and by the activities of the enzyme system. The eicosanoids produced from AA, the principal precursor under most conditions, appear to be more proinflammatory than those formed from EPA (**Fig. 103**).

Ingestion of oils containing omega-3 fatty acids results in a decrease in membrane levels of AA because the omega-3 fatty acids replace AA in the substrate pool and reduce the capacity to synthesize inflammatory eicosanoids. Inflammatory eicosanoids produced from AA are, therefore, depressed when dogs consume foods with high levels of omega-3 fatty acids. In addition, EPA is thought to exert its therapeutic effect on OA by reducing expression of genes encoding cartilage degrading enzymes (aggrecanase) within the chondrocytes[93]. *In vitro*

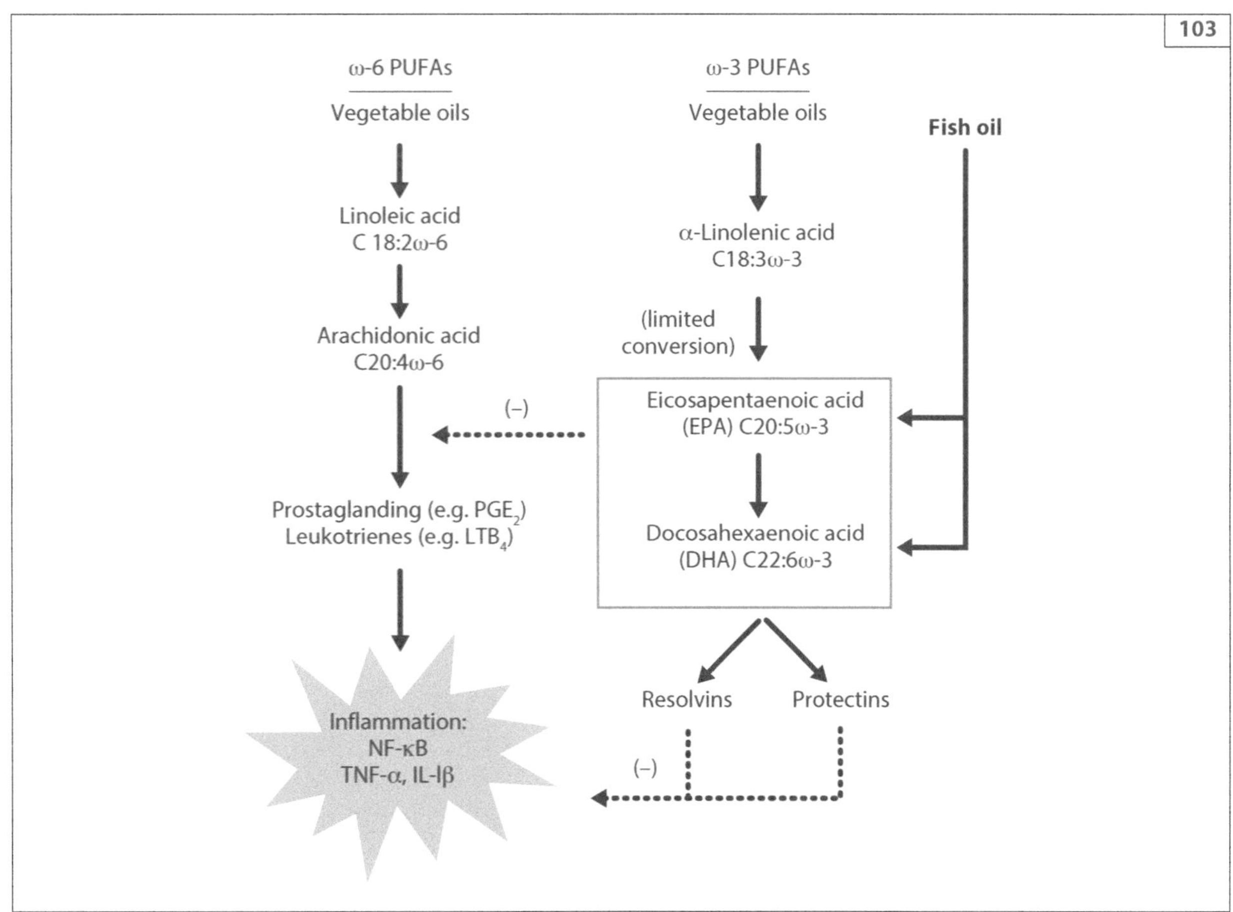

Fig. 103 Whereas arachidonic acid-derived eicosanoids tend to be proinflammatory, eicosapentaenoic acid (EPA)-derived eiosanoids tend to be less inflammatory (suppress the inflammatory process). IL: interleukin; NF-κB: nuclear factor kappa B; PUFA: polyunsaturated fatty acid; TNF: tumor necrosis factor.

studies revealed that by exposing normal canine cartilage to EPA before addition of the catabolic agent, oncostatin M, to initiate processes that mimic the cartilage damage that occurs during the pathogenesis of OA, cartilage degeneration was abrogated[94]. Food containing high concentrations of total omega-3 fatty acids and EPA, as well as a low omega-6:omega-3 ratio, appears to decrease the severity of OA clinical signs as early as 21 days after initiation of implementation (**Fig. 104**).

The optimal **omega-6:omega-3 ratio** is under debate, but is approximately 5:1.

Flaxseed oil and fish oil are both rich in omega-3 fatty acids. Fish oil is rich in EPA and DHA, while flaxseed oil contains alpha-linolenic acid (ALA). For ALA in flaxseed oil to have an anti-inflammatory effect, it must be converted to EPA. Efficiency of ALA conversion to EPA is very low (<10%), with most ALA being used for energy. Accordingly, a small amount of fish oil is more effective at providing EPA and DHA than a large quantity of flaxseed oil containing ALA.

Eicosapentaenoic acid within reputable commercial pet food diets is routinely more credible than over-the-counter sources because of consistent quality assurance testing.

S-ADENOSYLMETHIONINE

S-adenosylmethionine (SAMe) is a nucleotide-like molecule synthesized from methionine and adenosine triphosphate (ATP) by all living cells. SAMe is particularly important to hepatocytes (liver cells) and plays a pivotal role in the biochemical pathways of transmethylation, transulfuration, and aminopropylation. A therapeutic application of SAMe in joint disorders is derived from pain reduction and improved joint function[95,96], based on potential antioxidant and anti-inflammatory activity[97]. There are very few studies reporting the effect of SAMe on articular cartilage matrix or chondrocytes. One study in dogs reported an *in vitro* detrimental effect[98], while one study in humans showed an *in vitro* positive effect[99]. Lippiello *et al.*[100] has reported that the enzymatic inhibition of proteoglycan synthesis by MMP-3 *in vitro* is reversed by the combination of glucosamine and SAMe, but not with either agent alone.

CURCUMINOIDS

Studies to support existing *in vitro* evidence for curcuminoid alleviation of OA clinical signs are lacking. To date, green tea extract and other Asian herbal remedies have not been evaluated in companion animal models or in animals with spontaneous disease. Curcuminoids, types of phytonutrients extracted from turmeric, have been found to exert some anti-inflammatory effects in certain animal models and *in vitro* assays. A curcuminoid extract administered to dogs with OA was found to yield no treatment effect using the objective assessment of force plate analysis, although subjective assessment by the observer was positive.

NEW ZEALAND GREEN LIPPED MUSSEL (*PERNA CANALICULUS*) (LYPRINOL)

The starting point for the interest in green lipped mussel (GLM) as therapy for inflammation was folklore. This folklore was that coastal dwelling Maori in New Zealand, who regularly consumed mussels as part of their diet, suffered far less from arthritis than their inland dwelling relatives. Studies of GLM efficacy in the treatment of canine OA show varied results. Some studies show a positive result[101,102], while others (Dobenecker, 2002) show no effect[103], and still others show an equivacol response[104].

QUALITY OF EVIDENCE

Evidence-based medicine has been defined as 'the conscientious, explicit and judicious use of current best evidence in making decisions about the individual patients'. This means integrating individual clinical expertise with the best available clinical evidence from systematic research[105]. In veterinary medicine a broader, simpler definition may be appropriate: evidence-based veterinary medicine (EBVM) is the use of current best evidence in making clinical decisions.

A veterinary surgeon has a moral and ethical obligation to provide treatment for which there is good evidence of its efficacy. Society expects that safe and effective treatments are provided. Further, that most all the resources available for our decision making are also available to our clients (and their lawyers). When making clinical decisions that are questioned by clients following poor outcomes, we need accountability for our decisions. It is not enough that a veterinary surgeon declare that s/he knows an unproven treatment works on the basis of his or her own personal experience. Finally, the veterinary profession gains respect and trust from clients through its dedication to objective diagnosis and validation of treatments.

Scientific validation is the gold standard by which we can make sound judgments. Scientifically validated treatments and procedures are more likely to be safe and effective than nonvalidated ones and their risks are better understood than nonvalidated ones. In addition these treatments guarantee the most consistent and predictable outcomes. Accordingly, scientifically validated treatments and procedures should be preferred when available, while appreciating that data are often unavailable.

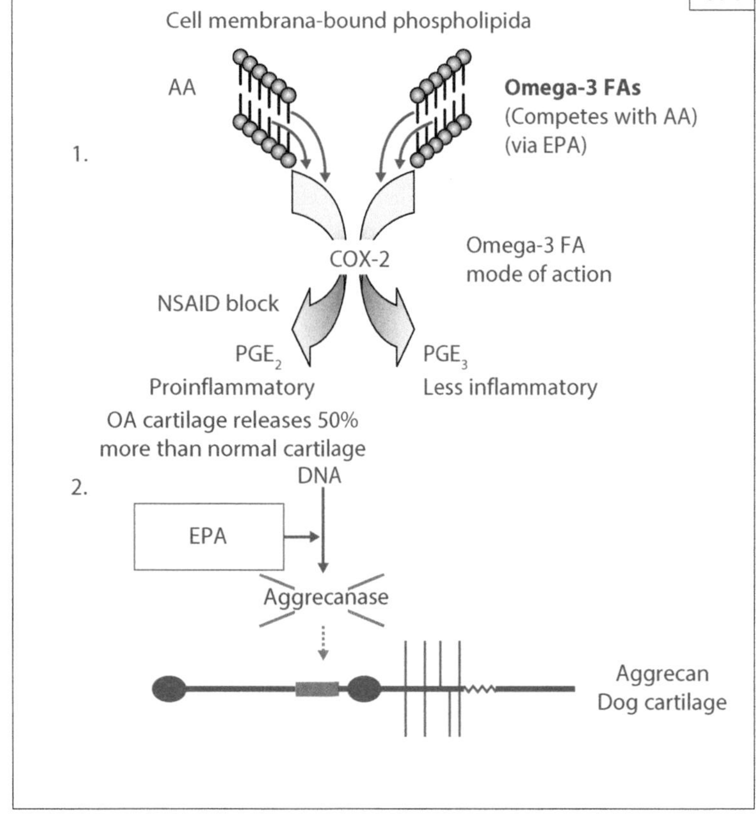

Fig. 104 Two therapeutic modes of action of eicosapentaenoic acid (EPA) for patients with osteoarthritis: 1) by replacing arachidonic acid substrate with EPA, fewer inflammatory eicosanoids are produced, and 2) EPA enhances the integrity of the cartilage matrix by decreasing the production of aggreganase–an enzyme that destroys the aggregan aggregate (the structural unit of cartilage). AA: archidonic acid; COX: cyclo-oxygenase; DNA: deoxyribonucleic acid; FA: fatty acid; NSAID: nonsteroidal anti-inflammatory drug; OA: osteoarthritis; PG: prostaglandin.

Within EBVM, the quality of information is graded, based on the probability that the data source will generate reliable conclusions and recommendations (**Fig. 105**):

- Class A (grade 1): evidence is best and is derived from well designed, properly randomized, double-blinded, placebo-controlled clinical trials. (The most reliable predictor of results likely to be seen in clinical practice.)

Double blind: typically used in randomized controlled trials. A design where both the animals/owners and the investigators do not know and cannot work out which animals are receiving treatment and placebo.

- Class B (grade 2): evidence is derived from high quality, well designed, randomized, controlled clinical trials using historical controls. (A good predictor of results likely to be seen in clinical practice.)
- Class C (grade 3): evidence is from uncontrolled case series; well designed, nonrandomized clinical trials, epidemiologic studies (cohort, case–control), and models of disease.

Cohort study: in which two groups (cohorts) of animals are identified. One group represents a cohort of animals exposed to a putative cause of an outcome, while the other is a cohort free from this exposure. The cohorts are examined for the outcome of interest in order to test the association of the putative cause with the outcome.

- Class D (grade 4): evidence is derived from anecdotal clinical reports, or expert opinion, descriptive studies, studies in other species, pathophysiology based on *in vitro* studies, or extrapolated from benchtop experiments.

The seven nutraceuticals listed have been examined for evidence of support for canine OA[103,106].

- GLM.
- ASU.
- Glucosamine and chondroitin sulfate (GS/CS).
- P54FP (tumeric extract).
- Special milk protein concentrate (SMPC).
- Homeopathic combination preparation-Zeel (HCP-Zeel).
- Elk velvet antler (EVA)

As of early 2010, EVA, HCP Zeel, SMPC, and P54FP have one published study each, while ASU and GS/CS have two studies each, and GLM has four studies (**Fig. 106**). Four products have a single randomized, controlled, clinical trial for assessing efficacy in canine OA (*Table 62*). Although based on very small sample size, these data suggest EVA and HCP Zeel are most likely to provide the best clinical improvement in dogs with OA.

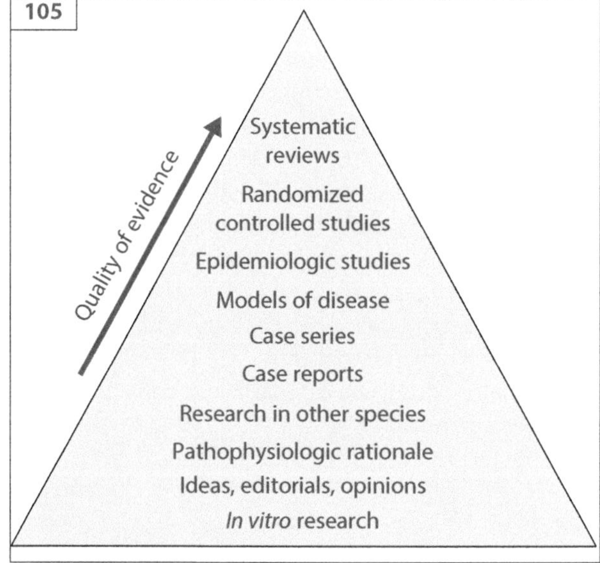

Fig. 105 The quality of evidence pyramid delineates the origin of confidence a clinician would have in a given treatment protocol.

TABLE 62: Nutraceutical products with a single randomized, controlled, clinical trial for assessing efficacy in canine osteoarthritis

Product	Evidence grade	# client owned dogs	Comments
EVA	1	28	Subjective and objective (force plate analysis) improvement at 60 days
HCP-Zeel	1	44	Subjective and objective (force plate analysis) improvement at 8 weeks
SMPC	1	50	Subjective improvement by both owner and veterinarian
P54PF	1	61	No effect by subjective owner and objective (force plate analysis) assessment at 8 weeks Veterinary subjective assessment was favorable

EVA: elk velvet antler; HCP-Zeel: homeopathic combination preparation-Zeel; P54FP: turmeric extract; SMPC: special milk protein concentrate.

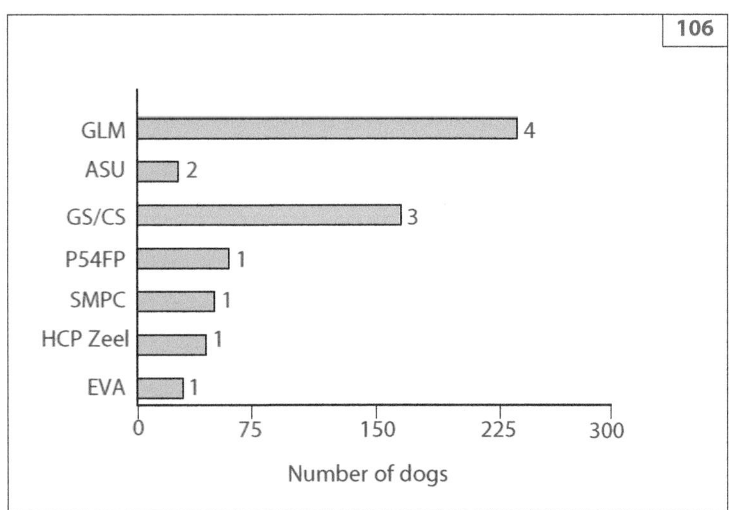

Fig. 106 Published studies supporting evidence for seven nutraceutical products used to manage canine osteoarthritis (number of studies). ASU: avocado and soybean unsaponifiable extracts; EVA: elk velvet antler; GLM: green lipped mussel; GS/CS: glucosamine and chondroitin sulfate; HCP-Zeel: homeopathic combination preparation-Zeel; P54FP: tumeric extract; SMPC: special milk protein concentrate.

Glucosamine and chondroitin supplements are quite popular; however, there are few studies documenting clinical efficacy in companion animal target species (*Tables 63,* and *64*). In human medicine there are conflicting reports (**GAIT** and **STOPP** trials) of efficacy.

Consumerlab.com is an independent organization providing evaluation of a variety of supplements. Over the past decade they have evaluated chondroitin sulfate products on four occasions (*Table 65*).

One feature of nutraceutical joint health products (JHPs) that is frequently overlooked is the use of these products in young, healthy animals before musculoskeletal trauma, injury, or the onset of OA clinical signs. This is particularly the case in breeds of animals predisposed to joint diseases or in athletic dogs prior to initiating a training program. The prophylactic use of these JHPs is a consideration that warrants discussion with the pet owner.

FELINE JOINT HEALTH PRODUCTS

Dietary modulation for the dog with OA has been advocated and commercially available for some time. There has been particular interest in diets rich in long-chain fatty acids of the 'n3' series (EPA, DHA, and eicosatetraenoic acid)[101, 107–110]. GLM extract has also been identified as beneficial for dogs with OA[101,102,104,111,112]. DJD in cats is an emerging area of interest, and although the etiology of feline DJD is poorly understood, some work has been reported on the effect of several 'wellness' foods on markers in geriatric cats with and without arthritis[113]. Further assessing the impact of a therapeutic diet for feline DJD, Lascelles *et al.*[114] reported that a diet high in EPA and DHA, supplemented with GLM extract and GS/CS, improved objective measures of feline mobility.

JOINT SUPPLEMENT GUIDELINES AND SAFETY

JHPs are commonly dispensed by veterinarians, and veterinary health professionals are also relied on to recommend such products to their clients. The ACCLAIM system has been developed to help clinicians rapidly evaluate a JHP for identification of safety and efficacy (*Table 66*).

The National Animal Supplement Council's (NASC) adverse event reporting system reports the incidence of adverse events to be 0.08/1 million administrations of all products sold for companion animals[115]. Recently, eight companies formed an animal supplement organization: the National Alliance of Animal Supplement Manufacturers and Marketers (NAASM), which aims to ensure the quality of animal supplement ingredients and products. The NAASM, together with the NASC, offers guidelines for product quality assurance and adverse event reporting.

TABLE 63: Overview of evidence-based studies for ASU, GS/CS, and GLM

Product	Evidence grade	# dogs	Comments
ASU	3 Model	8 laboratory dogs	Surrogate (markers of cartilage damage and repair) endpoint at 8 weeks
ASU	3 Model	24 laboratory dogs	Surrogate (markers of cartilage damage and repair) endpoint at 3 months
GS/CS	1	35 client owned	Mixed results at 70 days by subjective assessment
GS/CS	1	71 client owned	No effect by subjective and objective assessment at 60 days
GLM and GS/CS	1	58 client owned	No effect by subjective assessment at 12 weeks

ASU: avocado and soybean unsaponifiable extracts; GLM: green lipped mussel; GS/CS: glucosamine and chondroitin sulfate.

TABLE 64: Overview of evidence-based studies for GLM and GS/CS

Product	Evidence grade	# dogs	Comments
GLM	2	32/33 laboratory dogs	Subjective improvement at 6 weeks. ('top dressing' powder performed better than 'treat')
GLM	2	70 client owned	No effect at 28 days by subjective assessment, but at end of open label extension at 56 days, improvement was noted by owners' subjective assessment
GLM	1	40 client owned	Positive result in 8 weeks with subjective assessment
GLM & GS/CS	1	58 client owned	No effect in 12 weeks with subjective assessment

GLM: green lipped mussel; GS/CS: glucosamine and chondroitin sulfate.

TABLE 65: Consumerlab.com evaluation of commercially available chondroitin sulfate (CS) products

Year tested	Failed own label claim	%CS content of failed products
2000	53%	40% had <10% of claim
2003	16%	50% had no detectable CS
2007	39%	60% had <10% of claim
2009	20%	63% had no detectable CS

TABLE 66: The ACCLAIM system includes assessment of manufacturer information, label claims, and ease of calculation of recommended doses for the determination of recommending a joint health product (JHP)

A = A name you recognize?	Products manufactured by an established company that provides educational materials for veterinarians or other consumers are preferable to JHPs manufactured by a new company
C = Clinical experience	Companies that support clinical research and have their products used in clinical trials (e.g. safety, efficacy, or bioavailability studies) that are published in peer-reviewed journals to which veterinarians have access are more likely to have a quality product
C = Contents	All ingredients should be clearly indicated on the product label
L = Label claims	Label claims that sound too good to be true probably are. Products with realistic label claims based on results of scientific studies, rather than testimonials, are more likely to be reputable. Products with illegal claims (i.e. claim to diagnose, treat, cure, or prevent a disease) should be avoided
A = Administration recommendations	Dosing instructions should be accurate and easy to follow: it should be easy to calculate the amount of active ingredient administered per dose per day
I = Identification of lot	A lot identification number or some other tracking system indicates that a premarket or postmarket surveillance system (or both) exists to ensure product quality. In addition, companies that have voluntarily instituted current good manufacturing practices and other quality-control or quality-assurance techniques (e.g. tamper-resistant packaging or identification, or individual tablets or caplets) provide evidence of a long-term investment in their product and company
M = Manufacturer information	Basic company information should be clearly stated on the label. Preferably, this should include a web site or details for contacting customer support

SUMMARY

Clearly, credible *in vivo* evidence-based support for most nutraceuticals is meager. Arguably, the success of nutraceuticals is being driven by consumers' desire to 'do no harm', and the role of nutraceuticals is shrouded with vagaries, innuendo, and misinformation. Preliminary information guiding nutraceutical use should be considered with care. Results should be gathered in the target species (i.e. the dog or cat) and not in small laboratory animals, in man, bovine, or from *in vitro* studies. Dosage, duration, and route of the agent should be taken into account for product assessment. Since most of these products are not pharmaceuticals, neither purity nor content is controlled, although the package or informational materials may suggest otherwise.

Hyaline articular cartilage harvested from joints of different animal species responds very differently to a variety of catabolic stimulants that are commonly used by researchers to establish *in vitro* models of cartilage degradation that are believed to mimic mechanisms of cartilage degradation in the pathogenesis of DJDs. Innes *et al.*[116] has pointed out that exposure to IL-1 α or β, tumor necrosis factor-α, oncostatin M, and retinoic acid can all cause significant increases in cartilage proteoglycan degradation when bovine articular cartilage explant culture systems are used, but similar results are not always seen with the canine. Species differences may be due to species variability of catabolic stimulants themselves, which may have different affinities for receptors and other down-stream regulators that manifest their metabolic effects on cartilage metabolism. Differences in catabolic responses to cytokines in dogs highlight the difficulty in extrapolating results between species.

Perhaps the best advice for pet owners is to spend their money where the science is strong. Adding a nutraceutical will, likely, do no harm, but evidence-based endorsement is weak. Perhaps, variability in testimonials for various nutraceutical efficacies resides in genetic predisposition of as yet unidentified subpopulations for their activity. Many nutraceuticals are least-cost formulations and quality assurance is lacking or nonexistent. As a matter of record, in 2005 the FDA rejected 12 model claims related to products reducing the risk of OA, joint degeneration, cartilage deterioration, and OA-related joint pain, tenderness, and swelling.

Controversy remains over mechanisms by which nutraceuticals may lead to modulation of disease signs and cartilage degradation in OA, and which product is preferred for treatment. Perhaps our scientific community lacks the expertise or financial support to identify how these products might work. Nevertheless, as a class of agents, nutraceuticals fall short in evidence-based efficacy, lack dose titration studies to validate appropriate doses of individual products, and have shown inconsistencies of product quality assurance. Good intentions of the few have been clouded by many! A sound recommendation for consumers is, therefore, buyer beware. One might argue that the most responsible advice for recommending a nutraceutical is as an adjunct to a 'science-based' medicinal, in that the nutraceutical may, or may not, help. Recommending that the pet owner administer a nutraceutical as the first line of treatment lacks convincing scientific underpinning, and product selection should be determined by the ACCLAIM criteria, considering that all nutraceuticals are not created equal. Nutramax Laboratories Inc. (Edgewood MD) consistently meets these criteria.

Chapter 8

Multimodal Pain Management

INTRODUCTION

In addition to preventive (pre-emptive) analgesia, multimodal (or balanced) analgesia has changed the way we treat pain[1]. Multimodal analgesia denotes simultaneous administration of two or more analgesic drugs belonging to different classes (**Fig. 107**). Less commonly appreciated, multimodal can also denote different delivery methods and modality therapies.

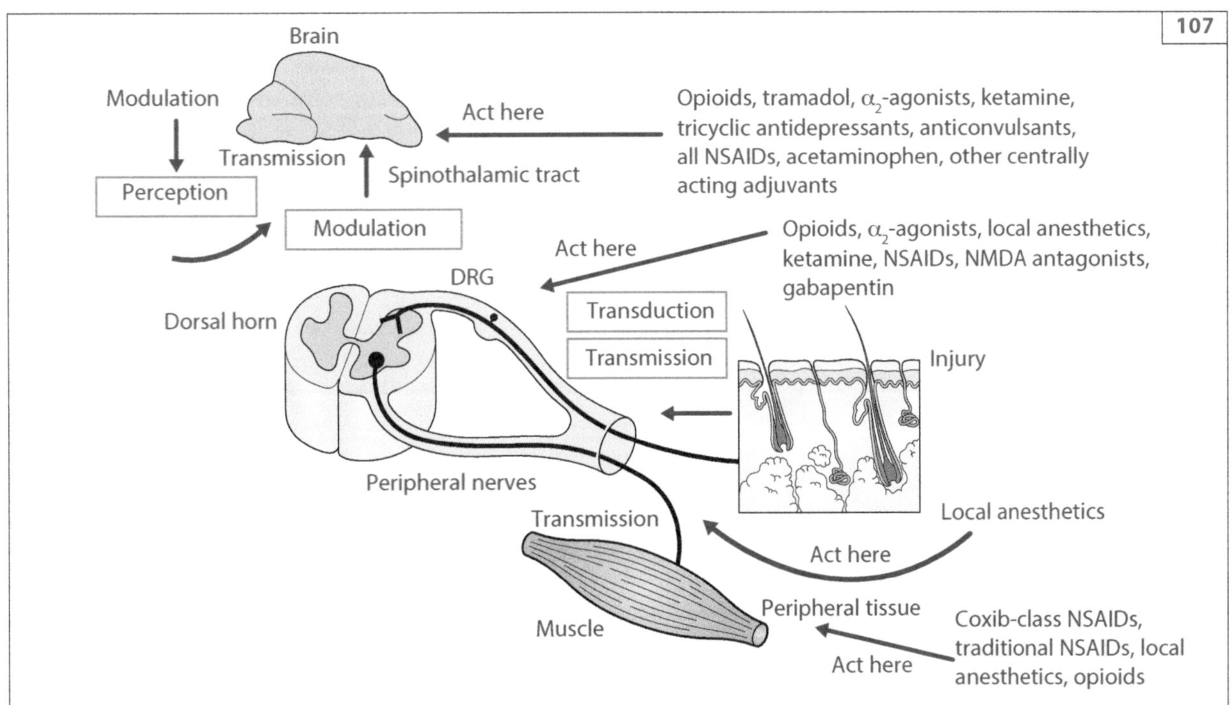

Fig. 107 Multimodal analgesia denotes the simultaneous administration of different classes of drugs, attempting to block the four physiologic processes of transduction, transmission, modulation, and perception. DRG: doral root ganglion; NMDA: N-methyl-D-aspartate; NSAID: nonsteroidal anti-inflammatory drug.

Dosages of each drug can typically be reduced because various classes of drugs have additive or synergistic analgesic effects when given together (e.g. opioids, α_2-agonist, and nonsteroidal anti-inflammatory [NSAID])[2,3]. As a result, adverse side-effects from each of the drugs in the combination can be anticipated to be less due to the lower dosing of each respective drug. For nearly two decades, the concept of 'multimodal analgesia' has created important advances in the approach to providing analgesia for both acute[4,5] and chronic pain in humans[6]. Nociception results in pain via multiple pathways, mechanisms and transmitter systems[7] , and it is naive to consider a single drug therapy would be as effective as several different drugs acting on multiple components of the nociceptive system (**Fig. 108**).

Contrary to widespread recommendations in human medicine, analgesic regimens administered prior to surgery are 'multimodal' less than 25% of the time. The majority of responders (45.1%) to a survey in human medicine, used two nonopioid analgesics, despite evidence that a combination of three or more compounds has been shown to improve postoperative pain control significantly. Only 12.2% used more than two drugs at a time. An exception was orthopedic surgery, where 87.7% said they use a multimodal regimen[8].

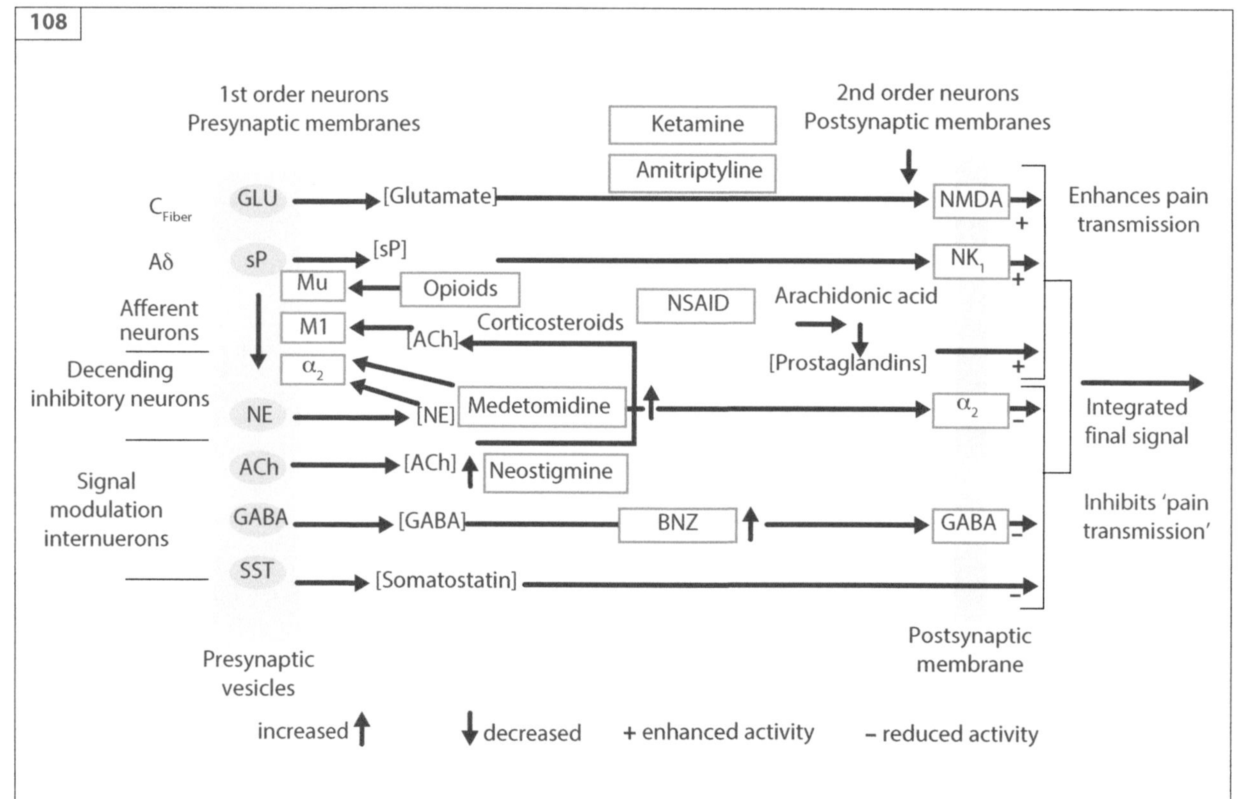

Fig. 108 Simplistic diagram of nociceptor transmission from the first- to second-order neuron. Most analgesics act via a single pathway, transmitter, or receptor; pain is the result of a complex nociceptive network. Therefore, it is naive to expect a single drug to block the entire 'network'. ACh: acetylcholine; BNZ: benzodiazepine; GABA: γ-aminobutyric acid; NE: norepinephrine; NK: neurokinin; NMDA: N-methyl-D-aspartate; NSAID: nonsteroidal anti-inflammatory drug; sP: substance P; SST: somatostatin. (Adapted from Tranquilli WJ, *et al.* [2004]. *Pain Management for the Small Animal Practitioner*, 2nd edn. Teton New Media.)

Although there is little published evidence that multimodal drug therapy is of benefit over monomodal therapy in veterinary patients suffering from chronic painful conditions, such as osteoarthritis and cancer, implementation seems implicit[9–14].

Herein arises the question: 'what drugs should go into a multimodal cocktail?' Drugs comprising the cocktail should be from different classes (so they can work by different modes of action and not compete for the same substrates or receptor sites) that block as many as possible of the four physiologic processes underlying pain; transduction, transmission, modulation, and perception (*Table 67*, **Fig. 109**).

TABLE 67: Pain recognition processes

Physiologic process	Definition
Transduction	Conversion of energy from a noxious stimulus (mechanical, thermal, or chemical) into nerve impulses by sensory receptors (nociceptors)
Transmission	Transference of neural signals from the site of transduction (periphery) to the central nervous system (spinal cord and brain)
Modulation	Alterations of ascending signals initially in the dorsal horn and continues throughout the central nervous system; this includes descending inhibitory and facilitatory input from the brain that influences (modulates) nociceptive transmission at the level of the spinal cord
Perception	Receipt and cognitive appreciation of signals arriving at higher central nervous system structures as pain

109

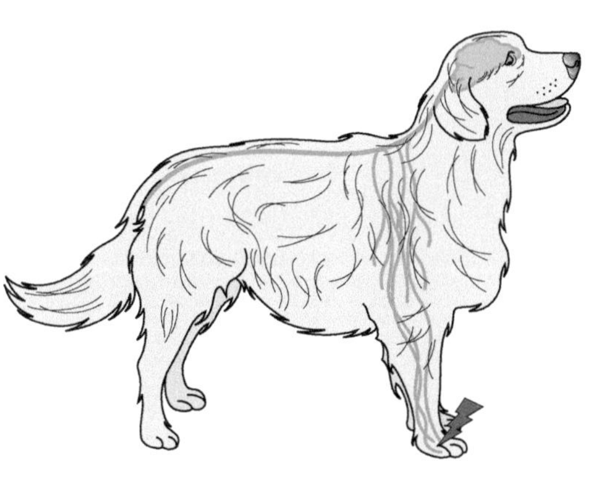

Perception (cerebral cortex)
- Anesthetics
- Opioids
- α_2-antagonists
- Benzodiazepines
- Phenothiazines
- NSAIDs

Modulation (spinal cord)
- Local anesthetic
- Tricyclic antidepressants
- Cholinesterase inhibitors
- NMDA antagonists
- Opioids
- NSAIDs
- α_2-antagonists
- Anticonvulsants

Transmission (sensory nerves)
- Local anesthetics
- α_2-antagonists

Transduction (sensory nerve endings, nociceptors)
- Local anesthetics
- Opioids
- NSAIDs
- Corticosteroids

Fig. 109 Drug classes listed are more effective than others in blocking each of the physiologic processes of transduction, transmission, modulation, and perception. NMDA: N-methyl-D-aspartate; NSAID: nonsteroidal anti-inflammatory drug.

DRUG CLASSES FOR MULTIMODAL USE

A popular combination for multimodal use consists of drugs from the opioid and NSAID classes. This combination is commonly used postoperatively and for addressing the World Health Organization's cancer pain ladder recommendation for mild-to-moderate and moderate-to-severe pain (*Table 68*). There are several opioid/NSAID combination drugs commercially available for human use (*Table 69*).

Fig. 110 shows a comparison of numbers needed to treat human patients, comparing single drug administrations to combinations[15]. Increased efficacy is obvious when paracetamol (acetaminophen) is combined with various opioids.

Delivery techniques

Local and regional administration techniques are re-emerging in popularity. Analgesic infiltration at a nerve trunk or regional administration via spinal injection provide regional analgesia. The principal benefit of regional analgesia is reduced sedation and other side-effects compared with those seen following parenteral administration of some analgesic agents.

TABLE 68: Comparison of opioid and nonsteroidal anti-inflammatory drug (NSAID) pharmacology

	Opioids	NSAIDs
Mechanism	Predominantly central	Predominantly peripheral
Availability	Controlled substances	Noncontrolled/ some available OTC
Therapeutic ceiling	No	Yes
Tolerance	Yes	
Addiction	Possible	Not possible
GI side-effects:		
Nausea and vomiting	More frequent	Less frequent
Constipation	Frequent	No
Gastric ulceration	No	Possible
GI bleeding	No	Possible
Respiratory side-effects	Depression	Infrequent
Effects on pupil	Yes	No
Cognitive impairment	Yes	No

GI: gastrointestinal; OTC: over-the-counter.

TABLE 69: Some nonsteroidal anti-inflammatory drug (NSAID)*–opioid commercial drug combinations available for human use

Combination	USA Trade name	Strength (mg)
Aspirin + caffeine + dihydrocodeine	Synalgos	356.4 + 30 + 16
Aspirin + carisoprodol + codeine	Soma compound w/codeine	325 + 200 +16
Aspirin + codeine	Empirin w/codeine #3 Empirin w/codeine #4	325 + 30 325 + 60
Aspirin + hydrocodone	LortabASA	500 + 5
Aspirin + oxycodone	Persodan-Demi Percodan	325 + 2.25 325 + 4.5
Ibuprofen + oxycodone	Combunox	400 + 5
Ketoprofen + hydrocodone	Vicoprofen Darvon compound –65	200 + 7.5 389 + 32.4 + 65

* Acetaminophen is not included in this table because acetaminophen is not technically a NSAID: it has analgesic properties, but not anti-inflammatory properties.

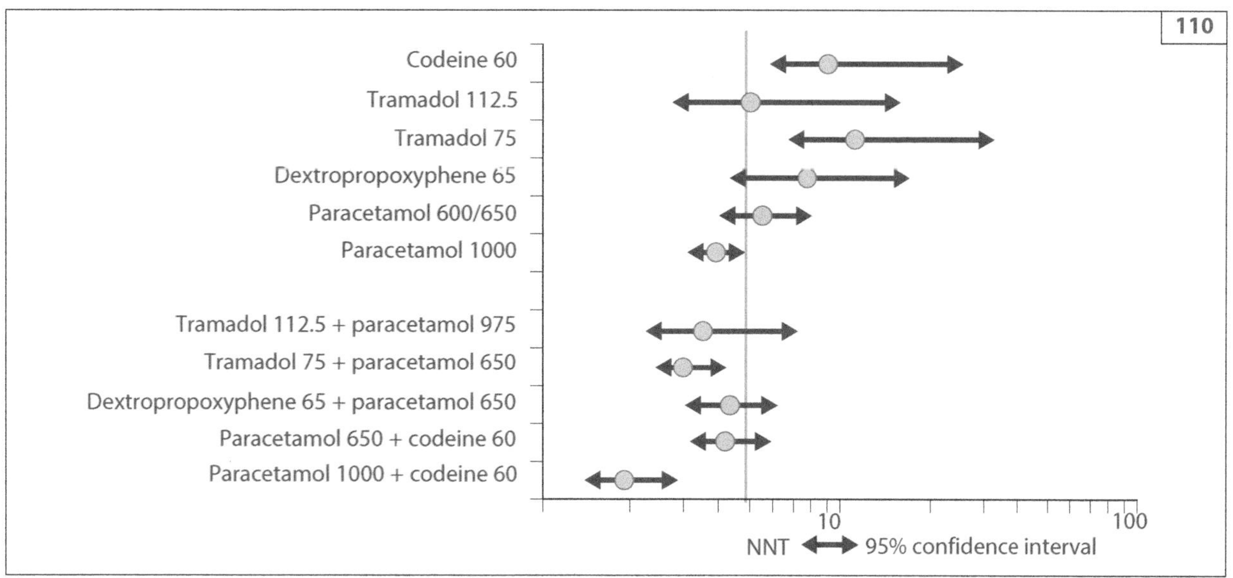

Fig. 110 Number needed to treat (NNT) demonstrates the increased efficacy when paracetamol (acetaminophen) is administered together with a different class of drug. (McQuay HJ, Moore A [2006][15].)

Many traditional analgesic drugs, including opioids and α_2-agonists, have a short duration of action and the potential to produce systemic side-effects, including emesis, respiratory depression, drowsiness, and ileus. In contrast, local anesthetics are comparatively safe. They are effective and relatively inexpensive. Local anesthetics have the unique ability to produce complete blockade of sensory nerve fibers and suppress the development of secondary sensitization to pain. Therefore, local and regional anesthetic/analgesic techniques are often used with opioids, α_2-agonists, N-methyl-D-aspartate antagonists and NSAIDs as part of a multimodal strategy.

LOCAL ANESTHETICS

During the generation of an action potential, voltage-gated sodium channels open and allow sodium ions to flow into the cell, which depolarizes the cell membrane. Local anesthetics bind to a hydrophilic site within the sodium channel on the cell membrane inner surface, and block activation of the channel, thereby preventing depolarization of the cell membrane. Small nerves and myelinated fibers tend to be more responsive to local anesthetics than are large nerves and unmyelinated fibers. Commonly, autonomic fibers (small unmyelinated C-fibers and myelinated B-fibers) and pain fibers (small unmyelinated C-fibers and myelinated Aδ-fibers) are blocked before other sensory and motor fibers (differential block). Local anesthetics are also more effective at sensory fibers because they have longer action potentials and discharge at higher frequencies than other types of fiber (frequency-dependent blockade). In addition, some local anesthetics, such as bupivacaine, selectively block sensory rather than motor function[16].

The practice of adding vasoconstrictors, such as epinephrine, to local anesthetics so as to reduce the rate of systemic absorption and prolong the duration of action, has fallen from favor with the availability of longer-acting local anesthetics, such as bupivacaine and ropivacaine.

Adverse side-effects of local anesthetics are rare if appropriate dosage recommendations are followed and are most commonly associated with inappropriate IV delivery. Central nervous system (CNS) and cardiovascular disturbances are the most common side-effects. With excessive dosing, the rate of depolarization of individual cardiac cells is reduced, leading to prolonged conduction of the cardiac impulse, arrhythmias, or bradycardia and asystole[17]. Rapid IV administration of local anesthetics can decrease vascular tone and myocardial contractility, resulting in the acute onset of hypotension. CNS effects can range from mild to full-blown seizure activity. The toxicity of most local anesthetics reflects potency, and in dogs, the relative CNS toxicity of lidocaine, etidocaine, and bupivacaine is 1:3:5, respectively[18].

Local anesthetics can be used in a variety of clinical settings to manage or pre-empt pain. Common uses include digital blocks for feline onychectomy, dental blocks for tooth extraction, local infiltration for cutaneous procedures, intra-articular analgesia, body cavity infusion before or after abdominal surgery, soaker catheters for wound analgesia, and epidural deposition for abdominal and/or hind limb procedures. Most nerves can be blocked with 0.1–0.3 ml of 2% lidocaine or 0.5% bupivacaine solution using a 25-gauge needle. Doses of local anesthetics, especially for cats and small dogs, should always be calculated carefully, and are best administered with the animal under general anesthesia or heavy sedation.

Onychectomy

Approximately 24% of owned cats in the USA are declawed[19], and postoperative pain is a generally accepted consequence[20]. Effective analgesia for onychectomy can be provided by blocking the radial, ulnar, and median nerves, although one study refutes this clinical observation[21] (**Fig. 111**). A combination of both lidocaine and bupivicaine (1.5 mg/kg of each) apparently provides both a quicker onset and longer duration of analgesic effect than when using either drug alone for blockade.

Dental

Sensory nerve fibers that innervate the bone, teeth and soft tissues of the oral cavity arborize

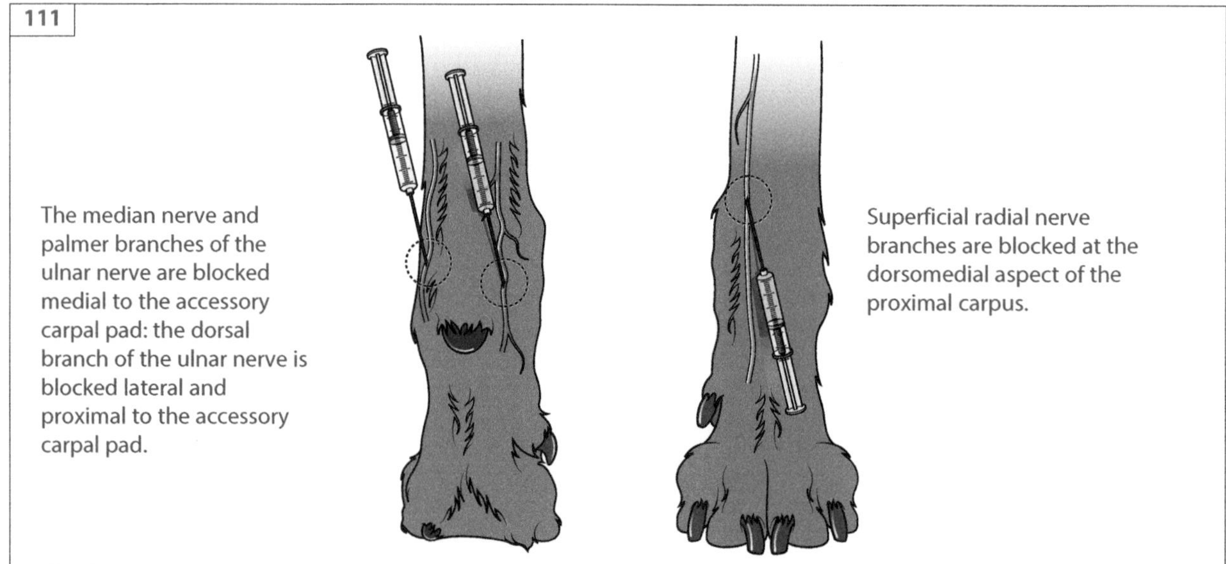

Fig. 111 Onychectomy is an excellent example of where analgesia is markedly improved by preventive local anesthetic blockade. Three sites of local anesthetic deposition effectively blocks the distal extremity.

from the maxillary or mandibular branches of the trigeminal nerve. Four regional nerve blocks can be easily performed to provide analgesia for dental and oral surgical procedures (*Table 70*, **Fig. 112**).

Dermal

Local anesthetic infiltration is often implemented for removal of tumors or dermal lesions, superficial lacerations, and as preincisional blocks.

TABLE 70: Dental nerve blocks with local anesthetic

Block	Mental	Mandibular (inferior alveolar)	Infraorbital	Maxillary
Effect	Anesthetizes all oral tissues rostral to the second premolar on the ipsilateral side	Affects the bone, teeth, soft tissue, and tongue on the ipsilateral side	Anesthetizes the bone, soft tissue, and dentition rostral to, but not including, the upper fourth premolar	Blocks the bone, teeth, soft tissue, and palatal tissue on the ipsilateral side
Location	Mental foramen ventral to the rostral (mesial) root of the second premolar	Lingual side of notch on caudal ventral mandible cranial to the angular process, midpoint between ventral and dorsal borders of the mandible	Infraorbital foramen of the maxilla dorsal to the caudal (distal) root of the upper third premolar	In the open mouth: notch where the zygomatic arch meets the bone surrounding the last maxillary molar

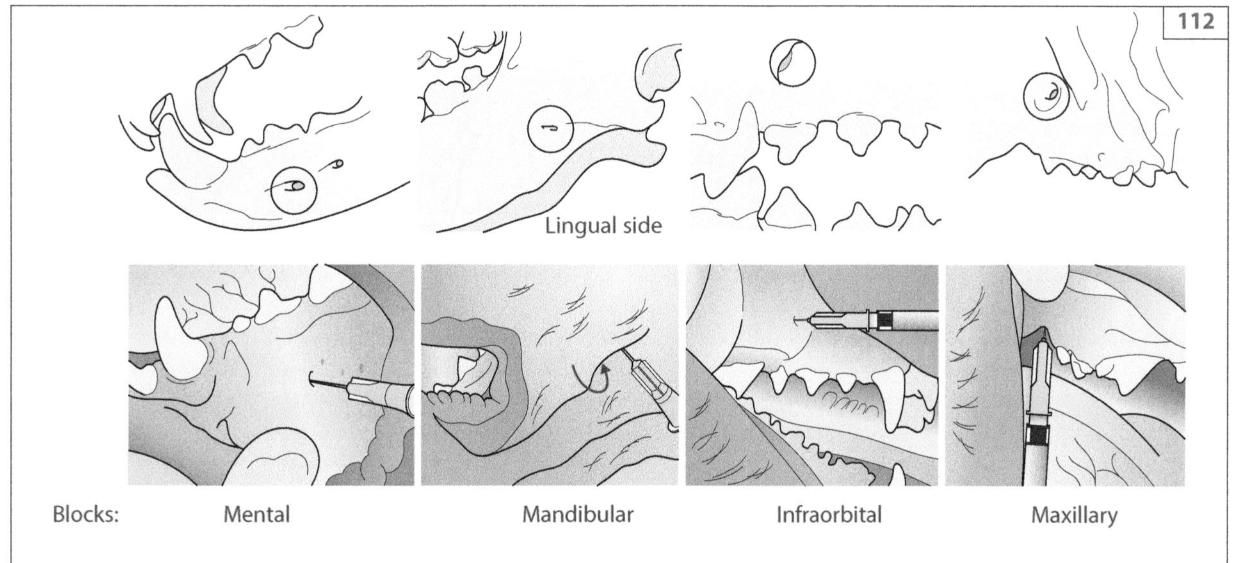

Fig. 112 Local anesthetic blocks are very effective in providing analgesia for oral cavity procedures. Anatomic area blocked is rostral to the injection site.

A small subcutaneous bleb (0.5–2.0 ml) is often sufficient for small lesion removal in the dermis. Infiltrative blocks for removal of subcutaneous masses requires a deeper area of desensitization and an inverted pyramidal area of infiltration works well (**Fig. 113**).

Body cavities

Intrapleural administration of bupivacaine has been described to manage pain in dogs undergoing intercostal or sternal thoracotomy[22,23], as has peritoneal administration for pancreatitis[24] and canine ovariohysterectomy[25]. In the conscious animal, pleural infusion of bupivacaine can be painful; therefore, sodium bicarbonate is added. In either case, 0.02 mEq/kg of sodium bicarbonate is added to 0.2 ml/kg of 0.5% bupivacaine solution; then, saline is added to produce a final volume of 10–20 ml for administration via a thoracostomy tube or abdominocentesis. The mechanism of analgesia has been suggested to be due to diffusion of local anesthetic through the parietal pleura, causing intercostal nerve block, blockade of the thoracic sympathetic chain and splanchnic nerves, and diffusion of the anesthetic into the ipsilateral brachial plexus, resulting in blockade of the parietal peritoneum[26–28]. Since cranial abdominal nerves enter the spinal cord at the level of the thorax, this technique is useful for acute pancreatitis or cranial abdominal surgery[16].

There is evidence for a reduction of postoperative pain after intra-articular local anesthesia in human patients undergoing arthroscopic knee surgery[29]. In dogs, intra-articular bupivacaine provided pain relief after stifle surgery better than intra-articular morphine[30] (**Fig. 114**).

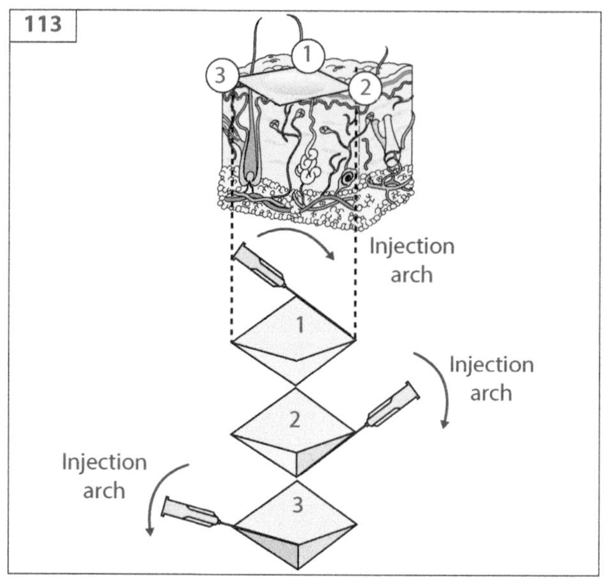

Fig. 113 Local anesthetic, administered through three injection site arches, will adequately infiltrate an area to be desensitized for procedures such as dermal mass removal. A 1:1 mixture of lidocaine and bupivacaine, not to exceed 3.0 mg/kg of lidocaine and 2.0 mg/kg of bupivacaine, takes advantage of the more rapid onset of action of lidocaine with the longer duration of effect from bupivacaine.

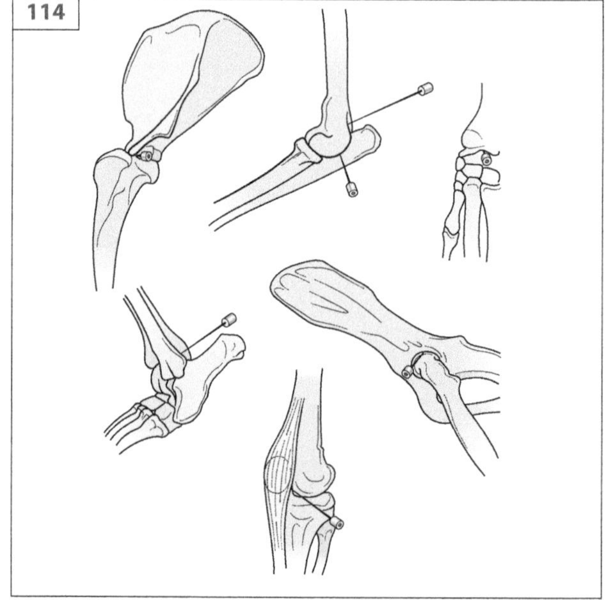

Fig. 114 Intra-articular analgesia. Many investigators suggest a combination of morphine (0.1–0.2 mg/kg) and bupivacaine (or lidocaine) (~1 ml/10 kg). Note: evidence exists that intra-articular local anesthetics are chondrotoxic[56–60].

Intercostal block

Patients undergoing thoracotomy, chest tube placement, or with traumatic rib injury benefit from intercostal block. A minimum of two adjacent intercostal spaces, both cranial and caudal to the incision or injury site, should be blocked due to overlapping nerve supply (**Fig. 115**). The anesthetic is inserted percutaneously at the caudal border of the rib, near the level of the intervertebral foramen.

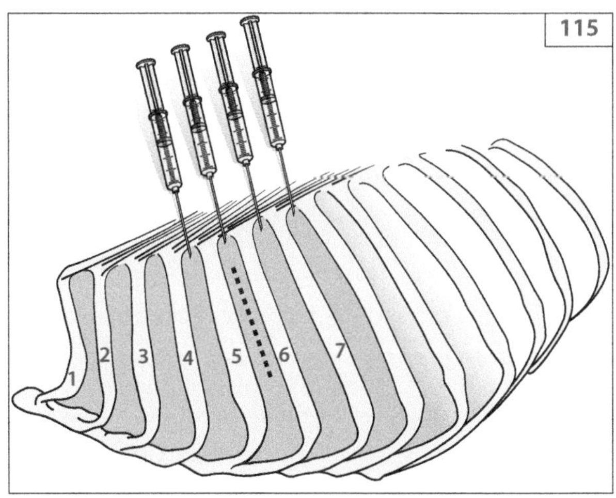

Fig. 115 Intercostal block. Local anesthetic is injected at the level of the intervertebral foramen two spaces in front of, and two spaces behind, the incision line (dotted line).

Epidural administration

In the 1970s it was discovered that epidural administration of opioids produced profound analgesia in animals with minimal systemic effects[31]. Since that time, interest has increased in the epidural route for administration of analgesics, particularly in the delivery of opioids, where the motor paralysis of local anesthesia administration can be avoided. The most frequently administered drugs are the local anesthetics and opioids, but α_2-agonists (xylazine and medetomidine) and combinations of these drugs have also been used.

Epidural drug administration and catheter placement for repeated administration have several advantages: 1) require lower drug doses than systemic injection, and therefore less risk for dose-related side-effects; 2) decreased perioperative injectable and inhalant agent requirement; and 3) decreased procedural costs due to the long duration of action and decreased dose of adjunctive drugs. It has been suggested that epidurals are best utilized together with general anesthesia as part of a balanced (multimodal) analgesia protocol, and likely play a noteworthy role in blocking CNS wind-up. The technique is frequently used for perianal, hind limb, and abdominal surgery; however, analgesia as far rostral as the thoracic limb (using morphine) can be provided in a dose-related manner[32]. Epidural morphine, with or without long-lasting bupivacaine, has been used to relieve pain associated with pancreatitis and peritonitis[33].

Urine retention and pruritus are reported as possible complications of this technique, although their occurrence is rare. The procedure is contraindicated in animals with bleeding disorders because of the potential for hemorrhage into the epidural space with inadvertent puncture of an epidural vessel.

Due to the potential for blockade of regional sympathetic nerves, epidurals should not be performed on **hypovolemic** or **hypotensive** animals. Injection site skin infection is also a contraindication.

The procedure should be performed in a sterile setting. The site for spinal needle insertion is on the dorsal midline at the lumbosacral space. In the adult dog the spinal cord ends at approximately the 6th vertebra, rostral to the injection site. The site for injection is just caudal to the 7th dorsal spinous process, which can be easily identified because it is shorter than the others. Confirmation of correct needle placement can be done by either the 'hanging drop' or 'loss of resistance' technique[33]. Following correct needle placement (**Fig. 116**), the drug(s) is slowly injected to ensure even distribution at doses shown in *Table 71*.

Epidural anesthesia at-a-glance

- Neurolepanalgesia or general anesthesia is usually required to perform an epidural.
- Needed supplies:
  Spinal needle (22 or 20 gauge, 1.5–3 inches) (because they have a stylet).
  Fenestrated drape (eye drape).
  Sterile gloves.
  Appropriate dose and volume of drug in a syringe.
  Air and saline syringe (3 ml): glass offers the least resistance.
  3 ml syringe for 1 ml of 2% lidocaine and a 23 gauge needle to desensitize the skin (in a conscious patient).
- Clip hair.
- Aseptic preparation of skin.
- Patient in sternal recumbency with rear limbs flexed and pulled cranially; this tends to 'open' the L–S space (lateral recumbency can be used).
- Block the spinal needle placement area with local anesthetic (if required).
- With thumb and middle finger on the ilial wings, the index finger of the palpating hand palpates L–S intervertebral space, caudal to dorsal spinal process of L7.
- Introduce the spinal needle, on the midline and perpendicular to the skin, staying close to L7.
- Advance the needle through the subcutaneous tissues, the supraspinous ligament, the interspinous ligament, the ligament flavum, and into the epidural space. A 'pop' or change in resistance to the passage of the spinal needle is usually apparent as the ligamentum flavum is penetrated
- Observe needle hub for egress of blood or spinal fluid to check for correct placement. Gentle aspiration may be performed and no fluid should be detected if the needle is in the epidural space. There should be no resistance to an injection of air or 0.5 ml of saline with a test syringe.
- 'Hang drop' technique may be used to confirm correct placement by removing the stylet before the needle penetrates the ligamentum flavum and placing a drop of sterile saline or local anesthetic in the hub. Once in the epidural space, the fluid is aspirated into the needle shaft by the subatmospheric epidural pressure. This is about 88% effective in medium sized dogs, and ineffective in lateral recumbency.
- False negatives are most commonly associated with tissue plugs during insertion; therefore, it is advised to remove the stylet only in close proximity to the flavum ligamentum or once it has been pierced.

In the dog, the spinal cord variably ends at L6–7; the dural sac ends at L7–S1. In the cat, the cord and the sac usually extend one vertebra more caudal (cord termination may be as caudal as S3). To facilitate catheter placement, a Touhy needle is used. NEVER withdraw a catheter through the needle, so as to avoid cutting the catheter and leaving it *in situ*.

Forelimb anesthetic blocks

The rostral limit of an epidural is approximately T11–13. Therefore, the forelimbs are not blocked by the epidural technique. The traditional axillary block is relatively easy to perform; however, it requires large volume of local anesthetic, onset time is slow (20-30 minutes), structures proximal to the elbow are not anesthetized, and incomplete blockade of the brachial plexus is relatively common. Paravertebral blockade of the brachial plexus provides analgesia and muscle relaxation for surgical procedures of the shoulder and brachium.

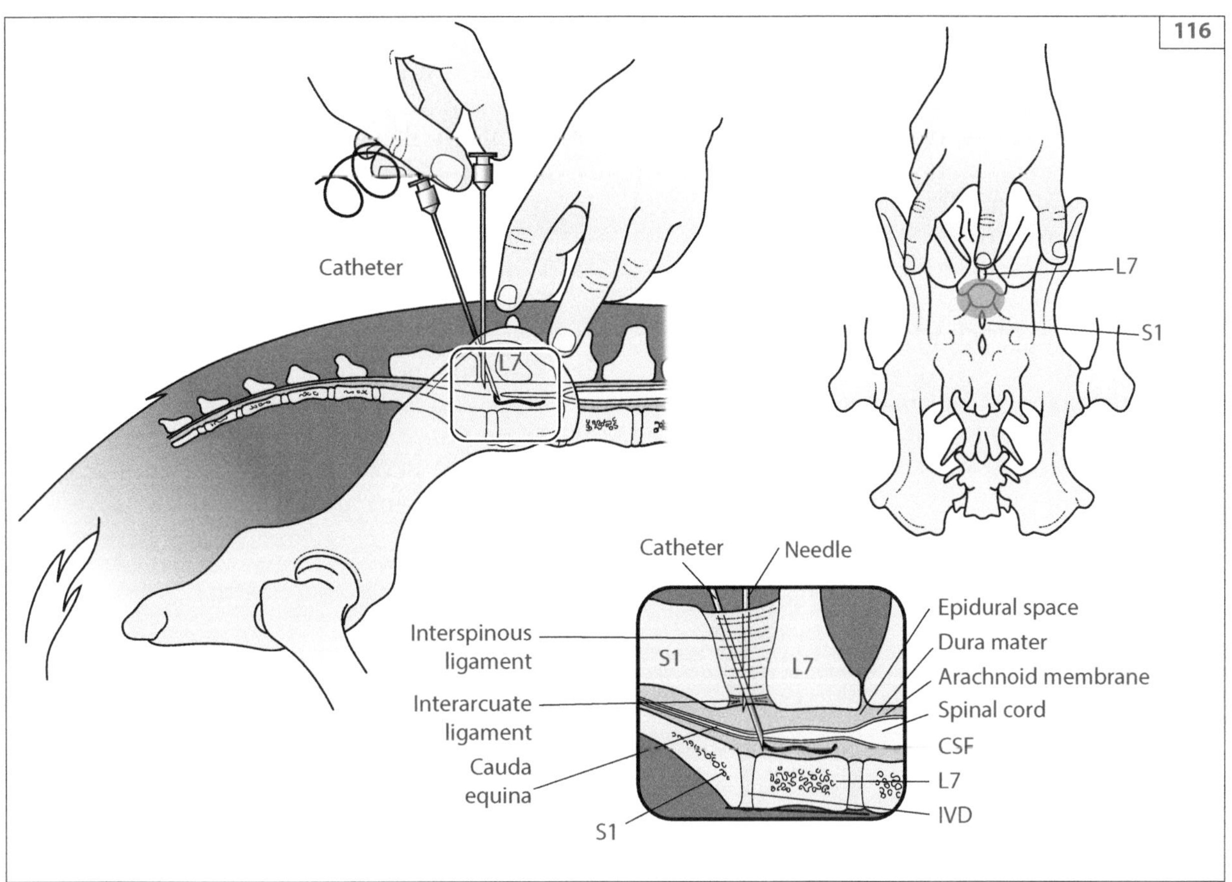

Fig. 116 Lumbosacral epidural needle and catheter placement. (Adapted from: Thurmon JC, Tranquilli WJ, Benson GJ (1996). *Lumb & Jones' Veterinary Anesthesia,* 3rd edn. Williams & Wilkins, Philadelphia.) CSF: cerebrospinal fluid; IVD: intervertebral disk.

TABLE 71: Drug dose and duration of action following epidural administration.

Drug	Dose (Dog)	Approximate onset (minutes)	Approximate duration (hours)
Lidocaine 2%	1 ml/3.4 kg (to T5) 1 ml/4.5 kg (to T13–L1)	10	1–1.5
Bupivacaine (0.25% or 0.5%)	1 ml/4.5kg	20–30	4.5–6
Fentanyl	0.001 mg/kg	4–10	6
Oxymorphone	Dog and cat: 0.05–0.1 mg/kg	15	10
Morphine	Dog and cat: 0.1 mg/kg	23	20
Buprenorphine	Dog: 0.005 mg/kg	30	12–18
Medetomidine	Dog and cat: 0.01 mg/kg	15	4

It is relatively easy to perform, provided anatomy of the brachial plexus is appreciated and key anatomic landmarks are accurately identified (**Fig. 117, Fig. 118**). It is, however, difficult to perform in obese dogs and dogs with heavy cervical musculature. It should not be performed if the transverse process of C6 and head of the first rib cannot be identified.

Paravertebral blockade of the brachial plexus

- After clipping and aseptic preparation of the site, the scapula is shifted caudally to expose the transverse process of C6 and the head of the first rib.
- The index finger is placed on the large ventral wing of the transverse process, isolating the cranial and caudal processes.
- Insert the needle dorsal to the cranial and caudal margins of the process, directed medially.
- Local anesthetic is injected along the nerve above the dorsolateral surface of the transverse process at each site (for blocking C6 and C7).
- With the scapula still shifted caudally, the first rib is palpated medial to the cranial margin of the scapula.
- Place the index finger just ventral to the rib head, and isolate the cranial and caudal margins.
- Insert the needle dorsal to the cranial and caudal margins, directed medially.

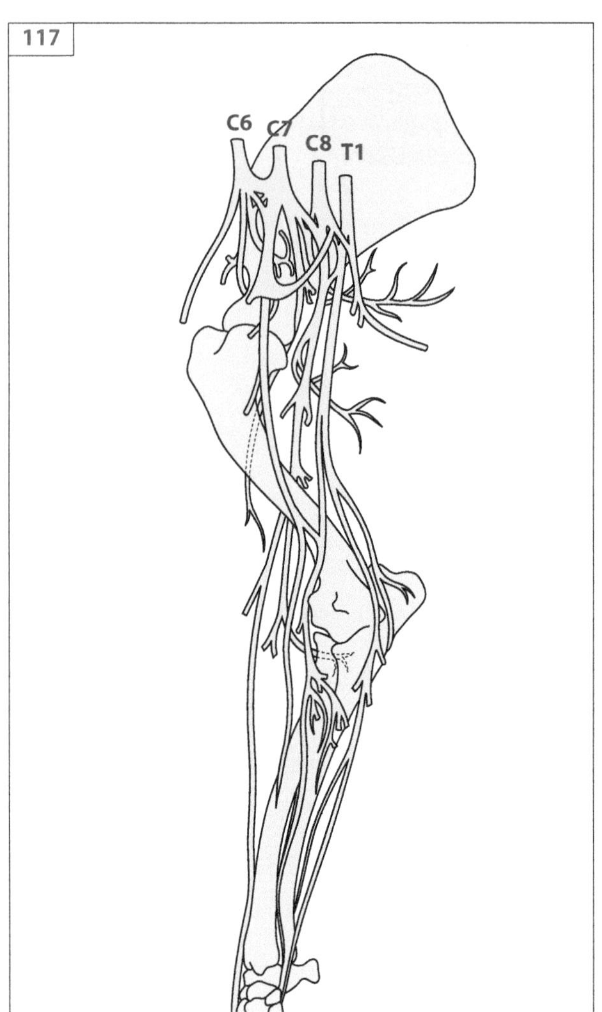

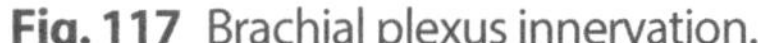
Fig. 117 Brachial plexus innervation.

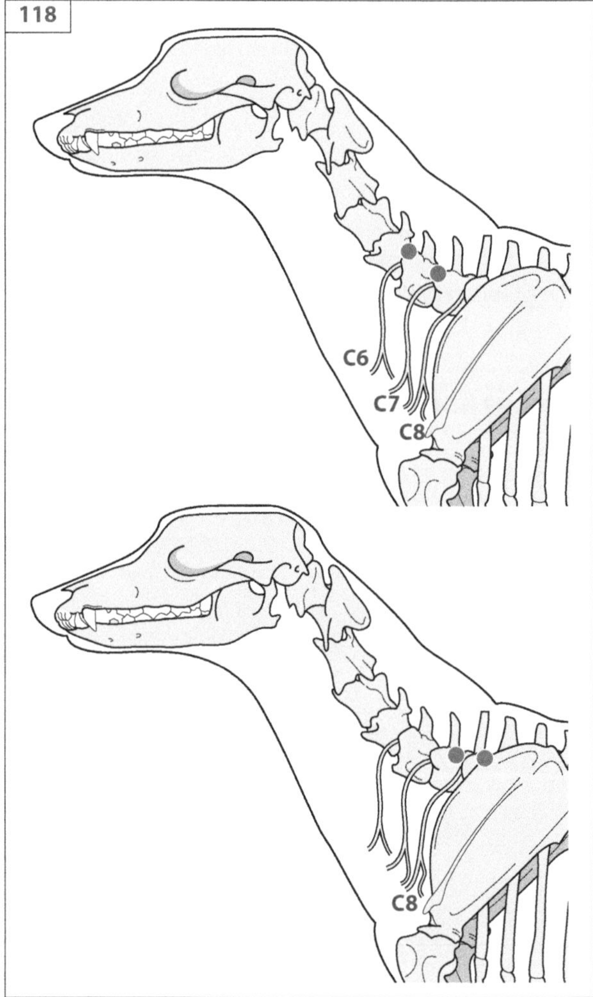

Fig. 118 Paravertebral blockade of the brachial plexus.

- Local anesthetic is injected dorsal to the head of the rib at each site (for blocking C8 and T1).
- Take care to avoid intravascular injection.

MUMR block

Modification of the brachial nerve block is the MUMR block, which blocks the median, ulnar, musculocutaneous, and radial nerves, desensitizing the area of the forelimb below the elbow (**Fig. 119**). The median, ulnar, and musculocutaneous nerves are blocked above the medial epicondyle of the humerus next to the brachial artery, proximal to the epicondyle, between the biceps and triceps. Note: the location of the brachial artery and vein along the medial surface of the humeral shaft. The radial nerve is blocked above the lateral epicondyle of the humerus, between the lateral head of the triceps and brachialis.

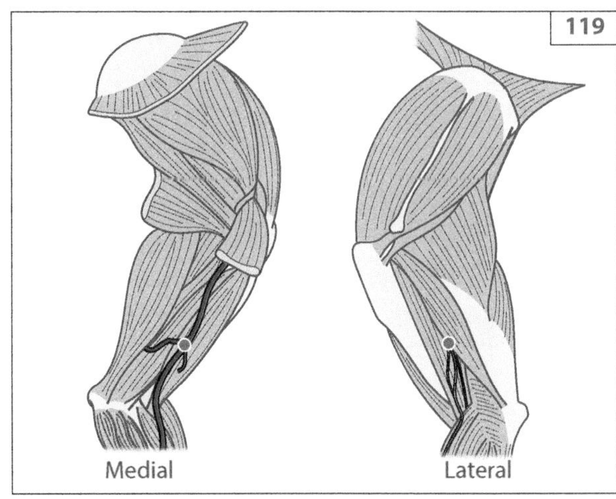

Fig. 119 MUMR distal limb block.

Nerve location

The success rates of nerve blocks may be improved by use of a nerve locator, which helps to locate the peripheral nerves accurately. Such a device consists of a constant current generator, a grounding patient electrode, an electrode attached to an insulated stimulating needle, and an extension set attached to a syringe for injection of local anesthetic. The use of nerve stimulators to locate peripheral nerves is routine in human surgery, and efficacy of the technique has been demonstrated in the dog[34–37].

Ultrasound (US) guidance uses anatomical landmarks, including the target nerves themselves, rather than a neurophysiologic end point as with electroneurostimulation. Sonographic guidance offers several potential advantages: direct visualization of the target nerves may reduce the need for multiple needle passes and thereby reduce tissue damage; a reduced risk of vascular laceration; target accuracy which reduces the volume of local anesthetic solution necessary; and minimized block performance time. Although electrostimulation has been considered the 'gold standard' technique for peripheral nerve localization[38], US-guided techniques are gaining popularity to facilitate peripheral nerve blocks as this technique provides the ability to both manipulate the needle under direct guidance and see the spread of the local anesthetic solution as it is being injected[39,40]. Success rates of 80% have been reported for peripheral nerve blocks performed using conventional techniques compared to almost 100% using US guidance[38]. The combination of US guidance and electrolocation offers the advantage of the anatomical as well as electrophysiologic confirmation of nerve identification and needle placement.

Ocular block

Effectiveness of local anesthetic injection into the retrobulbar space for postoperative analgesia following eye enucleation in dogs has also been reported[41].

Other local anesthetic techniques

Constant rate infusion (CRI) of lidocaine is also an effective method of delivering local anesthetic. Dog: 2–4 mg/kg IV bolus, then 25–80 g/kg/min; Cat: 0.25–0.75 mg/kg slow IV, then 10–40 g/kg/min (Note: efficacy and safety are not yet convincing). Finally, lidocaine is available in a topical patch (Lidoderm®), 2% jelly, and in a 10% spray formulation.

Specially designed catheters can be utilized for longer-term (days) continuous infiltration of local anesthetic[42], particularly following procedures such as ear canal ablation (efficacious findings[43], non-efficacious findings[44]), amputations, and after large soft tissue excision, such as fibrosarcoma removal in cats[45]. Commercial devices are available (Pain Buster®) that include a local anesthetic reservoir connected to a fenestrated catheter, or catheters can be constructed from red rubber or polyethylene tubing. Bupivacaine, 0.25%, is diluted to volume and can be given as a bolus: 2 mg/kg (cat: 1 mg/kg) first dose, then 1 mg/kg (cat: 0.5 mg/kg) doses can be given thereafter at intervals >6 hours for 1–2 days.

Other drug delivery routes

Oral transmucosal (OTM) drug administration is a relatively new delivery system used in humans, e.g. fentanyl lozenges. As noted in chapter 6, the NSAID meloxicam is now available as a transmucosal oral mist for dogs. This same route has been investigated by Robertson *et al.*[46] as it applies to the efficacy of buprenorphine in cats. Because, in part, the Pk_a of buprenorphine (8.24) is similar to the pH of the cat's mouth (9.0), buprenorphine is readily absorbed across the oral mucous membranes. Absorption by this route, rather than gastrointestinal, avoids hepatic first-pass elimination, because venous drainage is systemic. As a result, the onset of analgesic action is as early as 30 minutes and lasts up to 6 hours. This response in the cat is similar to the IV administration as assessed by a validated nociception thermal model. OTM administration is easy and avoids multiple injections, making it an excellent delivery form for both in-hospital and take-home use. Apparently, buprenorphine is odorless and tasteless, as cats do not resist OTM administration and do not hypersalivate in response.

ACUPUNCTURE

Acupuncture falls under the categorization of complementary (and, therefore, multimodal) and alternative medicine (AM) as part of traditional Chinese medicine (TCM), and is utilized in humans in at least 78 countries worldwide[47]. From a historical perspective, little information about acupuncture was available in the USA until after President Richard Nixon's visit to China in 1972. However, in 1826 Benjamin Franklin's grandson, a Philadelphia physician, published that acupuncture was an effective treatment for pain associated with rheumatism and neuralgia among prisoners at the Pennsylvania state penitentiary[48]. It is a safe, low-cost modality which is easy to administer and has no side-effects if performed by a trained practitioner; it can be administered stand-alone or as a complement to other medical therapeutics. It is misleading to refer to a single universal form of traditional Chinese acupuncture, as there are more than 80 different acupuncture styles in China alone, in addition to many Japanese, Korean, Vietnamese, European, and American styles.

Theory of acupuncture

TCM places emphasis on function rather than structure. Accordingly, in such practice it is more important to understand the relationships between variables and the functional 'whole' of the patient than to identify the specifics of a single pathology. Basic to the practice of acupuncture is the yin–yang theory, where yin and yang are interdependent but possess similar characteristics (**Fig. 120**)[49]. They can transform into each other, and can consume each other. In this regard, physiology and pathology are variations along a continuum of health and illness.

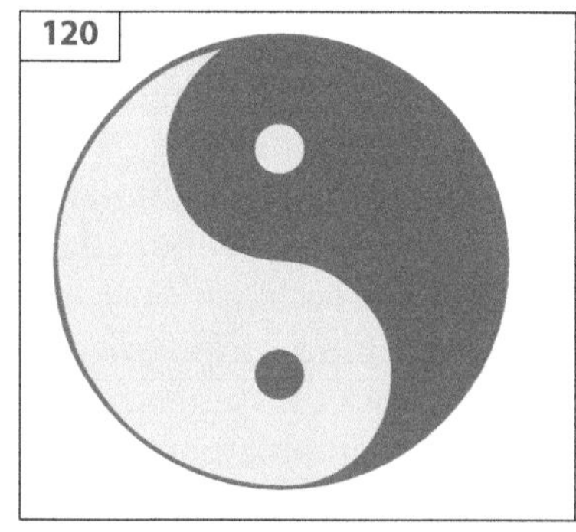

Fig. 120 The graphic which has come to represent the yin–yang theory.

A common feature shared by all different types of acupuncture is using needles to initiate changes in the soft tissue. Needles and needle-induced changes are believed to activate the built in survival mechanisms that normalize homeostasis and promote self-healing. Herein, acupuncture can be defined as a physiologic therapy co-ordinated by the brain which responds to the stimulation of manual or electrical needling of peripheral sensory nerves, where acupuncture does not treat any particular pathologic system, but normalizes physiologic homeostasis and promotes self-healing[50]. Acupuncture can be effective for both peripheral soft tissue pain and internal disorders, but in the case of peripheral soft tissue pain the result appears more predictable because of the local needle reaction.

Hypotheses of acupuncture mechanisms

The leading hypotheses include the effects of local stimulation, neuronal gating, the release of endogenous opiates, and the placebo effect. It is further proposed that the CNS is essential for the processing of these effects via its modulation of the autonomic nervous system, the neuroimmune system, and hormonal regulation. Clinical observation suggests that acupuncture needling achieves at least four therapeutic goals:

- Release of physical and emotional stress.
- Activation and control of immune and anti-inflammatory mechanisms.
- Acceleration of tissue healing.
- Pain relief secondary to endorphin and serotonin release.

Keeping in mind that acupuncture therapy is considered to activate built-in survival mechanisms, that is, self-healing potential, it is effective for those symptoms that can be completely or partially healed by the body. Additionally, each individual has a different self-healing capacity influenced by genetic makeup, medical history, lifestyle, and age, all of which may be dynamically changing.

Eastern perspectives meet western perspectives

Ancient Chinese thought holds that Qi is a fundamental and vital substance of the universe, with all phenomena being produced by its changes. It is considered a vital substance of the body, flowing along organized pathways known as acupuncture channels, or meridians, helping to maintain normal activities. TCM suggests that a balanced flow of Qi throughout the system is required for good health, and acupuncture stimulation can correct imbalances.

As of the mid-1990s, stimulation of acupuncture points is believed to cause biochemical changes that can affect the body's natural healing. The primary mechanisms involved in these changes include enhanced conduction of bioelectromagnetic signals, activation of opioid systems, and activation of autonomic and central nervous systems causing the release of various neurotransmitters and neurohormones[51]. Approximately 30 years ago it was discovered that acupuncture analgesia could be reversed by naloxone, a pure antagonist to all known opioids[52]. Acupuncture can change concentrations of serotonin and biogenic amines, including opioid peptides, met-enkephalin, leu-enkephalin, β-endorphin, and dynorphin.

Acupuncture can also be explained, in part, by Melzack and Wall's Gate Theory (see **Fig. 27**). When large, unmyelinated Aδ- and Aβ-fibers are stimulated by acupuncture, impulses from small unmyelinated C-fibers, transmitting ascending nociceptive information, are blocked by a gate of inhibitory interneurons.

The strongest evidence for acupuncture efficacy in human cancer has been in the areas of nausea, vomiting, and pain control[53,54].

SUMMARY

The term multimodal has come to denote the co-utilization of different delivery modes as well as a variety of different drug-class agents, the objective of which is to provide the patient a minimal effective dose of each agent and therefore render optimal pain relief with the minimal risk for adverse response (*Table 72 overleaf*).

TABLE 72: Various drugs commonly used in multimodal protocols

Drug	Dose	Species	Route	Duration	Comments
Morphine	0.5–1.0 mg/kg	Canine	IM, SC, IV	3–4 h	Caution with IV administration: histamine release–give slowly
	0.05–0.1 mg/kg	Feline	IM, SC	3–4 h	
	0.2 mg/kg: loading, IM	Canine: 0.1–0.5 mg/kg/h. Feline: 0.05–0.1 mg/kg/h	IM then CRI-IV		
	0.1 mg/kg preservative-free	Canine/feline	Epidural	12–24 h	
	1–5 mg in 5–10 ml saline	Canine	Intra-articular		
Meperidine	3–5 mg/kg	Canine/feline	IM, SC	1–2 h	Do *not* give IV (histamine release)
Methadone	0.1–0.5 mg/kg	Canine/feline	IM, SC, IV	2–4 h	NMDA antagonist activity
Oxymorphone	0.05–0.1 mg/kg	Canine	IM, IV, SC	3–4 h	Minimal histamine release
	0.03–0.05 mg/kg	Feline	IM, SC	3–4 h	
Hydromorphone	0.1–0.2 mg/kg	Canine/feline	IM, IV, SC	2–4 h	Minimal histamine release. Hyperthermia may be seen in cats
Fentanyl	5 μg/kg + 3–6 μg/kg/h	Canine	IV	Infusion	
	2–3 μg/kg + 2–3 μg/kg/h	Feline	IV	Infusion	
Fentanyl patch	25 μg/h	Canine: 3–10 kg		1–3 days	24 h to reach peak concentrations
	50 μg/h	Canine: 10–20 kg		1–3 days	
	75 μg/h	Canine: 20–30 kg		1–3 days	
	100 μg/h	Canine: >30 kg		1–3 days	
	25–50 μg/h	Feline		+ 6 days	6 h to reach peak concentrations
Butorphanol	0.1–0.2 mg/kg	Canine/feline	IM, IV, SC	Dog: 1h; Cat: 2–4 h	Low oral bioavailability
	0.2–0.4 mg/kg IV; then 0.1–0.2 mg/kg/h	Canine/feline	CRI		
Pentazocine	1–3 mg/kg	Canine/feline	IM, IV, SC	2–4 h	
Nalbuphine	0.03–0.1 mg/kg	Canine/feline	IM, IV, SC	2–4 h	
Buprenorphine	10–30 μg/kg	Canine/feline	IM, IV, SC	4–10 h	15–30 minute onset. Excellent buccal mucosa absorption in cats and dogs

Drug	Dose	Species	Route	Duration	Comments
Tramadol	2–10 mg/kg 5 mg/kg (suggested)	Canine Feline	PO PO	12–24 h	Nonscheduled. μ-agonist activity. Serotonin and norepinephrine reuptake inhibitor. NMDA antagonist at lower doses, GABA receptor inhibitor at high concentrations
Codeine	1–2 mg/kg	Canine	PO		
α_2-agonist					
Medetomidine/ dexmedetomidine	2–15 μg/kg	Canine	IM, IV	0.5–1.5 h	Sedation, bradycardia, vomition
	5–20 μg/kg	Feline	IM, IV	0.5–1.5 h	
	1 μg/kg IV, then 1–2 μg/kg/h 1–5 μg/kg 2–5 μg/kg	Canine/feline Canine/feline Canine/feline	CRI Epidural Intra-articular		
Xylazine	0.1–0.5 μg/kg	Canine/feline	IM, IV	0.5–1.0 h	
(Antagonist) yohimbine	0.1 mg/kg IV; 0.3–0.5 mg/kg IM	Canine/feline			
(Antagonist) atipamezol	0.05–0.2 mg/kg IV	Canine/feline			2–4 times the medetomidine dose
NMDA antagonist					
Ketamine	0.5 mg/kg; IV then 0.1–0.5 mg/kg/h	Canine/feline	CRI		
Amantadine	3–5 mg/kg	Canine/feline	PO	24 h	Neuropathic pain
Dextromethorphan	0.5–2 mg/kg	Canine	PO, SC, IV		D-isomer of codeine; weak NMDA antagonist
				NOT RECOMMENDED due to side-effects[ss]	
Methadone	0.1–0.5 mg/kg	Canine/feline	IM, SC	2–4 h	Opioid derivative
Tricyclic antidepressant					
Amitriptyline	1.0 mg/kg	Canine	PO	12–24 h	Enhanced noradrenergic activity
	0.5–1.0 mg/kg	Feline	PO	12–24 h	
Calcium channel modulator					
Gabapentin	5–10 mg/kg	Canine/feline	PO	12–24 h	VGCC inhibitor
Adjunct					
Acepromazine	0.025–0.05 mg/kg	Canine	IM, SC, IV	8–12 h	3 mg maximum total dose; used to potentiate or prolong analgesic drug effect
	0.05–0.2 mg/kg	Feline	IM, SC	8–12 h	

(continued)

TABLE 72: Various drugs commonly used in multimodal protocols (continued)

Drug	Dose	Species	Route	Duration	Comments
Diazepam	0.1–0.2 mg/kg	Canine/feline	IV	2–4 h	Used to potentiate or prolong analgesic drug effect
	0.25–1.0 mg/kg	Canine/feline	PO	12–24 h	
Local anesthetics					
Lidocaine (1–2%)	6.0 mg/kg	Canine	Perineural	1–2 h	Onset: 10–15 minutes. Maximum dose: 12 mg/kg (canine); 6 mg/kg (feline)
	+ 3.0 mg/kg	Feline	Perineural	1–2 h	
	2–4 mg/kg IV, then 25–80 µg/kg/min	Canine	IV: CRI		
	0.25–0.75 mg/kg slow IV, then 10–40 µg/kg/min	Feline	IV: CRI		*NOTE: efficacy and safety are not yet proven*
Bupivacaine (0.25–0.5%)	2.0 mg/kg	Canine	Perineural	2–6 h	Onset: 20–30 min. Maximum dose: 2 mg/kg (canine or feline)
	+ 1.0 mg/kg	Feline	Perineural	2–6 h	
Mepivacaine (1–2%)	+ 6.0 mg/kg	Canine	Perineural	2–2.5 h	
	+ 3.0 mg/kg	Feline	Perineural	2–2.5 h	

CRI: continuous rate infusion; GABA: γ-aminobutyic acid; NMDA: N-methyl-D-aspartate; VGCC: voltage-gated calcium channel.

Chapter 9

MultiModal Management of Canine Osteoarthritis

INTRODUCTION

In a review of related causes of dog deaths in North America, Fleming *et al.*[1] noted that degenerative processes ranked sixth overall, with increasing proportionate frequency correlated to increasing age. Further, it is appreciated that approximately 20% of dogs over 1 year of age are afflicted with osteoarthritis (OA)[2]. The hallmark clinical manifestation of OA is pain. It is, therefore, appropriate to focus on this disease, as it is arguably the most frequent cause of pain in the canine population. (Author's note: this may also be true of the feline population.)

There are no known cures for OA and it is often managed by combinations of therapy, such as nonsteroidal anti-inflammatory drugs (NSAIDs), and analgesics, nutraceuticals, functional foods, physical therapies, adjunctive agents, and alternative therapies, such as acupuncture (*Table 73*, **Fig. 121**).

TABLE 73: Evidence for various therapeutic approaches to osteoarthritis

Modality	Selected references/ establishing evidence
NSAID	3–6
Chondroprotectant	7–10
Adjuncts	11–13
Weight control/exercise	14–19
EPA-rich diet	20–25
Physical rehab	26–29

EPA: eicosapentaenoic acid; NSAID: nonsteroidal anti-inflammatory drug.

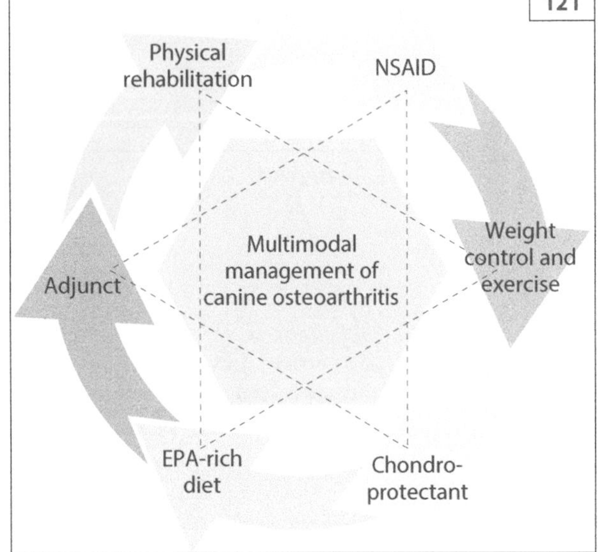

Fig. 121 The multimodal management of canine osteoarthritis integrates six different elements: nonsteroidal anti-inflammatory drugs (NSAIDs), weight control and exercise, chondroprotectant, eicosapentaenoic acid (EPA)-rich diet, adjunct, and physical rehabilitation. Three elements represent the pharmacologic management, while three others represent nonpharmacologic management.

Surgery has also been used, either to try to slow the progression of OA or to replace entire joints. Most often surgery is implemented to stabilize an arthritic joint.

The diversity of OA treatments makes it difficult for practitioners to choose the most appropriate. Studies of the efficacy of different treatments have been published in many different journals, and to assess these reviews critically, one must consider them in the light of evidence-based medicine, that is, the 'conscientious, explicit, and judicious use of the current best evidence' in making decisions about the care of individual patients. Sanderson *et al.*[30] have reported a systematic review of various OA treatment modalities with a focus on the clinical setting.

QUALITY OF EVIDENCE

Although contemporary experience precedes published literature, there is a growing evidence base for the multimodal management of OA. This evidence is a collation of clinical expertise, client/patient preferences, available resources, and research evidence, positioned on the evidence pyramid (**Fig. 122**). Quality of evidence is an important consideration when making a therapeutic decision, and can be graded from 1 to 4. Grades 1 and 2 compose the highest level of evidence, consisting of systematic reviews (meta-analyses) and well designed, properly randomized, controlled, patient centered clinical trials. Grade 3 notes a moderate level of evidence, consisting of well designed, nonrandomized clinical trials, epidemiologic studies (cohort, case–control), models of disease, and dramatic results in uncontrolled studies. Grade 4 is the lowest level of evidence encompassing expert opinions, descriptive studies, studies in nontarget species, pathophysiologic findings, and *in vitro* studies.

Quality of evidence is an important consideration when making a therapeutic decision, in that it is the best predictor of clinical outcome. Very few reports have been made reviewing the quality of evidence of treatments for OA in dogs[30,31], a leading cause of chronic pain.

The evidence-base for each modality of this multimodal management approach is substantial, and impacts the tenet of determining the minimal effective dose (MED) to maximize safety of pharmacologic therapy. NSAIDs will likely remain the foundation for treating canine OA, based on their anti-inflammatory, analgesic, and antipyretic properties. However, like all drugs, every NSAID has the potential for a patient-dependent intolerance.

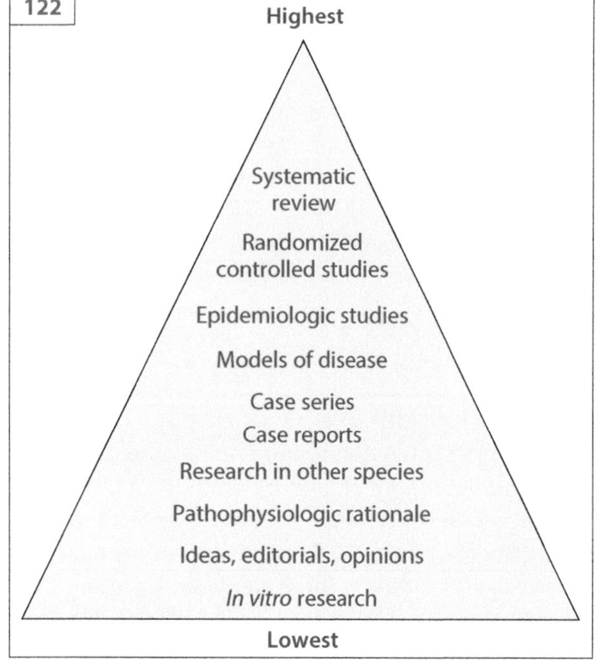

Fig. 122 Quality of evidence pyramid delineates the origin and level of confidence a clinician would have in a given treatment protocol.

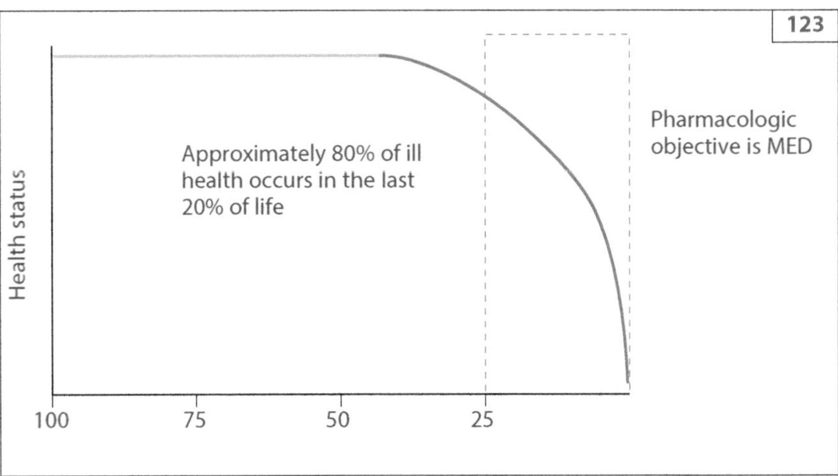

Fig. 123 During the later stages of life, when physiologic systems, such as renal and hepatic, begin to fail, a primary pharmacologic goal should be minimal effective dose (MED).

Further, NSAID adverse responses are overrepresented by excessive dosing and concomitant use of corticosteroids and/or different NSAIDs[32,33]. As OA patients age, and possibly experience renal and/or hepatic compromise, it is imperative that their maintenance NSAID administration be at the MED (**Fig. 123**). A multimodal OA treatment protocol is anchored on this tenet of NSAID MED.

BACKGROUND

For many years, pain was managed by administration of a single pharmacologic agent (if it was managed at all), and often only when the animal 'proved' to the clinician that it was suffering. Within the past 10–15 years advancements in the understanding of pain physiology, introduction of more efficacious and safe drugs, and the maturation of ethics toward animals have considerably improved the management of pain that our veterinary patients need and deserve.

Number needed to treat (NNT) is a common scheme for comparing human analgesic drug efficacy[34]. Edwards *et al.*[35] showed that the analgesic efficacy of nonopioid analgesics is improved (in humans) by combination with weak opioids.

Following the lead in human medicine, veterinarians have come to appreciate that the network of pain processing involves an incredibly large number of transmitters and receptors, all with different mechanisms, dynamics, and modes of action. From this appreciation comes the conclusion that it is naive to expect analgesia with a single agent, working by a single mode of action. Multimodal analgesia was initially understood as the administration of a combination of different drugs from different pharmalogic classes, such that they act by different, noncompeting modes of action. However, the concept has expanded to include different delivery forms, for example oral, systemic, transdermal, transbuccal, and epidural as well as nonpharmacologic modalities, such as acupuncture and physical rehabilitation. Intrinsic to the concept is that the drug combination will be synergistic (or at least additive), requiring a reduced amount of each individual drug, and therefore less potential for adverse response to each drug in the combination. Selection of drugs within the 'cocktail' would be optimal if they collectively blocked all four of the physiologic processes: transduction, transmission, modulation, and perception.

Perioperative multimodal analgesia is widely practiced today in veterinary medicine; however, monotherapy continues to be common practice for managing the chronic pain of OA. Since OA is recognized to be present in 1 out of 5 adult dogs, it is the most common chronic disease in the dog population. NSAIDs are the foundation for treating OA, and are likely to be so for some years to come. Many clinicians manage the elusive pain of OA simply by sequencing different NSAIDs until satisfactory patient results are found or unacceptable adverse reactions are experienced. However, optimal clinical results are most frequently obtained by implementing a multimodal protocol for managing OA, as has been proved for the multimodal perioperative analgesic scenario.

Although published documentation is only beginning to emerge, there is a growing evidence base for the multimodal management of OA. This evidence comprises a collation of clinical expertise, client/patient preferences, available resources, and research evidence, and credibility based on the 'Evidence Pyramid'. Case examples are presented in Appendix 2.

MEDICAL (PHARMACOLOGIC) MANAGEMENT

OA pain and NSAIDs

NSAIDs relieve the clinical signs of pain (**Fig. 124**). This is achieved by suppression of prostaglandins (PGs), primarily PGE_2, produced from the substrate arachidonic acid (AA) within the prostanoid cascade.

(Refer to Chapter 6 for details regarding NSAIDs. This section about NSAIDs emphasizes major issues associated with NSAID use.)

PGE_2 plays a number of roles in OA including: 1) lowering the threshold of nociceptor activation; 2) promoting synovitis in the joint lining; 3) enhancing the formation of degradative metalloproteinases; and 4) depressing cartilage matrix synthesis by chondrocytes. In contrast, PGs also play a positive metabolic role, such as enhancing platelet aggregation (to prevent excessive bleeding), maintaining integrity of the gastrointestinal (GI) tract, and facilitating renal function. Ecosanoid activity is tissue-dependent; therefore, maintaining an optimal balance of PG production is the 'NSAID challenge'.

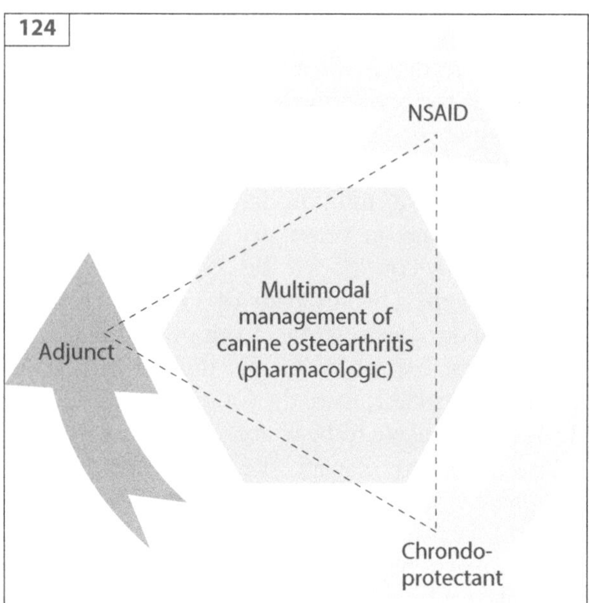

Fig. 124 The pharmacologic (medical) management of osteoarthritis is achieved with a nonsteroidal anti-inflammatory (NSAID), a chondroprotectant, and analgesic adjunct(s).

NSAID efficacy

To date, only one study has compared the relative efficacy of contemporary NSAIDs in dogs (n=8)[3]. This study received no commercial funding and utilized objective assessment (force plate gait analysis). It is noteworthy that each subject in the study responded to a NSAID, but each subject did not respond to each NSAID (**Fig. 125**).

Clinical implication: since nonsteroidal anti-inflammatory drug (NSAID) response is variable among patients, more than one NSAID should be stocked.

NSAID safety

The most common complications documented with NSAID use in the dog are associated with overdosing and the concurrent use with other NSAIDs and corticosteroids[39,40]. Because corticosteroids have their mode of action at a location higher in the arachidonic cascade than do NSAIDs, it is redundant to use them concurrently, and doing so markedly increases the severity of adverse reactions[41–43]. Data from humans[44] show that the risk of NSAID-induced GI complications are doubled when a NSAID is used concurrently with a corticosteroid.

As a class of drug, NSAIDs are most commonly associated with adverse drug events (ADEs) to the GI tract (64%), renal system (21%), and liver (14%)[45]. There is no published information relating to similar feline ADEs. GI problems associated with NSAIDs can be as benign as regurgitation, or as serious as gastric ulceration, perforation, and death. Vomiting has been identified as the most frequent clinical sign associated with gastric perforation[41].

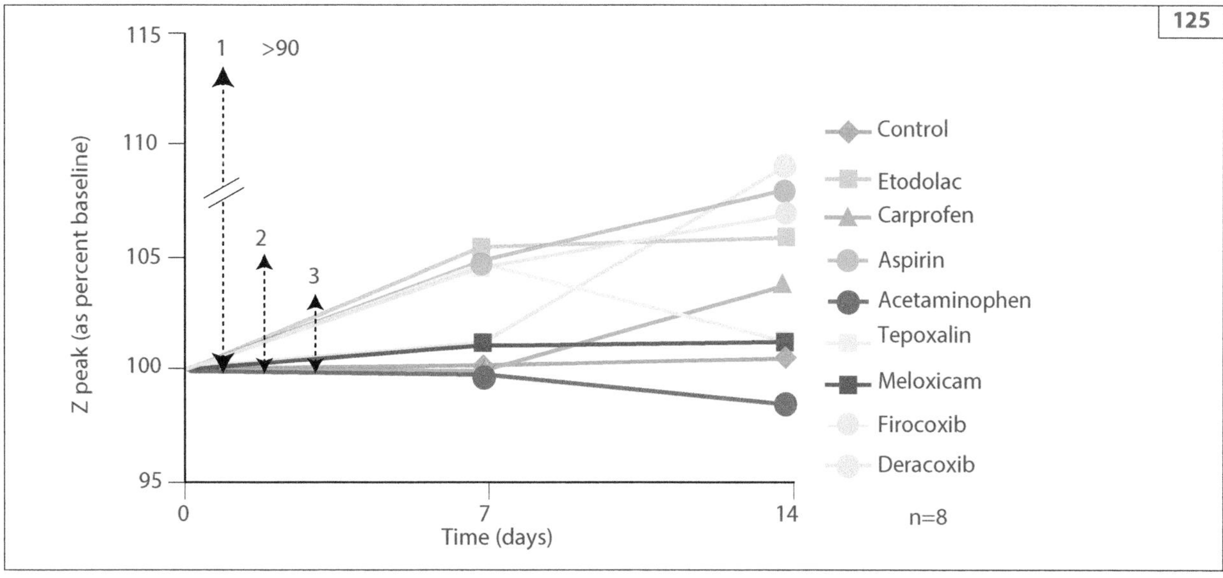

Fig. 125 Relative efficacy of several contemporary nonsteroidal anti-inflammatory drugs (NSAIDs) used in veterinary medicine to treat osteoarthritis[36–38]. Assessment is made by Z-peak of force plate gait analysis. Each dog in the study was given each separate NSAID, with a washout period between different NSAIDs. Every dog responded to a NSAID, but not every dog responded to each NSAID. Comparative Z-peak values are noted in response to weight loss (1), high eicosapentaenoic acid (EPA) diet (2), and an avocado/soybean unsaponifiable nutraceutical, Dasuquin (3).

Pet owners should be informed that if their pet experiences vomiting while taking an NSAID, the drug should be stopped and the patient should promptly be examined. This is a conservative approach since dogs are considered a 'vomiting species' and some NSAIDs are associated with more vomiting than others.

Enhancing responsible NSAID use

(Also see Chapter 6.)

Every pet owner who is discharged with medication, including NSAIDs, should have the following questions addressed:

- What is the medication supposed to do?
- What is the proper dose and dosing interval?
- What potential adverse response(s) are possible?
- What should I do if I observe an adverse response?

Both verbal and written instructions should be given.

Clinical implication: although it is a veterinarian's responsibility to address these questions with the client, it should be an assumed responsibility of the animal health technician and receptionist to ensure these questions are satisfactorily answered and understood prior to all patient discharges.

Preadministrative urinalysis and blood chemistries are well advised prior to dispensing NSAIDs for two primary reasons. Firstly, the pet may be a poor candidate for any NSAID, in that it may be azotemic or have decreased liver function. (These physiologic compromises may not preclude the use of NSAIDs, but such a determination must be justified.)

Secondly, a base-line status should be established for subsequent comparison, should the patient show clinical signs suggestive of drug intolerance. For the patient on a long-term NSAID protocol, the frequency of laboratory profiling should be determined by clinical signs and age. MED should always be the therapeutic objective, and routine examinations of the animal constitute the practice of good medicine. Since alanine aminotransferase (ALT) is more specific than serum alkaline phosphatase (SAP) as a blood chemistry for liver status, an elevation 3–4 times laboratory normal should prompt a subsequent liver function test. Because the kidney expresses both cyclo-oxygenase (COX) isozymes constitutively, no one NSAID can be presumed safer than another for renal function, and any patient that is hypotensive or insufficiently hydrated is at risk with NSAID administration.

NSAIDs play a major role in a perioperative protocol for healthy animals, due to their features as anti-inflammatories, analgesics, and antipyretics. NSAID inclusion helps prevent central nervous system (CNS) 'wind-up' and show synergism with opioids[46]. Surgery cannot be performed without resultant iatrogenic inflammation, and the best time to administer the anti-inflammatory drug is pre-emptively, before the surgery. It is imperative that surgical patients be sufficiently hydrated if NSAIDs are used perioperatively. Under the influence of gaseous anesthesia, renal tissue may suffer from under-perfusion, at which point PGs are recruited to assist with this perfusion, and if the patient is under the influence of an anti-PG (NSAID), the patient may be at risk for acute renal failure. However, in human medicine, some suggest that NSAIDs should not be withheld from adults with normal preoperative renal function because of concerns about postoperative renal impairment[47].

Improving safety

The following guidelines provide minimal risk factors for NSAID ADEs:

- Proper dosing.
- Administer MED.
- Dispense in approved packaging together with owner information sheets.
- Avoid concurrent use of multiple NSAIDs and NSAIDs with corticosteroids.
- Refrain from use of aspirin (acetyl salicylic acid).
- Provide pet owners with both oral and written instructions for responsible NSAID use.
- Conduct appropriate patient chemistry/urine profiling.
- Conduct routine check-ups and chemistry profiles for patients on chronic NSAID regimens. Do not fill NSAID prescriptions without conducting patient examinations.
- Caution pet owners regarding supplementation with over-the-counter NSAIDs.
- Administer GI protectants for high at-risk patients on NSAIDs.
- Avoid NSAID administration in puppies and pregnant animals.
- NSAIDs may decrease the action of angiotensin-converting enzyme inhibitors and furosemide, a consideration for patients being treated for cardiovascular disease.
- Geriatric animals are more likely to be treated with NSAIDs on a chronic schedule, therefore their 'polypharmacy' protocols and potentially compromised drug clearance should be considered.
- Provide sufficient hydration to surgery patients administered NSAIDs.
- Report ADEs to the product manufacturers.

Chondroprotectants

Chondroprotectants are agents that 'protect' the cartilage against destruction. They are available as both drugs (DMOAD: disease-modifying osteoarthritic drug) and nutraceuticals (DMOAA: disease-modifying osteoarthritic agents). (See Chapter 7 Nutraceuticals.)

A polysulfated glycosaminoglycan (PSGAG) (Adequan Canine®), as well as a pentosan polysulfate (PPS) (Cartrophen V®) are available as a chondroprotectant, as is a hyaluronic acid product (Legend.™). Other products (Chondroprotec™, IChON®) often considered nutraceuticals, are neither a nutraceutical nor a chondroprotectant. Such agents are licensed as topical wound devices.

The PSGAG is characterized as a DMOAD, which has met the rigors of USA Food and Drug Administration (FDA) registration. Experiments conducted *in vitro* have shown PSGAG to inhibit certain catabolic enzymes, which have increased activity in inflamed joints, and to enhance the activity of some anabolic enzymes[48] (**Figs. 126, 127**).

Catabolic enzymes are associated with **destruction**, while anabolic enzymes are associated with **building**, e.g. anabolic steroids.

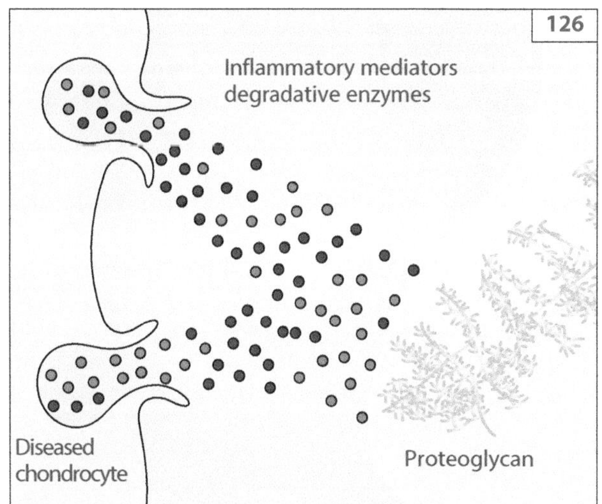

Fig. 126 Chondrocytes within the cartilage matrix (far left) generate all components of the matrix. In the osteoarthritis disease state, they also produce enzymes which degrade matrix aggrecan (pink structure). The polysulfated glycosaminoglycan, Adequan Canine®, helps to protect cartilage against the catabolic activity of these degradative enzymes.

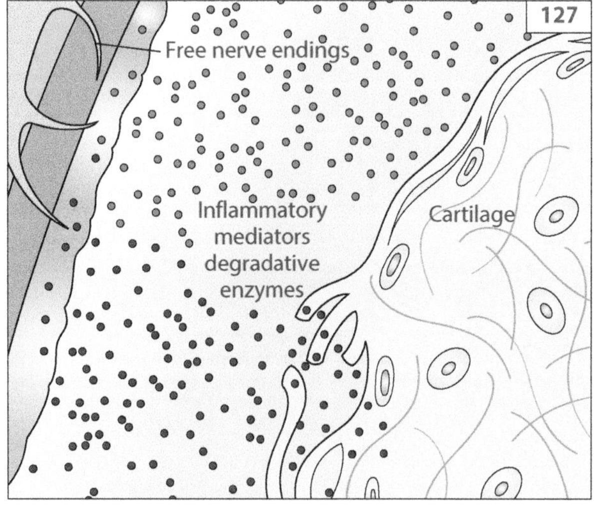

Fig. 127 As degradative enzymes are released from arthritic cartilage (right), they change the composition of joint fluid. Synoviocytes of the joint lining, sensing these inflammatory mediators, act as macrophages and release even more inflammatory agents into the joint. As weight bearing loads and unloads the cartilage, it acts as a sponge, absorbing and releasing these inflammatory agents within the joint. Hence, the worse it gets, the worse it gets! Polysulfated glycosaminoglycan acts to dampen this catabolic activity.

PSGAG has been shown to inhibit serine proteinases significantly, which play a role in the interleukin (IL)-1-mediated degradation of cartilage proteoglycans and collagen[49]. PSGAG has further been reported to inhibit some catabolic enzymes, such as elastase, stromelysin, matrix metalloproteinases (MMPs), cathepsin G and B1, and hyaluronidases, which degrade collagen, proteoglycans, and hyaluronic acid[50,51] (**Fig. 128**). It is also reported to inhibit PGE synthesis[52]. PSGAG has shown a specific potentiating effect on hyaluronic acid synthesis by synovial membrane cells *in vitro*[53].

Hyaluronic acid contributes to the viscosity, or 'slipperyness' of synovial fluid.

Clinical data from Millis, *et al.* (unpublished, 2005) showed that comfortable angle of extension and lameness scores were both improved following PSGAG (Adequan®) administration at both 4 and 8 weeks following anterior cruciate ligament transection, while the concentration of neutral metalloproteinase was reduced relative to controls. In an era where evidence-based treatment is being emphasized, the separation between patient response to FDA-approved drugs and unlicensed agents is widening.

Clinical implication: polysulfated glycosaminoglycan apparently has analgesic properties, although that is not a label claim.

The licensed PSGAG (Adequan®) is most appropriately administered in the early stages of OA, since once hyaline cartilage is lost, it is lost forever! The strategy in administering this chondroprotective is to delay the time during progression of OA at which medically aggressive treatment is required (**Fig. 129**).

Summary of the licensed PSGAG activity

- Reduction in proteoglycan degradation.
- Inhibition of synthesis and activity of:
  - Aggrecanases.
  - MMPs.
  - Nitric oxide (NO).
  - PGE_2.
- Stimulates glycosaminoglycan synthesis.
- Increases hyaluronan concentrations.

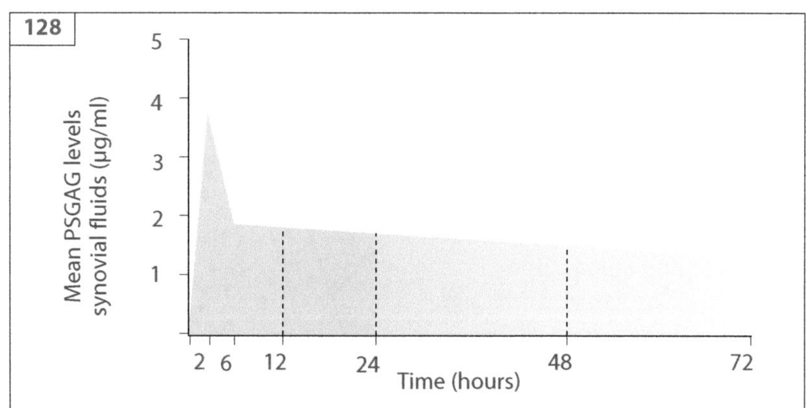

Fig. 128 Within 2 hours of administration, the polysulfated glycosaminoglycan (PSGAG) enters cartilage where it reduces proteoglycan degradation, inhibits synthesis and activity of degradative enzymes, stimulates glycosaminoglycan synthesis, and increases hyaluronan concentrations. Activity lingers for several days.

PPS has been used in human medicine as an antithrombotic/lipidemic agent and has become a popular DMOAD in a number of countries outside the USA. The sodium derivative of PPS has marketing approval for the treatment of canine OA in Australia, New Zealand, Canada, and much of the European Union. Ghosh *et al.*[54,55] have reviewed the many pharmacologic properties of PPS that support its classification as a DMOAD. In contrast to the animal origin of Adequan, Cartrophen Vet (PPS) is of plant origin (*Table 74*).

In animal models of OA, PPS modulates cytokine action and preserves proteoglycan content, and in humans with rheumatoid arthritis, it stimulates hyaluronan synthesis by synovial fibroblasts and increases the molecular weight of hyaluron in synovial fluid. In the Pond–Nuki model, PPS resulted in significantly decreased articular cartilage damage based on gross and histologic evaluation and maintenance of normal articular cartilage proteoglycan content[56]. Budsberg *et al.*[57] have reported that PPS-treated dogs improved significantly faster in breaking ground reaction forces than placebo-treated dogs following extracapsular stabilization of cranial cruciate ligament surgery. The estimated incidence of ADEs associated with PPS is 0.074% on an individual dose basis[58].

TABLE 74: DMOAD doses[59]

DMOAD	Dog dose	Cat*
Adequan Canine	2 mg/lb (4.4 mg/kg) IM, 2×/week for 4 weeks	Off label
Cartrophen Vet	3 mg/kg SC, Q5–7 days for 4 injections	No data

*Cat administration of Adequan is off-label; however, SC administration of the dog dose was found to reach joint tissues.
DMOAD: disease-modifying osteoarthritic drug.

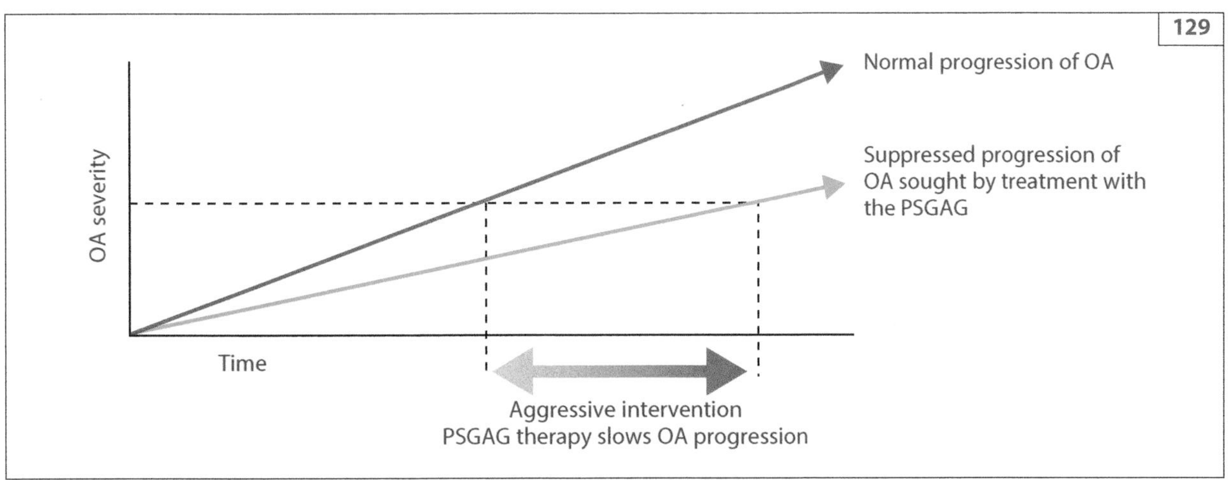

Fig. 129 The strategy of early polysulfated glycosaminoglycan (PSGAG) treatment is to delay the point in time when 'agressive' treatment is required to keep the patient comfortable. OA: osteoarthritis.

Adjuncts

OA is both a chronic disease and an acute disease, with intermittent flare ups that may render an NSAID ineffective as the sole analgesic because of 'breakthrough pain' (**Fig. 130**). Further, maladaptive pain is not just a prolonged version of adaptive pain. As pain signals are repeatedly generated, neural pathways undergo physiochemical changes that make them hypersensitive to the pain signals and resistant to antinociceptive input. In a very real sense, the signals can become embedded in the spinal cord, like a painful memory, 'which keeps on giving'.

Amantadine and gabapentin

The main neurotransmitter used by nociceptors synapsing with the dorsal horn of the spinal cord is glutamate, a molecule that can bind to a number of different receptors and initiate activity of the N-methyl-D-aspartate (NMDA) receptor. When activated, the NMDA receptor site allows a massive intracellular influx of Ca^{++}, and subsequent neuronal release of neurogenic transmitters. Discovering the role of the NMDA receptor in chronic pain has given rise to the (empirical) implementation of NMDA-antagonists, such as amantadine, which is occasionally administered together with voltage-gated ion channel modulator gabapentanoids (gabapentin, pregabalin) as adjuncts in a multimodal OA protocol (also finding efficacy in other maladaptive pain diseases).

Tramadol

(See also Chapter 5)

The synthetic codeine analogue, tramadol, is widely used (although not approved) in dogs and cats. Approximately 40% of its activity is at the mu-receptor, giving it some behavior as an opioid. Forty percent of tramadol activity is as a norepinephrine (noradrenaline) reuptake inhibitor and 20% is as a serotonin (5-HT) reuptake inhibitor (SRI), likely accounting for its efficacy in managing the neuropathic musculoskeletal pain of chronic OA. Since tramadol has SRI features, its use can be associated with increased bleeding, especially when used in combination with an NSAID. Since

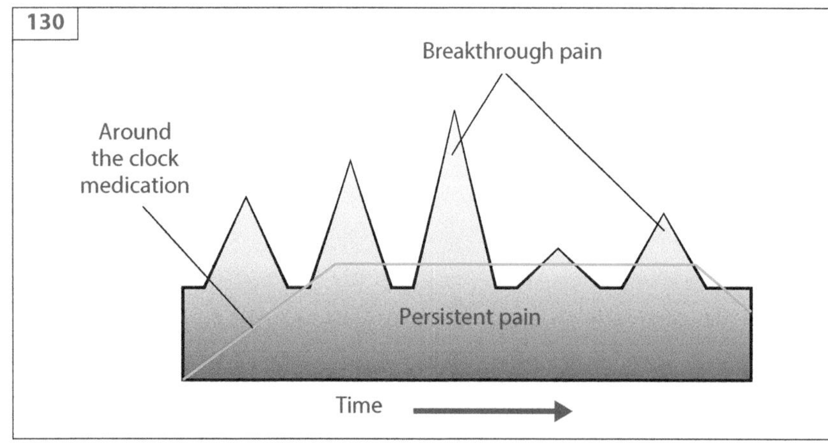

Fig. 130 Although medication may be given on a continuum to control pain, circumstances arise where the pain 'breaks through' analgesia provided by the medication, and an adjunct is necessary to control the pain once again.

the majority of tramadol activity is other than at the mu-receptor, it is a poor substitute for the 'pure' opioids. However, it can be an effective adjunct to an opioid or an NSAID[60]. In humans, tramadol is able to reduce the amount of substance P in synovial fluid as well as IL-6, which seems to correlate with the stage of OA[61]. The American College of Rheumatology and the American Medical Directors Association support the addition of tramadol to an NSAID for the management of chronic pain in humans[62,63]. Despite its wide use, there is little-to-no safety or efficacy data on the use of tramadol in veterinary patients. Published data suggest caution with its cavalier use, pending further studies assessing its effects in cats and dogs[64,65].

The serotonin, norepinephrine (noradrenaline) reuptake inhibitor, **duloxetine**, has recently (late 2010) been given an additional Food and Drug Administration approval for chronic musculoskeletal pain in humans.

Substance P and **interleukin-6** might be considered as markers, suggesting the progression of osteoarthritis.

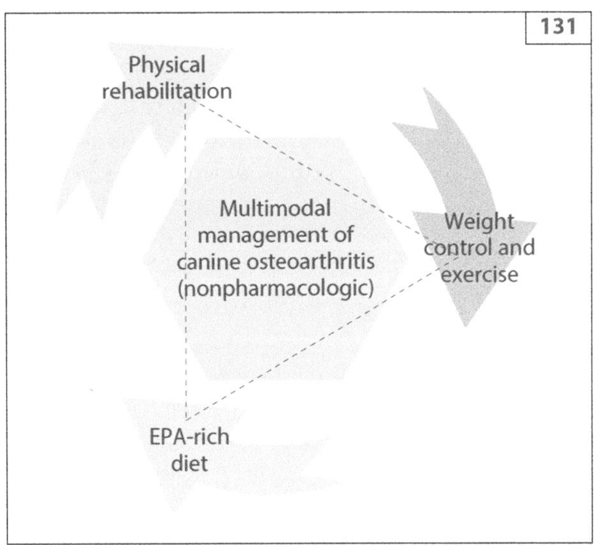

Fig. 131 The nonpharmacologic management of osteoarthritis comprises weight control/exercise, eicosapentaenoic acid (EPA)-rich diet, and physical rehabilitation.

NONMEDICAL MANAGEMENT (FIG. 131)

Diet

Diet is arguably one of the most important environmental factors influencing health and disease. Although genes are critical for determining predilections, nutrition modifies the extent to which different genes are expressed and thereby modulates whether individuals fully express the promise established by their genetic background. New genomic technologies, the so called '-omics tools', are now elucidating the basis of the associations between diet and health. These technologies monitor the activity of multiple genes simultaneously at the level of ribonucleic acid (RNA) by transcriptomics, the level of the proteins by proteomics, and ultimately the level of metabolites by metabolomics. The science of nutrigenomics employs all of these tools to explore how nutrients influence health and disease by altering the expression of an individual's genetic makeup[66]. The application of nutrigenomics to specific veterinary conditions is opening new avenues of disease prevention and therapy[67]. The role of n-3 fatty acids in canine OA is one example of application of nutrigenomic principles to clinically important conditions in veterinary medicine.

Weight control

Impellizeri, *et al.*[18] showed that in overweight dogs with hind limb lameness secondary to hip OA, weight reduction alone may result in a substantial improvement in clinical lameness. Further, from the Labrador Retriever life-long Nestlé Purina study, Kealy and others[14,17] showed that the prevalence and severity of OA in several joints was less in dogs with long-term reduced food intake, compared with control dogs, and that food intake is an environmental factor that may have a profound effect on development of OA in dogs (**Fig. 132**). Dogs on a restricted diet showed a significant reduction in progression of OA hip scores and lived longer (**Fig. 133**).

Over the life-span of investigated dogs, the mean age at which 50% of the dogs required long-term treatment for clinical signs attributable to OA was significantly earlier (10.3 years, $p<0.01$) in the overweight dogs as compared to the dogs with normal body condition scores (13.3 years)[17].

Traditionally the mechanical stress of excess weight has been thought to be a primary perpetrator of the pathophysiology and progression of OA. However, recent studies have documented metabolic activity in adipose tissue (fat) that may be of equal or greater importance. Adipocytes (fat tissue cells) secrete several hormones including leptin and adiponectin, and produce a diverse range of proteins termed adipokines (**Fig. 134**). Among the currently recognized adipokines are a growing list of mediators of inflammation: tumor necrosis factor-α (TNF-α), IL-6, IL-8, IL-10. These adipokines have been documented in both human and canine adipocytes[68,69]. Production of these proteins is increased in obesity suggesting that obesity is a state of chronic low-grade inflammation. The presence of low-grade inflammation may contribute to the pathophysiology of a number of diseases commonly associated with obesity, including OA. This might explain why relatively small reductions

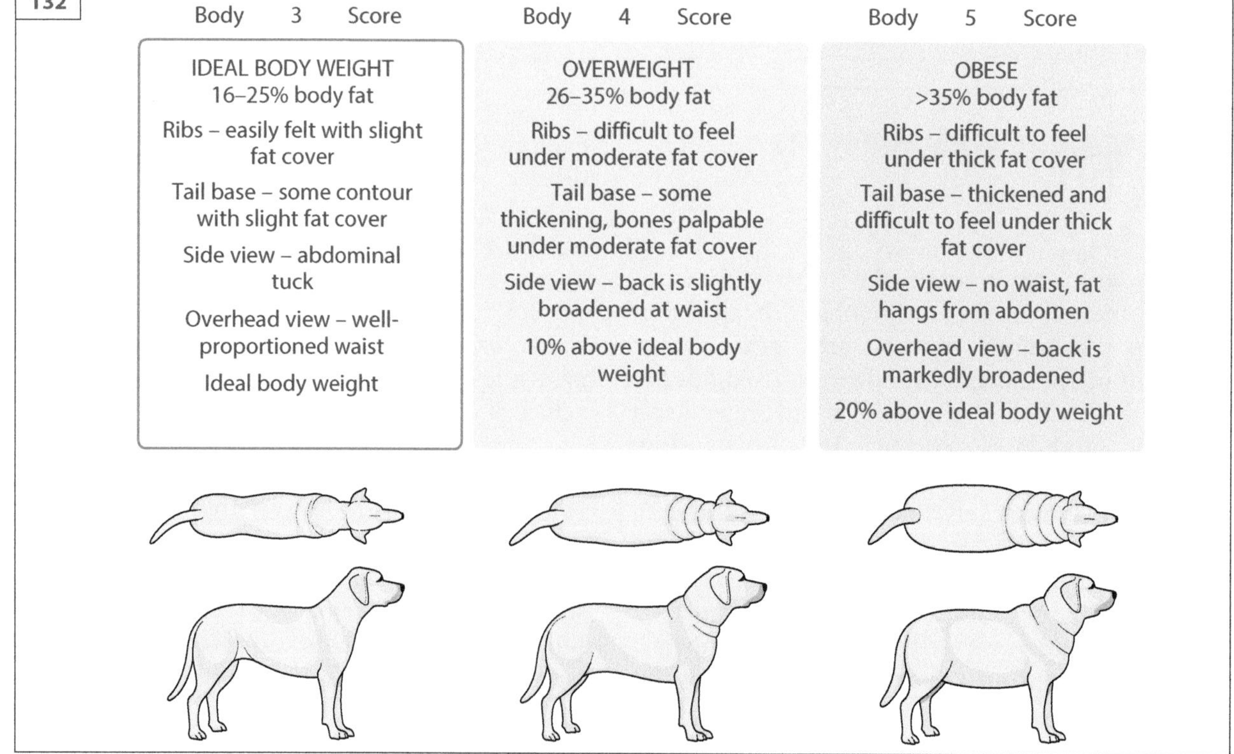

Fig. 132 Dogs with body condition scores >3/5 are at increased risk for developing clinical signs of osteoarthritis.

in body weight can result in significant improvement in general health. The overproduction of inflammatory mediators in obese individuals is associated with changes in the genome. These changes enhance the phenotypic expression of OA compared to genetically similar dogs that remain lean their entire lives.

A **phenotype** is any observable characteristic or trait of an organism. Phenotypes result from the expression of an organism's genes as well as the influence of environmental factors and possible interactions between the two.

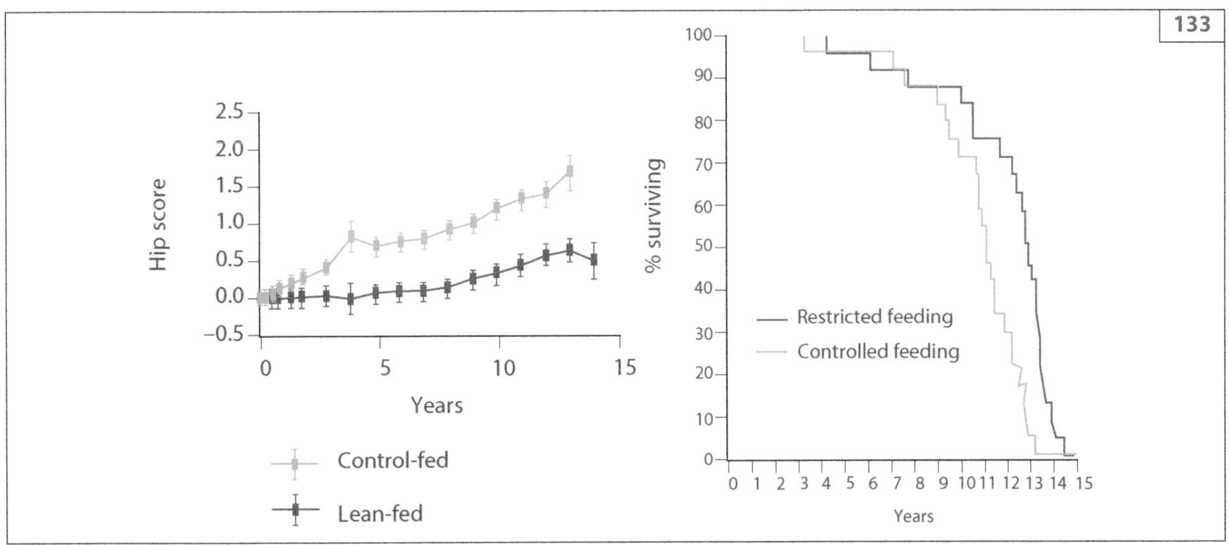

Fig. 133 Dogs on a diet of restricted caloric intake not only demonstrate a significant reduction in progression of osteoarthritis hip scores, but also live longer.

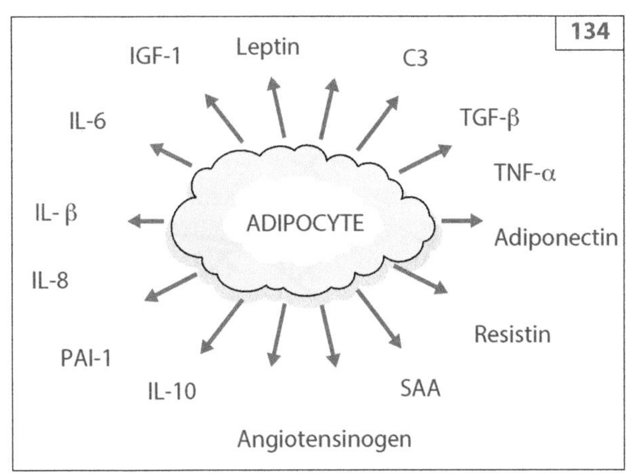

Fig. 134 Hormones, cytokines, and other substances secreted from adipose tissue. This list continues to grow as new substances are identified:
C3: complement protein 3; IGF-1: insulin-like growth factor-1; IL: interleukin; PAI-1: plasminogen activator inhibitor-1; SAA: serum amyloid A; TNF-α: tumor necrosis factor-α; TGF-β: transforming growth factor-β.

Eicosapentaenoic acid-rich diet

Aggrecan is the major proteoglycan (by mass) of articular cartilage, consisting of the proteoglycan monomer that aggregates with hyaluronan. Many aggrecan monomers attach to a hyaluronic acid chain to form an aggrecan aggregate. Aggrecan aggregates, type II collagen fibrils, water, and chondrocytes comprise the cartilage matrix wherein structure reflects function (**Fig. 135**). When structure is altered, so too is function.

A disruption in the normal relationship of collagen and proteoglycans in the articular cartilage matrix is one of the first events in the development of OA. Compared with normal cartilage, OA-affected cartilage behaves like an activated macrophage, with up-regulation of IL-1, IL-6, and IL-8 gene expression. Also up-regulated in arthritic chondrocytes are PGE_2, TNF-α, NO, and MMP-2, -3, -9, and -13.

These enzymes, MMPs and aggrecanases, destroy collagen and proteoglycans faster than new ones can be produced, transitioning the cartilage from an anabolic (constructive) state to a catabolic (destructive) state. Imbalance of tissue inhibiting metalloproteinases (TIMPs) and MMPs contributes to the pathologic breakdown of cartilage.

AA and eicosapentaenoic acid (EPA) act as precursors for the synthesis of these inflammatory cytokines. The amounts and types of eicosanoids synthesized are determined by the availability of the

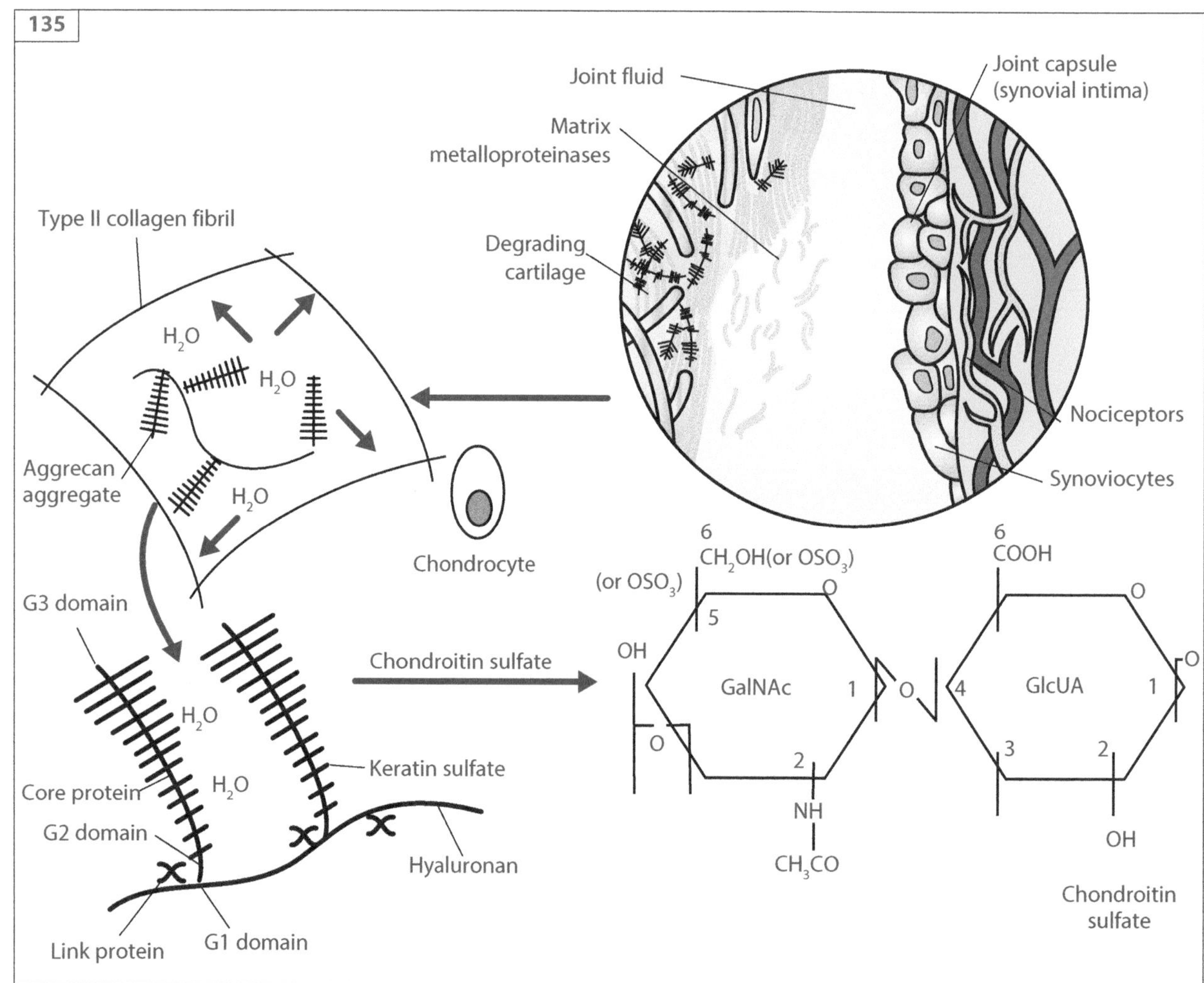

Fig. 135 Structure of cartilage.

fatty acid precursor and by the activities of the enzyme systems which synthesize them (**Fig. 136**). In most conditions the principal precursor for these compounds is AA, although EPA competes with AA for the same enzyme systems. The eicosanoids produced from AA are proinflammatory. In contrast, eicosanoids derived from EPA promote minimal to no inflammatory activity. Ingestion of oils containing n-3 fatty acids results in a decrease in membrane AA levels. This produces an accompanying decrease in the capacity to synthesize eicosanoids from AA. Studies have documented that inflammatory eicosanoids produced from AA are depressed when dogs consume foods with high levels of n-3 fatty acids[70] (**Fig. 137**).

Reducing the production of proinflammatory mediators is only one mechanism by which n-3 fatty acids promote the termination of inflammation and return to homeostasis. In people, failure of inflammation to come to an end has emerged as a central component of many diseases in modern western civilization (e.g. arthritis, periodontal disease, cardiovascular disease, cancer and Alzheimer's disease)[71]. Recent work has demonstrated that resolution of inflammation is an active endogenous process aimed at protecting the individual from an excessive inflammatory response. The first endogenous local counter-regulatory mediators recognized were the lipoxins, which are derived from AA[72]. More recently, two new families

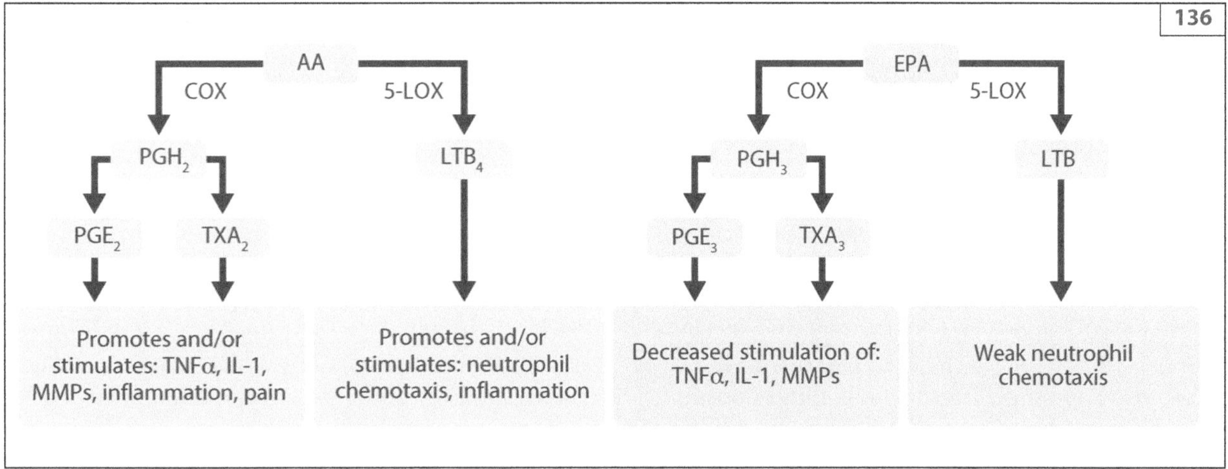

Fig. 136 Types of eicosanoids synthesized are determined by the availability of the fatty acid precursor. AA: archidonic acid; COX: cyclo-oxygenase; EPA: eicosapentaenoic acid; IL: interleukin; LOX: lipoxygenase; LT: leukotriene; MMP: matrix metalloproteinase; PG: prostaglandin; TNF: tumor necrosis factor; TX: thromboxane.

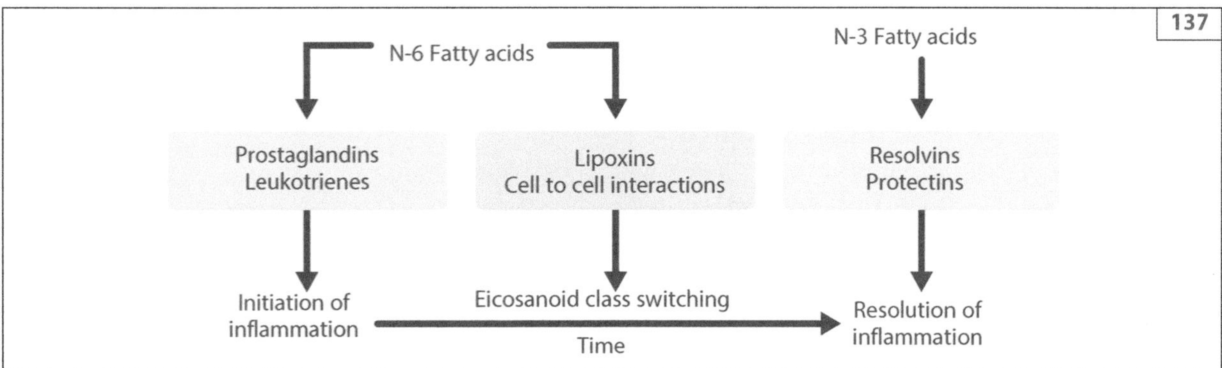

Fig. 137 Proposed mechanism for n-6 and n-3 fatty acid-derived mediators in the initiation, transition, and resolution of acute inflammation.

of lipid mediators derived from omega-3 fatty acids, resolvins and protectins, have been identified. These bioactive mediators have potent anti-inflammatory, neuroprotective, and proresolving properties[70]. Further discovery of the molecular actions of these previously unappreciated families of lipid-derived mediators may shed light on the clinically recognized beneficial effects of omega-3 fatty acids. Although the molecular mechanisms for controlling the resolution of inflammation through resolvins and protectins have not been fully elucidated, it is conceivable that omega-3 fatty acids modulate this process at the level of the genome or proteome.

The end result is that when the omega-3 fatty acid EPA replaces AA in cell membranes, the inflammatory cascade is decreased. Further, dog chondrocytes selectively store EPA (and no other omega-3 fatty acid) in the chondrocyte membrane which turns off signal-mRNA that prompts production of degradative aggrecanase (**Fig. 138**).

Clinical studies indicate that nutritional management using a therapeutic food supplemented with n-3 fatty acids helped improve the clinical signs of OA in dogs as noted by pet owners, clinical orthopedic examination, and gait analysis of ground reaction forces. Based on these studies, a food designed to aid in the management of OA in dogs should provide levels of total omega-3 fatty acids between 3.5% and 4.5% (dry matter), and specifically 0.41–1.1% (dry matter) EPA. The n-6 to n-3 fatty acid ratio should be less than 1:1. Dogs consuming the therapeutic food should receive an average of 55–100 mg EPA/ kg body weight/day. These results demonstrate that therapeutic foods developed through the application of nutrigenomic principles can result in clinically significant improvements in patients suffering from OA.

Clinical trial results from feeding EPA-rich diets have demonstrated increased serum EPA concentrations, improved clinical performance as assessed by both the veterinarian and pet owner, improved weight bearing as measured by force plate gait analysis, and shown potential for NSAID dose reduction[38].

In summary, EPA diets have two principal modes of action: 1) by providing an alternative substrate for COX metabolism, the resultant prostanoids are less inflammatory; and 2) EPA diets help suppress the degradative enzymes associated with cartilage destruction (of aggrecan). EPA helps maintain the integrity of hyaline cartilage, and subsequently its function.

Understanding the relationship between genes, nutrients, and health is the central tenet of nutrigenomics. As this emerging field matures, it is reasonable to envision an era where dietary intervention, based on knowledge of nutritional requirements, nutritional status, and genotype can be used to prevent or cure chronic disease. It has been suggested that, in the future, nutrigenomics may well hold the key to ensuring optimal health and longevity for both humans and animals regardless of their genetic predispositions.

Physical rehabilitation

(See Chapter 10)

Physical rehabilitation is fast becoming an important component of a multimodal approach to treating OA. Physical rehabilitation is a term that defines a broad spectrum of methods from the most advanced techniques used in complex orthopedic surgery recoveries, to the simple techniques that can be taught to pet owners for use at home with their pets. The goal is to restore, maintain, and promote optimal function, optimal fitness, wellness, and quality of life as they relate to movement disorders and health.

The chronic OA patient is often reluctant to exercise. This reluctance may be due to the patient's unwillingness or inability. Unwillingness is frequently due to pain, which can be managed pharmacologically. However, the inability is often a consequence of decreased muscle mass and decreased joint range of motion, both the sequelae of OA. Physical rehabilitation focuses on the patient's inability to exercise, providing a resultant 'freedom of movement' and serves as a palliation of the disease progression. Frequently, physical rehabilitation together with weight control can be as effective as pharmacologic intervention.

Nutraceuticals

(See Chapter 7)

Next to NSAIDs, nutraceuticals are the fastest growing group of healthcare products in both human and animal health. Yet, many do not understand the definition and constraints of a nutraceutical. A nutraceutical is defined as a food additive that is given orally. As such, nutraceuticals are not under regulation by the

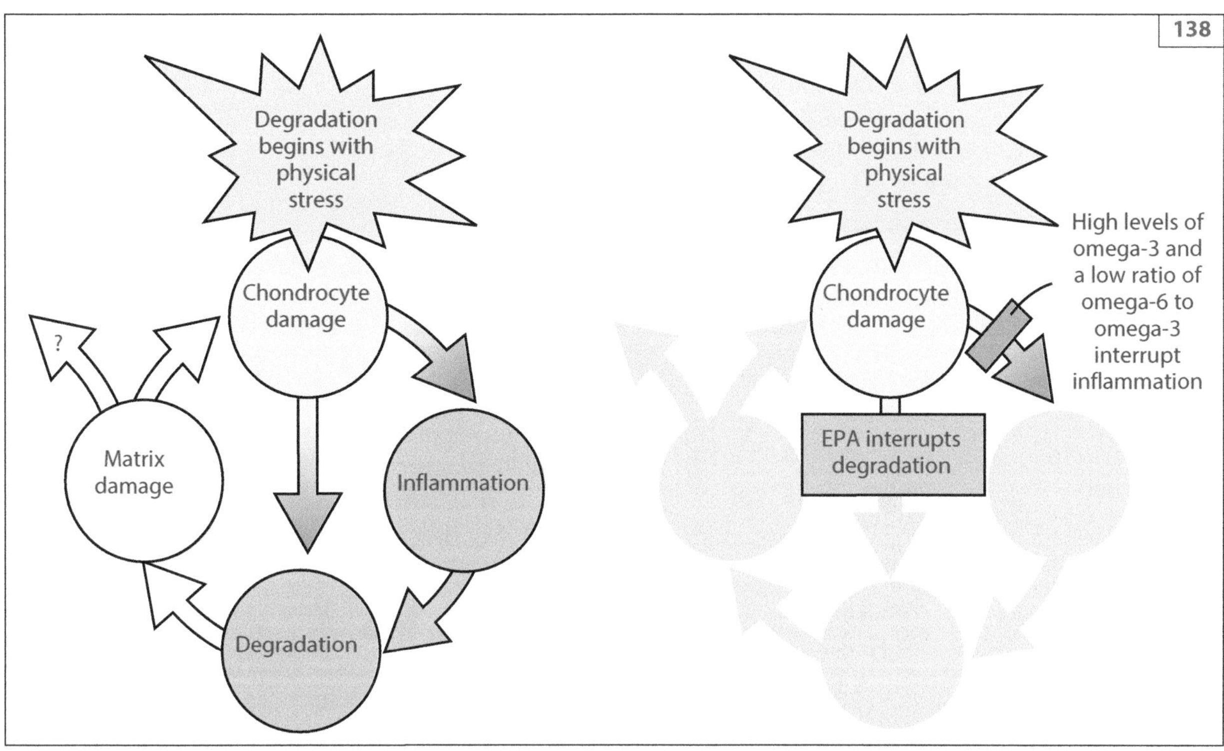

Fig. 138 The common pathways that lead to the destruction of articular cartilage begin with the loss of proteoglycans (aggrecans). Damage to chondrocytes causes up-regulation of catabolic enzymes, particularly aggrecanases. Aggrecanase enzymes destroy proteoglycans faster than new ones can be synthesized. This imbalance leads to deterioration of the extracellular matrix, cartilage's normal physiologic properties, and ultimately to structural and functional failure of the joint. In canine cartilage, eicosapentaenoic acid (EPA) has been shown to inhibit the up-regulation of aggrecanase enzymes by blocking the signal at the level of the messenger RNA, thereby interrupting the self-perpetuating cycle of degradation. By replacing arachadonic acid in cell membranes, EPA modulates the inflammatory response as well.

FDA. In contrast, (injectable) chondroprotectives are FDA-regulated. Together, chondroprotectants and nutraceuticals are considered DMOAAs, whereas nutraceuticals are not considered DMOADs. More than 30 nutraceutical products have been listed as potentially active in OA (*Table 75 overleaf*)[73]. Avocado/soybean unsaponifiables (ASU) is a recent entry to the nutraceutical pool. It is suggested that this compound may promote OA cartilage repair by acting on subchondral bone osteoblasts. ASU has been observed to prevent the inhibitory effect of subchondral osteoblasts on aggrecan synthesis, while having no significant effect on MMP, TIMP-1, COX-2, or inducible nitric oxide synthase expression[74].

TABLE 75: Nutraceuticals used for osteoarthritis

Ascorbic acid	Hyaluronic acid
Avocado/soybean unsaponifiables	Hydrolysate collagen Methylsulfonylmethane
Boswellia serrate	Milk and hyperimmune milk
Bromelain	n3-PUFAs
Cat's claw	Phycocyanin
Chondroitin sulfate	*Ribes nigrum*
Cetyl myristoleic oil	*Rosa canina*
Collagen hydrolysate	S-adenosylmethionine
Curumin	Selenium
Chitosan	Strontium
Devil's claw	Silicium
Flavonoids	Turmeric
Glucosamine SO4/	Vitamin D
Acetyl/HCl	Vitamin E
Green lip mussel	Willow
Ginger	

PUFA: poly unsaturated fatty acid.

Controversy remains over mechanisms by which nutraceuticals may lead to modulation of disease symptoms and cartilage degradation in OA, and which product is preferred for treatment. Perhaps our scientific community lacks the expertise to identify how these products might work. Nevertheless, as a class of agents, nutraceuticals fall short with *in vitro* evidence-based efficacy, lack dose titration studies to validate appropriate doses, and have shown inconsistencies of product quality assurance. Good intentions of the few have been clouded by many! A sound recommendation for consumers is, buyer beware. One might argue that the most responsible advice for recommending a nutraceutical is as prophylaxis to a high-risk disease condition or as an adjunct to a 'science-based' medicinal, in that the nutraceutical may, or may not, help. Recommending the pet owner spend resources on a nutraceutical as the first line of treatment lacks convincing scientific underpinning.

MESENCHYMAL STEM CELL THERAPY

Mesenchymal stem cell (MSC) therapy in regenerative medicine is a growing area of research, and (adipose-derived) stem cell therapy is being used to treat OA[75–77]. Adipose tissue is an accessible source of MSCs, and because adipose-derived MSC (AD-MSC) are 'minimally manipulated' for therapy, this particular autologous stem cell therapy does not require regulatory approval.

The mechanisms responsible for the efficacy of AD-MSC therapy in canine OA are not known. However, several theories have been proposed. From the work of Ortiz and colleagues[78] has come the proposal that mesenchymal cells secrete an IL-1 receptor antagonist (IL-1ra). IL-1 is known to play a major role in joint disease, and inhibiting IL-1 with IL-1ra has been shown to play a beneficial role in equine OA[79]. Another postulate is that stem cells also promote tissue recovery through the local delivery and secretion of cytokines and growth factors[80].

MSCs can be isolated from a variety of adult tissues, including bone marrow, adipose tissue, and synovial membrane[81]. They are able to differentiate *in vitro* into at least three mesenchymal lineages, such as osteoblasts, adipocytes, and chondrocytes[82]. In addition, Toghraie *et al.*[83] showed that MSCs could be obtained from rabbits, and that injection of these MSCs resulted in a significantly better quality of cartilage at 20 weeks after administration in an iatrogenically-induced rabbit model of stifle OA. This study suggests the MSCs may require time to differentiate and proliferate, and that infrapatellar fat pad derived MSCs are a promising cell source for cartilage engineering.

Studies are emerging that show the improvement gained by AD-MSC therapy[84,85]. Black *et al.*[85] have shown that the greatest improvements in elbow joint function (30–40%) were detected in functional disability and lameness, whereas pain on manipulation of the joints was not as prominent a feature of the involved joints and showed less change. Moreover, the duration of effect was at least 180 days. AD-MSC therapy is in its infancy of clinical application, yet early results suggest it may have efficacy as an adjunct in the management of canine OA.

PLATELET-RICH PLASMA THERAPY

Platelet-rich plasma therapy (PRP) is an emerging treatment in a new health sector known as 'orthobiologics'. Such therapy offers a promising solution to accelerate healing of tendon injuries and OA naturally, without subjecting the patient to significant risk[86]. The concept is to merge cutting edge technology with the body's natural ability to heal itself. Platelets are known to be responsible for blood clotting; however, over the past 20 years it has been observed that when activated in the body, platelets release a number of growth factors. PRP, therefore, involves the concentration of platelets that delivers a powerful cocktail of growth factors that can stimulate tissue repair and regeneration. Some proteins included in PRP can selectively be isolated that promote anti-inflammatory effects and pain reduction.

Canine platelet enhancement therapy (C-PET) is a filter-based system that utilizes a unique technology to concentrate platelets and their associated growth factors from a small volume of a dog's own blood. This system does not require a centrifuge or power supply, a purported advantage over other platelet enrichment techniques. Investigators representing Western University CVM, Pall Corporation, and The Ohio State University reported clinical outcome using C-PET at the 39th Annual Conference of the VOS, 2012. A measurable reduction in lameness associated with OA was reported at 12 weeks in a cohort of dogs: elbow (n=5), stifle (13), tarsus (1), and shoulder (1)[87].

SURGICAL INTERVENTION

The focus of this work is on the 'conservative' management of pain associated with degenerative joint disease. However, it must be recognized that surgical intervention is necessary for some patients. Surgery most often involves extraction of inciting causes (e.g. ununited anconeal process, fragmented coronoid, joint mouse osteophytes, osteochondrosis dissecans [OCD] lesions) and/or attempts to stabilize an affected joint. Clear indications for surgery include, but are not limited to:

- Cruciate ligament deficient stifle and/or meniscal tears.
- Symptomatic medial or lateral patellar luxation.
- Fragmented medial coronoid process and ununited anconeal process.
- Hip dysplasia that is nonresponsive to 'conservative management'.
- End-stage: tarsal or carpal disease, stifle disease, hip disease, and elbow disease.
- Chronic shoulder luxation.
- OCD lesions.

SUMMARY

The term multimodal has come to denote the co-utilization of different delivery modes, a variety of different drug-class agents, and various techniques, the objective of which is to provide the patient with a MED of each agent and therefore render optimal pain relief with the minimal risk for adverse drug response. Specifically regarding NSAIDs, the cornerstone of treatment for OA, a multimodal approach encourages responsible use. 'Best medicine' dictates the clinician's responsibility to achieve a MED for each patient. Registered label dosing makes this more easily achieved with some NSAIDS than with others.

Following adoption of the multimodal scheme (**Fig. 139** *overleaf*), the question at hand is sequencing the different modalities. Herein, there appears to be two different suggestions. Some suggest starting the patient on nonpharmacologic modalities (such as nutraceuticals), weight loss, and diet modifications. Thereafter, the pharmacologic agents are integrated. However, this approach is challenged by two well-founded arguments. First, it is recognized that most of the nonpharmacologic modalities take 3–4 weeks before a clinical response is observed, and pet owners want to see a response sooner than that. Second, it is in the patients' best interest to provide analgesia as soon as possible. Anything less could be argued as inhumane, not providing immediate relief to the patient, which it needs and deserves. Accordingly, starting the protocol with an NSAID would appear to be the most ethical approach.

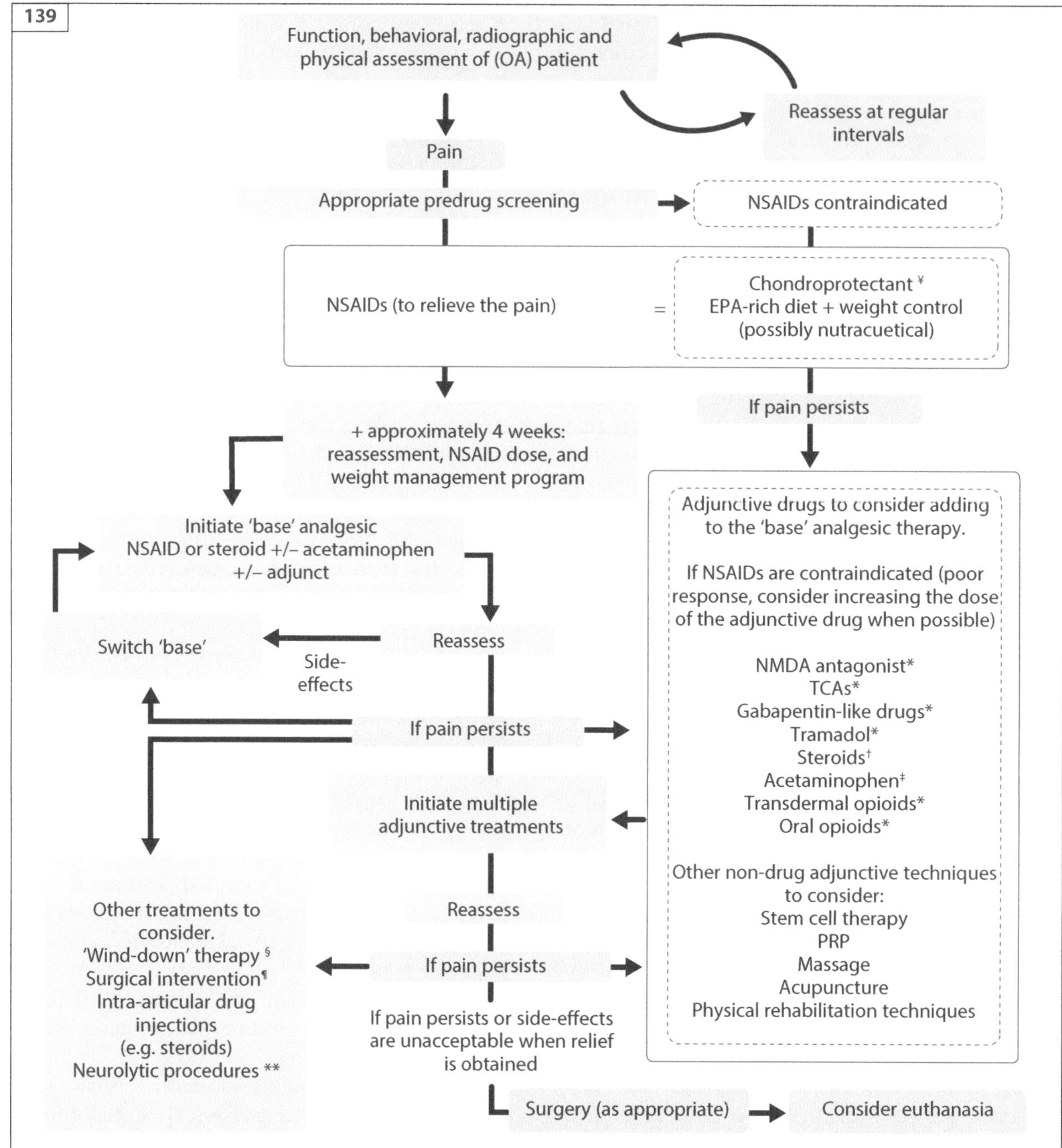

Fig. 139 Algorithm for implementing a multimodal approach for OA patients. *These drugs may be used in combination without an NSAID, acetaminophen, or a steroid base, but are likely to be less effective. †Steroids should not be used in combination with a NSAID, ‡Acetaminophen has been used in combination with NSAIDs, but it probably increases the risk of gastrointestinal ulceration. §'Wind-down' therapy refers to an unproven technique of using combinations of IV analgesics over a 48–72 hour period in OA cases that are refractory to oral treatment in an attempt to 'Wind-down' the central nervous system changes and allow oral treatment to be more effective. Surgical intervention refers to total hip or other joint replacement and arthrodesis. **'Neurolytic' is used to refer to surgical denervation and also neuroablative procedures. ¥Adequan®Canine (polysulfated glycosaminoglycan). (Modified from Lascelles 2009 Merial Pain Management Symposium 2009 NAVC Conference and 2009 Western Veterinary Conference.) EPA: eicosapentaenoic acid; NMDA: N-methyl-D-aspartate; NSAID: nonsteroidal anti-inflammatory drug; OA: osteoarthritis; PRP: platelet-rich plasma; TCA: tricyclic antidepressant.

Chapter 10

Physical Rehabilitation in the Management of Musculoskeletal Disease

INTRODUCTION

Historically, the management of musculoskeletal disease has focused on pharmacologic intervention, managing the pain. Unquestionably, pain management is a primary focus of managing degenerative joint disease (DJD); however, there are other modalities that appear to be efficacious in treating the pain of DJD. Canine physiotherapy/rehabilitation is a discipline that encompasses the application of physical therapy techniques to patients whose comfort and function have been compromised. Commonly used techniques include cryotherapy, thermotherapy, physical rehabilitation and therapeutic exercises, transcutaneous electrical nerve stimulation (TENS), low-level laser, magnets, and pulsed acoustic cellular excitation (extracorporeal shock wave treatment: ESWT). Acute response to treatment is most pronounced, while long-lasting results have been acknowledged for many modalities.

The very term 'physical rehabilitation' suggests previous trauma or significant compromise, yet the overall goal of physiotherapy/rehabilitation is to restore, maintain, and promote optimal function, optimal fitness, wellness, and quality of life as they relate to movement disorders and health. Techniques implemented are as broad-reaching as are compromises to the patient's functions. Some modalities are as simplistic as leash walking, which can easily be administered by the pet owner. On the other hand, some modalities are complex, requiring administration by trained, professional personnel. Those administering more sophisticated techniques should be sufficiently trained with inclusive knowledge of risks and precautions for these modalities. Suggestions for physical rehabilitation for selected patient conditions are presented in Appendix 3.

ENVIRONMENTAL MODIFICATION

It is difficult to overstate the positive difference that simple environmental changes can make for the maladaptive pain patient. Yet, this is one area that is easy to overlook because it does not involve as much 'hard science' as choosing a pharmacologic regimen or calculating an appropriate nutritional profile. With a few simple questions, it is fairly straightforward to determine if the rehabilitation patient will benefit from environmental modification. It does mean taking the initiative to gather information about the home, floor surfaces, stairs, placement of food and water dishes, type of bedding, location of bedding, and so on.

One of the simplest environmental modifications that can have a positive effect on the chronically painful rehabilitation patient is to protect the dog from slippery floor surfaces.

Aging patients, particularly those with osteoarthritis (OA), experience a loss of proprioceptive function in joint receptors versus younger patients. Nonskid area rugs, flooring used in children's play areas, and rubber-backed mats are some examples of ways a dog owner can make the home more comfortable for the painful patient.

Raising food and water dishes to between elbow and shoulder height makes for more comfortable meal times. Be sure the dog is able to stand on a nonskid surface while eating and drinking. Have the client explore the home for potential 'problem spots'. Steps in and out of the house, patio stones, and garage floors can create unintentional challenges for the painful dog. Recommend ramps for getting into and out of vehicles. Likewise, have the client consider ramps or steps if the dog is used to getting onto and off furniture. It may be best to use child restraint gates at the top and bottom of staircases to prevent unsupervised access. Memory foam or 'egg-shell' foam may make for a more comfortable sleeping surface for the painful dog. Assistive devices, such as slings and 'walking wheelchairs', can sustain mobility during the initiation of appropriate multimodal pain management strategies. Finally, it is best for the dog to receive moderate exercise every day than to do excessive exercise on the weekend, requiring the rest of the week to recover.

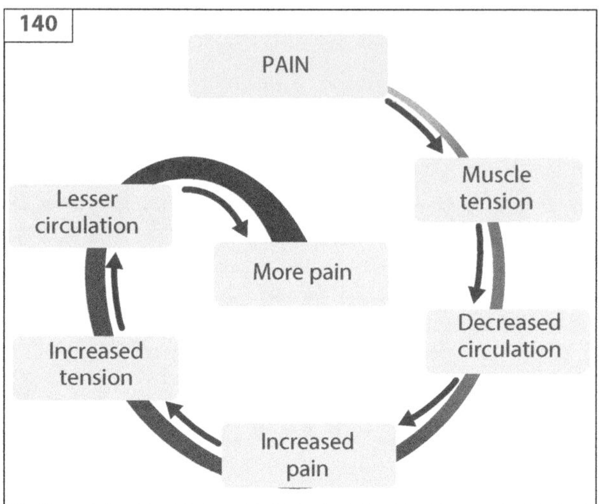

Fig. 140 The cyclic nature of the pain–spasm–pain process.

PAIN PATHOPHYSIOLOGY RELATED TO PHYSICAL REHABILITATION

In response to injury, specialized nerve endings (nociceptors) are activated, which transmit nerve signals through the spinal cord to the brain, where the sensations of pain are cognitively recognized. Almost simultaneously, neurotransmitters initiate a spinal reflex that increases muscle motor activity and tonicity at the site of injury, leading to a reflexive muscle contraction. If persistent, the increase in muscle tone can cause painful muscle spasms, which may lead to further tissue damage due to decreased blood flow and oxygen (hypoxia) in the surrounding tissues. This precipitates cyclic pain, and the injury process is called the pain–spasm–pain cycle (**Fig. 140**). To reduce the pain or unpleasant sensation, this cycle must be broken or interrupted.

Many of the physical modalities used for the management of OA in veterinary patients are derived from use in human OA patients. However, there is great variability in the recommended implementation of various modalities. In 2007, the Osteoarthritis Research Society International Treatment Guidelines Committee reported on a critical appraisal of published guidelines and systematic review of recent evidence for relevant therapies for the management of hip and knee OA in humans[1]. Among the 1,462 published guidelines reviewed that met the inclusion/exclusion criteria, 23 guidelines were developed for the treatment of hip and/or knee OA. Twenty of 51 modalities of therapy were universally recommended by these guidelines.

Optimal management of human patients with hip or knee OA requires a combination of nonpharmacologic and pharmacologic modalities of therapy. Recommendations cover the use of 12 nonpharmacologic modalities: education and self-management, regular telephone contact, referral to a physical therapist, aerobic, muscle strengthening and water-based exercises, weight reduction, walking aids, knee braces, footwear and insoles, thermal modalities, TENS, and acupuncture.

Eight recommendations cover pharmacologic modalities of treatment including acetaminophen (paracetamol), cyclo-oxygenase (COX)-2 non-selective and selective oral nonsteroidal anti-inflammatory drugs (NSAIDs), topical NSAIDs and capsaicin, intra-articular injections of corticosteroids and hyaluronates, glucosamine and/or chondroitin sulfate for symptom relief, glucosamine sulfate, chondroitin sulfate, and diacerein for possible structure-modifying effects, and the use of opioid analgesics for the treatment of refractory pain. There are recommendations covering five surgical modalities: total joint replacements, unicompartmental knee replacement, osteotomy and joint preserving surgical procedures, joint lavage and arthroscopic debridement in knee OA, and joint fusion as a salvage procedure when joint replacement has failed.

Thermoreceptors, special temperature-sensitive nerve endings, which are activated by changes in skin temperature, initiate nerve signals that block nociception within the spinal cord. Another type of specialized nerve endings, called proprioceptors, detect physical changes in tissue pressure and movement. Proprioceptor activity can also inhibit the transmission of nociception signals to the brain. Activity of these receptors within the spinal cord reduces muscle tone, relaxes painful muscles, and enhances tissue blood flow (**Fig. 141**).

Topical hot and cold modalities have been used since antiquity for the treatment of musculoskeletal injuries; however, only recently has there been an understanding of the complexity of their physiologic actions. Although cold and hot treatment modalities both decrease pain and muscle spasm, they have opposite effects on tissue metabolism, blood flow, inflammation, edema, and connective tissue extensibility (*Table 76*).

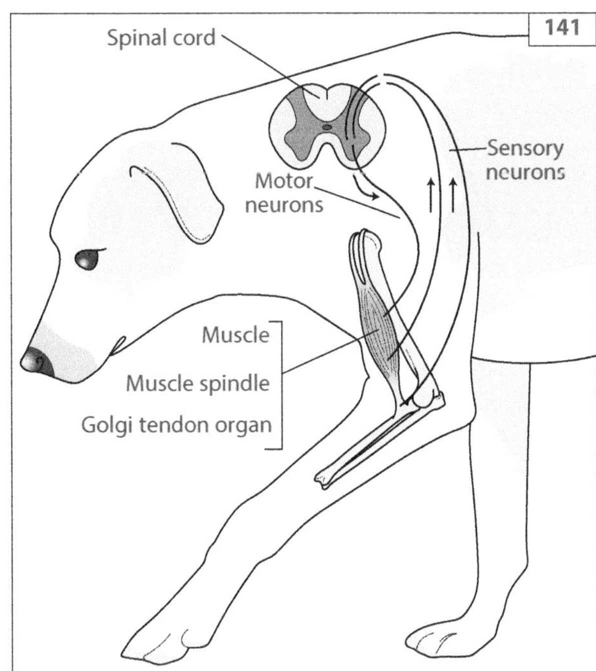

Fig. 141 Skeletal muscle hosts the neuromuscular spindles. There are more of these in muscles of the limbs than elsewhere. The proprioceptors are responsible for sending information back to the brain that determines the increase or decrease in muscle tension, which is determined by the lengthening or stretching of individual fibers. This relays information regarding the rate of muscle contraction as well as the speed of muscle contraction. The endings of the sensory neurons spiral around particular muscle fibers in order to sense the changes in each individual muscle fiber, which in turn permits them to discern this information.

TABLE 76: Effects of temperature on physiologic actions

	Cold	Heat
Pain	↓	↓
Spasm	↓	↓
Metabolism	↓	↑
Blood flow	↓	↑
Inflammation	↓	↑
Edema	↓	↑
Extensibility	↓	↑

CRYOTHERAPY

Cryotherapy decreases tissue blood flow by causing vasoconstriction, and reduces tissue metabolism, oxygen utilization, and muscle spasm[2–4]. As a result of the decreased circulation, cold penetrates deeper and lasts longer than heat. At joint temperatures of 30°C (86°F) or lower, the activity of cartilage degrading enzymes, including collagenase, elastase, hyaluronidase, and protease, is inhibited[5]. Cold raises the activation threshold of tissue nociceptors, increases the duration of the refractory period, and reduces nerve conduction velocity of pain nerves. The result is a local anesthetic effect called cold-induced neuropraxia[6,7].

Cryotherapy works by both neurologic and vascular mechanisms to yield effects both locally and at the level of the spinal cord. Topical cold treatment decreases the temperature of the skin and underlying tissues to a depth of 2–4 cm, decreasing the activation threshold of tissue nociceptors and the conduction velocity of nerve signals[8]. Various methods, such as ice packs[9], ice towels, ice massage[10], gel packs, refrigerant gases, and inflatable splints, can be used. Cold is used to reduce the recovery time as part of the rehabilitation program both after acute injuries and in the treatment of chronic injuries.

A bone scanning study[11] demonstrated that the application of an ice wrap to one (human) knee for 20 minutes decreased arterial blood flow by 38%; soft tissue blood flow by 26%; and bone uptake, which reflects changes in bone blood flow and metabolism, by 19%. From a Cochran Database of Systematic Reviews[12] authors reviewed three randomized controlled trials involving 179 human patients, revealing that in one trial administration of 20 minutes of ice massage, 5 day per week, for 3 weeks, compared to controls demonstrated a clinically important benefit for knee OA on increasing quadriceps strength (20% relative difference). There was a statistically significant improvement in knee flexion, range of motion (ROM), function, and strength. Additionally cold packs were shown to decrease swelling. One study has shown that ice massage reduces the appearance of plasma creatine kinase following muscle damage[13] (*Table 77*).

Precautions and contraindications

Frostbite is a potential complication of cryo therapy, therefore signs of frostbite should be monitored throughout and following treatment. Caution should also be taken when applying cryotherapy in the vicinity of superficial nerves and areas of decreased perfusion[7,14–16]. One might intuitively think that the animal's hair coat acts as an insulating barrier to the application of cold; however, this may not be the case[17].

Drygas *et al.*[18] have demonstrated the efficacy of cold compression therapy on postoperative pain, swelling, ROM, and lameness following tibial plateau leveling osteotomy in dogs.

THERMOTHERAPY

Thermotherapy is the therapeutic application of any substance to the body that adds heat to the body, resulting in increased tissue temperature. Heat therapy can be either superficial (up to approximately 2 cm) or deep (3 cm or more), and like cryotherapy, it provides analgesia and decreased muscle tonicity. In contrast to cryotherapy, thermotherapy increases tissue temperature, blood flow, metabolism, and connective tissue extensibility, and heat is carried away by circulation more rapidly than cold. Nevertheless, both heat and cold relieve pain and muscle spasm[19]. Heat causes general relaxation of painful muscle spasms, and may inhibit motor neurons, helping to break the pain–spasm–pain cycle. Heat therapy is delivered in three modalities: radiant (infrared lamp), conduction (hot pack), and convection (whirlpool) (*Table 78*).

A 1°C (1.8°F) increase in tissue temperature is associated with a 10–15% increase in local tissue metabolism[20]. Resultant increased blood flow facilitates tissue healing by supplying proteins, nutrients, and oxygen to the site of injury. Conductive topical heat treatment of the knees of healthy human subjects increased popliteal artery blood flow by 29%, 94%, and 200% after 35 minutes of treatment with heating pad temperatures of 38°C (100.4°F), 40°C (104°F), and 43°C (109.4°F), respectively[21]. Erasala *et al.*[22] demonstrated that deep tissue blood flow was found to increase by 27%, 77%, and 144% in the trapezius muscle of healthy human volunteers with heating pad treatments, resulting in skin temperature increases to 38°C (100.4°F), 40°C (104°F), and 42°C (107.6°F), respectively.

TABLE 77: Cryotherapy application

Modality	Comments
Ice packs	Covering ice packs with a single layer of wet towel can enhance heat exchange Apply ice packs for up to 10–20 minutes 15 minutes on : 15 minutes off (empirical) Ice packs can consist of crushed ice or a bag of 'frozen peas' can be substituted 1/3 part isopropyl alcohol with 2/3 part water placed in a resealable plastic bag can be kept in a freezer
Commercially available cold packs	Often made of silica gel in plastic or canvas covers Most are less efficient than ice
Iced towels	Soaked in ice-water slush Towels warm quickly, therefore alternate a two-towel 'exchange'
Ice wrap bandages	Often marketed for horses and humans May be maintained in refrigerator
Ice gels	Variable retention of cold (material dependent)
Ice massage	'Popsicle'-like ice Rubbed over small area, provides massage while cooling; pressure from massage stimulates mechanoreceptors more than other forms of cryotherapy Applied parallel to muscle fibers, for 5–10 minutes or until the affected area is erythematous and numb
Cold/compression	As with a circulating coolant boot Efficacy established in horses
Cold bath	Immersion of body part in cool or icy 'slush' water Cool, cold, or very cold bath
Vapocoolant sprays	Highly volatile liquids that cause evaporative cooling
Contrast baths	Alternating immersion in warm and cold water Vascular exercise producing vasodilation and vasoconstriction Support for efficacy appears anecdotal Research has demonstrated the superior effects of continuous cryotherapy and thermotherapy in the treatment of pain as opposed to intermittent treatment

TABLE 78: Thermotherapy application

Modality	Comments
Heat	Generally applied for 15–30 minutes, with equal time off
Hot packs	Heat is absorbed mostly by skin and subcutaneous fat Most packs retain heat for approximately 30 minutes
Heat wraps	Commercially available for non canine species May retain low level heat for up to 8 hours
Whirlpool	Patients with chronic conditions may use warmer water (range: 27°C–35°C) (80.6–95°F) Provides advantage of hydrostatic pressure
Warm water hosing	More commonly used for equine patients

Further, functional brain imaging has revealed that non-noxious skin warming increases activation of the thalamus and posterior insula of the brain, contributing to pain relief[23]. There are no scientific data supporting the contention that moist heat is therapeutically superior to dry heat.

Nadler *et al.*[24] showed that heat, topically applied to the skin, was superior to both acetaminophen and ibuprofen in the treatment of acute lower back pain for all therapeutic measurements, including pain relief, muscle stiffness, lateral trunk flexibility, and disability. Two days after treatment was discontinued, extended pain relief was significantly greater for the heat wrap than for either acetaminophen or ibuprofen.

In a human rheumatoid arthritis model, investigators demonstrated that fibroblast-like synoviocytes exposed to hyperthermia showed reductions in interleukin (IL)-1β-induced prostaglandin (PG) E_2 release and suppressed activation of the vascular cell and intracellular adhesion molecules-1, the cytokines tumor necrosis factor-α, IL-1α and IL-8, as well as COX-2 protein synthesis[25]. These investigators demonstrated by Western blot that fibroblast-like synoviocytes exposed to hyperthermia were suppressed in the phosphorylation and subsequent degradation of IκBα, thereby retaining the nuclear factor κB complex in the cell cytoplasm; the clinical relevance being that there was suppressed phosphorylation and decreased production of inflammatory cytokines.

The implications of these findings for OA are unknown because rheumatoid arthritis and models stimulating this condition are quite inflammatory relative to OA.

Precautions and contraindications

As with cryotherapy, the greatest concern is with excessive application, in the case of heat therapy, burns. *Electric heating pads must be closely monitored!* Contraindications include: cardiac insufficiency, malignancy, fever, areas of hypoperfusion, acute inflammation, and hemorrhage. Caution the use of superficial heat treatment in areas of edema and open wounds.

THERAPEUTIC EXERCISES

Active and passive exercise programs are beneficial for the OA patient through improvement of muscle strength, joint stability, ROM, and aerobic fitness. Improving these functions is intended to reduce pain and disability. Therapeutic exercise should include stretching and ROM, aerobic conditioning, muscle strength and endurance training, and correction of gait abnormalities. Increasing intensity and duration per session should be implemented in a stepwise fashion until aerobic activity is maintained for 25–30 minutes per treatment session.

Treatment to enhance joint mobility consists of ROM and stretching. Passive ROM is implemented with the patient in lateral recumbency in a quiet and comfortable area. The target joint(s) is slowly and gently flexed and extended until the patient shows initial signs of discomfort, such as tensing the limb, moving, vocalizing, turning the head toward the therapist, or trying to pull away. The therapist should 'challenge' the ROM limits, but not cause undue discomfort. Typically, 15–20 repetitions, performed 2–4 times daily, are adequate.

Stretching is actually a distention of ROM exercises, designed to increase flexibility of tissues. Application of superficial heat or therapeutic ultrasound (US) before stretching may be advantageous, as less damage to the tissues may occur if the tissues are warmed first. The stretch should be a prolonged limit to the patient's functional ROM for at least 15 seconds. Each targeted muscle group should be stretched 3–5 times per session, and 2–4 sessions per day is common.

Active ROM exercises include walking and swimming. More 'demanding' walking activities include walking in snow, sand, tall grass, and crawling through a play tunnel. Climbing stairs and walking over Cavaletti rails further develops joint excursions and increases strength. As the patient demonstrates continued improvement with therapeutic exercises, strength and endurance are developed. Generally, endurance, cardiovascular fitness, and obesity are addressed through endurance activities. With progression, activities are modified first by increasing the frequency of activity, then by modifying the length of activities, and finally by increasing the speed. A reasonable rule of thumb is to increase the length of activity by 10–15% per week. Further, it is better to provide multiple short-duration sessions rather than one extended session.

Leash walking

Leash walking is commonly performed incorrectly. Walking an animal slowly encourages the use of all limbs in a sequenced gait pattern (**Figs. 142, 143**). However, the walk must be slow enough to allow weight bearing; if too fast, the animal tends to simply hold the compromised limb up in a flexed, nonweight-bearing position. Slow leash walks encourage placement of each limb on the ground, increasing stance time and weight bearing. When appropriate, exercise on a leash can be altered to include fast walking, slow jogging, and running on a long lead. Faster walks further challenge balance, coordination, proprioception, and cardiorespiratory endurance, as well as functional muscle strengthening and endurance (**Fig. 144**).

Walking through a field of tall grass enhances muscle strengthening and endurance, because of the resistance provided by the grass, as well as coordination to navigate varying terrain (**Fig. 145**).

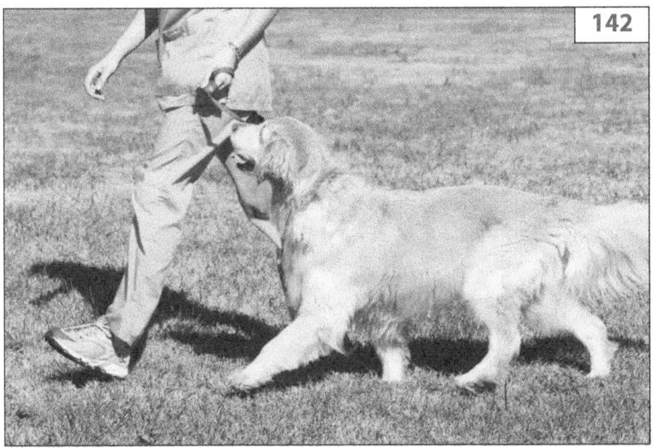

Fig. 142 Slow leash walking encourages limb placement, increased stance time, and weight bearing.

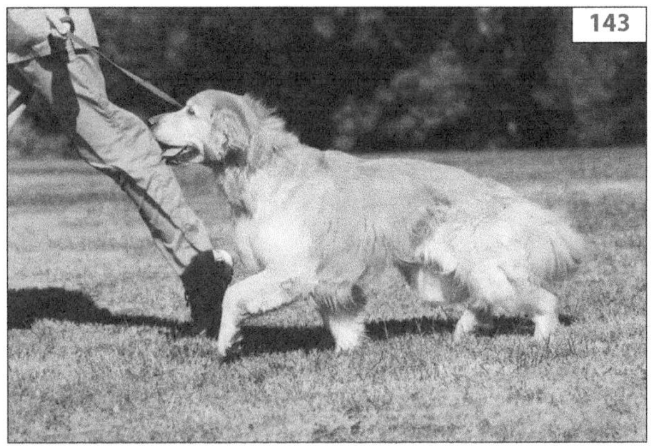

Fig. 143 Faster leash walking promotes muscle strengthening and endurance.

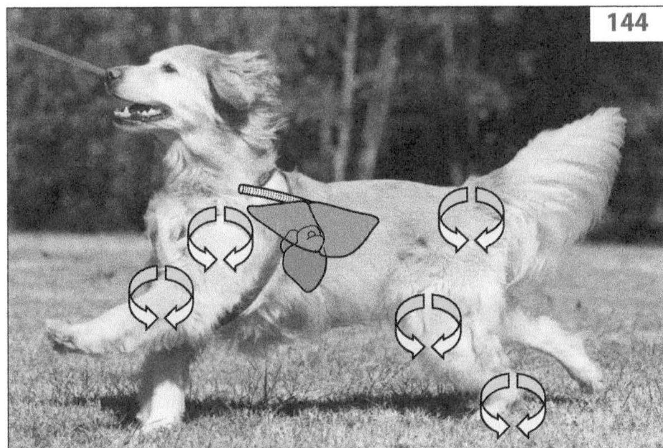

Fig. 144 Fast leash walking promotes cardiorespiratory conditioning and general minor-to-moderate extended range of motion for all joints.

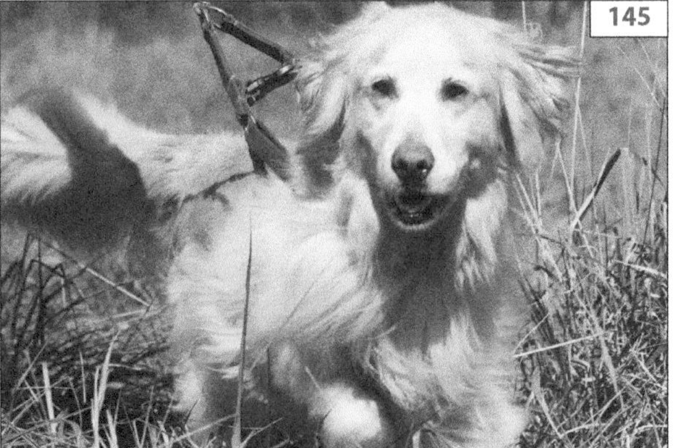

Fig. 145 Leash walking in tall grass, sand, or snow encourages an increased range of joint motion as the animal accomodates to the terrain.

Further, dogs have a tendency to flex their joints to a greater extent as they negotiate the grass. Walking on a gradient is also beneficial for developing strength (**Fig. 146**). Exercising in sand and snow minimizes concussive forces placed on arthritic joints, while allowing strengthening of supporting periarticular muscles.

Weight shifting

Static balance refers to the animal's ability to maintain balance while the body is stationary, such as while standing. Dynamic balance refers to the animal's ability to maintain balance while the body is moving, such as while walking. Exercises performed to challenge the animal's dynamic balance include encouraged weight shifting, manual up-loading of a single limb, balance board, and exercise balls and rolls. The goal is to disturb the animal's balance just enough so the animal can recover, being careful not to force the animal to fall.

With a rebound-weight shift, the animal is gently pushed toward the affected side. When the animal shifts its weight to resist the movement, pressure is suddenly released, and gentle pressure is simultaneously applied toward the unaffected side. This results in a sudden unbalancing; the animal initially shifts its weight toward the unaffected side, but to keep from falling, it immediately shifts its weight back toward the affected side. Weight shifts may also be performed during walking. As the animal is walked in a straight line, the handler gently bumps or pushes the animal to one side to challenge the dog to maintain its balance.

When a limb is lifted and held, the animal shifts its body weight in response to this alteration in center of gravity. To maintain the unassisted

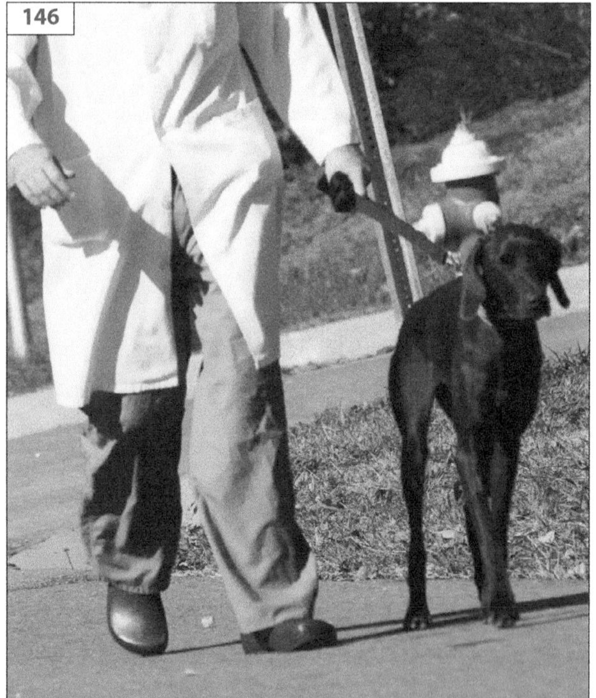

Fig. 146 Leash walking on a gradient promotes balance, proprioception, strengthening, and proper limb placement.

position, the animal is required to use strength, coordination, and balance. The handler may lift each leg separately to see where the animal is weakest, and focus on that area in subsequent treatment sessions.

A platform on rockers (balance platform or biomechanical ankle platform system) may be used to rock a patient forward and backward, side to side, diagonally and 360° (**Figs. 147, 148**). With these apparatus, it is important to have one person help support the patient while another person slowly and gently rocks the platform to allow the animal an opportunity to shift its weight and exercise its proprioceptive mechanism (**Figs. 149, 150**).

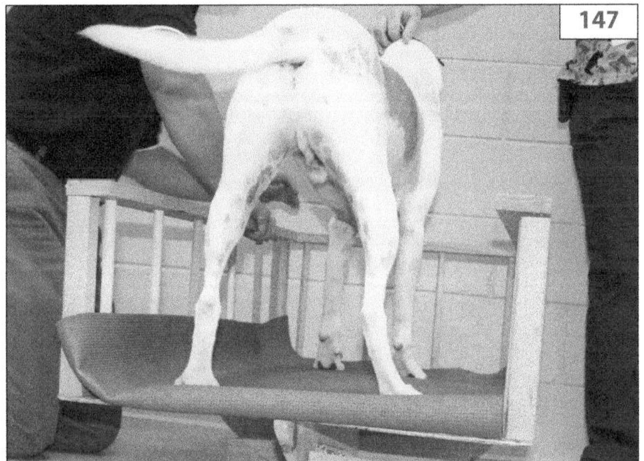

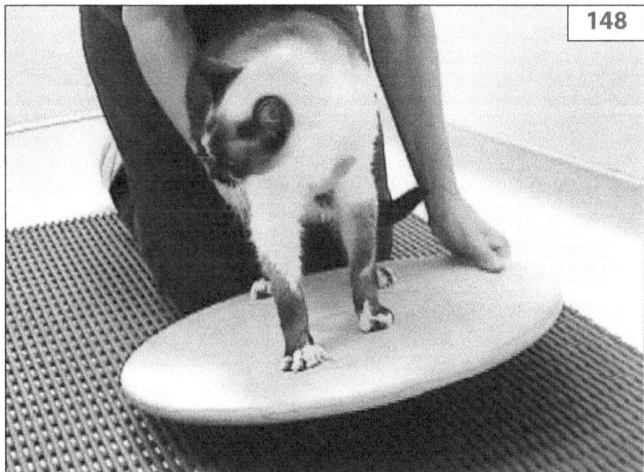

Fig. 147,148 A rocker (teeter board) can be used to rock the patient into a number of positions that help develop its balance and proprioception. (Courtesy of Dr. Darryl Mills and Sandra Hudson.)

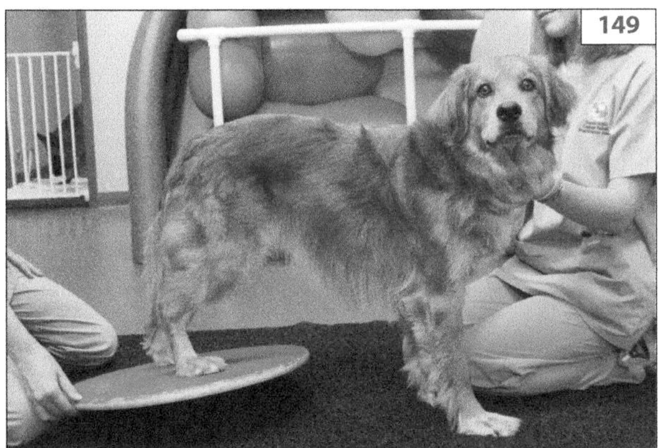

Fig. 149 When using a balance board, one person is attendant to the animal's head, while the other person manipulates the apparatus and assists limb placement.

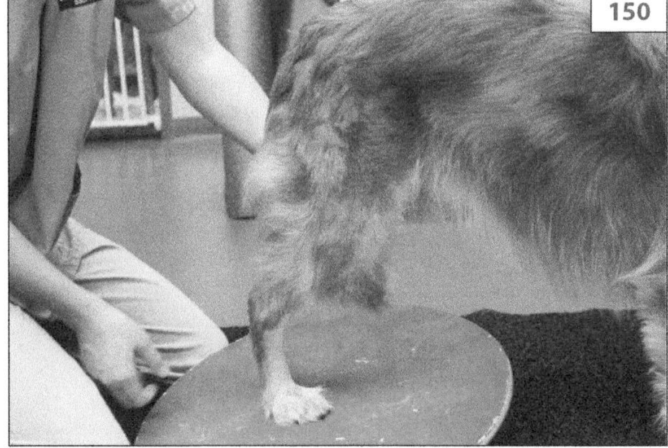

Fig. 150 Balance boards can be used to focus on each individual limb.

Human exercise balls and rolls are easily adapted to animal use (**Figs. 151–153**). The animal's forelimbs are placed on the ball and supported by the handler, requiring the patient to maintain static balance of the caudal trunk and rear limbs. Dynamic balance is challenged as the ball or roll is slowly moved forward, backward, and side to side, challenging the rear legs to maintain balance while movement occurs. In a similar manner, the rear limbs can be placed over the ball to challenge the forelimbs and cranial trunk.

Sit-to-stand exercise

Sit-to-stand exercises help strengthen hip and stifle extensor muscles and improve active ROM. The act of sitting, then standing up requires muscle strength of the quadriceps, hamstring, and gastrocnemius muscle groups. This exercise may be particularly beneficial for dogs with OA of the hips. The sit-to-stand exercise allows active contraction of the gluteal muscles, but the hip joint is not generally extended to the point that results in pain. This allows strengthening without creating undue pain.

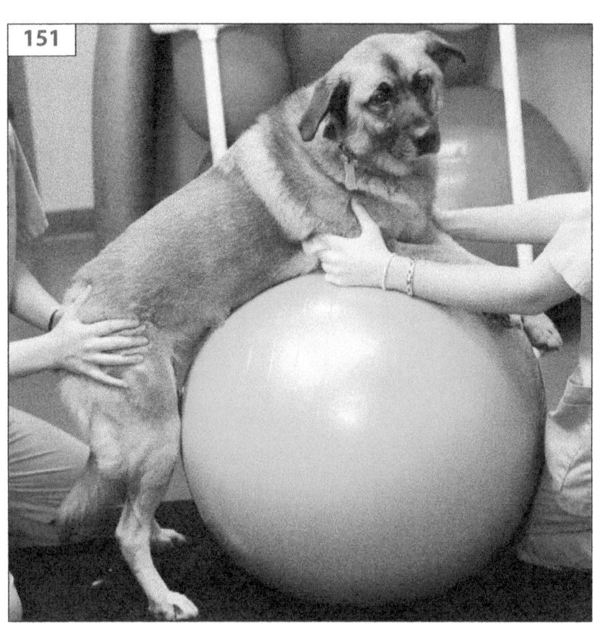

Fig. 151 Physioballs and rolls are excellent aids for balance and proprioception development.

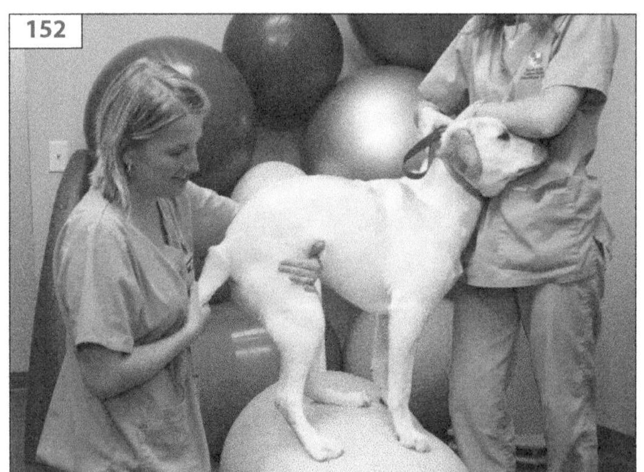

Fig. 152 With appropriate assistance, the physioroll will accommodate standing of small and medium-sized dogs.

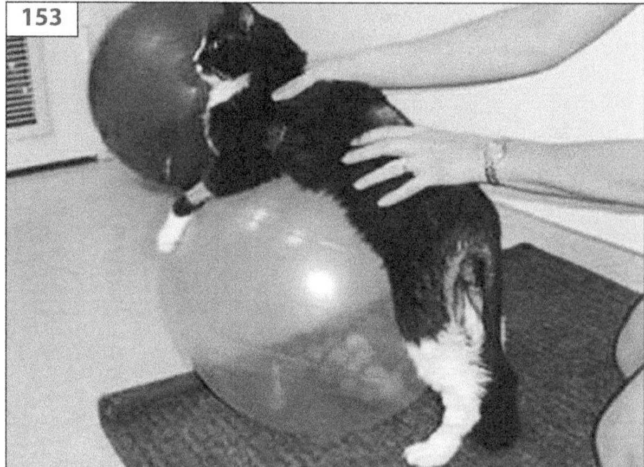

Fig. 153 Physioballs are equally valuable in the rehabilitation of cats as they are with dogs. (Courtesy of Sandra Hudson.)

Attention should be paid to sitting and standing straight, with no leaning to one side, and the joints of both rear limbs should be symmetrically flexed so that the dog sits squarely on its haunches. The exercise may be repeated a number of times before the dog is allowed to rest. In some cases it may be easier to back the dog into a corner, with the affected limb next to a wall so that the dog cannot slide the limb out while rising or sitting. Start with 5–10 repetitions once or twice daily, then work up to 15 repetitions 3–4 times daily, using 'empty calorie treats' as required as an incentive (**Figs. 154–157**).

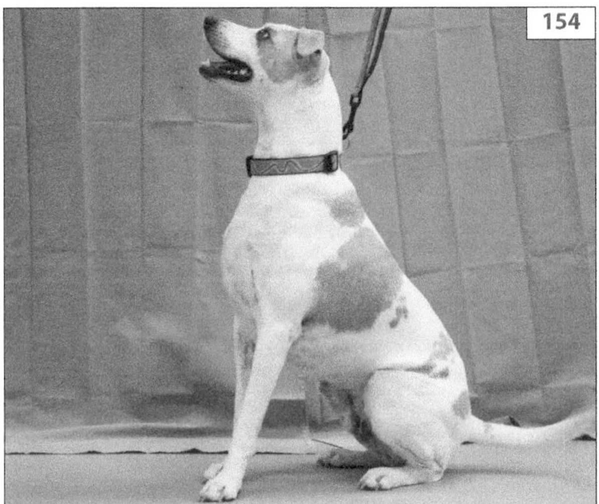

Fig. 154 The sit-to stand exercise focuses on hind limb muscle group conditioning. Commencing the exercise with the dog positioned in a corner may be helpful if the patient has difficulty controlling its limbs.

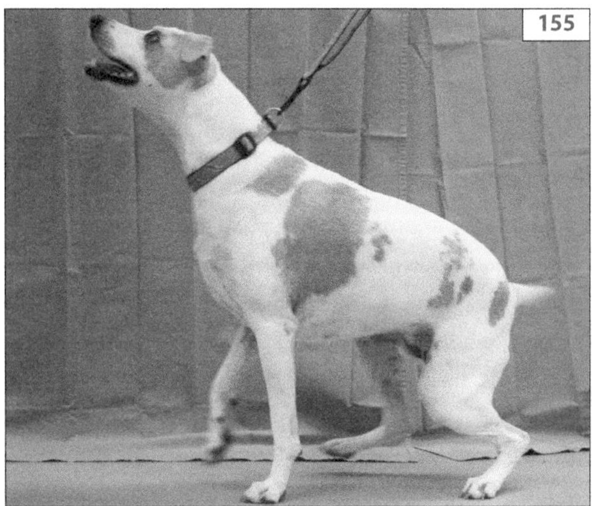

Fig. 155 As the dog begins to rise, contraction is focused on the sartorius, vastus, adductor, and gastrocnemius muscle groups.

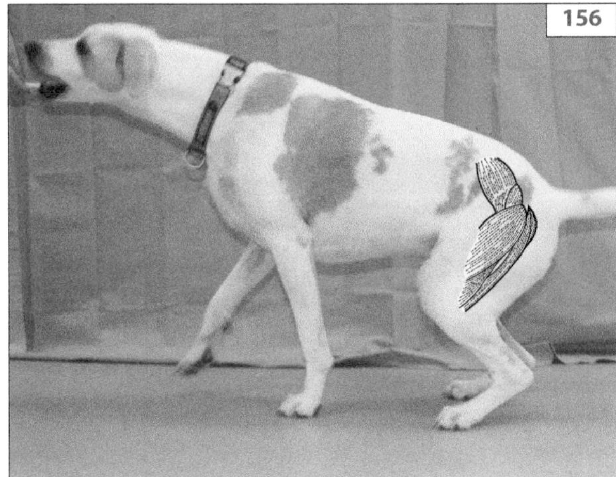

Fig. 156 As the dog continues to rise, the biceps, gluteal, and semitendenosis/membranosus muscle groups are strengthened.

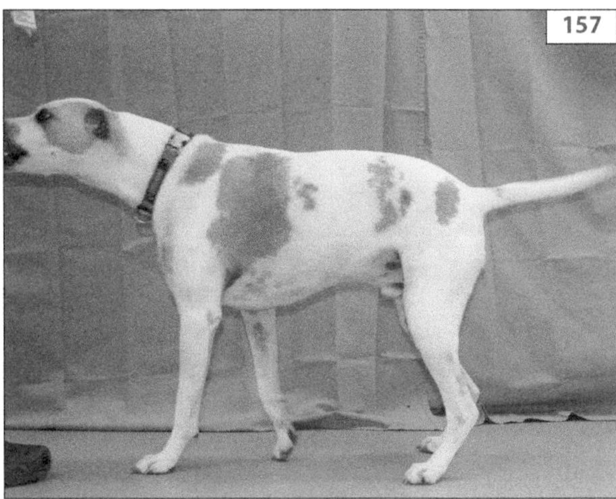

Fig. 157 The dog finishes this exercise in the standing position. 'Empty calorie' treats may be helpful in persuading the dog to perform the sit-to-stand exercise.

Stairs and steps

Climbing stairs is useful to improve power in the rear limb extensors, ROM, coordination, and balance. Quadriceps and gluteal muscle groups are strengthened as the animal pushes off, extending both hips and knees while propelling the body weight up the steps. Begin with 5–7 steps, and gradually increase to 2–4 flights of stairs once or twice daily (**Figs. 158, 159**).

Inclines and declines

Weight bearing while climbing, promotes extension of the knee and hip joints. Inclines and declines should be introduced slowly, beginning with gradual slopes, progressing to longer, steeper slopes and increasing the duration and speed of the exercise. Walking down slopes is typically more difficult because it requires the animal to reach under its body with the hindlimbs, which requires flexion of the hock, stifle, and hip (**Figs. 160, 161**).

Exercising on slopes aids in strengthening of the quadriceps, semitendinosus, semimembranosus, and gluteal muscles with relatively low-impact activity. Muscle strength in the hips and stifles is required for the dog to propel itself up an incline. Further, if the animal's head is held up slightly during the exercise, weight is shifted caudally, requiring the animal to drive up the hill with its rear limbs and challenge these muscles to a greater extent (**Figs. 162, 163**).

Dancing and wheelbarrowing

Dancing is a technique to increase weight bearing and force on the rear limbs, while also challenging proprioception, coordination, and balance. When the dog's front legs are lifted off the ground, this shifts the weight to the hindlimbs and also promotes stifle, hock, and hip extension. The higher the dog is elevated off the ground, the more extension is required in the rear limb joints. Once the dog is capable of using its affected limb consistently at a walk with minimal lameness, it may begin dancing exercises.

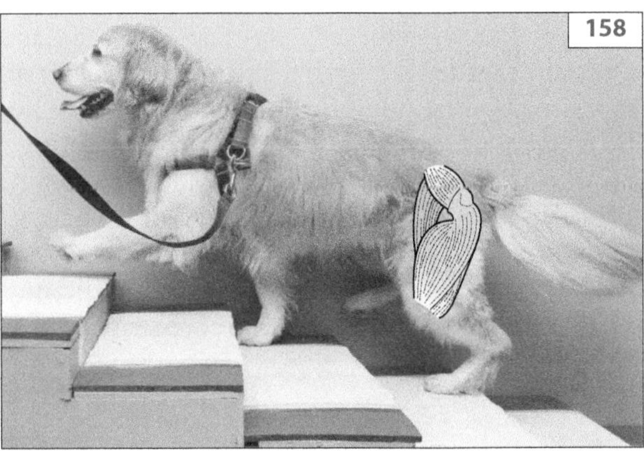

Fig. 158 Ascending steps is a rather complex exercise that conditions the quadricep, hamstring, and gluteal muscle groups.

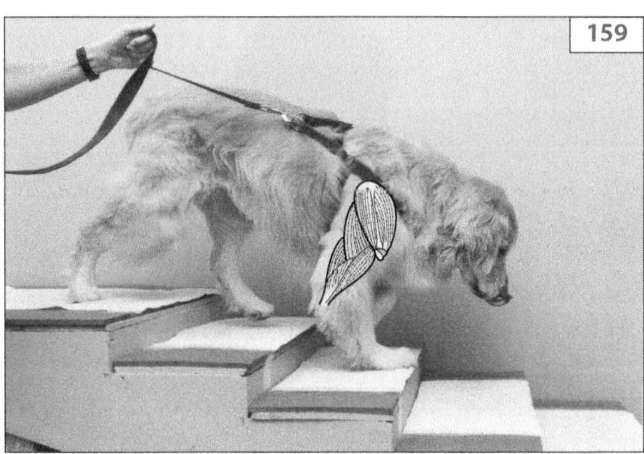

FIg. 159 Descending steps requires balance and proprioception as well as a focus on the forelimb muscle groups. When performing step exercises, ensure a nonskid surface and harness/leash control.

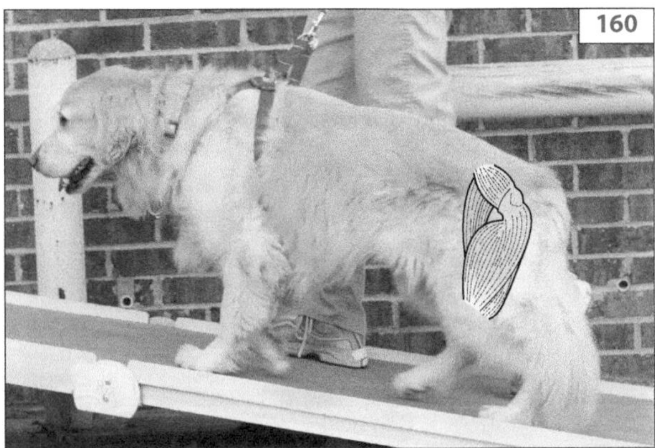

Fig. 160 Inclines focus on extension of both the hip and tarsal joints.

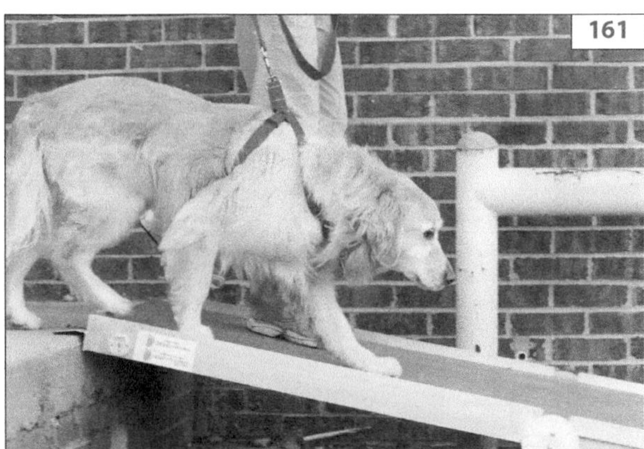

Fig. 161 The 'decline' exercises focus on flexion of the stifle and tarsal joints as the dog reaches under its body with the hindlimbs.

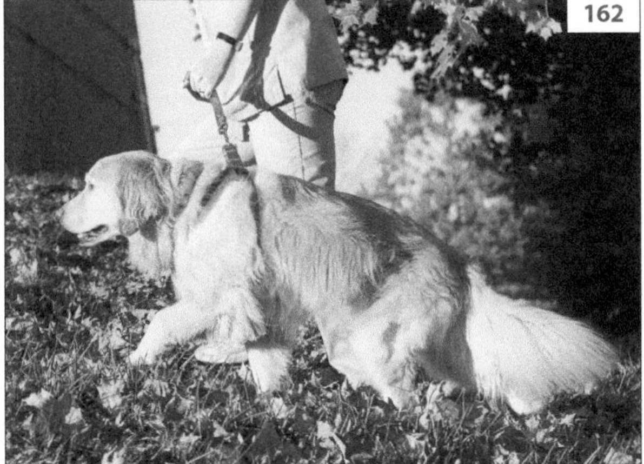

Fig. 162 The 'incline' exercise can be integrated into a leash walk by ascending hills of various gradients.

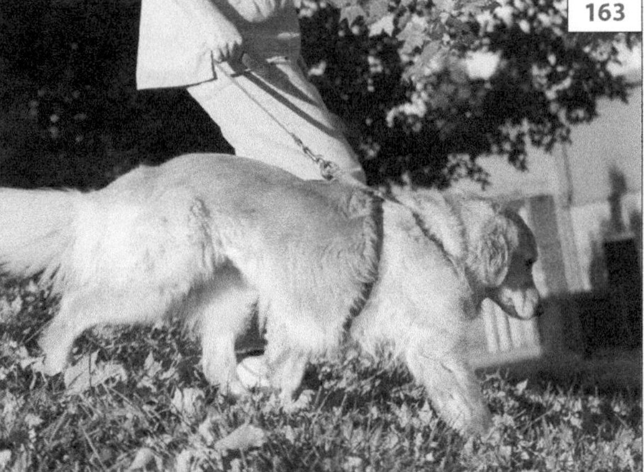

Fig. 163 The 'decline' exercise can be integrated into a leash walk by descending hills of various gradients.

How far the dog is elevated off the ground depends on the amount of stress the animal is able to handle comfortably on the hindlimbs. Dogs with normal proprioception will naturally move the rear limbs as the handler moves and the animal 'dances' forward and backward. Dogs may be elevated as high as possible and also dance up and down inclines or hills to place additional stress on the hindlimbs (**Figs. 164–166**).

Wheelbarrowing is an exercise similar to dancing, except that the forelimbs are targeted for therapy. For wheelbarrowing, the handler places the hands under the caudal abdomen and lifts the rear limbs of the dog off the ground, and the dog is moved forward. This exercise encourages increased use of the forelimbs and challenges proprioception, coordination, and balance (**Figs. 167, 168**). For both dancing and wheelbarrowing, it is advised to muzzle the dog, until the dog demonstrates receptivity to the exercise.

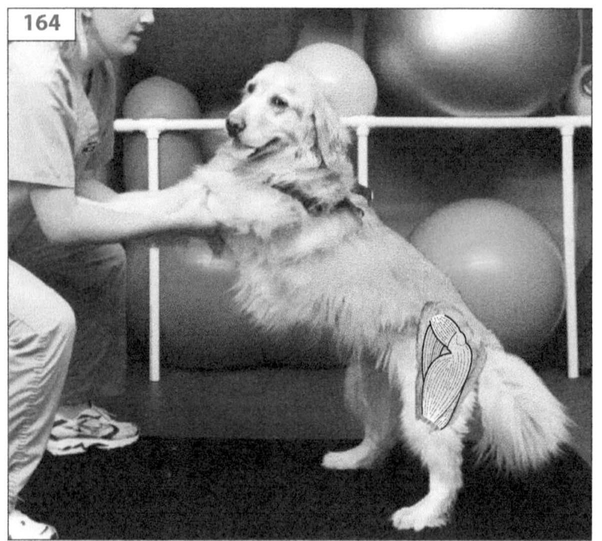

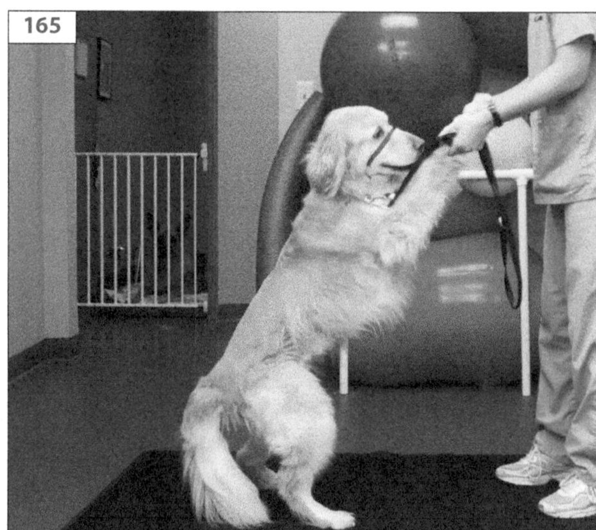

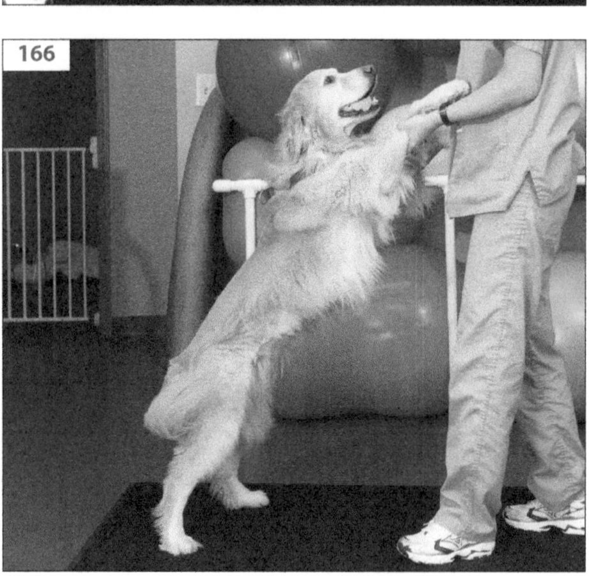

Figs. 164–166 Dancing increases weight bearing and force on the hind limbs. Dancing at a lower height requires less extension of the hip joint (**164**), while dancing at a more medium height can be performed if the dog has a greater range of motion in the hip joint (**165**). Dancing in a stretched position (**166**) requires maximum extension of the hind limb joints.

Treadmill activities

Treadmill walking is easily accommodated by dogs that will leash walk. However, they are not used to the ground moving under them, so proprioception, coordination, and balance may be challenged during the first couple of sessions (**Figs. 169, 170**). Treadmills may be useful during initial rehabilitation for conditions in which extension of the hip or stifle is painful, such as hip dysplasia or postoperative recovery from cruciate ligament surgery. Normally, patients are reluctant to perform activities such as climbing stairs because extension of these joints is painful. Treadmill walking is less painful in some patients because the belt provides assistance with hip and stifle extension by helping to pull the rear limb back. There is less need for active contraction of the gluteal and quadriceps muscles for joint extension when walking on a treadmill than when walking on land. For patients with neurologic conditions, the therapist may stand beside the patient and manually advance a foot during the normal gait sequence to encourage gait cadence.

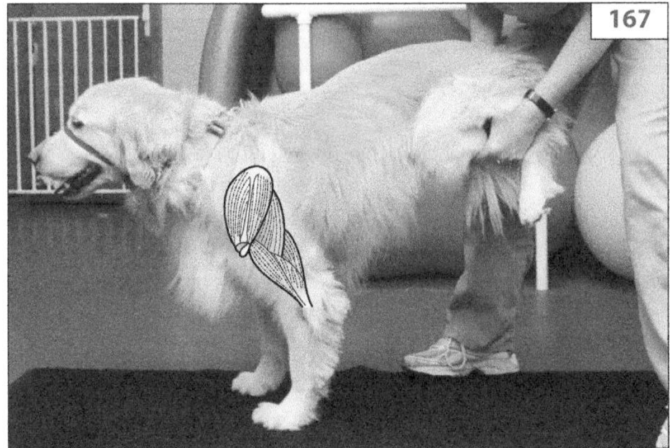

Fig.167 Wheelbarrow exercises focus on development of the triceps, infra-, and supraspinatus muscle groups.

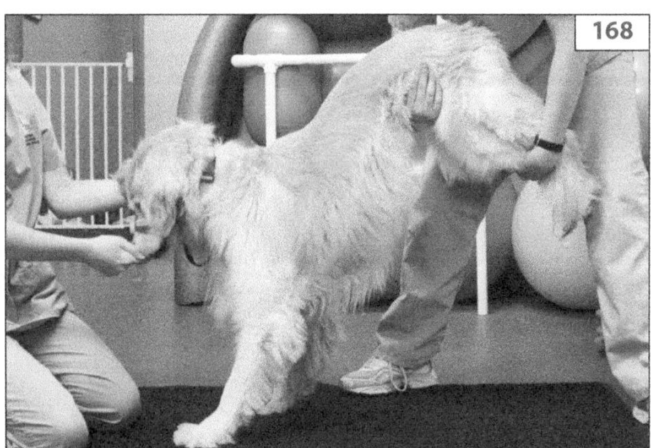

Fig. 168 Administering a 'high' wheelbarrowing exercise challenges the dog's forelimb balance and proprioception.

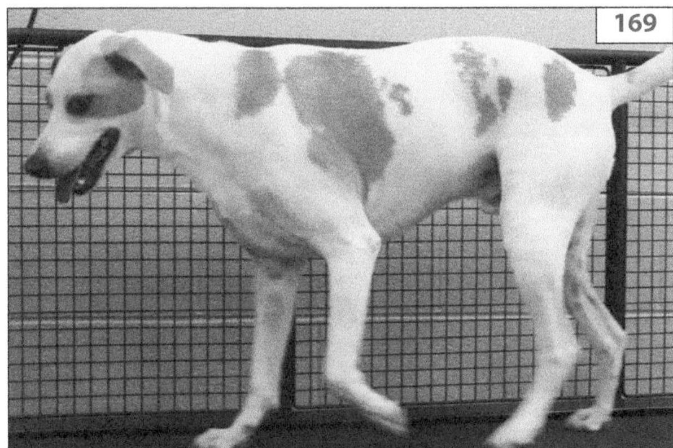

Fig. 169 Treadmill exercise develops proprioception, coordination, and balance. The moving belt assists in hindlimb extension.

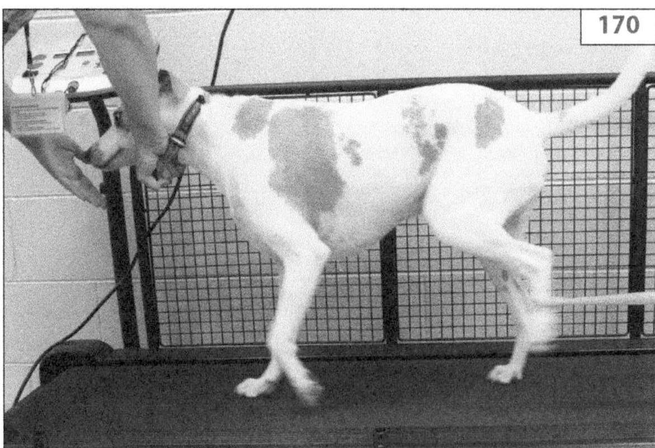

Fig. 170 By attaching an elastic band to the limb, the amount of resistance to forward limb placement can be increased.

Human-use treadmills may be modified for canine use by adding an overhead bar with a support system to which a canine harness can be attached. The harness helps support the dog in the event it stumbles or falls. Finally, the treadmill may be angled up or down to reduce or increase the forces placed on the forelimbs or hindlimbs.

Cavaletti rails

Cavaletti rails are poles that are spaced apart on the ground at a low height. Cavaletti rails may be used to encourage greater active ROM and lengthening strides in all limbs. Exercises can be helpful for either orthopedic or neurological patients in need of improved voluntary motor control and accuracy in placement of their limbs, challenging proprioception, balance, and coordination (**Figs. 171, 172**).

After initial Cavaletti rail adaptation, the handler can further challenge the dog by making simple modifications, such as adding more poles, increasing the height of all the poles to encourage greater active flexion and extension of joints, and altering the heights of alternating poles to encourage dogs to negotiate different situations (**Figs. 173, 174**). After achieving progress with walking Cavaletti rails, trotting may be introduced.

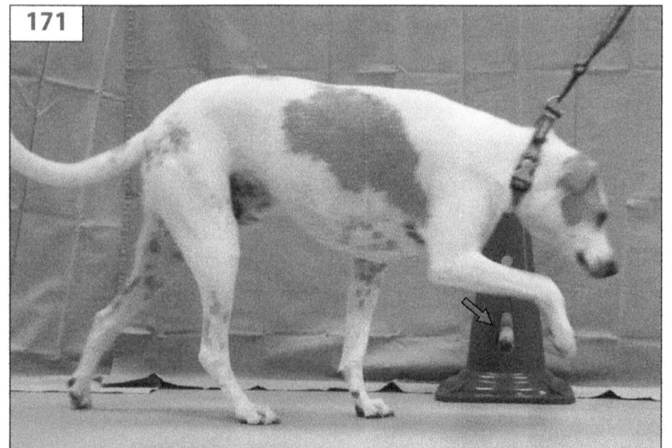

Fig. 171 Cavaletti rails (arrow) encourage a greater range of motion and lengthening stride.

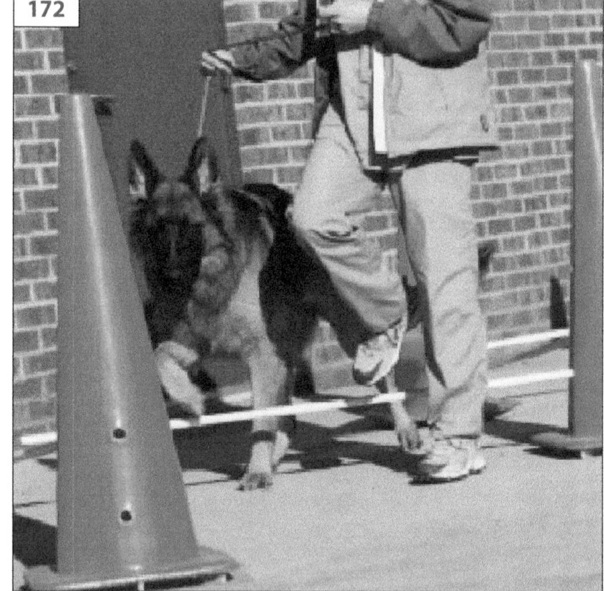

Fig. 172 Exercises using Cavaletti rails encourage development of balance, coordination, and proprioception.

Pole weaving

Weaving between vertical poles helps to promote side bending of the dog's trunk and also challenges proprioceptive functioning and strengthening of limb abductor and adductor muscles. The handler must lead the animal so that the head, neck, and body actually flex as the poles are negotiated. The distance between poles should be adjusted so that sufficient side bending results; in general, the distance between poles should be slightly less than the body length of the dog (**Figs. 175, 176**).

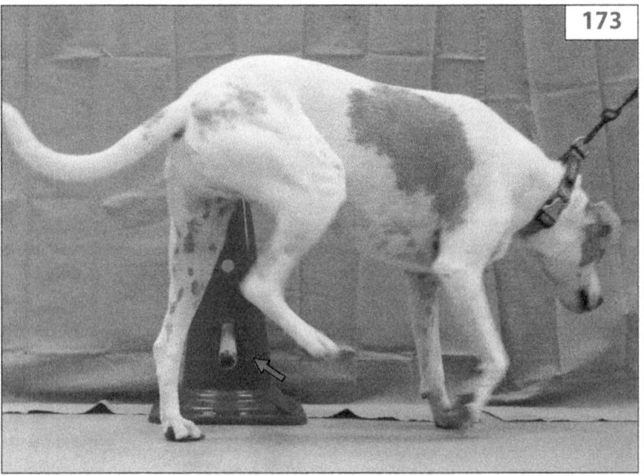

Fig. 173 Cavaletti rails require an increased range of motion in both the forelimbs and hindlimbs.

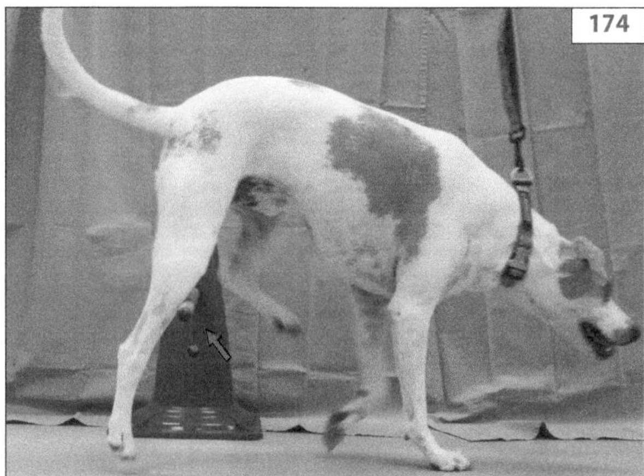

Fig. 174 Cavaletti rails can be raised or lowered to accommodate a desired amount of limb flexion.

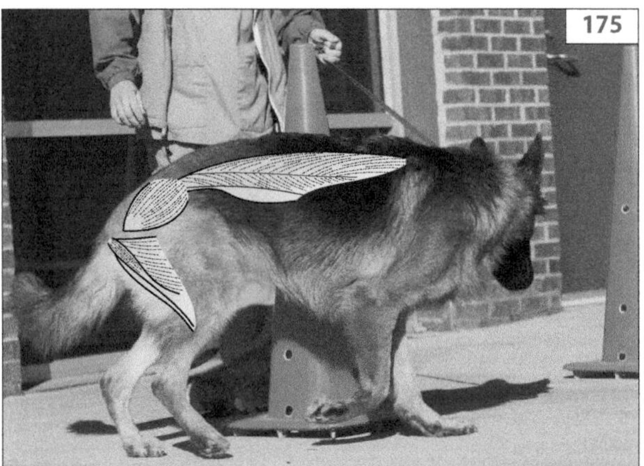

Fig. 175 Pole weaving challenges proprioceptive functioning and strengthens limb abductor and adductor muscles.

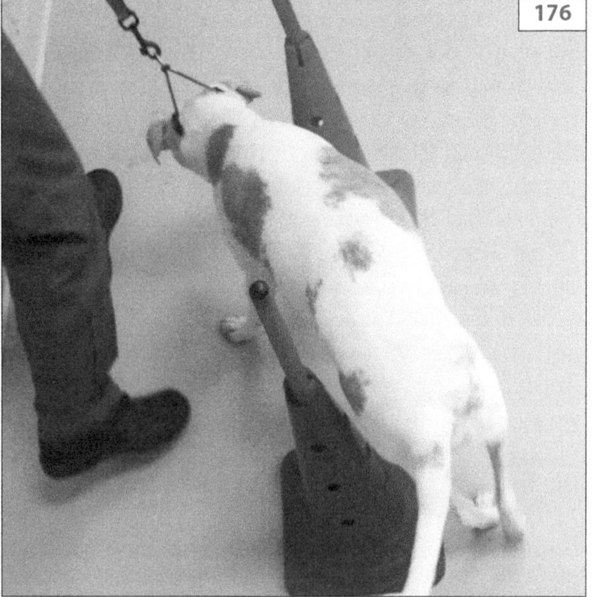

Fig. 176 A dorsal view of pole weaving allows appreciation of the bending of the dog's trunk while navigating the poles.

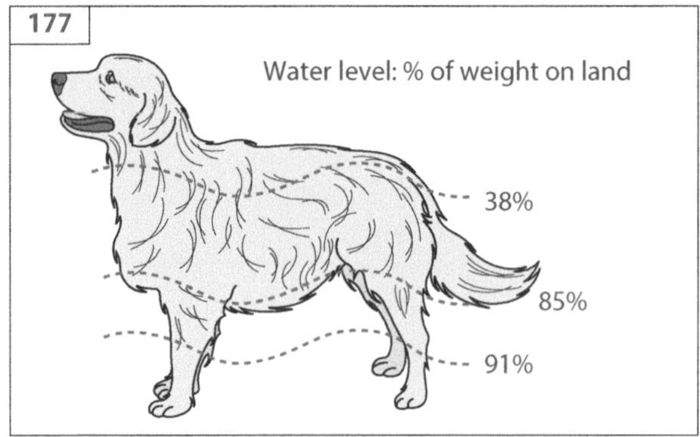

Fig. 177 The depth of patient immersion within water determines the amount of 'relative' weight bearing.

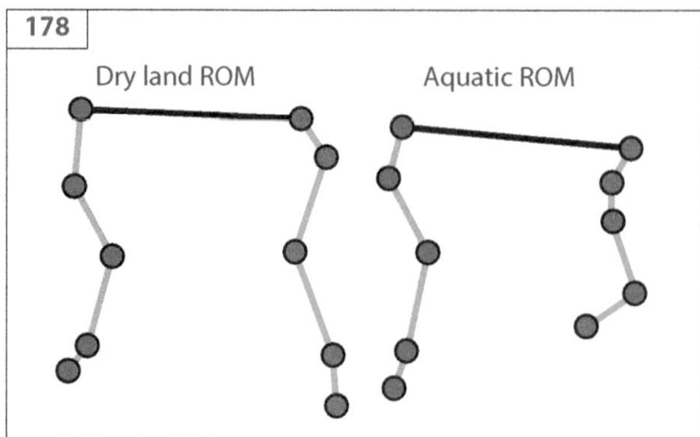

Fig. 178 Kinematic tracings from dogs ambulating both on dry land and immersed in water. An increased range of motion (ROM) is most apparent for the hindlimbs from this particular tracing. (Courtesy of Dr. Mike Conzemius.)

Aquatic exercises

Aquatic therapy takes advantage of several basic principles associated with water: relative density, buoyancy, viscosity, resistance, hydrostatic pressure, and surface tension.

Buoyancy is defined as the upward thrust of water acting on a body that creates an apparent decrease in the weight of a body while immersed. Further, the amount of buoyancy is determined by how deeply the patient is immersed. Therefore, water allows the patient to exercise in an upright position and may decrease pain by minimizing the amount of weight bearing on joints. Levine *et al.*[26] have shown that vertical ground reaction force decreases as the depth of immersion increases (**Fig. 177**).

Fluid (hydrostatic) pressure is exerted equally on all surfaces of an immersed body at rest at a given depth in accordance to Pascal's law. This fluid pressure is directly proportional to both the depth and the density of the fluid (the deeper a body is immersed in water, the greater the pressure exerted). Hydrostatic pressure opposes the tendency of blood and edema to pool in the lower portions of the body and can therefore aid in reducing swelling.

The viscosity, or resistance to fluid flow, is significantly greater in water than in air, making it harder to move through water than to move through air. Water can therefore provide resistance that may strengthen patient muscles and improve cardiovascular fitness.

Surface tension becomes a factor when a limb breaks the surface of the water. Resistance to movement is slightly greater on the surface of water because there is more cohesion on the surface. Therapeutically, if a patient is extremely weak, movements may be performed more easily in the water just beneath the surface rather than at or on the surface.

Studies indicate that pain decreases with aquatic therapy, and active ROM as well as functional ability increases (**Figs. 178–183**)[27]. There are many physiologic effects resulting from exercise in heated water: increased circulation to muscles, increased joint flexibility, and decreased joint pain[27]. If the water temperature is low, peripheral vasoconstriction occurs, blood moves centrally, venous return is enhanced, and stroke volume increases.

Summary

The key to a successful therapeutic exercise program is to have site- and condition-specific exercises whenever possible, to use a variety of exercises and techniques to keep the therapy team and patient from becoming bored, and to allow the animal to appropriately progress so that tissues are adequately challenged for strengthening, but not so rapidly as to result in complications and tissue damage.

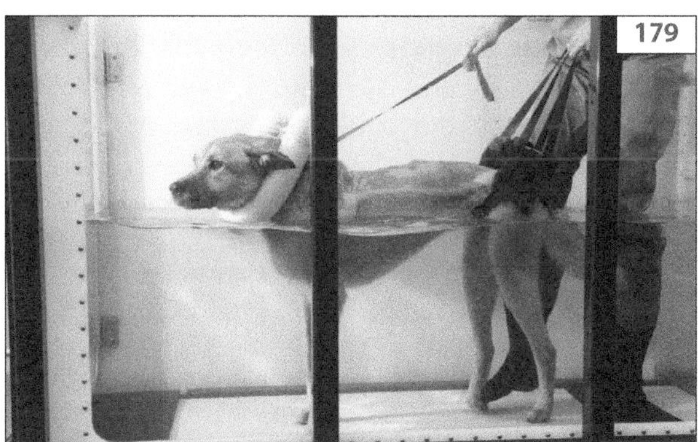

Fig. 179 Buoyancy provided by an underwater treadmill allows excellent facilitation of proprioception training.

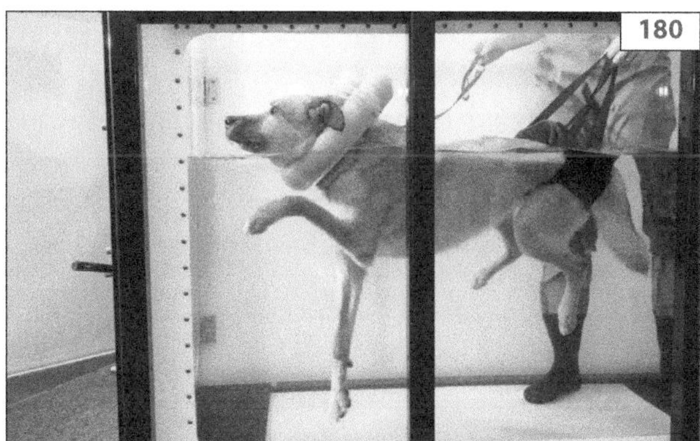

Fig. 180 Increasing the water level to force swimming encourages a much greater range of motion from all limbs.

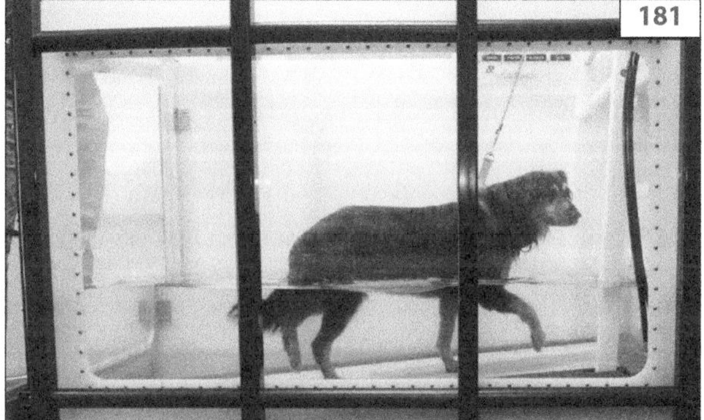

Fig. 181 Underwater treadmills with a variable incline feature take advantage of both the buoyancy and inclined plane features.

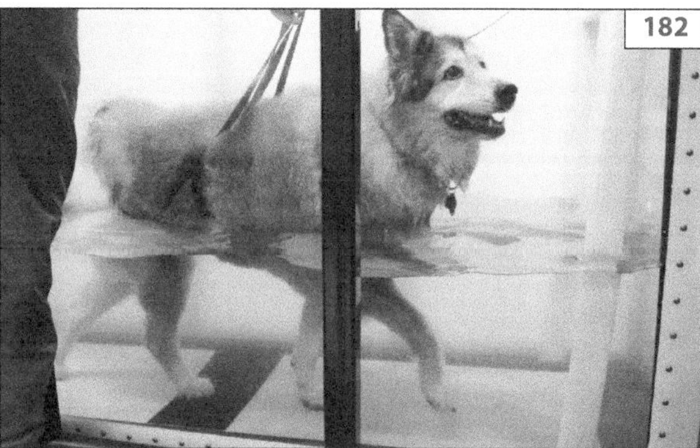

Fig. 182 Underwater treadmill exercising is effective not only for rehabilitation, but also for 'routine fitness'.

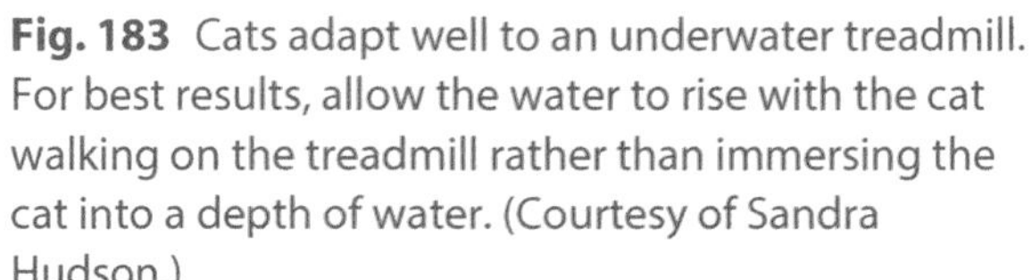

Fig. 183 Cats adapt well to an underwater treadmill. For best results, allow the water to rise with the cat walking on the treadmill rather than immersing the cat into a depth of water. (Courtesy of Sandra Hudson.)

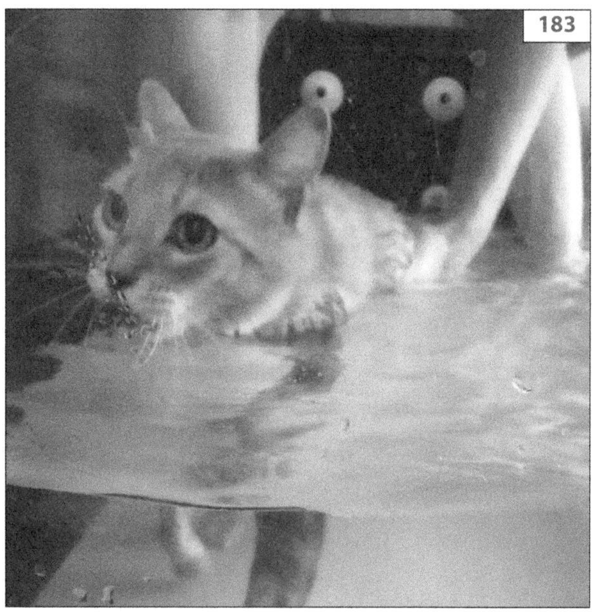

OTHER REHABILITATION TECHNIQUES

Deep heat: shortwave diathermy: ultrasound

Diathermy involves the use of high-frequency oscillating current and US (inaudible sound wave vibrations >20 KHz) to create deep heating. US is a deep-heating modality, effective in heating structures that superficial heat cannot reach. It is useful for improving the distensibility of connective tissue, which facilitates stretching. It is not indicated in acute inflammatory conditions where it may serve to exacerbate the inflammatory response and typically provides only short-term benefit when used in isolation.

US absorption is high in tissues with a high proportion of protein (muscle); however, US waves do not penetrate through air, so it is recommended to clip the hair coat to ensure optimal tissue heating. The duration of US therapy is short, but the dosage is difficult to monitor. Tissue burns can occur if the intensity is too high or the transducer is allowed to concentrate energy in a small area by stationary positioning. US has been effective for tendonitis[28,29], joint contraction[30], wound healing[31], and bone healing[32]. Physes of immature animals should be avoided.

Electrical stimulation

The goal in using electrical stimulation (ES) for neuromuscular dysfunction is to depolarize a motor nerve (neuromuscular electrical stimulation: NMES) and cause a muscle contraction, whereas the goal for pain management is to depolarize sensory nerves (TENS) to suppress the pain. NMES is used to maintain muscle mass/tone in nonweight-bearing patients. ES electrodes should be applied to clipped skin.

Transcutaneous electrical nerve stimulation

TENS is a noninvasive therapy mainly used for pain relief for a variety of pain syndromes. Theoretically, high frequency (>50 Hz) and low intensity TENS (HFT) are assumed to work through segmental pain inhibition processes (Gate Control Theory[33]). Low frequency (<10Hz) and high intensity TENS (LFT) are assumed to be effective by the release of endogenous opioids (suprasegmental effect[34]). Pulse duration and stimulus intensity differ in HFT and LFT and could be a decisive factor in efficacy. Both animal and human studies have shown higher analgesic effects by increasing the stimulus intensity or longer pulse duration[35]. Conventional TENS stimulators most commonly used in animals are high frequency (40–150 Hz, 50–100 µsec pulse width, low to moderate intensity) because they are more comfortable and create less anxiety in small animal patients.

According to the Gate Control Theory, nociceptive information from small diameter afferents is overridden by stimulation of large diameter fibers, and the pain stimulus is prevented from reaching supraspinal centers. Endogenous opioids released in the central nervous system have also been implicated in the analgesic mechanism of TENS by various investigators. Sluka *et al.*[36] have shown that low frequency TENS produces antihyperalgesia by activating central µ-opioid receptors, while high frequency TENS activates δ-opioid receptors both spinally and supraspinally in the rostral ventromedial medulla. Further, in rats, repeated application of low or high frequency TENS can lead to development of tolerance of spinal µ- and δ-opioid receptors, respectively[37].

In the year 2000, a review of seven trials of TENS and acupuncture-like TENS for the treatment of human knee OA concluded that this treatment is effective in managing pain[38]. Levine *et al.*[39] showed, using force plate analysis, that there was a significant improvement in limb loading of dogs after application of TENS to knees with chronic arthritic impairment. Significant improvement in ground reaction forces was found 30 minutes after treatment, and these differences persisted for 210 minutes after TENS application.

Precautions and contraindications for TENS

High intensity stimulation should be avoided directly over the heart, over areas of impaired sensation, near the pelvic region during pregnancy, over the carotid sinus, or where electrical stimulation might interfere with other electronic sensing devices, such as electrocardiogram monitors.

TENS application

Only trained personnel should administer TENS treatment. Patients should be placed in lateral recumbency, muzzled, and may require sedation. Hair is clipped, or the hair is wetted to accommodate fine wire electrodes. Up to four electrodes may be placed over a treatment area. Treatment protocols are empirical; however, application to the desired area(s) for 30 minutes, 3–7 times/week is a common practice. Amperage (intensity) may be slowly increased to the animal's tolerance level, but should be reduced if the patient shows any signs of distress/intolerance.

Acupuncture (See Chapter 8)

Low-level laser therapy

Low-level laser therapy (LLLT) affects photochemical reactions in the cell (photobiomodulation), exploring the concept that sources of light, such as infrared and ultraviolet light, have therapeutic attributes. Many different types of laser (light amplification by stimulated emission of radiation) are used both industrially and for medical purposes. Lasers used for rehabilitation techniques, LLLT, are also called cold lasers (<100 mW), as contrasted to high-power surgical lasers (3,000–10,000 mW) designed for thermal destruction of tissues.

Laser light is collimated, coherent, and monochromatic. These properties allow low-level laser light to penetrate the skin surface without causing damage to the skin or any heating effect.

Three basic types of laser are used for LLLT: gaseous HeNe and gallium–arsenide (GaAs) or gallium–aluminum–arsenide (GaAlAs) semiconductor or diode lasers. HeNe lasers emit a visible red light with a wavelength of 632.8 nm, whereas GaAs and GaAlAs emit invisible light near the infrared band with a wavelength of 820–904 nm. Longer wavelengths are more resistant to scattering than are shorter ones; accordingly, GaAs and GaAlAs lasers penetrate more effectively (direct effect at up to 2 cm, indirect effect to 5 cm) than HeNe lasers (direct effect up to 0.5 cm, indirect effect up to 1 cm) due to less epidermal and dermal absorption or scattering.

Three variables determine the use of lasers for LLLT: 1) wavelength (typically in the infrared or near-infrared range of 600–1,000 nm); 2) number of watts or milliwatts (typically between 5 and 600 mW); and 3) number of seconds to deliver joules of energy (1–8 J of energy are typically applied to treat various conditions). Given these variables, the time needed to hold the laser probe perpendicular to the treatment area can be calculated[40]. Unfortunately, optimal wavelengths, intensities, and dosages have not been studied sufficiently in animals to determine optimal treatment regimens.

The area of treatment should be clipped free of hair; however a coupling medium is not necessary, as in US, because the laser beam is not attenuated by air. LLLT should be administered by a trained therapist wearing eye protection.

LLLT has been used for the treatment of OA[41–44]; cartilage healing[45]; muscle, ligament, and tendon injuries[46], wound repair[47,48]; bone healing[49]; and pain relief[50]. Although results from LLLT treatment for pain have been contentious, 635 nm low-level lasers for the management of chronic minor pain, as in OA and muscle spasms, has been approved by the USA Food and Drug Administration.

Extracorporeal shock wave therapy

ESWT therapy uses very short acoustic waves emitted at low frequency (infrasound) and under very high pressure. They have very high energy and are characterized by a peak of very high overpressure (up to 100 times atmospheric pressure), followed by a trough. This occurs very rapidly, within microseconds. Energy is released into tissues when a change in tissue density is encountered, and this energy release is thought to stimulate healing.

Mechanisms explaining the clinical response to ESWT are lacking; however, reported effects include reduced inflammation and swelling, short-term analgesia, improved vascularity and neovascularization, increased bone formation, realignment of tendon fibers, enhanced wound healing, and perhaps, analgesia[51–54]. Research has revealed that ESWT is associated with an increase of bone morphogenetic proteins at fracture sites, as well as induction of cytokines and growth factors, such as transforming growth factor $\beta1$, substance P, vascular endothelial growth factor, proliferating cell nuclear antigen, and osteocalcin[52].

Francis *et al.*[55] reported the effects of ESWT on hip and elbow OA in dogs. Improvements in weight bearing and comfortable joint ROM were similar to what is typically expected with the use of NSAIDs. Favorable results with ESWT have been reported in dogs by other authors[56–58].

Shock waves should not be focused on gas-filled cavities or organs due to potential damage to surrounding tissues from energy release, and should not be administered over open growth plates. Heavy sedation or anesthesia is required for most ESWT patients. Because petechiation/bruising is not an uncommon sequelae, concurrent treatment with a COX-1-selective NSAID is inappropriate. Since ESWT is a localized treatment, a complete understanding of the treatment area anatomy is critical. Only well-trained professionals should administer ESWT. The optimal energy level and the number of shocks for various conditions is unknown. Generally, treatments should be repeated no more frequently than twice weekly, and most conditions are treated two or three times.

Dogs with immune-mediated joint disease or neurologic deficits should not be treated with ESWT because the effects are unknown on these conditions. Neoplastic joint disease, infectious arthritis, and diskospondylitis should not be treated with ESWT because of the risk for spreading the disease.

Static magnet field (SMF)

The application of permanent magnets for treating specific human medical problems, such as arthritis, chronic pain syndromes, wound healing, insomnia, and headache, have steadily increased. Magnets marketed directly to consumers are considered safe by the USA National Center of Complementary and Alternative Medicine (NCCAM)[59]. Pet owners can purchase magnets that are embedded in wraps, collars, or pet beds.

Results from basic science research demonstrate certain biologic effects attributed to SMF, suggesting clinical benefits[60–64] , namely increased local blood flow, release of endorphins, and anti-inflammatory effects. One study on the effect of SMF on relative blood flow to the metacarpus of horses refutes such benefits[65]. Therapeutic magnets range in strength from 2,500 to 6,000 gauss. (By comparison: the earth's magnetic field is 0.5 gauss, magnetic resonance imaging [MRI] produces magnetic fields that are 2–4 times that of therapeutic magnets, and common refrigerator magnets are 50–200 gauss.)

In 2007 a critical review of treatment parameters was made for SMF therapy in humans[66]. Among 56 studies reviewed, 61% failed to provide sufficient detail to permit protocol replication by other investigators. This finding illustrates that there are few well-designed, blinded, placebo-controlled studies to evaluate the clinical value of SMF. At present, there is little evidence that this treatment modality has beneficial clinical effects.

Adipose-derived mesenchymal stem cell therapy (See also Chapter 9)

Adipose-derived mesenchymal stem cells (AD-MSCs) have recently been introduced as another modality for the treatment of OA in dogs. AD-MSCs have been used in horses for tendon and ligament injuries, and have been used in animal cartilage defect studies. Mesenchymal stem cells 'communicate' with the cells of their local environment, can suppress immunoreactions, inhibit apoptosis, and improve mitochondrial function in damaged cells to enhance aerobic metabolism[67]. One study evaluated dogs with chronic OA of the hip. Dogs treated with AD-MSC therapy had significantly improved scores for lameness, as well as improved compiled scores for lameness, pain, and ROM compared with control dogs[68].

There are few precautions or contraindications for AD-MSC therapy. Dogs should not have infectious or inflammatory arthritis, and dogs must be healthy enough to undergo general anesthesia for harvesting the stem cells. People performing AD-MSC therapy are advised to undergo a brief certification process.

Approximately 50 g of fat are aseptically obtained from the lateral thorax, the inguinal region, or the falciform ligament. Harvested fat is processed to separate the AD-MSCs, and the appropriate number of cells for each desired joint of administration are prepared for injection. (This may be carried out through a commercial laboratory.) It is recommended that the patient be heavily sedated or lightly anesthetized for injection. The hair is clipped and the site is aseptically prepared for injection. If possible the injections should be done under fluoroscopic guidance because chronic joints may not have adequate synovial fluid to allow flashback into the hypodermic needle after insertion into the joint (dry joint), making it difficult to be certain that the cells are being injected directly into the joint. Once certain that the needle is in the joint, the cells are injected and the patient is recovered. Improvement typically occurs in 7–14 days. On occasion, after injecting cells into the most affected joints, cells may also be injected IV through a special filter in the event that multiple other joints are affected.

Canine platelet enhancement therapy (See Chapter 9)

Canine platelet enhancement therapy (C-PET) is a filter-based system involving the injection of concentrated platelets and their associated growth factors. It includes sedating the dog, drawing blood, filtering the blood, recovering the platelet concentrate, and delivering the cell therapy. In most cases, the process can be completed in 30 minutes or less.

The prevailing mechanism of action of platelet therapy stems from the belief that the growth factors they secrete serve as a homing signal for the recruitment of stem cells from other parts of the patient's body to the site of application of the platelets.

In concept, regenerative medicine and acupuncture share the common tenet of simply 'assisting' the body to heal itself.

Chapter 11

Cancer Pain

INTRODUCTION

The word cancer means 'crab' and was given to the disease because of its tenacity, a singular ability to cling to its victim like a crab's claws clinging to its prey. The all-important reality of cancer pain is witnessed in John Steinbeck's book, *The Grapes of Wrath*, where the character Mrs. Wilson, who is dying of cancer, states, 'I'm jus' pain covered in skin'[1].

Frank Vertosick, MD, states, 'From the Darwinian point of view, cancer is an unimportant disease. Since it preferentially afflicts animals beyond their child-bearing years, cancer poses no threat to animals in the wild, since natural populations experience death in other ways long before they are old enough for cancer to be a concern. We feel the sting of advanced prostate cancer because we are fortunate enough to live into our seventh decade and beyond, a feat rarely achieved even a hundred years ago. During the evolution of the nervous system, we developed pain to help us heal reversible insults: cracked vertebrae, pinched nerves, temporarily blocked colons, broken legs. To our great sorrow, this same pain also works against us when irreversible diseases like cancer strike; consequently, death becomes a painful affair. We die with all of our pain alarms impotently sounding. It is said that we are all born in another's pain and destined to die in our own'[2].

Clinical implication: cancer has become a frightening diagnosis in our culture, and when pets are diagnosed with cancer, the owner's first concern is usually pain.

TAXONOMY

In 1994 the International Association for the Study of Pain (IASP) revised a classification for chronic pain[3]. This classification includes five axes: 1) location of the pain; 2) involved organ or tissue system; 3) temporal pattern of pain; 4) pain intensity and time since onset of pain; and 5) etiology of pain. A distinct group of syndromes, therapies, and other etiologies of pain occur in cancer patients[4], such that neither the IASP nor any other diagnostic scheme distinguishes cancer pain from nonmalignant causes of chronic pain. Because the classification of cancer pain may have important diagnostic and therapeutic implications, a promising concept is a mechanism-based treatment approach, determining the sequence of analgesic agents based on the underlying causative pathology of cancer pain.

SCHEMES FOR CLASSIFYING CANCER PAIN

Etiologic classifications

Four different etiologies of cancer pain are that which: 1) is directly produced by the tumor; 2) is due to the various treatment modalities; 3) is related to chronic debility; and 4) is due to unrelated, concurrent disease processes (*Table 79*)[5]. Identification of these etiologies is important, as they reflect distinct treatment options and prognoses.

Pain relief from debulking tumors suggests that mechanical distortion of tissues is a component of tumor pain. Compression of a peripheral nerve can cause local demyelination, Wallerian degeneration of the nerve, secondary axon sprouting, and neuroma formation. Physiologic studies have demonstrated that dorsal root ganglion (DRG) compression can initiate a continuous afferent barrage that becomes self-sustaining. When tumors are identified as a foreign body, they can give rise to paraneoplastic neuropathy.

Wallerian degeneration refers to the degeneration of a nerve fiber and its myelin sheath that has been severed from its nutritive source.

It is proposed that expression of onco-neuronal antigens by cancer cells result in an autoimmunity. When the tumor develops, the body produces antibodies to fight it, by these binding to and helping the destruction of tumor cells. Such antibodies may cross-react with epitopes on normal nervous tissue, resulting in an attack on the nervous system. Neoplasms of the spinal cord may be either intramedullary or extramedullary, and primary tumors affecting the paravertebral area may spread and compress the cord, particularly within the intervertebral foramena (**Fig. 184**). An enlarging cancerous lymph node can compress the cord, and cancer that metastasizes to the vertebrae or surrounding tissues may also cause spinal cord compression.

Pain generating mediators are often released from certain tumors or from surrounding tissues

TABLE 79: Classification of cancer pain

Etiologic	Primarily caused by cancer Treatment of malignancy Debility Concurrent pathology
Pathophysiologic	Nociceptive (somatic, visceral) Neuropathic Mixed pathophysiology
Location of cancer pain syndromes	Head and neck Chest Vertebral and radicular pain Abdominal or pelvic Extremity
Temporal	Acute Breakthrough Chronic
Severity-based	Mild Moderate Severe

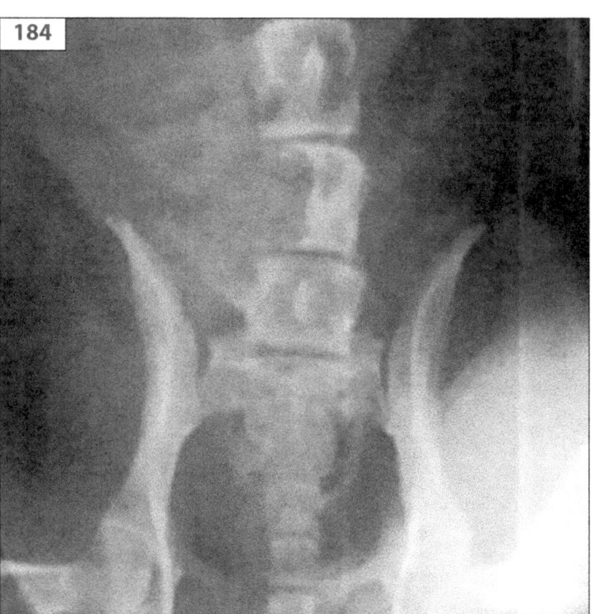

Fig. 184 Paravertebral mass identified as a chondrosarcoma in the body of L6.

involving invasion or metastasis, thereby producing pain itself[6]. Paradoxically, various cancer therapies may result in pain. Chemotherapeutic agents have been associated with peripheral neuropathies and acute pain in humans[7], and radiation therapy may injure soft tissue or neuronal structures. Furthermore, immunosuppressive therapy may render some patients at increased risk for secondary infection and complications.

Although psychogenic pain in animals is controversial, nociceptive and neuropathic types of cancer pain are recognized. Stimulation of afferent nociceptive pathways in visceral or somatic tissue leads to nociceptive pain. Neuropathic pain is caused by dysfunction of, or lesions involving, the peripheral or central nervous systems (CNS). Differentiating the two may influence the selection of a specific therapy. Nociceptive somatic cancer pain arises from soft tissue structures that are non-neurologic and nonvisceral in origin, including skin, muscle, bone, and joints, and often correlates with the extent of tissue damage. Nociceptive visceral cancer pain arises from the deep organs of the abdomen, thorax, or pelvis, and is often difficult to localize. Obstruction of hollow viscera, distention of organ walls, stretching of the pancreas or liver capsule, or extension of metastasis into mesentery may induce visceral pain.

Neuropathic cancer pain

Neuropathic pain affects the nervous system, and may have multiple etiologies, including nerve compression, deafferentation injury, and a sympathetically-induced origin[8]. Nerve compression has been identified as the most common cause of neuropathic pain in human cancer patients (79%), followed by nerve injury (16%), and sympathetically mediated pain (5%)[9]. Neuropathic pain is considered to be relatively less responsive to opioids[10]. Nonopioid adjuncts, such as antiepileptic, antidepressant, and antiarrythmic agents or combinations of these, should be considered[11,12].

Noteworthy pain and neurologic deficits result from tumor infiltration or compression of the peripheral nervous system. This may include infiltration of spinal nerve roots, producing radicular symptoms, and invasion of neuronal plexuses. Such invasion or compression may involve a perineural inflammatory reaction that accentuates the nerve pain[13]. Degenerative changes and deafferentation are a consequence of prolonged tumor infiltration or compression[14]. Resultant peripheral sensitization is associated with an increased density of sodium channels in the damaged axons and associated DRG[15]. Ectopic foci of electrical activity arise in injured axons and stimulus thresholds are decreased. Activated peripheral nociceptors release mediators for central sensitization, for example, the amino acid glutamate and neuropeptides, such as substance P (sP) and neurokinin A. In turn, these neurotransmitters cause an increase of intracellular calcium and up-regulation of N-methyl-D-aspartate (NMDA) receptors.

Associated with this increased intracellular calcium comes activation of enzymatic reactions causing expression of genes that ultimately lower the excitatory threshold of dorsal horn neurons, exaggerate their response to noxious stimuli, and enlarge the size of their receptor fields (secondary peripheral sensitization).

Deafferentation is the state of having an incomplete afferent connection with the central nervous system.

Clinical implication: tumors of the peripheral nervous system can lead to a state of 'wind-up' and a 'spread' of painful response to neighboring tissues.

Sympathetically-mediated cancer pain

Sympathetically-mediated cancer pain may result from direct or indirect involvement of the sympathetic chain. This pain is perceived in alignment with the pattern of sympathetic vascular innervation, rather than localization to the area of distribution for a specific peripheral nerve or dermatome[6]. Although pathophysiologic classification of cancer pain is informative for treatment insight, one study in humans has revealed that 70% of patients showed two or more pathophysiologic classes of pain in the advanced stages of cancer[16].

Anatomically-based cancer pain

Anatomic classification of cancer pain has limited applications since it lacks specificity as to the mechanism of pain; however, it does provide guidance for certain invasive therapies, such as external radiation, neurolytic blocks, electrical stimulation, or perhaps, targeted drug delivery.

Severity-based cancer pain

Severity-based classification of cancer pain reflects the extent of tissue destruction, size of the tumor, or its location. In human patients, metastatic bone lesions and injury to nerves are typically more painful than soft tissue tumors. The severity of cancer pain is dynamic, reflecting the course of the disease and different therapies administered; therefore, it is prudent to review the severity of the pain over time.

The WHO cancer pain ladder

In 1986 the World Health Organization (WHO) developed a simple three-stage analgesic ladder for treatment of cancer pain that relies on widely available and inexpensive analgesic agents[17]. The WHO analgesic ladder provides clinical guidance from a severity-based pain classification system (**Fig. 185**). Although the quality of evidence for the WHO ladder approach has been challenged, it has been globally distributed and is considered the standard for cancer pain management in human patients. Contemporary thinking, however, is to use 'stronger' analgesics earlier.

Mechanism-based treatment

A mechanistic-based treatment strategy for managing cancer pain in humans has been studied[18]; neuropathic pain was treated with antidepressants and anticonvulsants, while opioids were integrated into the treatment protocol only after these drugs were considered ineffective. Interestingly, all human patients studied required concurrent therapy with a mean of three drug classes, including an opioid, to control their pain. This illustrates the heterogeneity of cancer pain mechanisms and the subsequent value of a 'balanced or multimodal analgesia' approach to treatment.

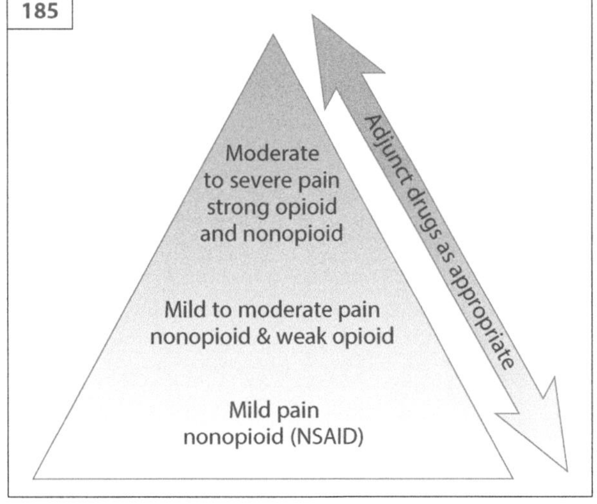

Fig. 185 World Health Organization Ladder was adopted in 1986 to give guidance for managing human cancer pain. It has been adopted in veterinary medicine and also provides guidance for noncancer pain. NSAID: nonsteroidal anti-inflammatory drug.

PREVALENCE

Prevalence of cancer in animals

The frequency of cancer pain in animals is difficult to identify, as is the prevalence of cancer itself in the pet population. Not all cancers are painful, sensitivity to pain varies between individuals, and the degree of pain may vary during the course of the cancer. The most comprehensive effort to estimate cancer incidence rates was a survey of veterinary practices in Alameda and Contra Costa counties (California, USA) from 1963 to 1966, and remains as the seminal study for estimating the incidence of canine and feline cancers (*Table 80*)[19]. This survey revealed an annual incidence rate of 381/100,000 among dogs living in households that used veterinary services, while the incidence rate for cancer in cats was 155.8/100,000. Intuitively, these data are only estimates as not all cases of cancer are diagnosed equally, considering the many special procedures, diagnostic tests, and costs involved. In a study of 2002 dogs that underwent necropsy at the Angell Memorial Animal Hospital, cancer accounted for 20% of the deaths at 5 years and increased to over 40% in dogs 10 years of age[20].

Prevalence of animal cancer pain

Currently, there are no estimates for the numbers of animals with cancer pain, and sparse data on the efficacy of various therapies. Cancer-related pain has been estimated to afflict 30–60% of human patients at the time of diagnosis, and 55–95% of human patients during the advanced stages of disease[21]. Some authors have indicated that approximately 28% of human cancer patients die without adequate pain relief [22]. (Likely, this figure is less now than in 1984 when these data were published.) Several authors[23,24] have reported the under-use of perioperative analgesics in animal patients, suggesting the likelihood that analgesic management of cancer pain is similarly quite low. Although inappropriate, under-treatment is not surprising since the medical profession (both human and veterinary) have historically been slow to administer analgesics. Reasons for this include:

- Under utilization of clinical staff for assessing cancer pain during the course of the disease.
- Lack of good or validated methods for assessing animal pain.
- Failure to include the owner's input into their pet's ongoing assessment.
- Failure to appreciate the high frequency with which cancer patients experience pain.
- Lack of knowledge regarding analgesic therapies and the probable need to alter these therapies, during the course of the cancer.

TABLE 80: Annual crude incidence rates of cancer per 100,000 population for humans, dogs, and cats (Alameda County, 1960–1966)[19]

Cancer site	Humans	Dogs	Cats
All sites	272.1	381.2	155.8
Skin, nonmelanoma	31.8	90.4	34.7
Malignant melanoma	8.3	25.0	ND
Digestive	74.5	25.2	11.2
Respiratory	32.9	8.5	5.0
Connective tissue	2.4	35.8	17.0
Mouth and pharynx	10.3	20.4	11.6
Breast	37.3	198.8	25.4
Lymphoid tumors	13.3	25.0	48.1
Bone	1.2	7.9	4.9
Testis	2.6	33.9	ND

ND: not determined

Considering that an overall average of about 70% of humans with advanced cancer suffer pain[25], and that many biologic systems are common between man and animals, a conservative estimate might be that 30% of animal cancers are painful[26]. As a rule, pain is more frequently associated with tumors arising in noncompliant tissue (e.g. bone) (*Table 81*). It should not be overlooked that some treatment therapies for cancer may create pain (*Table 82*).

CANCER PAIN ASSESSMENT IN ANIMALS

The assessment of cancer pain in animals is particularly challenging, and few reports have been made in this area. Yazbek and Fontana[28] suggest that a simple questionnaire may be useful in assessing health-related quality of life (QOL) in dogs with pain secondary to cancer, in that dogs with cancer had significantly lower scores than did healthy dogs. A number of animal pain scales have been proposed (e.g. visual analog scales [VAS], numerical rating scales, simple descriptive scales, multifactorial pain scales, and composite measure pain scale [CMPS]); however, these are applied to the assessment of acute pain, where some are more valid than others. Physiologic variables, such as heart rate, respiratory rate, cortisol levels, temperature, and pupil size, are unreliable measures for assessing acute pain[29,30], and behavioral changes are now considered the most reliable indicator of pain in animals[31,32]. Any change in an animal's normal behavior may be associated with pain. Herein lies the value of integrating the pet owner's observations into the patient's assessment on a continuum of follow-ups. In fact, some studies show that the owner was a better assessor of their animal's chronic pain than a veterinarian.

Certain behaviors are worth noting:

- Painful animals are less active.
- Animals in pain do not groom as frequently, especially cats.
- Dogs, in particular, may lick a painful area.
- Both painful dogs and cats may show decreased appetites.
- Painful cats tend to seek seclusion.
- Dogs in pain tend not to yawn, stretch, or 'wet dog shake'.
- Animals in pain often posture differently.

One of the most reliable methods for identifying pain is the animal's response to analgesic intervention.

TABLE 81: Tumors frequently associated with pain

Tumor	Remarks
Bone	Noncompliant tissue tumors are typically painful
Central nervous system	Tumors arising from neural tissue are not usually painful until late into the course of the disease; extradural tumors are associated with pain
Cutaneous (invasive)	Ulcerative, invasive cutaneous tumors tend to be painful
Gastrointestinal	Distention of the esophagus, stomach, colon, and rectum are painful Colonic and rectal pain often presents as perineal discomfort
Intranasal	Bone and turbinate destruction leads to pain
Intrathoracic and abdominal (e.g. mesothelioma, malignant histiocytosis)	Response to intracavity analgesics, such as local analgesics, suggests that these conditions are painful
Mammary carcinoma (inflammatory)	Dogs consistently show abnormal behavior considered to be pain-induced
Oral and pharyngeal	Soft tissue tumors of the pharynx and caudal oral cavity are particularly painful, perhaps due to constant irritation from eating Soft tissue tumors of gingival origin are relatively nonpainful, but become very painful with invasion of bone
Prostate	Quite painful, particularly with bone metastasis
Surgery	Postoperative pain associated with tumor removal can be greater than anticipated, perhaps due to the presence of neuropathic pain

TABLE 82: Chemotherapy-induced dysfunction and pain syndromes (humans)

Chemotherapeutic agent	Toxicity	Impact on pain
Vinca alkaloids (vincristin, vinblastin)	Neurologic	Peripheral neuropathy, autonomic neuropathy
Paclitaxel/docetaxel	Bone marrow suppression, neurologic	Neutropenia, mucositis
Platinum complexes (cisplatin, carboplatin)	Renal, bone marrow suppression, neurologic	Decrease creatinine clearance, peripheral neuropathy (cisplatin)
Ectoposide	Bone marrow suppression	Leukopenia, thrombocytopenia, mucositis
Nitrogen mustards (mechlorethamine, chlorambucil, cyclophosphamide, ifosphamide)	Bone marrow suppression	Leukopenia, thrombocytopenia, hemorrhagic cystitis (cyclophosphamide)
Anthracycline antibiotics	Bone marrow suppression, cardiac	Leukopenia, thrombocytopenia/anemia, stomatitis, cardiac arrhythmias, congestive heart failure
Mitoxanthrone	Bone marrow suppression	Mucositis
Cytarabine	Bone marrow suppression, neurologic	Granulocytopenia/thrombocytopenia, peripheral neuropathy
Methotrexate	Bone marrow suppression, renal	Pancytopenia, mucositis, chronic renal failure
Bleomycin	Pulmonary	Mucositis, lung fibrosis

Source: Miguel RV (2006)[27].

CANCER PAIN MECHANISMS

Bone cancer model

Periosteum, mineralized bone, and bone marrow are highly innervated by Aβ-, Aδ-, and C-fibers, all of which conduct sensory input from the periphery to the spinal cord (**Fig. 186**).

Recently, the first animal models of bone cancer pain have been developed. In the mouse femur model, bone cancer pain is induced by injecting murine osteoclytic sarcoma cells into the intramedullary space of the femur. These tumor cells proliferate, and ongoing, movement-evoked, and mechanically-evoked pain-related behaviors develop that increase in severity over time. These models have allowed elucidation of how cancer pain is generated and how the sensory information is processed when molecular architecture of bone is changed by disease (**Fig. 187**).

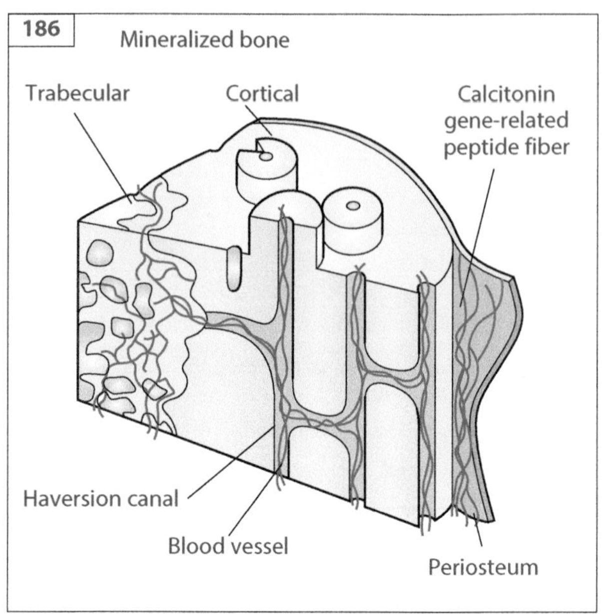

Fig. 186 Bone histology: bone marrow, mineralized bone, and periosteum are highly innervated, sending sensory input to the spinal cord.

Afferent sensory neurons

Sensory neurons are also highly 'plastic', in that they can change their phenotype in response to a sustained peripheral injury. Altering patterns of signaling peptide and growth factor expression underlies peripheral sensitization, lowering the activation threshold and creating a state of hyperalgesia. Peripheral tissue damage also activates previously 'silent' nociceptors, which create a state of hyperalgesia and allodynia.

In mice with bone cancer, normally nonpainful palpation of the affected femur induces the release of sP from primary afferent fibers that terminate in the spinal cord. Substance P, in turn, binds to and activates the neurokinin-1 receptor that is expressed by a subset of spinal cord neurons[33]. A similar activity is noted with c-fos[34]. Peripheral sensitization of nociceptors may be involved in the generation and maintenance of bone cancer pain.

Nociceptor excitation

Tumor and tumor-associated cells, including macrophages, neutrophils, and T-lymphocytes, secrete a wide variety of factors including prostaglandins (PGs), endothelins (ETs), interleukin-1 and -6, epidermal growth factor, transforming growth factor, and platelet-derived growth factor, which directly excite primary afferent neurons. Each of these factors may play an important role in the generation of pain associated with various cancers. Pharmaceutical targeting of these factors provides opportunities for pain relief, while anti-PGs and anti-ETs are already commercially available.

Tumor-associated macrophages and several tumor cells express high levels of cyclo-oxygenase-2 (COX-2), producing large amounts of PGs[35,36]. Although all nonsteroidal anti-inflammatory drugs (NSAIDs) are anti-PGs, the new COX-2 inhibitors, or coxibs, preferentially inhibit COX-2 and avoid many of the COX-1 inhibition side-effects. Additionally, some experiments have suggested that COX-2 is involved in angiogenesis and tumor growth[37,38]. Although further research is required to characterize the effect of coxib-class NSAIDs on different types of cancer, in addition to blocking cancer pain, COX-2 inhibitors may have the added advantage of reducing the growth and metastasis of tumors.

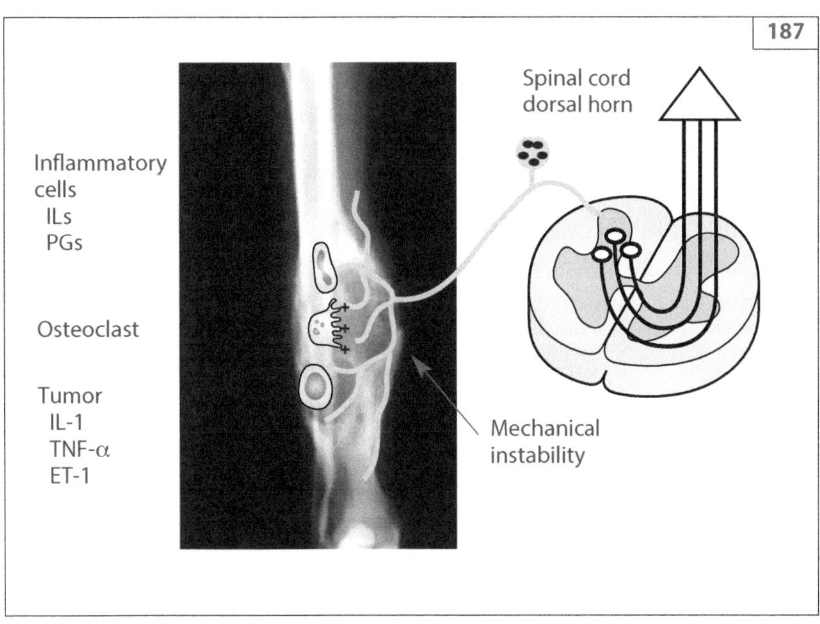

Fig. 187 Bone cancer changes the molecular architecture and bioneurologic status of the diseased bone. ET-1: endothelin-1; IL: interleukin; PG: prostaglandin; TNF: tumor necrosis factor.

A PubMed search for the terms NSAID and cancer conducted in February 2005 generated 7, 513 abstracts. The same search conducted in December 2007 generated 9,624 abstracts, and 14,019 in December 2011. A similar search for the terms NSAID and COX-2 revealed 1,907 abstracts in February 2005, compared to 3,529 abstracts in December 2007, and 8,306 in December 2011. The role of NSAIDs, and particularly coxib-class NSAIDs, in cancer research is an area of intense interest[39].

An (incomplete) listing of canine patient tumors expressing COX-2 includes:

- Transitional cell carcinoma[40].
- Renal cell carcinoma[41].
- Squamous cell carcinoma[42].
- Prostate carcinoma[43].
- Rectal polyps[44].
- Nasal carcinoma[45].
- Osteosarcoma[46].
- Mammary carcinoma[47].
- Intestinal adenocarcinoma[44].
- Oral melanoma[48].

In contrast to dogs, the absence of COX-2 expression in most feline neoplasms might suggest that COX-2 inhibitors would have a lower potential as anticancer agents in this species[49].

The peptide ET-1 is another pharmacologic target for treating cancer pain. A number of small unmyelinated primary afferents express receptors for ETs[50], and ETs may well sensitize or excite nociceptors. Several tumors of humans, including prostate cancer, express high levels of ETs[51], and clinical studies have shown a correlation between the severity of the pain in human patients with prostate cancer and ET plasma levels[52].

Tumor-induced local acidosis

Tumor burden often outgrows its vascular supply, becoming ischemic and undergoing apoptosis. Subsequently, an accumulation of acid metabolites prevails, resulting in an acidotic local environment. This is relevant to cancer pain, in that subsets of sensory neurons have been shown to express different acid-sensing ion channels[53], sensitive to protons or acidosis. Two major classes of acid-sensing ion channels expressed by nociceptors, both sensitive to decreases in pH, are the transient receptor potential (TRP) V1 and the acid-sensing ion channel-3 (ASIC-3). As tumors grow and undergo apoptosis, there is a local release of intracellular ions and inflammatory-mediated protons that give rise to a local acidic environment. This neurobiologic mechanism is particularly relevant in bone cancer where there is a proliferation and hypertrophy of osteoclasts. Osteoclasts are multinucleated cells of the monocyte lineage that resorb bone by maintaining an extracellular microenvironment of acidic pH (4.0–5.0) at the interface between osteoclast and mineralized bone[54]. Experiments in mice have shown that osteoclasts contribute to the etiology of bone cancer pain[55], and that osteoprotegrin and a bisphosphonate[56], both of which induce osteoclast apoptosis, are effective in decreasing osteoclast-induced cancer pain. TRPV1 or ASIC antagonists would act similarly, but by blocking excitation of acid-sensitive channels on sensory neurons.

Growth factors from tumor cells

Different patients with the same cancer may have vastly different symptoms. Metastases to bone in the same individual may cause pain at one site, but not at a different site. Small cancer deposits in one location may be more painful than large cancers at an unrelated site. Why the variability? One explanation may be that changes in the periphery associated with inflammation, nerve injury, or tissue injury are reflected by changes in the phenotype of sensory neurons[57]. Such changes are, in part, caused by a change in tissue levels of several growth factors released from the local environment at the injury site, including nerve growth factors (NGFs)[58], and glial-derived neurotrophic factor[59]. Likely, the milieu of growth factors to which the sensory neuron is exposed will change as the developing tumor invades the tissue that the neuron innervates.

The mouse sarcoma cell model has also demonstrated that growing tumor cells destroy both the hematopoietic cells of the marrow and the sensory fibers that normally innervate the marrow[60]. This neuronal damage can give rise to neuropathic pain. Gabapentin is a drug originally developed as an anticonvulsant, but is effective in treating several forms of neuropathic pain, and may be useful in treating cancer-induced neuropathic pain[61].

Summarizing the contributors to bone cancer pain:

- Release of cytokines, PGs, and ETs from hematopoetic, immune, and tumor cells.
- Osteoclast activity ⇑s ⇒ lowered pH ⇒ activation of TRPV1-receptor.
- Bone erosion ⇒ release of growth factors e.g. NGF.
- Tumor growth ⇒ compression of afferent terminals.
- Neurochemical changes in DRG and spinal cord.

Central sensitization

If local neuropathic pain is a sequel to cancer, do the spinal cord and forebrain also undergo significant neurochemical changes? The murine cancer pain model revealed extensive neurochemical reorganization within the spinal cord segments receiving input from primary afferent neurons innervating cancerous bone[62]. Up-regulation of the prohyperalgesic peptide, dynorphin, and astrocyte hypertrophy, contribute to the state of central sensitization maintained by cancer pain.

THE MOVING TARGET OF CANCER PAIN

As cancer progresses, changing factors may complicate the pain state. In the mouse model of bone cancer, as the tumor cells begin to proliferate, pain-related behaviors precede any noticeable bone destruction. This is attributed to prohyperalgesic factors, such as active nociceptor response in the marrow to PGs and ET released from growing tumor cells. At this point, pain might be managed by a coxib-class NSAID or ET antagonist. With continued tumor growth, sensory neurons innervating the marrow are compressed and destroyed, giving rise to neuropathic pain, possibly responsive to gabapentin. Once the tumor becomes invaded by osteoclastic activity, pain might be largely blocked by antiosteoclastogenic drugs, such as biphosphonates or osteoprotegerin. As the intramedullary space becomes filled with dying tumor cells, generating an acidic environment, TRPV1 or ASIC antagonists may attenuate the pain. In the later stages of bone destruction, antagonists to the mechanically gated channels and/or adenosine triphosphate (ATP) receptors in the highly innervated periosteum may alleviate movement-evoked pain. This scenario illustrates how a mechanistic approach to designing more effective therapies for cancer pain should be created based on the understanding of how different stages of the disease impact tumor cell influence on nociceptors, and how phenotype of nociceptors and CNS neurons involved in nociceptive transmission change during the course of advancing cancer.

Clinical implication: because cancer is not a static condition, but rather a neurobiologic changing state, effective management of associated pain must be continually assessed and possibly changed.

Clearly, the mechanisms associated with cancer pain are complex. However, only through the understanding of these mechanisms can we best manage our patient's pain with evidence-based confidence. The murine bone cancer model has given us insights as to the progressing, dynamic neurobiologic changes associated with cancer. These insights further lead us to the conclusion that effective treatment must be multimodal and dynamic.

Visceral cancer pain

Many cancers involve internal organs and symptoms are silent until ischemia, compression, or obstruction reach a given stage, at which time visceral pain is manifest. Pain of visceral cancer origin can be divided into four groups: (1) acute mechanical stretch of visceral structures; (2) ischemia of visceral structures; 3) chemical stimuli from an infiltrating tumor or the body's reaction to infiltration; and (4) a compressive form of neuropathic pain that occurs due to direct invasion of nervous structures involving the viscera. Visceral pain can also result from treatment damage of viscera and associated nerves from surgery, chemotherapy, or radiation.

CHEMOTHERAPY

Chemotherapy is a common treatment modality for cancer patients. Human cancer patients can complain of a wide range of cancer-related side-effects, such as pain, fatigue, depression, nausea, vomiting, diarrhea, constipation, cardiac arrhythmias, vascular and pulmonary toxicity, skin changes, mucositis, and sensory-motor disturbances[63]. Chemotherapy-induced peripheral neuropathy (CIPN) symptoms can present as pure sensory or motor disturbances, or as mixed sensory–motor neuropathy[64]. Cranial nerve neuropathy has been reported in humans treated with cisplatin or carboplatin[65]. Muscle pain is a symptom reported in human patients with CIPN, and is occasionally reported as muscle spasms. It is unclear if the cramps are a direct toxic effect of the antitumor agent on the muscle fiber or manifestations of a sensory neuropathy. To date there is no specific drug or method for prevention of CIPN.

Chemotherapeutic neuropathies

Several antitumor agents can lead to neuropathies[64]. Paclitaxel (Taxol™) has cytotoxic activity through its ability to interfere with microtubule function by inducing the polymerization of tubulin[66], and induces peripheral neuropathy in a dose-dependent manner[67]. Platine-compound cytotoxic agents (e.g. cisplatin and carboplatin) also cause peripheral neuropathy in a dose-dependent manner in humans[68], and cisplatin is deemed more neurotoxic than carboplatin[69]. Prevalence of platine-compound neuropathy is approximately 50% in human studies[70]. Vincristine is a microtubule-interfering agent that is administered to patients with hematologic malignancies. The incidence of vincristine-induced peripheral neuropathy is between 50% and 100% in humans[71]. Ifosfamide is a cyclophosphamide-related drug with toxic effects on the CNS, and in humans these are manifest by hallucinations, confusion, and cranial nerve dysfunction[72].

These are but a few of the cytotoxic drugs used to treat animals with cancer whose neuropathic toxic potential has been described in humans. Clinical manifestations of these drugs in veterinary patients may be more subtle or less severe since many animals undergo therapy for a shorter period of time than humans. Nevertheless, these neuropathic consequences from cytotoxic agents should be understood by the caregiver, and it should be appreciated that administration of two or more cytotoxic agents, which is a common practice, can aggravate or accelerate the induction of neuropathic manifestations.

RADIATION THERAPY

Radiation kills cells by causing irreversible deoxyribonucleic acid (DNA) damage[73], and there is a direct relationship between the amount of physical energy deposited, the degree of DNA damage, the number of cells killed, and the extent of tissue injury. Cell death by radiation is either by apoptosis or necrosis. With apoptosis, cells break down into apoptotic bodies and become resorbed by neighboring cells[74]. With necrosis, cells break down into fragments, release lysosomal enzymes, and generate inflammatory responses that can lead to fibrosis, atrophy, and ulceration at the local tissue level. Adverse response to radiation can be divided into early and late effects. Early effects are most often seen in cell populations that have high turnover rates, for example, gastrointestinal (GI), oropharyngeal, and esophageal mucosa, bone marrow, and skin. Late radiation effects more often involve tissues that are nonproliferating or slowly proliferating, such as oligodendroglia, Schwann cells, kidney tubules, and vascular endothelium. Radiation-induced peripheral neuropathies result from late effects of radiation treatment. The actual axons of peripheral nerves are less likely affected, but supporting cells, such as Schwann cells, are vulnerable to ionizing radiation. Radiation can also affect tissues surrounding peripheral nerves, leading to development of fibrosis around nerve trunks. This fibrosis with subsequent compression of nerve bundles is suspected to be the primary etiology of peripheral radiation neuropathies[75].

Carsten *et al.*[76] have demonstrated that skin acute radiation score (ARS) in dogs with cancer of the forelimb undergoing curative intent radiation therapy was a highly statistically significant predictor of pain as reflected in VAS and the Glasgow CMPS (short form). Skin ARSs increased prior to the increase in pain scores, but not simultaneously. The investigators concluded that it is optimal to combine daily ARSs with use of a pain scale to achieve optimal pain management in the radiation therapy patient.

Although cancer pain is associated with both tissue injury/inflammation and nerve injury, it is unlikely that the pain is just the sum of these two mechanisms, but rather, is a unique neurochemical pain state (*Table 83*). Analgesics commonly used in cancer pain are presented in Appendix 1 *Tables 5* and *6*.

TABLE 83: Effects of therapy and disease on tissue and nerve injury

Iatrogenic:	**Tissue injury**	**Nerve injury**
Chemotherapy		X
Radiation		X
Surgery	X	X
Disease:		
Tumor compression		X
Release of active factors	X	
Immune response	X	X

NUTRITIONAL MANAGEMENT

Many types of cancer are influenced by nutrition, diet, and nutritional status of the patient. In humans, cachexia is seen in 32–87% of cases, commonly associated with cancers of the upper GI tract[77]. Weight loss can be detrimental to the patient's QOL and prognosis, as well as dramatically impacts on the pharmacokinetics and pharmacodynamics of chemotherapeutics and contributes to increased treatment-related toxicity[78]. Malnutrition is arguably one of the most common causes of death in people with cancer. Association between documented metabolic abnormalities, actual weight loss, and poor prognosis in cats or dogs with cancer has not been convincingly demonstrated. One study from a referral oncology practice showed that only 4% of the dogs were cachectic and 15% of the dogs had detectable and clinically significant muscle wasting[79]. Nevertheless, nutritional assessment of the cancer patient should be part of every treatment plan, focusing on history, physical examination, and routine hematologic and biochemical parameters. For the under-nourished dog or cat, a liquid nutritional supplement (Recuperation™; Viyo Veterinary) has been found helpful to encourage water and food consumption[80].

The following five steps have been proposed to define the nutritional requirements for dogs or cats with cancer[81]:

- Estimate fluid requirements.
- Estimate energy requirements.
- Distribute calories (between protein, fat, and carbohydrates).
- Evaluate remaining nutrients (vitamins, minerals, essential nutrients, and so on).
- Select a method of feeding (voluntary intake being preferred).

End-of-life considerations

Reflecting on Dr. Vertosick's insight that we are all born in another's pain and destined to die in our own[2], part of our moral obligation as veterinarians is to relieve pain and suffering in terminally-ill cancer patients. Due to the strong human–animal bond built over the pet's lifetime, this obligation often involves assistance for both the pet and its owner. At this point a 'pawspice' – end-of-life care program, is a professional obligation. We can, with solidarity, offer pet owners supportive, palliative options for complete care and attention to their pet's special needs when death is imminent. Finally, veterinary medicine is entrusted with the responsibility and option of euthanasia to help animals die in a humane and pain-free manner.

Pet owners don't really care how much you know, they want to know how much you care.

An algorithm for treating cancer pain in dogs and cats is presented in **Fig. 188**. Clearly, the WHO three-step analgesic ladder should not be discontinued, but it may require refinement in light of clinical experience that has accumulated in the 20 years since the ladder was proposed. First and most importantly, just as was true for the original WHO recommendation, this algorithm requires the worldwide availability of various forms of 'strong' opioids.

An alternative algorithm[82] proposes the following three stages of treatment for cancer pain: (1) For mild pain, nonopioid analgesic treatment should be initiated. If pain is not adequately controlled, then low doses of 'strong' opioids should be added and titrated according to the individual patient's needs; (2) for moderate pain, low doses of 'strong' opioids should be initiated and titrated, with or without nonopioids; (3) the treatment of severe pain obviously requires the immediate use of 'strong' opioids, with or without nonopioids. Adjuvant drugs should be used for all stages when indicated. As a rule, 'weak' opioids should be dropped in the treatment of cancer, other than in countries where 'strong' opioids are not readily available or clinicians are not well trained in their use.

188

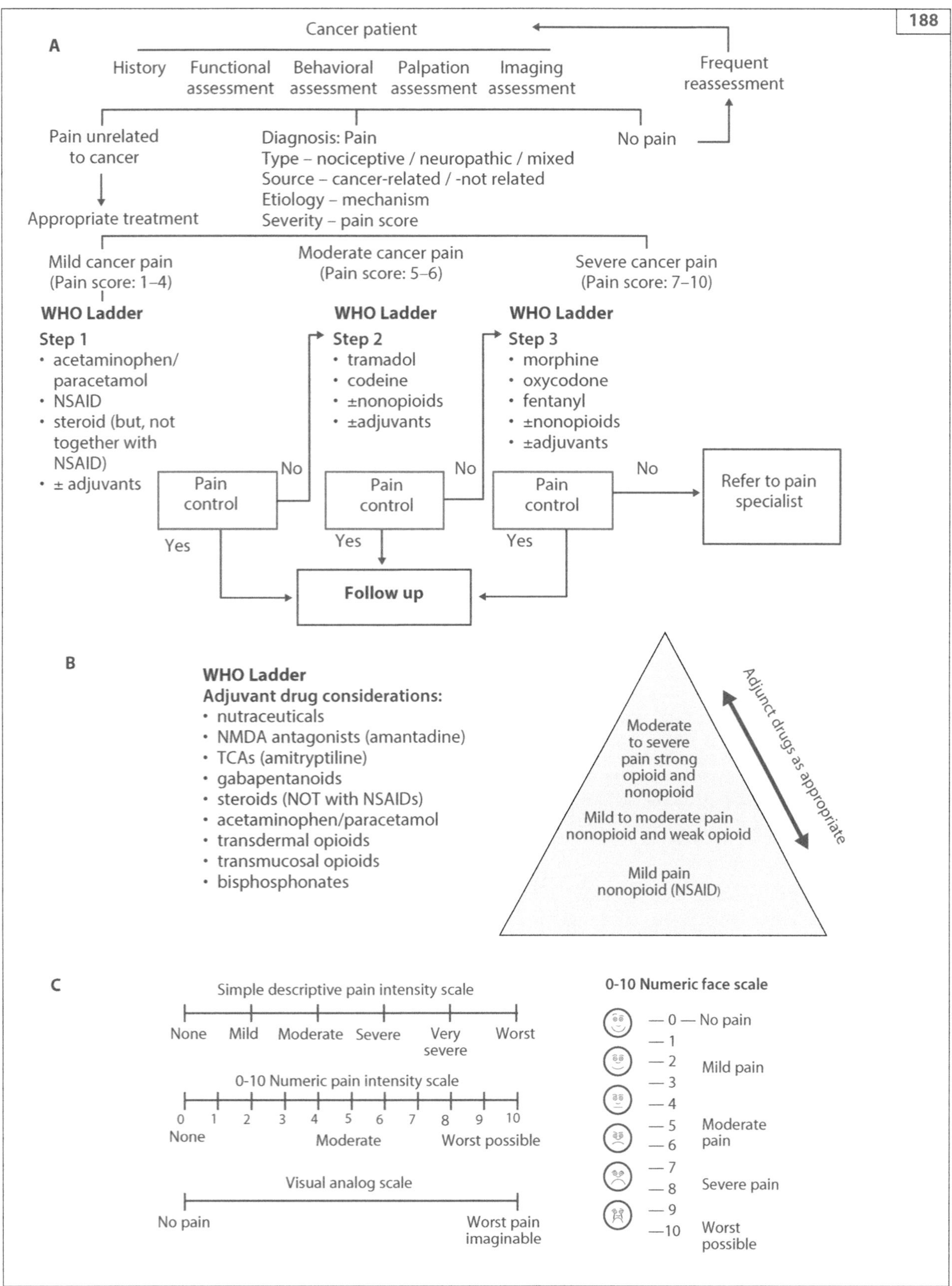

Fig. 188A: Algorithm for treating cancer pain in dogs and cats[82]; **B**: World Health Organization (WHO) ladder. **C**: pain scales; NMDA: N-methyl-D-aspartate; NSAID: nonsteroidal anti-inflammatory drug; TCA: tricyclic antidepressant.

Chapter 12

Pain Management Features Unique to the Cat

INTRODUCTION

In many countries, pet cats outnumber pet dogs. This includes the USA, the UK, and emerging growth countries in AustralAsia, such as China[1]. With the growth in cat numbers has come the demand from cat owners for 'best medicine'. In 1970 the American Association of Feline Practitioners (AAFP) was initiated with the goal of improving the health and welfare of cats by supporting high standards of practice, continuing education, and scientific investigation.

Only in recent years has the cat become a focus of investigations in clinical studies. Within the past 10 years there has been published an ever-increasing number of peer-reviewed papers in a variety of subjects related to the cat. It might be interesting to note that despite the 'late bloom' of interest in clinical anomalies of the cat, the cat has been a preferred laboratory animal (together with mice and rats) model for many disease processes, such as osteoarthritis (OA) pain. Accordingly, there are many published investigations outside the 'veterinary literature'.

A major driver for the growth of interest in feline pain management is economics. The increased number of cats has caught the economic interest of pet supply providers, veterinary clinicians, the pet food industry, and pharmaceutical manufacturers. For many years pharmaceutical manufacturers were constrained by the mentality that drugs were sold on a dose per kilogram of weight basis, suggesting that since the cat is a small mammal product sales are constrained. With the growth of cats in the pet population and acceptance of a 'premium price' positioning, the pharmaceutical industry is now, through extensive marketing efforts, making pain management in the cat a front-of-mind issue.

Cats require a species-specific approach as is expressed in the familiar aphorism 'cats are not small dogs'! Because most small animal veterinary practices focus principally on the cat and dog, it is important to understand species differences. Further, it is equally important to focus disease treatment upon a mechanism-based approach (See Chapter 4 Functional Physiology of Pain; Classifying pain: mechanism-based.)

Specific anatomic differences between the dog and cat have been described by Scott and McLaughlin as they influence orthopedic conditions and repairs[2]. Cats' expression of both adaptive and maladaptive pain is equally different.

It is much more difficult to identify a painful response in the cat, especially if the parameters of assessment are based on the dog. Interpreting a cat's pain response as equivalent to the dog's is likely a major reason cats are under-treated for pain[3].

Difficulty of recognizing pain in cats

A 'first rule' for recognizing pain would be an anthropomorphic recognition of anticipated pain associated with the injury or procedure. Signs suggestive of pain in cats include a hunched posture with the head held low, squinted eyes, sitting quietly and seeking no attention, trying to hide, or resentment of being handled (**Fig. 189**)[4,5]. Cats tend to withdraw and remain quiet through a wide range of painful experiences. Consequently, the painful cat that is immobile and withdrawn is often overlooked and goes untreated for its painful state (**Fig. 190**).

Behavior is the best means of assessing the presence and degree of adaptive pain[6].

Clinical implication: cats in acute traumatic or postoperative pain are usually depressed, immobile, and silent.

Brondani et al.[7] have provided initial evidence of construct validity and reliability of a multidimensional composite tool for use in assessing acute postoperative pain in cats undergoing ovariohysterectomy. Construction of the scale includes selection of behavioral and physiologic items supported by the relevant literature. Factor analysis revealed that four factors contributed to 78.8% of the total variance: psychomotor change, protection of wound area, physiologic variables, and vocal expression of pain. (See also Chapter 3, *Table 8*.)

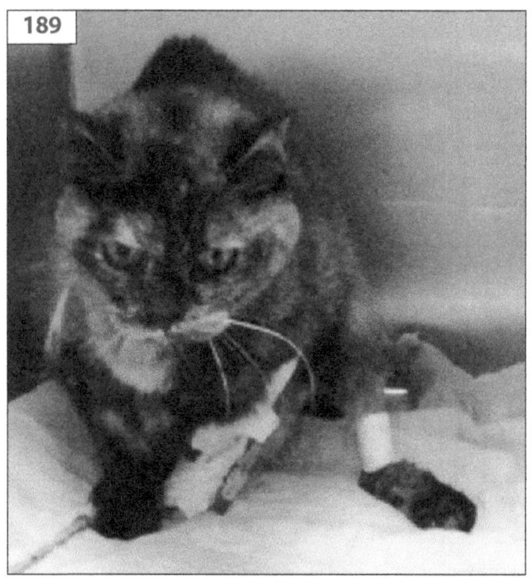

Fig. 189 Cat following surgery in a 'typical' posture of pain: hunched, head low, and sitting quietly. (After Reference 4.)

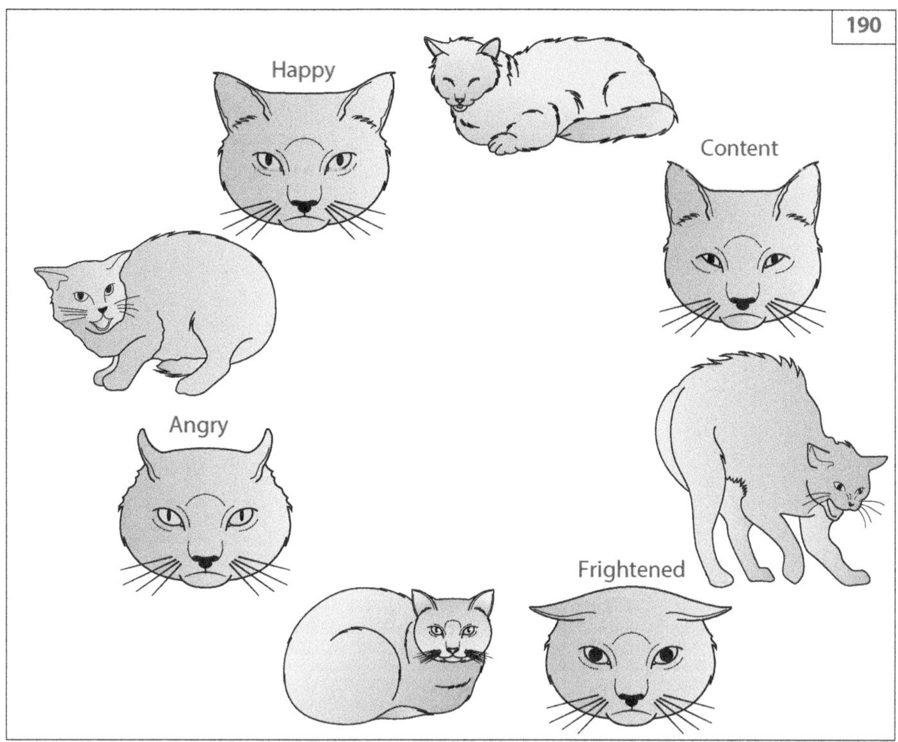

Fig. 190 Illustrations of facial expressions and body positions expressed by the cat.

It is proposed that four behavioral domains – mobility, activity, grooming and temperament – are particularly useful to both clinicians and owners in assessing chronic musculoskeletal pain and monitoring the response to therapy[8]. The owner is the best person to judge and track the cat's behavior and demeanor, which is the foundation of the client-specific outcome measures used in a recent study[9]. (See Chapter 3, **Fig. 14** Client specific outcome measures.)

Challenges of treating pain in cats

Only at glacial speed are we making progress in the area of feline-specific information, adverse side-effects, and research and development (R&D) in the feline species. Many constraints are presently compounded by recent economic pressures. (See also Chapter 1, *Table 3*.)

Summary of constraints in treating feline pain

- Difficulty in recognizing pain in cats.
- Unique feline metabolism of drugs.
- Paucity of drugs labeled for cats.
- Challenges of feline drug administration.
- Lack of feline-specific information.
- Adverse side-effects unique to the cat.
- Limited R&D resources.

PHARMACOLOGIC MANAGEMENT IN CATS

Opioids (*Table 84*)

- Many opioids with clear analgesic properties are not minimum alveolar concentration (MAC)-sparing.
- 'Morphine mania' in cats is a misconception:
  - Dose-dependent.
- Opioid-related hyperthermia (>40°C [104°F]) in cats (hydromorphone: 75% of cats) (0.05–0.1 mg/kg) and morphine (>1.0 mg/kg).
- Opioids cause marked mydriasis in cats:
  - Avoid bright light, and approach deliberately.
- Vomiting and salivation are common after morphine and hydromorphone, but uncommon after butorphanol, buprenorphine, fentanly, meperidine, or methadone.
- Cats on opioids should be well hydrated to avoid potential constipation.
- Individuals are unique with regard to the number, morphology, and distribution of genetically determined opioid receptors.
- Genetic variability is multifactorial, involving genes that code for metabolizing enzymes, the µ-opioid receptors, and blood–brain barrier transporters[10] : e.g. individual variability to butorphanol antinociception duration ranged from 0 to ≥360 minutes)[11].
- Effects may be dose-related:
  - Hydromorphone <0.1mg/kg had minimal effect[12].
  - Perhaps a minimal number of opioid receptors must be occupied before a response is measurable.

Routes of administration

- Route of hydromorphone affects onset time, intensity of effect, and duration of effect; SC is least effective[13].
- Fentanyl and buprenorphine are available as a transdermal patch (as is lidocaine).
- Transbuccal (oral transmucosal (OTM)) bioavailability of buprenorphine is nearly 100%.
- Morphine (16 h @100 µg/kg), buprenorphine (10 h @ 12.5 µg/kg), fentanyl, meperidine (pethidine), and methadone have been administered via epidural route in cats:
  - Morphine appears to be the most clinically useful epidural opioid.

Morphine in cats

- 0.1–0.2 mg/kg is effective in clinical cases and does not cause excitement.
- Slow onset of action (45–60 minutes).
- Less effective in cats than dogs[6,14]

Oxymorphone in cats

- Does not seem to be associated with hyperthermia, vomiting, and nausea, or adverse behavioral effects.
- Common feline dose: 0.05–0.2mg/kg IM, IV, or SC.
- 2–4 h duration of effect.
- Less effective than buprenorphine for postoperative analgesia[15].
- Costly, and sometimes difficult to procure.
- Low dose of oxymorphone (<0.2 mg/kg) and butorphanol (<0.2 mg/kg) in combination produces greater levels of antinociception than when used individually[16].

Hydromorphone in cats

- Has replaced oxymorphone (less costly) (**Fig. 191**).
- Common dose: same as oxymorphone (0.05–0.2 mg/kg IM, IV, SC.
- IV administration (0.1 mg/kg) produces the greatest intensity and duration of analgesia with least incidence of vomiting and salivation *vs*. SC or IM.
- Use is limited (by some) due to incidence of hyperthermia[17,18].

TABLE 84: Perioperative opioids for use in cats[33]

Opioid	Dose/Route	Indications	Duration*
Morphine	0.05–0.1 mg/kg IM, SC	Moderate to severe pain	3–4 h
Morphine continuous rate infusion	0.1 mg/kg loading dose IV, then 0.05–0.1 mg/kg/h IV	Moderate to severe pain	Infusion
Oxymorphone	0.05–0.1 mg/kg IV, IM, SC	Moderate to severe pain	2–4 h
Hydromorphone	0.05–0.1 mg/kg IV, IM, SC	Moderate to severe pain	2–4 h
Fentanyl	0.001–0.005 mg/kg IV, IM, SC	Mild to severe pain, inadequate duration of action from a single bolus injection	20–30 min
Fentanyl continuous rate infusion	0.002–0.003 mg/kg loading dose IV, then 0.001–0.005 mg/kg/h IV	Moderate to severe pain	Infusion
Fentanyl patch	0.005 mg/kg/h transdermal	Mild to severe pain	3–5 days
Butorphanol	0.2–0.4 mg/kg IV, IM, SC	Mild to moderate pain	1–3 h
Buprenorphine	0.005–0.015 mg/kg IV, IM, SC	Mild to moderate pain	3–8 h

*Duration of action varies with the dose and route of administration. In general, IV administration results in a more rapid onset and shorter duration of action than listed above. Use lower end of dose range for initial IV administration.
IM = intramuscular; SC = subcutaneous; IV = intravenous.

Butorphanol in cats

- μ-antagonist, producing analgesia through κ-agonist activity.
- Generally dosed at 0.2 mg/kg (0.1–0.4 mg/kg).
- 'Ceiling' effect, with analgesic properties questioned in both dogs and cats.
- Short-acting (<90 min) (~40 min in dogs).
- Better visceral than somatic effect.
- Poor analgesic choice for most situations.

The analgesic properties of butorphanol have been questioned in both cats and dogs. In one study of the IV administration of butorphanol to cats, no difference in either the intensity or duration of thermal antinociception for butorphanol at doses of 0.1, 0.2, 0.4, and 0.8 mg/kg was reported[19]. To date there have been no clinical dose titration studies of butorphanol performed in cats, and debate continues regarding optimal dose[20].

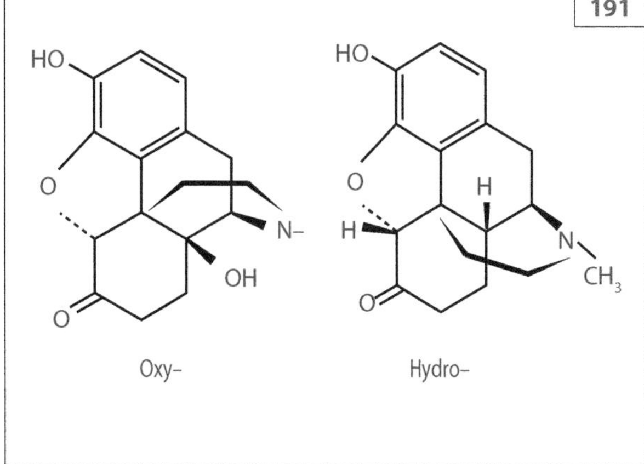

Fig. 191 Structure of oxymorphone and hydromorphone.

Buprenorphine in cats

- Most popular opioid in UK for small animal practice[3].
- Common feline dose: 0.005–0.02 mg/kg IV, IM, SC or OTM (6–8 h duration)[21].
- OTM administration has become very popular[22].
- IM dose of 0.01 mg/kg gives slow onset (2 h) with variable duration (4–12 h).
- IV or OTM gave similar response (dosed at 0.02 mg/kg): onset within 30 min, peak effect at 90 min, and duration of 6 h.
- Compared to other opioids:
  - Better analgesia than morphine for soft tissue and orthopedic procedures[23].
  - Better than oxymorphone for sterilization procedures[15].
  - Longer pain relief than meperidine for ovariohysterectomy.
- Transdermal (matrix) buprenorphine patch is available for human use (Transtec: Napp Pharmaceuticals, Cambridge UK):
  - Variable plasma concentrations with no effective analgesia noted @ 35 µg/h patch in cats[24].
  - Loading dose may be required, as with buprenorphine constant rate infusion (CRI), to achieve a steady-state plasma concentration.

Fentanyl in cats

- Fentanyl is a short-acting pure µ-agonist.
- Common dose: 0.001–0.005 mg/kg IM, IV, or SC.
- 10 µg/kg IV provided rapid onset (<5 min) lasting 110 min with no excitement, salivation, or vomiting[25].
- Transdermal fentanyl (TDF) patches have been used for acute perioperative pain in cats:
  - Plasma concentrations are variable.
  - Factors affecting concentrations include size of patch, skin permeability, and body temperature.
  - Steady-state plasma concentration achieved within 6–12 h, persisting for 18–20 h after patch removal[26,27].
  - Other opioids (except butorphanol, which may antagonize fentanyl) should be administered during the uptake phase.
- CRI is preferable to transdermal fentanyl:
  - 2–4 µg/kg/h, increased to 10 µg/kg/h as needed, is effective in the conscious cat.
- Transdermal fentanyl (Recuvyra™) should not be used in cats.

Methadone in cats

- Methadone is a synthetic opioid agonist, with mild N-methyl-D-aspartate (NMDA) activity and seretonin/norepinephrine reuptake inhibition.
- Common dose: 0.1–0.5 mg/kg SC/IM/IV.
- Pharmacokinetic profile in dogs is quite different from people (profile not available in cats)[28]:
  - Low oral bioavailability.
  - Rapid clearance.
  - Short elimination half-life.
- Levo-methadone (0.3 mg/kg, Q8 h, 5 days) was less effective than carprofen or buprenorphine in cats after major orthopedic surgery, and was associated with excitement in some cats[29].
- Antinociceptive effects after OTM administration were longer than by IV administration (≥4 h *vs.* ≥2 h) despite 2× higher IV dose[30].

Tramadol in cats

- Much of the information about tramadol is taken from its use in humans.
- One of the biggest drawbacks with oral tramadol is its bitter taste, which is difficult to mask for presentation to the cat.
- Cats metabolize tramadol slower than the dog, with a half-life of approximately 2.5 h.

- In a thermal threshold model for assessing tramadol's nociceptive effect in cats, a dose of 4 mg/kg Q6 h was proposed to be optimal[31].
- The magnitude of effect was related to dose, with lower doses yielding less intense analgesia.
- Perioperative administration of tramadol does not interfere with platelet aggregation, bleeding time, or biochemical variables in cats[32].

Alpha-2 agonists in cats

- Including xylazine, medetomidine, and dexmedetomidine, provide sedation, muscle relaxation, and analgesia in cats; they are sedative-analgesics, NOT anesthetics.
- Xylazine should be discouraged due to the risk factor for perioperative mortality in cats, in contrast to medetomidine[34].
- Medetomidine is not licensed for use in cats within the USA, while dextomidine is licensed in the USA for cat use.
- Dexmedetomidine (40 µg/kg) OTM yielded longer lasting analgesia than when given IM[35].
- Dexmedetomidine minimal effective dose to increase nociceptive thresholds is 40 µg/kg; but this is comparatively less effective than buprenorphine[36].

NMDA antagonists in cats

- Anesthetic protocols incorporating ketamine provide better postoperative analgesia in cats after ovariohysterectomy[37].
- Popular ketamine CRI dose: 0.5 mg/kg IV; 0.1–0.5 mg/kg/h.
- Anecdotal suggestion of amantadine at approximately 3–5 mg/kg PO daily for feline chronic pain[38].
- Toxic dose of amantadine is 30 mg/kg in cats[39].
- Often used together with NSAIDs or gabapentin.

Other analgesics in cats

- Amitriptyline (2.5–12.5 mg/kg PO *sid*) has been used to treat feline interstitial cystitis, with few side-effects[40].
- Gabapentin is thought to be an effective treatment for neuropathic pain.
- Suggested starting dose in the cat: 10 mg/kg *bid*[41].
- Sedation seen at higher doses.

DEGENERATIVE JOINT DISEASE IN THE CAT

Retrospective studies indicate that degenerative joint disease (DJD) is common in cats. The term DJD is more appropriate for the cat than is the term OA, in that less is known about the disease in cats than in dogs, and some of the criteria for classification of OA in dogs are not consistently found in the cat.

There are only a few experimental animal models of OA that have been followed over some years. Two such models are the anterior cruciate ligament (ACL) transected dog and cat[42,43]. Cats with transected ACLs have been followed for as long as 12 years.

It is held that the cat knee does not suffer from naturally-occurring OA; therefore, degenerative changes in joint structure, control, and movement can be associated directly with targeted interventions, even when animals are followed over years where age effects might play a role in other experimental models, such as the dog.

One reason the cat 'OA model' is popular is because the cat hind limb is arguably the best known mammalian system in terms of muscular anatomy, *in vivo* force production, and neurophysiologic movement control. Within approximately 4 months of ACL transection in the cat, joint stability in the anterior and internal rotation direction are fully re-established[44].

Tibial thrust at the instant of foot contact during locomotion, which is typically observed in ACL deficient humans, dogs, and sheep, is not seen in the cat[45,46]. The actual detailed adaptations responsible for the quick re-establishment of knee stability following ACL transection in the cat are not known. However, the cat knee continues to degenerate despite the quick recovery of anterior translation and medial rotation (**Fig. 192**).

Radiographic evidence of feline DJD suggests a prevalence ranging from 16.5% to 93%[47–51], and several studies propose that DJD can be associated with pain[9,52–54]. In addition to the above radiographic-based observations, Lascelles *et al.* conducted a cross-sectional study to evaluate the prevalence of feline appendicular and axial skeletal DJD within a randomly selecting subset of 100 cats from a single practice database of 1640. Among this group, 91% had at least one appendicular joint with radiographic DJD. From the same working group, Freire[55] reported that many joints of middle-aged cats that have significant cartilage damage have no radiographic signs of DJD. These data confirm that feline DJD may be associated with less tendency to form new bone than is canine OA, and that a nonbiased approach should be made to the diagnosis of feline musculoskeletal disease. Perhaps because there are no validated outcome measures to assess DJD-associated pain in cats, to date there are no approved treatments approved in the USA for treating this painful condition. (Meloxicam is approved in several countries outside the USA.)

There are no pathognomonic signs of DJD in cats; however, the following should prompt suspicion:

- Not able, or unwilling to jump.
- Decreased height of jump.
- Inappropriate elimination (i.e. missing the litter box).
- Increased time sleeping, reduced activity.
- Altered temperament or resentment of handling.
- Reduced grooming or appetite.
- Reduced play or stretching.
- ADR (ain't doin right).

Bilateral DJD is common in the cat, but difficult to diagnose. Whereas lameness in canine OA is common, lameness is not usually the principal sign of feline DJD (4–43% frequency). Thickening of the joints, reduced range of joint movement, and crepitus is often minimal in the cat, unless the disease is advanced.

Physical diagnosis of DJD in cats is difficult, even for experienced clinicians because:

- Cats can tolerate severe orthopedic disease due to their small size and agility.
- Cats generally resent physical handling or manipulation during physical exams.
- Cats are notorious for cowering on examination and remaining immobile.

Although various parameters have been proposed for identifying pain in various species, the real litmus test is the response of an animal to an analgesic. 'Veterinarians will rule out OA as a diagnosis by actually having the owners treat the cat for DJD and seeing if the owners note any improvement in their cat's quality of life'[56].

Nonsteroidal anti-inflammatory drugs (NSAIDs) are the cornerstone for treating canine OA. As a class, NSAIDs are less safe than opioids or α_2-agonists, and are not reversible. Further, because cats are poor at gluceronidation, drug accumulation is a potential problem with NSAIDs.

Overview of NSAIDs in cats (See Chapter 6):

- Cats seem to be particularly susceptible to the adverse renal effects of NSAIDs.
- Carprofen, meloxicam, and ketoprofen are widely used in cats:
  - Mean half-life of carprofen in cats is ~20 h (9–49 h range); about 2× that in dogs.
  - Meloxicam appears to be metabolized by oxidative enzymes, with potentially less variable results and fewer side-effects.
  - SC meloxicam is approved in the USA @ 0.3 mg/kg (1-time dose).
  - European Union (EU) has approved meloxicam for long-term use @ 0.05 mg/kg/d.
  - Ketoprofen is a potent cyclo-oxygenase (COX)-1 inhibitor: avoid preoperative use.
- Robenacoxib is labeled for postoperative pain in the cat: tablet in the USA; tablet and injectable in the EU.
- Proposed metabolism is by oxidative enzymes.

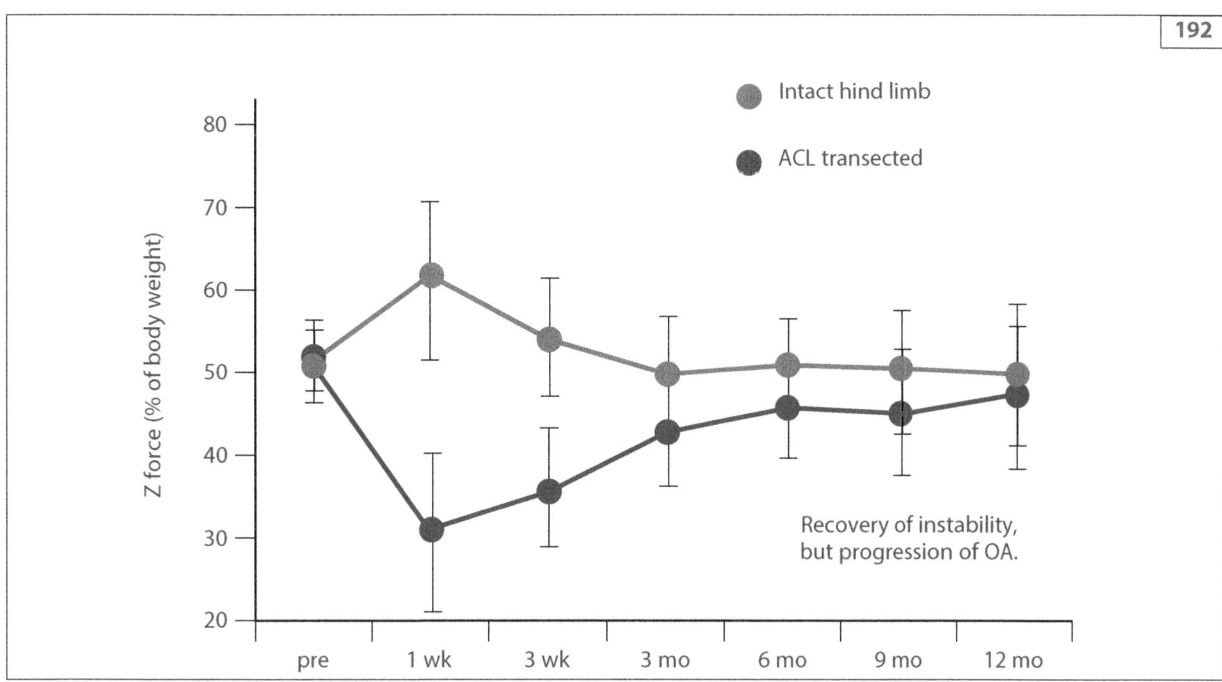

Fig. 192 Peak vertical ground reaction forces after feline anterior cruciate ligament (ACL) transection. Somewhere between 3 and 6 months postoperatively, cats 'regain' stifle stability, although the disease process progresses. (After Reference 44.) OA: osteoarthritis.

The International Society of Feline Medicine (ISFM) and the American Association of Feline Practitioners (AAFP) has published a set of guidelines for the long-term use of NSAIDs (*Table 85*): http://www.isfm.net/toolbox/info_sheets/NSAIDs_guidelines.pdf.

ISFM/AAFP recommendations summary:

- Using drugs with a greater COX-2 selectivity in cats will help avoid some of the potential adverse effects associated with COX-1 suppression.
- It is presumed that dual inhibition of COX and lipoxygenase may be associated with reduced gastrointestinal adverse effects over COX inhibition alone.
- Owners should be encouraged to titrate NSAID administration to the minimal effective dose (MED), understanding that this may change over time.
- In overweight cats, dose should be calculated according to lean or ideal body weight.
- In seeking the MED, it would be prudent to reduce the label dose but maintain the label frequency where possible.
- Intermittent therapy is better than no therapy at all, but may result in periods of suboptimal therapy (author's note: and may compromise compliance).
- Intermittent drug withdrawal or reduction may help owners assess drug efficacy.
- With few exceptions, 'pulse therapy' has little rationale.
- Liquid formulations provide the most accurate dosing and dose adjustment of NSAIDs in cats.
- Use of a dedicated and clearly marked syringe for NSAID administration of a liquid is encouraged over administration directly from a storage container.
- A washout period of 3–5 days between different NSAIDs is sensible; an exception being when switching from aspirin (acetyl salicyclic acid), where 7–10 days is suggested.
- The risk of acute renal failure during appropriate therapeutic NSAID use in cats is low. Risk factors for renal toxicity in humans are presumed to apply to cats.
- Monitoring serum renal analyses and urine parameters before and after commencement of NSAID therapy is highly recommended.
- NSAIDs should be administered with food, and therapy withheld if food is not eaten. Using wet rather than dry diet is a sensible precaution to optimize water intake.

TABLE 85: Nonsteroidal anti-inflammatory drugs (NSAIDs) licensed for systemic use in cats

NSAID	Cyclo-oxygenase (COX) selectivity*	Formulation	Dose	Route	Frequency	Licensing indications	Duration
Carprofen	COX-2 preferential	Injection, 50 mg/ml	4 mg/kg (~0.08 ml/kg)	SC, IV	Once	Postsurgical pain	Once only
Ketoprofen	None	Injection, 10 mg/ml	2 mg/kg (~0.2 ml/kg)	SC	q24h	Relief of acute pain and inflammation associated with musculoskeletal and other painful disorders	Up to 3 days
		Tablets, 5mg	1mg/kg (~1 tablet/5kg)	PO	q24h		Up to 5 days, ± can use injection instead on day 1
Meloxican	COX-2 preferential	Injection, 5mg/ml	0.3 mg/kg (~0.06 ml/kg)	SC	Once	Postoperative analgesia following overiohysterectomy and minor soft tissue surgery	Once only

(*continued*)

TABLE 85: Nonsteroidal anti-inflammatory drugs (NSAIDs) licensed for systemic use in cats (continued)

NSAID	COX selectivity*	Formulation	Dose	Route	Frequency	Licensing indications	Duration
		Injection, 2 mg/ml	0.2 mg/kg (~0.1 ml/kg)	SC	Once	Mild to moderate postsurgical pain	Can be followed by 0.05 mg/kg q24h PO for 4 days
		Oral suspension, 0.5 mg/ml	0.1 mg/kg (~0.2 ml/kg) day 1, then 0.06 mg/kg (~0.1 ml/kg)	PO	q24h	Inflammation and pain in chronic musculoskeletal conditions	Indefinite
Robenacoxib	COX-2 selective	Tablets, 6 mg	1 mg/kg (~1 tablet/ 6 kg)	PO	q24h	Pain and inflammation associated with musculoskeletal disorders (postoperative orthopedic surgery in USA)	Up to 6 days
		Injection 20 mg/ml	2 mg/kg (~1 ml/ 10 kg)	SC	Once	Pain and inflammation associated with soft tissue surgery	Once only
Tolfenamic acid	None?	Tablets, 6 mg	4 mg/kg (~1 tablet/ 1.5 kg)	PO	q24h	Treatment of febrile syndromes	3 days
		Injection, 40 mg/ml	4 mg/kg (~0.1 ml/kg)	SC	q24h	Adjuvant treatment of upper respiratory tract disease	2 days, or once, followed by tablets (above)
Acetylsalicylic acid†	*None*	*Tablets/caplets*	*1–25 mg/kg*	*PO*	*q72h*	*n/a*	*Indefinite*

†Aspirin is NOT licensed for use in oats, but is included here as it has commonly been recommended for use in cats as an antithrombotic agent to help prevent thromboembolism, particularly associated with cardiomyopathy. Wide ranging doses have been recommended (usually in the region of 5–75 mg/cat every 3 days) and its efficacy remains unproven

*COX-2 preferential – greater suppression of COX-2 than COX-1; COX-2 selective – virtually no COX-1 suppression at therapeutic doses

A variety of other (off-license) dose regimens have been advocated for a number of NSAIDs in cats, in addition to dose regimens for other analgesic agents

(NB not all drugs are licensed in all regions and veterinarians should refer to local information and regulations)

(ISFM and AAFP consensus guidelines. Long-term use of NSAIDs in cats. http://www.isfm.net/toolbox/info_sheets/NSAIDs_guidelines.pdf.)

- Specific risk factors, such as dehydration and hypovolemia, should always be addressed before therapy is administered. Take care to ensure good renal perfusion is maintained if anesthesia is required during therapy.
- At least some NSAIDs can be used safely in cats with stable chronic kidney disease, and this condition should not be reason for withholding analgesic therapy when it is indicated.
- Care is urged with the use of NSAIDs in patients with the combination of cardiac and renal disease.
- In the face of renal failure, potassium monitoring is recommended during therapy.
- Use of COX-1-sparing NSAIDs for long-term therapy in cats is preferable.
- NSAIDs should routinely be given with, or after, food in cats.

- Hypertensive cats receiving NSAID therapy should have their blood pressure monitored regularly.
- Routine biochemical monitoring, including liver enzymes, of cats receiving long-term NSAID therapy is recommended.
- Dose-reduction should be considered in cats with pre-existing liver disease, and in the face of severe liver dysfunction, NSAIDs should be used with extreme caution.
- Concurrent use of NSAIDs and glucocorticoids should be avoided whenever possible, and washout periods should be implemented between different NSAIDs and NSAID/corticosteroids.
- Caution the use of NSAIDs with other highly protein-bound drugs.
- The concomitant use of angiotensin-converting enzyme inhibitors and/or diuretics with NSAIDs will increase the risk of renal adverse effects.
- Abnormalities identified in the clinical examination and on laboratory testing do not necessarily preclude the use of NSAIDs, but the risks and benefits of NSAID therapy must be discussed with the owner.
- Involvement of owners in monitoring therapy is crucial. Owners need to be made aware of signs that should prompt cessation of therapy and/or the need for veterinary advice.
- A routine re-evaluation of all cats is recommended after the first 2–4 weeks of NSAID therapy.
- For 'low risk' patients, re-evaluations should take place every 2–6 months, depending on the perceived risks.

Other treatment modalities for feline DJD

There are very little data on the role of various drugs in alleviating chronic DJD-related pain in cats and most administration is anecdotal. Likely, this will not change for some time because of the development cost for new therapies, and the fact that most drugs used in cats are 'taken' from human medicine where the patent has expired. It is therefore of little financial return for a pharmaceutical company to pursue a feline label.

- Tricyclic antidepressants (TCAs), including amitriptyline, clomipramine, and imipramine, have been used to alter the actions of serotonin and norepinephrine both centrally and peripherally.
- Anecdotal reports suggest that amitriptyline (2.5–12.5 mg for an adult cat orally once a day) may be effective for feline DJD.
- Some individual case reports suggest that gabapentin shows promise in cats, and doses starting at 10 mg/kg given orally twice daily have been suggested.
- Cats tend to tolerate the tablet and capsule formulations better than the liquid oral form and they do not contain xylitol.
- Tramadol is basically a TCA/serotonin (5-HT) reuptake inhibitor with minimal opioid activity.
- To date there have been no studies of safety or efficacy of tramadol in cats (or dogs).
- A draw-back with tramadol is its unpleasant/bitter taste, making it difficult to administer to cats even within an otherwise palatable compounded carrier.
- Dosing of 1–4 mg/kg *bid* has been suggested.
- A diet high in eicosapentaenoic acid and docosahexaenoic acid, supplemented with green lipped mussel extract and glucosamine/chondroitin sulfate, improved objective measures of mobility in cats with DJD[57].
- Polysulfated glycosaminoglycan has been shown to reach the feline joint structures when administered SC at the labeled canine dose. (See Chapters 7 and 9.)
- Physical rehabilitation is equally effective for the cat as it is for the dog. (See Chapter 10.)

See Appendix 1, *Table 6* Analgesics commonly used for cancer pain in the cat, and *Table 86*.

The diagnosis and treatment of DJD in cats is quite possibly the most explosive growth opportunity in small animal practice.

TABLE 86: Example protocols for feline procedures

Procedure	Level of pain	Protocol A	Protocol B
Feline rear limb orthopedic procedure	Moderate to severe to excruciating	**Premedication** Acepromazine#, 0.05–0.2 mg/kg SC, IM + Morphine*, 0.25 mg/kg SC, IM ± Atropine, 0.01– 0.04 mg/kg SC, IM or Glycopyrrolate, 0.005–0.01 mg/kg SC, IM**	**Premedication** Medetomidine, 0.02 mg/kg IM (DexMed, 0.01 mg/kg IM) + Hydromorphone*, 0.05–0.1 mg/kg IM ± Atropine, 0.01–0.04 mg/kg SC, IM or Glycopyrrolate, 0.005–0.01 mg/kg SC, IM** + 25 µg/h fentanyl patch placed 8–12 h prior to surgery or at time of surgical preparation
		Intraoperative analgesia Consider epidural morphine, 0.1 mg/kg	**Intraoperative analgesia** Ketamine CRI (0.5 mg/kg IV followed by 10 µg/kg/min during surgery and 2 µg/kg/min for 24 h following surgery)
		Postoperative analgesia Buprenorphine, 0.01–0.02 mg/kg buccal every 8–12 h for 2–4 days beginning 4–6 h after initial dose of opioid ± NSAID for 5–7 days	**Postoperative analgesia** May need to repeat opioid dose 1–2 times to cover immediate postoperative pain or until fentanyl patch becomes effective ± NSAID for 5–7 days
Feline dentistry with extractions	Moderate to severe	**Premedication** Acepromazine#, 0.05–0.2 mg/kg SC, IM + Hydromorphone*, 0.05–0.1 mg/kg SC, IM ± Atropine, 0.01–0.04 mg/kg SC, IM or Glycopyrrolate, 0.005–0.01 mg/kg SC, IM**	**Premedication** Medetomidine, 0.02 mg/kg IM (DexMed, 0.01 mg/kg IM) + Buprenorphine*, 0.02 mg/kg IM + Ketamine, 2–4 mg/kg IM
		Intraoperative analgesia *Infraorbital, mandibular, or other regional nerve blocks:* Bupivacaine, 1.5 mg/kg maximum dose (± 1:200,000 epinephrine)	**Intraoperative analgesia** *Infraorbital, mandibular, or other regional nerve blocks:* Bupivacaine, 1.5 mg/kg maximum dose (±1:200,000 epinephrine)
		Postoperative analgesia ± NSAID for 5–7 days	**Postoperative analgesia** Repeat buprenorphine 6–8 h after initial dose Buprenorphine, 0.01–0.02 mg/kg buccal every 8–12 h for 2–4 days beginning 4–6 h after last IM dose ± NSAID for 5–7 days

(continued)

TABLE 86: Example protocols for feline procedures (continued)

Procedure	Level of pain	Protocol A	Protocol B
Feline onychectomy	Moderate Pain	**Premedication** Acepromazine#, 0.05–0.2 mg/kg SC, IM + Hydromorphone*, 0.05–0.1 mg/kg SC, IM ± Atropine, 0.01–0.04 mg/kg SC, IM or Glycopyrrolate, 0.005–0.01 mg/kg SC, IM**	**Premedication** Apply 25 μg/h fentanyl patch 6–12 h before surgery or at time of surgical preparation (may cover half of the absorptive surface of the patch in cats < 5 kg) Medetomidine, 0.02 mg/kg IM (DexMed, 0.01 mg/kg IM) + Morphine*, 0.2–0.5 mg/kg IM ± Atropine, 0.01–0.04 mg/kg SC, IM or Glycopyrrolate, 0.005–0.01 mg/kg SC, IM**
		Intraoperative analgesia *Declaw block:* Bupivicaine, 1.5 mg/kg maximum dose or lidocaine 2.0 mg/kg + bupivacaine 0.75 mg/kg (without epinephrine)	**Intraoperative analgesia** Declaw block: bupivacaine, 1.5 mg/kg maximum dose (without epinephrine)
		Postoperative analgesia *In hospital:* Hydromorphone*, 0.05 mg/kg IM or SC, 4–6 h after initial dose and repeat as needed	**Postoperative analgesia** May need to repeat opioid dose 1–2 times to cover immediate postoperative pain or until fentanyl patch becomes effective
		At home: Buprenorphine, 0.01–0.02 mg/kg buccal every 8–12 h for 2–4 days beginning 4–6 h after last hydromorphone dose ± NSAID for 5–7 days	Remove fentanyl patch in 3–5 days ± NSAID for 5–7 days
Feline OHE	Moderate pain	**Premedication** Acepromazine#, 0.05–0.2 mg/kg SC, IM + Hydromorphone*, 0.05–0.1 mg/kg SC, IM ± Atropine, 0.01–0.04 mg/kg SC, IM or Glycopyrrolate, 0.005–0.01 mg/kg SC, IM**	**Premedication** Medetomidine, 0.02 mg/kg IM (DexMed, 0.01 mg/kg IM) + Buprenorphine, 0.01–0.02 mg/kg IM + Ketamine, 2–4 mg/kg IM
		Intraoperative analgesia *Incisional block:* Bupivacaine (with 1:200,000 epinephrine), 1.5 mg/kg	
		Postoperative analgesia Repeat dose of opioid 4–6 h following the initial dose, or sooner if needed ± NSAID for 5–7 days	**Postoperative analgesia** Repeat buprenorphine 6–8 h after initial dose Buprenorphine, 0.01–0.02 mg/kg buccal every 8–12 h for 2–4 days beginning 4–6 h after last IM dose ± NSAID for 5–7 days

*Consult other references for dosages of other drugs from the same class.

**Anticholinergics (e.g. atropine and glycopyrrolate) have been listed as an option in a number of protocols. Use of anticholinergics should always be based on evaluation of the patient, the anesthetic protocol, and the experiences of the veterinarian. These agents should fit into the protocol on an individual patient basis and should not necessarily be a routine component of every premedicant protocol. Further, the lower end of the atropine dose may not always be effective in alleviating bradycardia.

#maximum dosage of acepromazine in cats is 1 mg total dose (3–4 mg total dose in dogs). Acepromazine dosages as low as 0.01 mg/kg may be effective in dogs, but higher dosages are generally required for adequate sedation in cats.

--Dexmedetomidine (DexMed) may be substituted for medetomidine (same volume: half the dose).

CRI: constant rate infusion; NSAID: nonsteroidal anti-inflammatory drug; OHE: ovariohysterectomy.

Chapter 13

Selected Bandages, Casts, and Splints

INTRODUCTION

Patient coaptation with bandages, casts, and splints is an everyday occurrence in veterinary practice. Often it is the animal health technician/ veterinary nurse who is entrusted with routine coaptation device checkups, and with giving pet owners advice on how to manage the apparatus. Bandages, casts, and splints are often administered to manage musculoskeletal pain; however, an improperly applied coaptation device can be very painful to a patient and potentially lead to catastrophic tissue damage. As such, it is important to be familiar with proper application and maintenance techniques.

Unstable injuries, particularly fractures and joint trauma, should be coapted following examination so as to reduce further soft tissue injury and to increase patient comfort. Coaptation bandaging is also frequently applied following orthopedic surgeries, particularly to extremities. Fracture or luxation support below the elbow and stifle are best managed with a padded bandage, while fractures above the elbow or stifle joints are more difficult to coapt. This is because a fundamental tenet is to immobilize *both* the joint above and the joint below the fractured bone(s) (**Fig. 193**).

Coapt means to approximate.

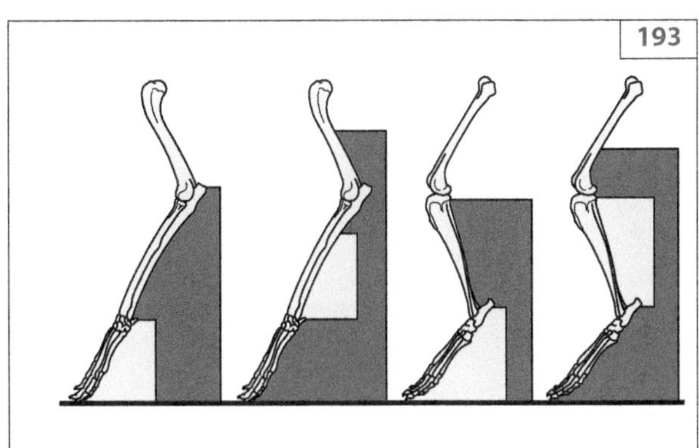

Fig. 193 Bandage/cast length relative to fracture site. The lightly shaded area represents the location of fracture, and the darker shaded area represents the appropriate length of bandage/cast. This applies the concept of immobilizing the joints both above and below the fracture site.

ROBERT JONES BANDAGE

Robert Jones bandages and their modifications are the external splints most often used in veterinary patients. It is effective for immobilization, but it is also effective in absorbing fluid, and decreasing or preventing edema which makes it very useful following arthrotomy surgeries and surgeries involving extensive soft tissue trauma. The bandage is best applied while the patient is still under anesthesia at the end of a surgery or with the patient under heavy sedation.

The classic Robert Jones bandage is a highly padded bandage, designed to be in place for 4–5 days. It consists of commercially available, 12-inch (300-mm), rolled cotton that is liberally applied to the limb to a thickness of 4–6 inches (100–150 mm). The 'modified' Robert Jones bandage uses less cotton, but still provides compression.

Materials needed:

- Adhesive tape.
- Cotton padding, (12-inch [300-mm] rolled cotton ('cotton wool') is simultaneously unrolled and split to provide 2 rolls of 6-inch [150-mm] width. This is easier than cutting the 12-inch roll in mid-section) (**Fig. 194, 195**).
- Gauze (4- to 6-inch [100–150-mm] width is optimal).
- Elastic tape or Vetrap.

Bandage application begins by placing porous tape 'stirrups' to the dorsal and ventral or medial and lateral surfaces of the paw (**Fig. 196**).

- Extend the stirrups 6–8 inches (150–200 mm) proximal to the digits, and the same distance distally. 'Dog ear' or place a tongue depressor between the distal extension of the stirrups for ease of separation later. Failure to integrate stirrups into a bandage is the most common reason for distal slippage of the bandage.
- With the stirrups being used to extend the limb, and the wound having been appropriately dressed, snugly wrap the rolled cotton from distal to proximal, as far as possible into the axilla or groin, overlapping about 1/3 the cotton width. Nail beds of digits 3 and 4 should be left visible at the distal limit of cotton wrapping (**Fig. 197**). A second layer of cotton wrapping may be applied over the first layer to obtain the depth of bandage thickness desired. Wrap the cotton as tight as possible without tearing the cotton (**Fig. 198**).
- The cotton is then over-wrapped with the gauze, leaving a small amount of cotton uncovered by the gauze at both the proximal and distal limits of the cotton. Wide gauze (6-inch [150-mm] width) allows for a more firm compression of the cotton than with narrower gauze. Wrap the gauze as tight as possible, overlapping about 50% (**Fig. 199**). Gauze wrap is not taken to the proximal and distal limits of the bandage so as to avoid it 'creeping' over the cotton and possibly chafing the skin.

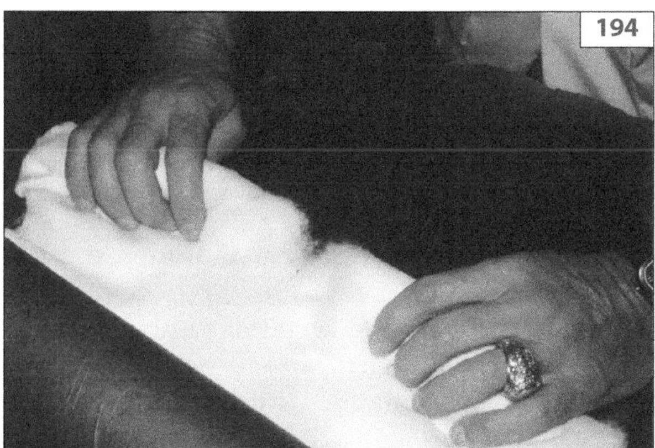

Fig. 194 Twelve-inch (300-mm) cotton is most easily divided by tearing it apart as it is unrolled.

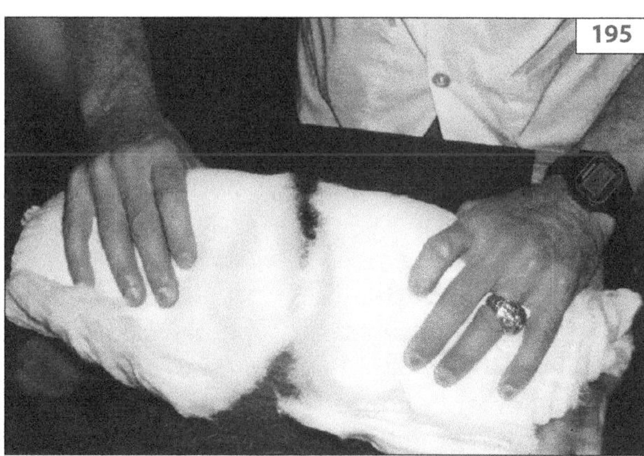

Fig. 195 Having separated the 12-inch (300-mm) roll of cotton, the 'half-rolls' are a convenient size for rolling onto the injured limb.

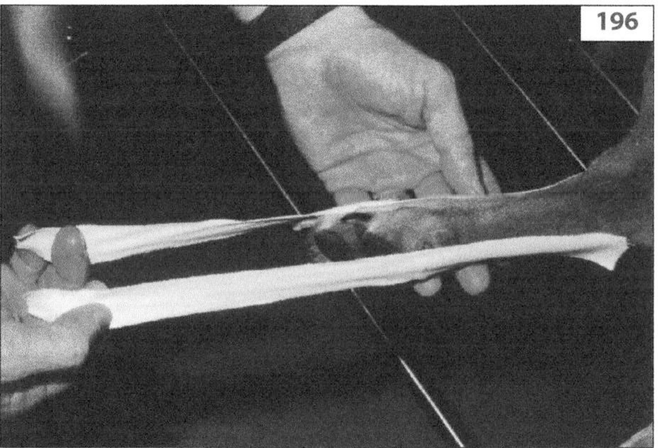

Fig. 196 Tape stirrups are the secret to preventing bandages and casts from slipping.

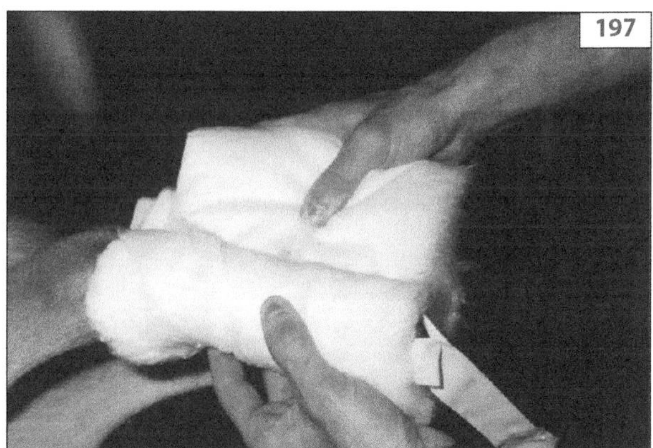

Fig. 197 Cotton is wrapped from distal to proximal over the stirrups leaving the distal portion of the digits visible.

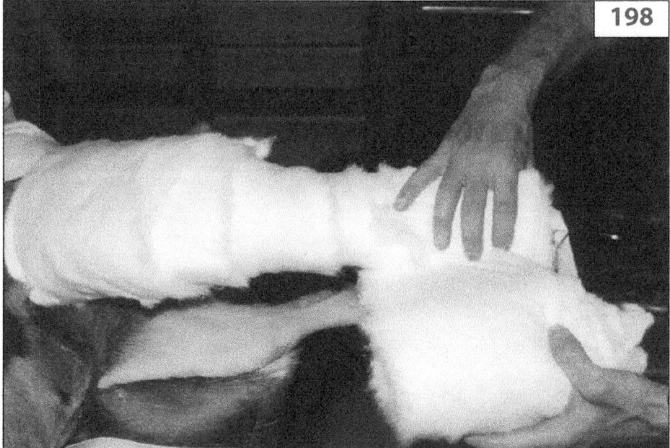

Fig. 198 As needed, a second layer of cotton padding is applied.

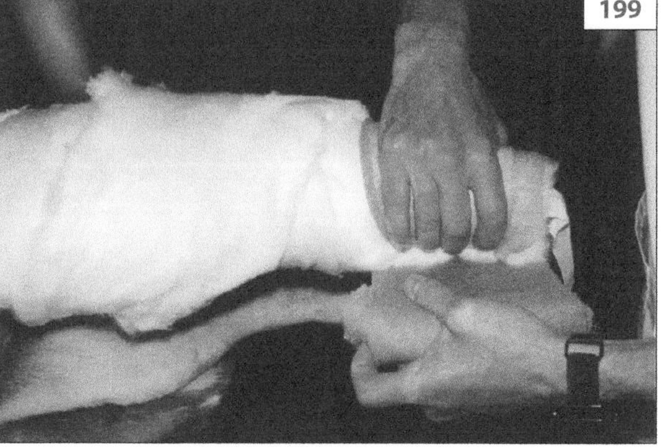

Fig. 199 Gauze over-wraps the cotton padding. Wide gauze is easier to apply and precludes 'bunching' of the underlying cotton.

- The tape stirrups are now separated from one another and reflected back into the bandage by rotating each piece of tape 180° and placing the sticky side onto the gauze wrapping (**Fig. 200**). This should make the toes protruding from the distal limit of the bandage even more visible.
- Finally, the extremity is wrapped from distal to proximal with elastic tape or Vetrap (**Figs. 201, 202**). Because the stirrups are now integrated into the wrapped layers of the bandage and the stirrup tape against the skin is being held in place by compression of the bandage itself, there is little likelihood that the bandage will slip (**Fig. 203**).

Because the Robert Jones bandage contains a large amount of cotton it easily absorbs and holds water. If the patient is taken outside for eliminating in wet or damp conditions, a plastic bag or impervious material should be temporarily placed over the foot to keep the bandage material clean and dry. Owners should be instructed to check the protruding toes twice daily for swelling. Swelling is often identified by toenails spreading apart. Foul odor or exudate from the bandage is

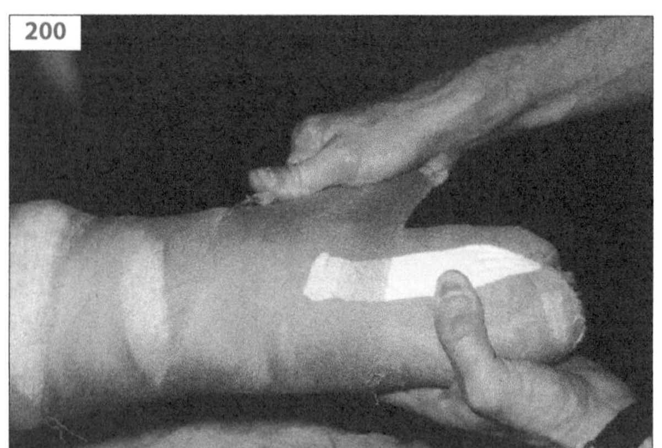

Fig. 200 The tape stirrups are reflected onto the first layer of gauze wrap and covered by the second wrapping of gauze.

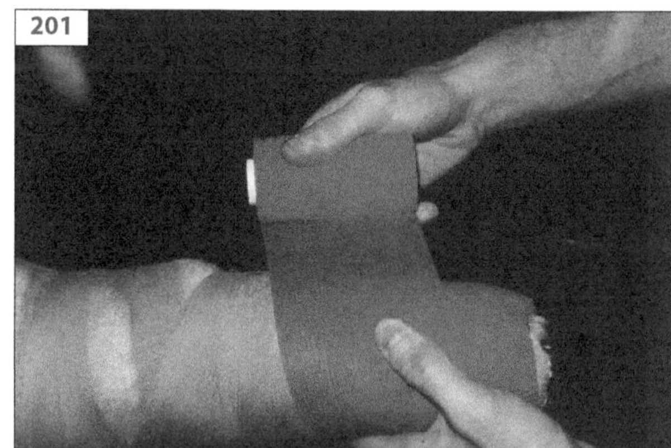

Fig. 201 Vetrap provides the final exterior layer.

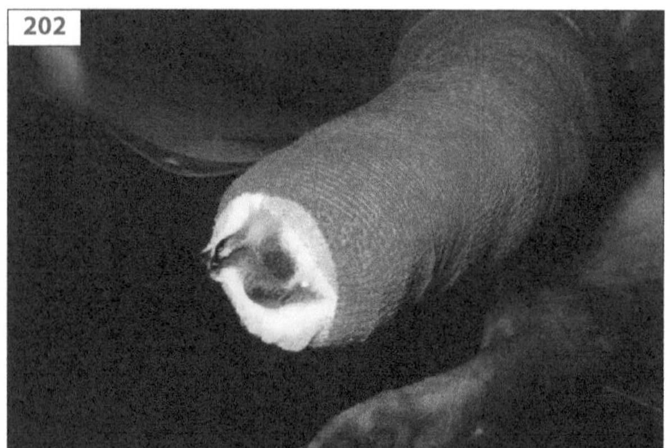

Fig. 202 The middle toes are left visible for assessment of underlying discharge or swelling.

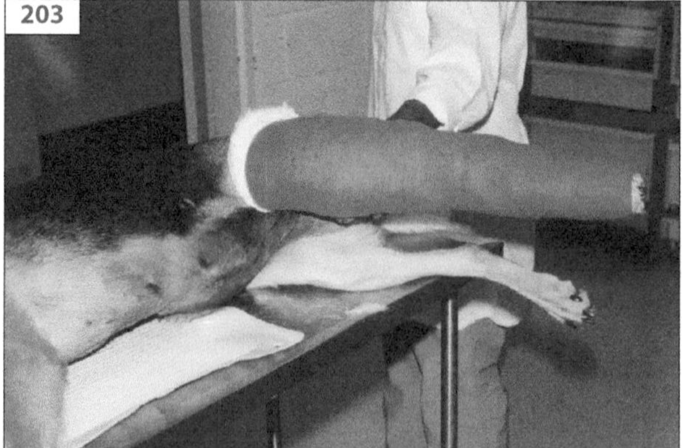

Fig. 203 The completed Robert Jones bandage should be firm (with the sound of a ripe melon when 'thumped' with a finger), and should have 'collars' of cotton padding both proximal and distal to the gauze/Vetrap wrappings.

reason for bandage removal and closer examination. Although ambulation may initially be awkward, the patient quickly adapts to the bandage, and a trouble-free Robert Jones bandage can be left in place for as long as 3 weeks. It is usually left in place for 3–5 days (**Fig. 204**).

The most common complications associated with the Robert Jones bandage are neglecting to heed the early warning of toe swelling, leaving a soiled bandage on too long, and gauze slipping over the top or through insufficiently layered cotton, thereby causing skin abrasions.

CASTING

Length of casts or splints for fractures should follow the same guidelines as for the Robert Jones bandage, that is to include immobilization of the joints above and below the fracture. Casts should also leave the distal limits of digits 3 and 4 exposed as aids to monitor circulatory stasis and swelling.

Plaster of Paris

There are many different types of casting materials. Traditional plaster of Paris is inexpensive, but it is relatively heavy, has a low porosity, requires a prolonged drying time, is susceptible to moisture damage and weakening, is brittle, and messy. Because it is inexpensive, it may be appropriate where multiple cast changes are anticipated. Plaster of Paris is also easily molded, but can be irritating to handle and protective gloves are advised during application. Plaster of Paris is made from dehydrated calcium sulfate crystals. Setting time is 3–8 minutes with an exothermic reaction, and this time can be somewhat extended by the use of cold water. Curing time is 8–48 hours, during which time excess water evaporates, making the cast lighter. Excessive weight bearing should be avoided during this period. The strength of a plaster of Paris cast is proportional to its thickness.

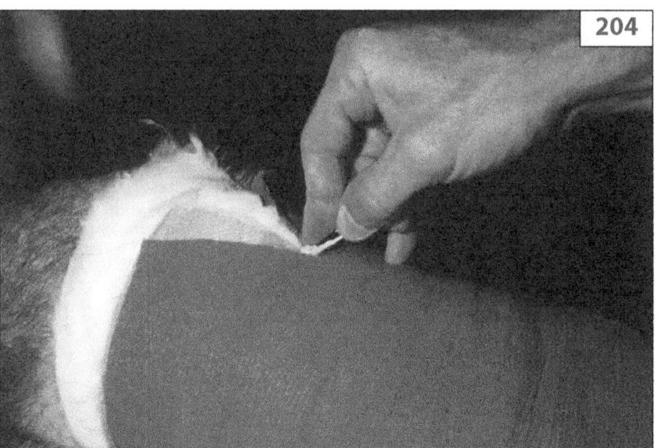

Fig. 204 Removal of the Robert Jones bandage is most easily performed by cutting the Vetrap and gauze layers with a blade, then tearing apart the cotton layer.

Synthetic casting materials

- Polyester-cotton (Cutter cast) is impregnated with a water-activated polyurethane impregnated resin. It is lightweight, water immersible, porous, relatively strong, and virtually radiolucent.
- Fiberglass casting can be activated by water (Delta Lite), ultraviolet light (Lightcast), or a urethane polymer (Ultracast). Fiberglass casts are strong, lightweight, radiolucent, permeable to water vapor, and immersible in water. Fiberglass bandages can interfere with radiographic observation of healing fracture because the weave pattern of the material is visible.
- Thermomoldable (Hexcelite, X-Lite, Veterinary Thermoplastic [VTP]) casting is often an open-weave cotton fabric coated with a high-density thermoplastic resin. VTP is a solid homogenous material rather than an open mesh. This material softens in hot water and becomes rigid in 10 minutes after application. The 'curing' process is minimally exothermic and the end result is an open weave, rough finish surface. This surface makes it easy for some dogs to get their teeth into and chew the casting. (Often, covering the cast with 'ducktape' precludes 'chewing off' the cast, because it does not allow the patient to secure a good bite into the casting material.) Polypropylene substrates impregnated with polyurethane resin are more radiolucent than fiberglass with less radiographic distracting pattern.

Although synthetic casting materials are convenient, strong, and lightweight, several advisements might be taken:

- Open one packaged roll at a time and use within 2–3 minutes.
- Humidity will cause hardening of the preapplied rolled material.
- Shelf-life is approximately 6 months.
- Shelf-life may be extended for sealed, unused rolls by refrigeration.
- Cost may be 3–10× that of plaster of Paris.
- May require special cast cutting blades.

Cast padding

Proper, commercial cast padding (e.g. polypropylene or synthetic) should be used because they shed water. These materials 'breathe' and since they do not retain water, their use results in fewer soft tissue problems, such as skin maceration. Use sufficient cast padding to protect the limb from developing cast sores, but do not use excessive padding that would prevent the cast from resting snugly against, and conforming to, the limb. Generally, cast padding should be only two layers thick.

Materials needed:

- Cast material (left sealed until time of application).
- Stockinette.
- Adhesive tape.
- Cast padding.
- Elastic tape or Vetwrap (optional).

Cast application

- Apply stirrups as with the Robert Jones bandage (**Fig. 205**).
- Place an over-sized length of stockinette over the limb (**Fig. 206**). Two to three inches (50–70 mm) of stockinette should extend from the groin or axilla (initially as a roll), and 2–3 inches (5–75 mm) of stockinette should extend distal to the digits (covering the stirrups).
- Cast padding is rolled diagonally from distal to proximal with 50% overlap. Two layers of cast padding are adequate, with additional turns (three or four) at both the top and bottom of the limb. Distal limits of digits 3 and 4 should be left uncovered as with the Robert Jones bandage.

Extremity casts and bandages should extend from as **proximal as is feasible to the limits of the toes**. This precludes the bandage/cast acting as a constraint to swelling at mid-section of the limb: a 'rubber band' effect, where swelling at either end of the bandage/cast can cause the edges of the bandage/cast to cut into the soft tissues.

- The first roll of casting material is now applied firmly as it is rolled from distal to proximal, leaving approximately 0.5–0.75 inches (10–15 mm) of uncovered cast padding both proximal and distal (**Fig. 207**).
- The proximal roll of cast padding is now unrolled and reflected onto the casting material. Distally, the stirrups are separated and reflected together with the excess stockinette back onto the casting material (**Fig. 208**). This step will provide a ring of cast padding to cushion against the sharp edges of the cured casting material both proximally and distally.
- The second roll of casting material is now applied from distal to proximal, rolled over the reflected stockinette, but short of the proximal and distal cast limits by approximately 0.5–0.75 inches (10–15 mm). This leaves approximately 0.5–0.75 inches (10–15 mm) of stockinette-covered cast padding, which serves as a comfortable 'collar' to guard against tissue abrasion from the edges of the cast. Further wrapping of the cast by elastic tape or Vetrap is optional. If the cast is intended to be in place for an extended period of time, intermittent replacement of Vetrap covering might maintain a more cosmetic appearance.

- If greater rigidity is desired for the cast, longitudinal splints can be added. These are cut from the cast material roll, molded/contoured, and applied over the spiraled cast material. Mechanical testing has revealed that these splints add more strength to fiberglass casts when applied cranially and caudally[1]. A walking bar can also be added to the cast if necessary (i.e. a heavy patient). Direct weight bearing on the cast may cause the cast material to erode, resulting in abrasion of the dorsal paw. Walking bars are easily fashioned in the form of a 'U' shape from aluminum alloy rods and applied cranial-to-caudal on the distal limits of the cast. Cranial to caudal orientation allows less risk for catching on objects, such as tree roots, and curb edges.

Casts should be checked approximately 3–5 days after application for general adaptation and owners should be advised to have the cast checked regularly at 7–10 day intervals or at any sign of foul odor, drainage, loosening, chafing, instability, or obsessive licking or chewing on the cast. These signs suggest removal of the cast and assessment of the underlying soft tissues.

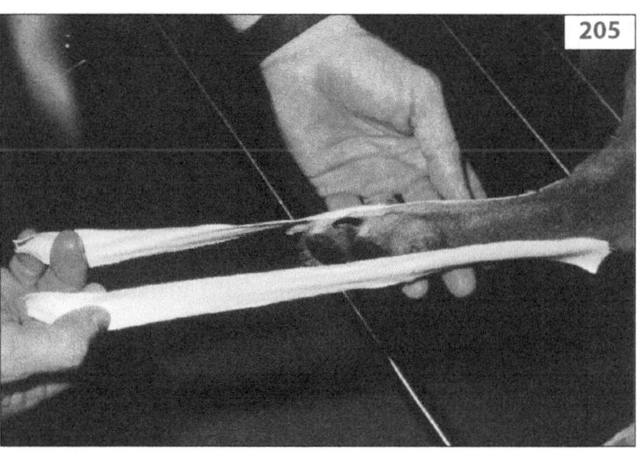

Fig. 205 Tape stirrups are applied as with the Robert Jones bandage.

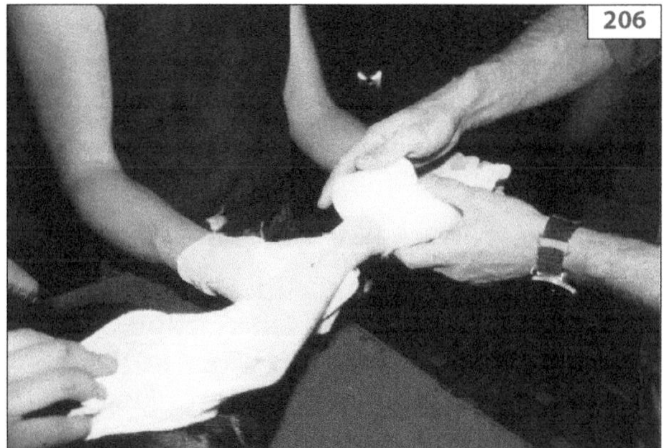

Fig. 206 Stockinette is applied from the distal limit of the stirrups to as far into the axilla or groin as possible, with additional length of stockinette rolled proximally.

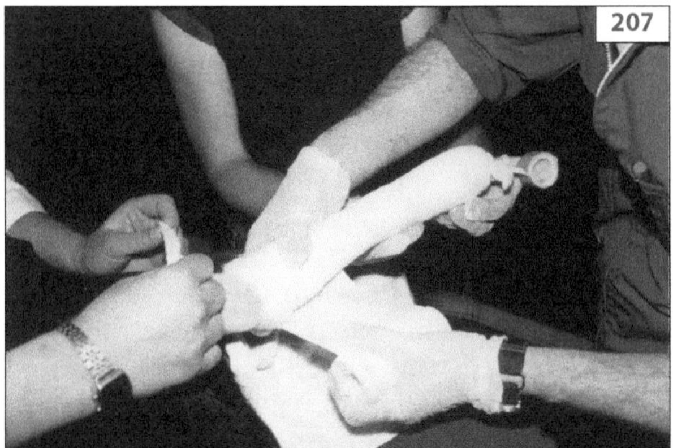

Fig. 207 Stockinette is reflected over the cast padding and integrated into the three to four layers of casting material at both the proximal and distal ends of the cast. This provides a soft collar at both ends of the cast, which precludes sharp edges of the hardened cast from cutting into the underlying tissues.

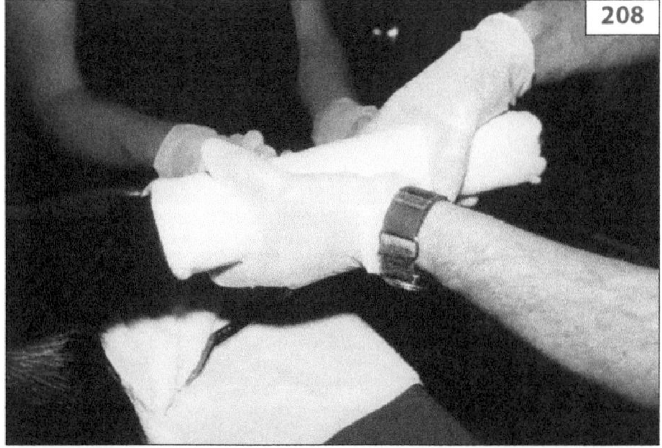

Fig. 208 After the layers of casting materials are applied, the cast is 'hand-rolled' to yield a smooth, molded appearance.

Cast removal

Casts must be removed with a cast-cutting oscillating saw whether they are made of plaster of Paris or other synthetic materials (**Fig. 209**). The process of cast removal is not painful, but patient sedation is advised because the noise and vibration of the saw is often frightening to the patient. Sedation with an opioid and or alpha-2 agonist works well. Bivalving the cast can be very useful, especially if frequent removal for inspection is necessary. Using the oscillating saw, make a full thickness cut of the cast material both medially and laterally for the full length of the cast. Then separate the two halves and cut the cast padding and stockinette for inspection. For reapplication, simply apply new stockinette and cast padding, replace the cast material halves, and secure them with nonelastic, adhesive tape. Care should be taken to apply approximately the same amount and type of padding as was originally used so as to prevent undue pressure or looseness.

SCHROEDER–THOMAS SPLINT

This splint is an aluminum alloy rod frame designed to place a limb in traction, thereby providing some immobilization of tibial or antebrachial (radius/ulna) fractures (**Fig. 210**).

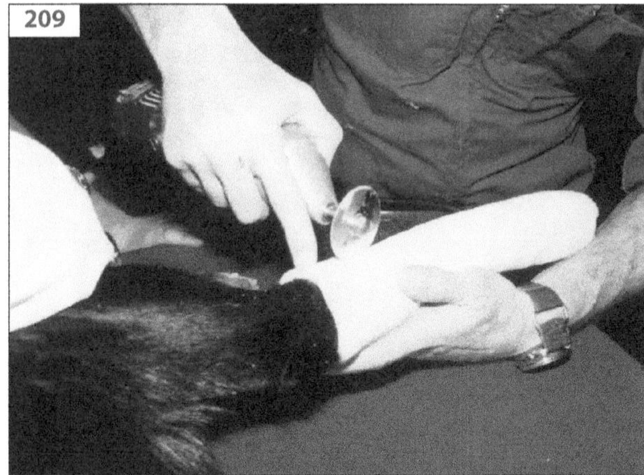

Fig. 209 Casts are cut with an oscillating saw. Although this saw will not cut tissue, the author finds that extending the index finger to contact the cast surface provides optimal saw control.

Widely used in the past, this splint has been largely replaced by molded splints and casts. It is effective *only* for immobilization of fractures below the elbow or stifle. Considerable artistry is required to construct a functional, well-tolerated, and effective Schroeder–Thomas splint. It is the author's experience that this splint is associated with the most frequently presented complications of all coaptation devices, and should be utilized only by personnel with extensive experience in its use. Complications most often arise when the device is applied in an attempt to stabilize a fracture of the humerus or femur. Under such circumstances, the lower half of the ring through which the limb is placed, continually distracts fractures of the humerus or femur, thereby leading to nonunions (**Fig. 211**). Additionally, anchorage points of the limb with adhesive tape are common sites for soft tissue injury. Although the Schroeder–Thomas splint is useful for some, alternative options are advised.

CARPAL FLEXION BANDAGE

This simple bandage is intended purely to discourage weight bearing, while maintaining passive motion of the shoulder and elbow joints. It is particularly useful following lateral shoulder luxation, supraspinatus and biceps brachii surgery, as well as protection for repairs of the scapula, shoulder, humerus, and elbow.

Materials needed:

- Wide white tape.
- ± Cast padding.
- ± Vetrap.

Application

With the carpus gently flexed, 2-inch (50-mm) white tape is applied to encircle the distal radius/ulna and the metacarpal region. A strip of more narrow tape is placed around the middle of this encirclement, between the metacarpals and radius/ulna. This step prevents the limb encirclement from slipping over the carpus. Finally, the entire limb distal to the elbow can be wrapped with Vetrap (optional) (**Fig. 212**). An alternative application is to wrap the limb distal to midradius with cast padding and tape, then flexing the carpus and holding it in flexion with tape extending from the distal limits of the toes to the proximal antebrachium.

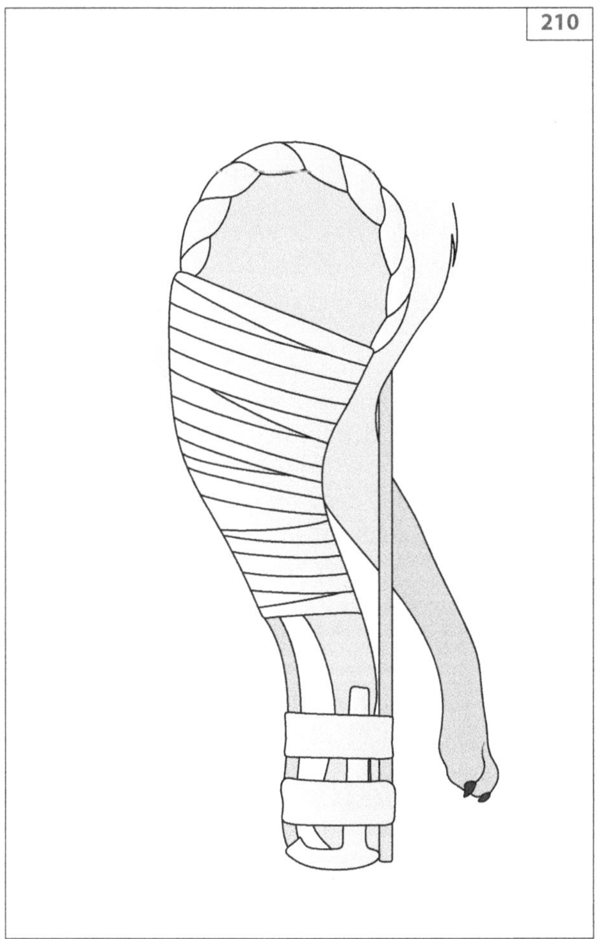

Fig. 210 The Schroeder–Thomas splint is intended for fracture stabilization below the elbow or stifle.

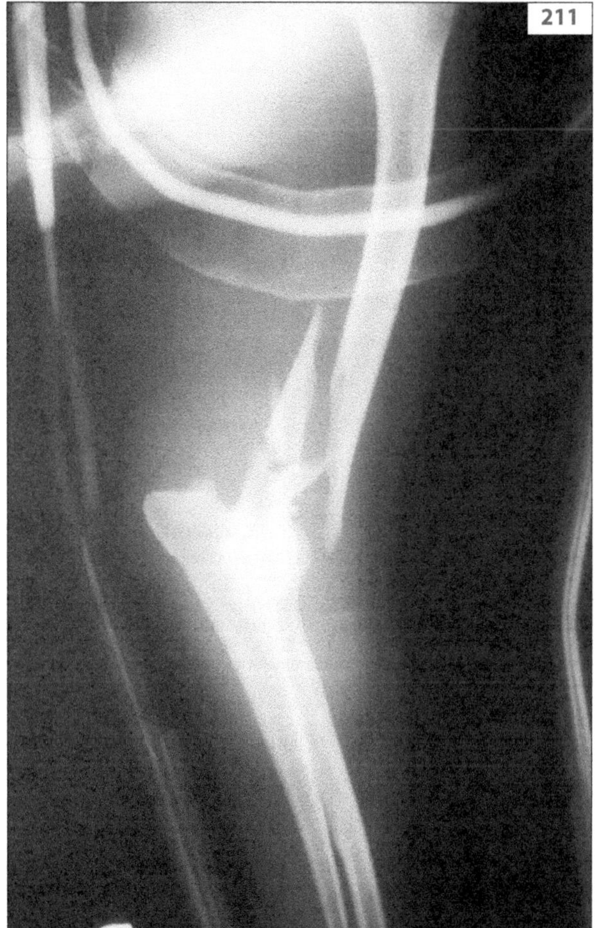

Fig. 211 This radiograph illustrates why the Schroeder–Thomas splint is inappropriate for fractures above the elbow (or stifle). As the forelimb moves, the ventral aspect of the aluminum ring continually distracts the fracture site.

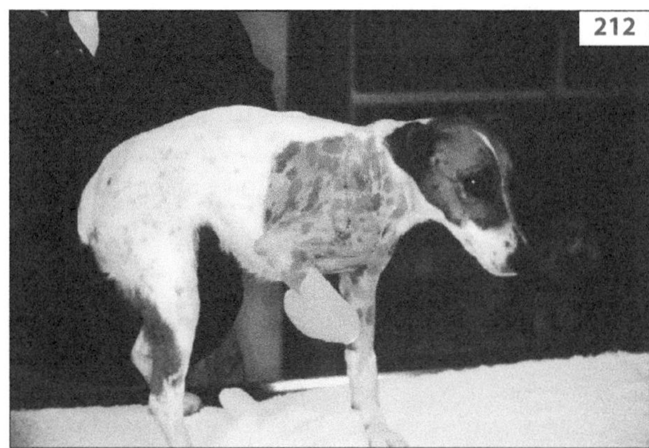

Fig. 212 Carpal flexion bandage, protecting against weight bearing of the forelimb.

VELPEAU SLING

The Velpeau sling is another device to prevent weight bearing of the forelimb; however, the carpal flexion bandage is more simple. The Velpeau sling is most often used to help maintain reduction of medial shoulder luxation and to support scapular fractures (**Fig. 213**).

Materials needed:

- Elastic gauze or kling.
- Elastic tape or Vetrap.

Application

With the carpus, elbow, and shoulder flexed, the forelimb is splinted against the thorax by wrapping layers of gauze around the affected limb and thorax and behind the opposite axilla. Covering the entire limb prevents the lower limb or elbow from being forced out of the bandage with an attempt to flex or extend the limb. Additional support is provided by adding an outer layer of elastic tape or Vetrap. The sling may be retained for approximately 2 weeks.

EHMER SLING

The Ehmer sling is primarily used to partially immobilize and stabilize the hip joint. It is commonly used to support closed or open reduction of hip luxations, in that it places the hock into abduction, which tends to 'drive' the femoral head into the acetabulum (**Fig. 214**).

Materials needed:

- Cast padding.
- 4- or 6-inch (100–150-mm) gauze (or kling) or elastic tape.

Application

- Clipping hair on the thigh helps to prevent bandage slippage.
- Avoid extreme hyperflexion of the hock, which can cause excessive pressure from the bandage wrap on the plantar surface of the metatarsus.
- Place three to four wrappings of cast padding around the metatarsus.
- Wrap several (two to three) layers of gauze or elastic tape around the midmetatarsal padding from medial to lateral.
- 'Smartly' flex the stifle, and carry the gauze (or elastic tape, with the tape rolled so that the sticky side now faces the medial side of the stifle) medial to the flexed stifle and over the cranial surface of the thigh. This abducts the hock, internally rotating the limb at the hip joint, 'driving' the femoral head into the acetabulum.
- The wrap is now brought medial to the tibia and tarsus and over the plantar surface of the tarsus to the lateral surface of the metatarsus.
- Several more 'circuits' (three to four) are made in a continued figure-of-eight fashion around the flexed stifle and hock.

Sling application may be made with gauze and then covered with elastic adhesive tape, or the sling may be applied without any gauze by starting with adhesive tape applied to the skin. The latter application keeps the sling from slipping, but may lead to skin irritation on the cranial thigh. It is difficult to keep the sling from slipping over the stifle on short-legged breeds of dogs and on cats. A possible solution of this slippage is to attach wide adhesive tape to the paw area of the completed sling, then carry the tape upwards over the back and then around the abdomen. The sling may remain in place for up to 3 weeks.

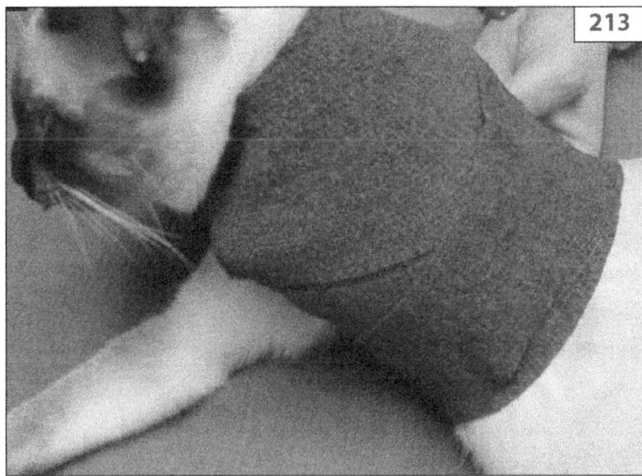

Fig. 213 Velpeau sling adapted to a cat[2].

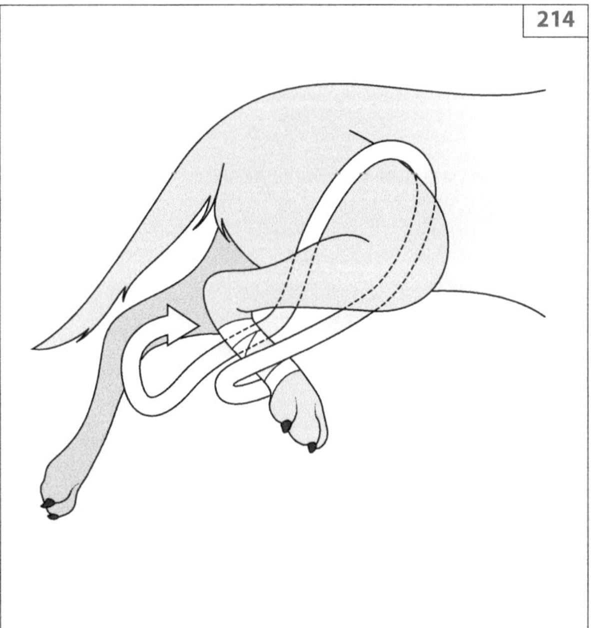

Fig. 214 The Ehmer sling forces the hock away from the body (abducts), thereby 'driving' the femoral head (ball) into the acetabulum (socket).

COAPTATION BANDAGE COMPLICATIONS

Most complications associated with coaptation bandages are minor (e.g. swelling of the limb distal to the bandage, slippage of the bandage, skin abrasions, edges of the cast or bandage cutting into the soft tissues). However, serious complications may occur (e.g. fracture nonunion, limb loss from ischemic necrosis) (**Figs. 215–217**). Application of a coaptation bandage or cast should not be considered a minor procedure or one requiring minimal follow-up observation.

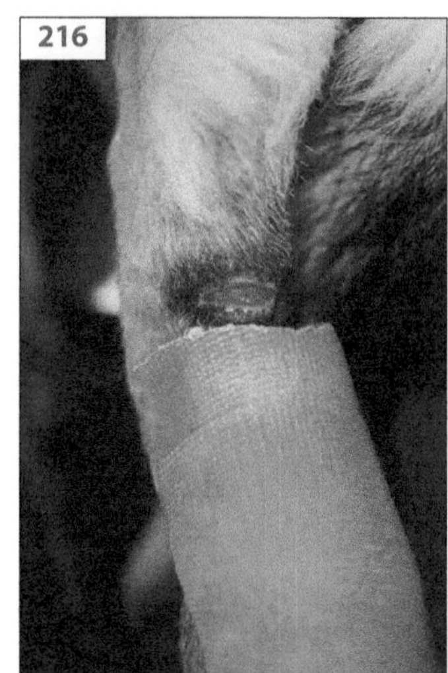

Fig. 216 Cast complication. The cast was bivalved for extended duration of support; however, a soft padding collar was not provided and the sharp edge of the casting material lacerated the skin.

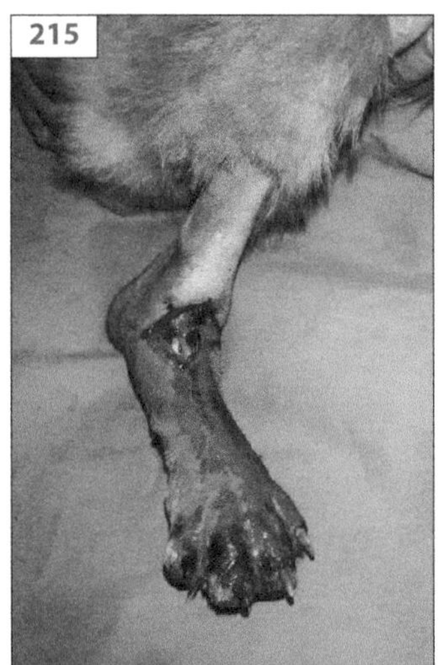

Fig. 215 Bandage/cast complication. Soft tissue necrosis occurred under the coaptation device, but was not caught early enough to avoid major damage, because the owner was not regularly checking the device as instructed.

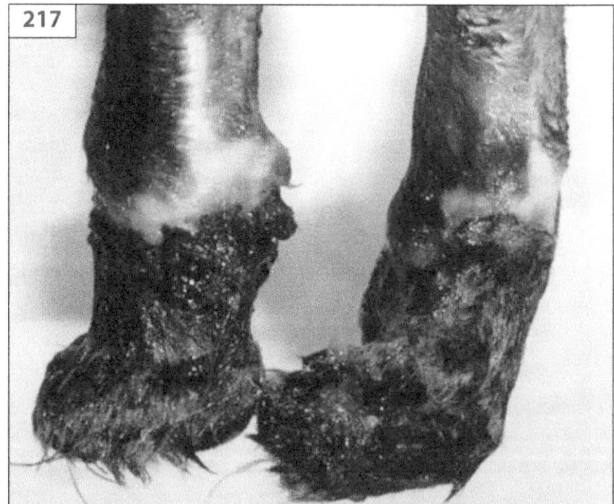

Fig. 217 Distal forelimb necrosis following feline onychectomy. The bandaging was too tight and inappropriately checked.

Chapter 14

Pain, Lameness, and the Orthopedic Examination

INTRODUCTION

One in five dogs over 1 year of age is proposed to be afflicted with osteoarthritis (OA)[1]. (Some propose that the prevalence of degenerative joint disease [DJD] in the cat is similar or higher.) Such recognition makes DJD the most common source of pain in small animal practice. Although every patient visit should be accompanied by a physical examination, inclusion of an orthopedic examination is often lacking. A cursory orthopedic examination can be conducted in approximately 5 minutes, provided the clinician is appropriately trained. For early detection of the inevitable pain associated with OA, it is, therefore, imperative that the clinician be familiar with the proper conduct of an orthopedic examination.

Pain

Pain is the clinical sign most frequently associated with DJD[2]. The clinical manifestation of this pain is lameness. When an animal presents with clinical lameness, a determination must be made whether the animal is *unable* to use the limb, or is *unwilling* to use the limb. Inability to use the limb may be attributable to musculoskeletal changes, such as joint contracture or muscle atrophy. These anomalies are best addressed with physical rehabilitation (see Chapter 10). On the other hand, unwillingness to use a limb is most often attributable to pain. Herein, lameness is an avoidance behavior.

Ironically, articular cartilage is frequently the focus of studies in OA – the most common cause of musculoskeletal pain. However, clinical treatment of the OA patient is most often focused on the alleviation of pain. Appreciating that articular cartilage is aneural (without nerves), the focus of OA pain management resides in the periarticular structures. No pain is elicited by stimulation of cartilage, and stimulation of normal synovial tissue rarely evokes pain[3].

OA pain is the result of a complex interplay between structural change, biochemical alterations, peripheral and central pain processing mechanisms, and individual cognitive processing of nociception (see Chapter 4) (**Fig. 218**).

The source of pain in the joint 'organ' is multifocal: direct stimulation of the joint capsule and bone receptors by cytokines/ligands of inflammatory and degradative processes; physical stimulation of the joint capsule from distention (effusion) and stretch (laxity, subluxation, abnormal articulation); physical stimulation of subchondral bone from abnormal loading; and (likely) physical stimulation of muscle, tendon, and ligaments.

Bony changes at the joint margins and beneath areas of damaged cartilage can be major sources of OA pain. Subchondral bone contains unmyelinated nerve fibers, which increase in number with OA[4]. Increased pressure on subchondral bone (associated with OA) results in stimulation of these nociceptors. This is thought to contribute to the vague, but consistent pain frequently associated with OA. In humans, OA is believed to be responsible for increased intraosseous pressure, which may contribute to chronic pain, particularly nocturnal pain. Human OA patients report pain, even at rest, associated with raised intraosseous pressure[5].

Lameness

Most often lameness in pets is identified by the owner, who subsequently seeks further consultation and advice from their veterinarian, or the lameness is identified by the veterinarian during routine examination. Most simply, dogs (and cats) are lame because they *cannot* or *will not* use one or more limbs in a normal fashion.

Pain associated with OA is recognized to become more persistent and intense as the disease progresses. The condition may be asymptomatic in the early stages. With progression of the disease, discomfort may be continuous, exacerbated by motion and weight bearing. In the later stages of OA, pain can become pervasive and affects nearly all activities and behaviors.

Diagnosis of musculoskeletal pain

A proper diagnosis depends on a complete history and full assessment of the patient, possibly including all of the below:

- A complete physical, orthopedic and neurologic examination.
- Radiographs of affected area(s)
- Advanced imaging, such as computerized tomography, magnetic resonance imaging, nuclear scintigraphy.
- Advanced gait analysis, such as force plate (kinetic) analysis of gait and motion (kinematic) analysis.
- Clinicopathologic examination, including hematology and serum chemistries, especially creatine kinase and electrolytes, and synovial fluid analysis.
- Electrodiagnostic testing: electromyography, nerve conduction velocity measurements, evoked potential recordings with repetitive nerve stimulation.
- Muscle biopsy examination, including histopathology and histochemical analysis.
- Special tests: muscle percussion, serology for pathogens (e.g. *Neospora*, *Toxoplasma*), measurement of acetylcholine receptor antibody, immunohistochemistry, and molecular diagnostic techniques.

Anamnesis

The medical history, signalment, and owner's complaint(s) comprise the process of anamnesis. Most canine patients do not vocalize from their musculoskeletal pain, and many pet owners do not believe their pet is painful if it does not vocalize. Nevertheless, signs suggesting animal discomfort include lameness, muscle atrophy, reluctance to exercise, general malaise, lethargy, inappetence or anorexia, change in temperament, licking or biting an affected joint, restlessness, insomnia, seeking warmth, seeking comfortable bedding, and difficulty posturing to toilet. Supraspinal influences are known to alter the behavior of humans with OA[2], and it is reasonable to presume the same occurs in dogs.

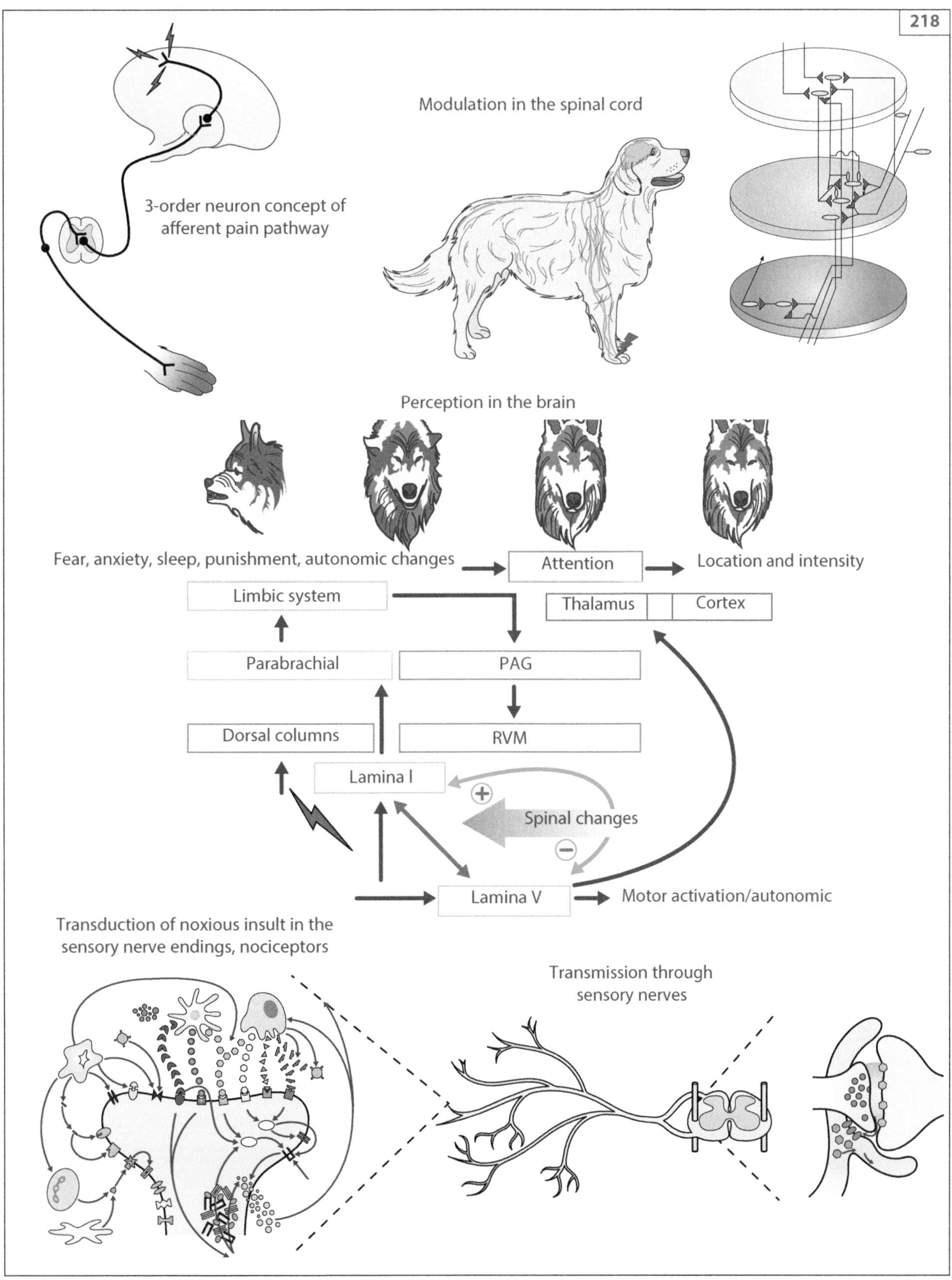

Fig. 218 The pain associated with osteoarthritis (OA) is far more complex than the 3-order neuron 'pathway'. Many sophisticated processes occur in the functions of transduction, transmission, modulation, and perception. PAG: periaqueductal gray; RVM: rostral ventromedial medulla.

Pet owners often recognize lameness only when there is gait asymmetry. However, dogs with bilateral OA, such as with hip or elbow dysplasia, have a symmetrically abnormal gait and do not favor a single limb. These patients shift weight from hind- to frontlimbs or *vice versa* with resultant muscle atrophy of the affected limbs and increased development in compensating limbs. Rarely are dogs nonweight bearing simply due to OA. Pet owners do often report that their dog is stiff after resting, particularly following strenuous exercise, but they report that the pet will 'warm-out' of the stiffness. The amount of time required to warm-out of this stiffness gradually increases with progression of the disease. Pet owners also frequently report a shortened stride and stiff gait. This is associated with a decreased range of motion (ROM) in the joint, often due to joint capsule fibrosis and osteophyte formation.

Examination

For many years DJD (often used interchangeably with the term OA) was considered a disease of the cartilage. DJD is most appropriately considered a disease of the entire joint, with the influence of multiple structures, including articular cartilage.

Clinical implication: pain is a hallmark of degenerative joint disease, provoked by instability, and therefore a comprehensive physical examination is an essential diagnostic tool.

An orthopedic examination should be part of every routine examination and should be conducted in conjunction with a neurologic examination (when appropriate) to identify differential neurologic causes for pain or lameness, such as a nerve root signature sign secondary to a laterally herniated intervertebral disk or brachial plexus pathology.

A consistent 'routine' for examining a patient is advised, and it is also recommended that the 'lame' limb be examined last. A consistent examination pattern (e.g. distal limb to proximal limb, and left side to right side or *vice versa*) is helpful to avoid missing a structure during the examination, and leaving the most painful limb for last in the examination avoids the early elicitation of pain which may render the patient noncompliant for further examination. A thorough examination also requires the aid of an animal health technician (AHT) who is adequately trained to hold and restrain the animal. The AHT plays an important role in identifying the animal's painful response to examination, such as body shifts and change of facial expression.

Animal restraint

Appropriate animal restraint by the AHT (with the patient standing on the examination table) is with one arm over or under the patient's thorax, while the other arm is placed under and around the patient's neck (**Fig. 219**). This constraint allows the AHT to tighten his/her grip quickly to control the animal and avoid the patient from harming anyone, should it become confrontational. In lateral recumbency the AHT should be at the animal's dorsum, 'lightly leaning' on the animal with his/her forearms while holding the rear and forelimbs. One forearm should be placed on the animal's neck, with that hand grasping the forelimb that is closest to the table, or the 'down limb'. The other arm is placed over the top of the abdomen and the hand grasps the 'down' rear limb (**Fig. 220**). With this restraint, the AHT can rapidly increase his/her amount of weight on their forearms, thereby controlling the animal's movements. Regarding constraint, large dogs are analogous to horses: if you control their head, you control their body.

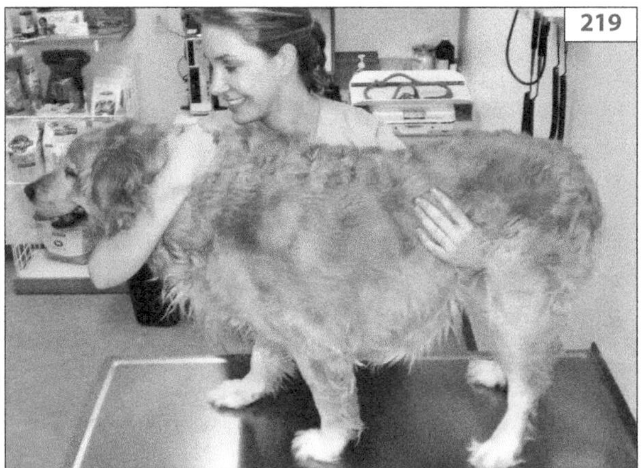

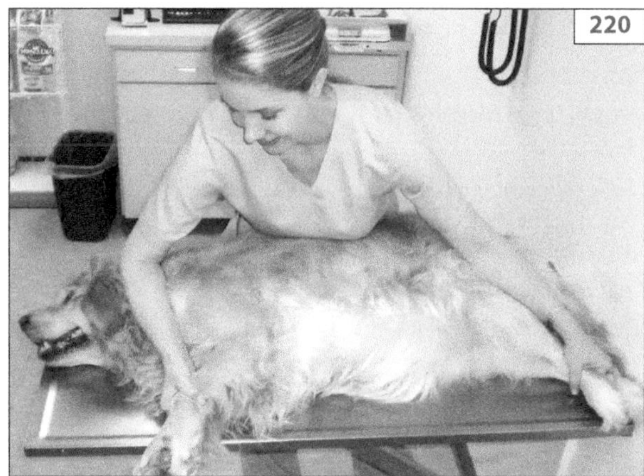

Fig. 219, 220 Restraint for examination. Standing restraint (**219**) of large dogs is done with the neck cradled close to the animal health technician (AHT)'s chest with one arm, while the other arm controls the patient's trunk by placement either under or over the trunk. If the patient struggles or becomes aggressive, the AHT holds the dog as tight as possible. Lateral restraint (**220**) of large dogs is done with the AHT's forearm over the dog's neck. If the patient struggles, more weight is applied on the forearm.

THE MUSCULOSKELETAL EXAMINATION

Forelimb examination

In the *growing dog*, forelimb lameness differentials mostly reflect abnormal stressors on normal bone or normal stressors on abnormal bone (excluding fractures and minor soft tissue injuries), and include:

- Osteochondrosis dissecans (OCD): shoulder.
- Luxation/subluxation shoulder: congenital.
- Avulsion: supraglenoid tubercle.
- OCD: elbow.
- Ununited anconeal process (elbow).
- Fragmented coronoid process (elbow).
- Ununited medial epicondyle (distal humerus).
- Elbow incongruity:
  - congenital.
  - physical injury.
- Premature closure of growth plates, such as with radius curves.
- Retained cartilaginous core (ulna).
- Panosteitis* (a disease of metaphyseal bone).
- Hypertrophic osteodystrophy*.

In the *adult dog*, forelimb lameness differentials mostly reflect abnormal stressors on normal bone or normal stressors on abnormal bone (excluding fractures and minor soft tissue injuries) and include:

- Arthritis.
- OCD: shoulder.
- Luxation /subluxation: shoulder.
- Avulsion: supraglenoid tubercle.
- Bicipital tenosynovitis*.
- Calcification of supraspinatus tendon*.
- Contracture of infra- or supraspinatus*.
- Medial glenohumeral laxity.
- OCD: elbow.
- Ununited anconeal process.
- Fragmented coronoid process.
- Ununited medial epicondyle.
- Elbow incongruity.
- Angular limb deformity.
- Hypertrophic osteopathy.
- Bone/soft tissue neoplasia*.
- Inflammatory arthritis.

(*Denote pathology/disease conditions which are not considered OA, but often manifest similar clinical presentations.)

For the purpose of examination, the forelimb can be anatomically segmented into the paw, antebrachium, brachium, scapula, and interpositional joints. Although the entire limb should be examined in every patient, the orthopedic examination can be focused more on areas prone to disease and signalment of the individual patient.

Paw

The paw should be thoroughly examined with flexion and extension of each digit, as well as inspection of each nail and nail bed. Findings incidental to those suggesting OA might include:

- Pad lacerations.
- Foreign bodies.
- Split nails.
- Overgrown nails.
- Nail bed tumors.
- Phalangeal luxations/fractures.

Some patients resist manipulation of the paws. Here, the AHT can be very helpful by talking to the patient or scratching the patient to distract it from the examination.

Carpus

The carpus should be placed under stress in flexion, extension, valgus, and varus. The normal carpus should flex comfortably until the palmar surface of the paw nearly touches the flexor surface of the antebrachium (**Figs. 221–224**).

Findings from the carpal examination may include:

- Young dog 'carpal laxity syndrome'.
- Carpal flexural deformity of young dogs.
- DJD.
- Hyperextension.
- Inflammatory arthritis.
- Luxation.
- Fracture (including an intra-articular fracture, possibly mistaken as OA).

Joint capsule distention is easily palpated and suggests joint inflammation.

Fig. 221 Carpus flexion. The carpus should be comfortably flexed with the palmar surface nearly touching the flexor surface of the antebrachium.

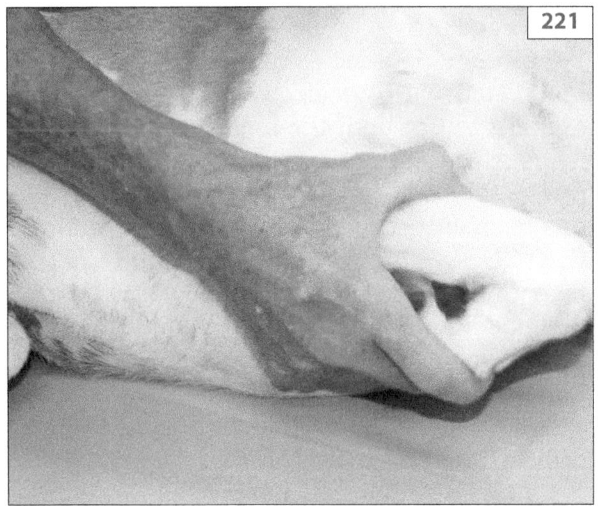

Fig. 222 The carpus should be stressed in extension, looking for signs of discomfort/pain.

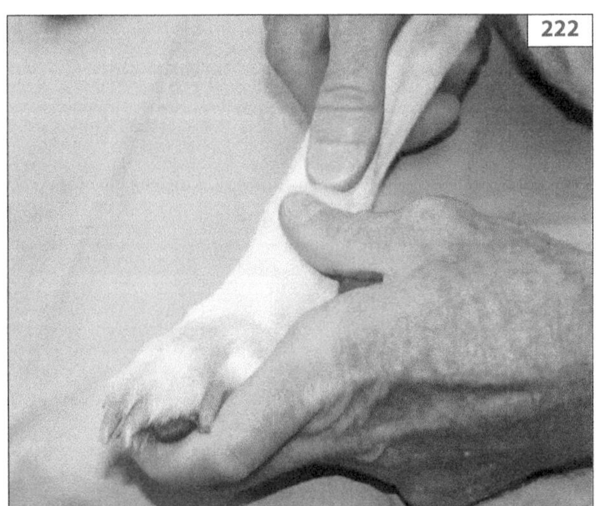

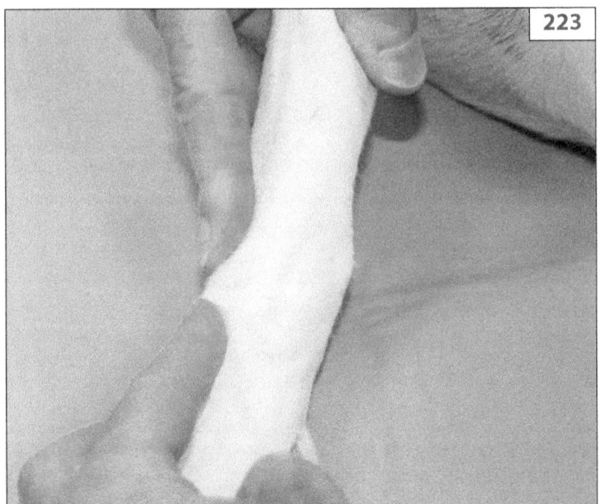

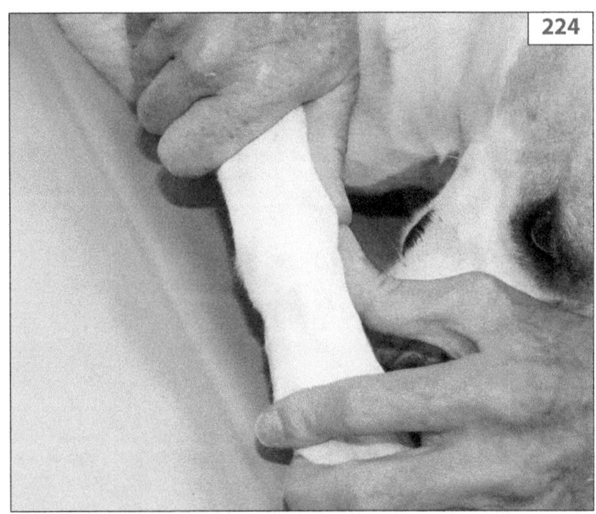

Figs. 223, 224 Placing a varus stress on the carpus challenges the integrity of the lateral ulnar collateral ligament.

Antebrachium

Periosteum of bone is a sensitive tissue, well innervated with nociceptive axons. Therefore, examination of both the radius and ulna should focus on deep palpation for a response of bone pain (**225**). Panosteitis is commonly revealed in this manner. Osteosarcoma is another condition that results in pain on palpation of the metaphyseal region of bones. Although an orthopedic examination would include assessment of the antebrachium, OA includes only diarthrodial joints. Nevertheless, joint pain should be localized and differentiated from the pain of long bones and soft tissues.

Physeal disturbances are relatively common in the growing dog, the severity of which depends on the amount of growth remaining following injury until physeal closure. Resultant aberrant growth is expressed as angular limb deformities of the carpus and/or the elbow. In general, the plane of the elbow joint should be parallel to the plane of the carpal joint. Sources of lameness within the radius/ulna include:

- Hypertrophic osteopathy.
- Angular limb deformities.
- Panosteitis.
- Neoplasia.
- Hypertrophic osteodystrophy.

Elbow

The elbow is the most common forelimb joint responsible for lameness, especially in growing dogs of predisposed breeds (i.e. large breeds, sporting dogs, and Rottweilers). The elbow should be manipulated through a complete ROM (**Fig. 226**), noting the abnormal presence of crepitus or painful response, particularly in full extension. In a normal dog, hyperextension of the

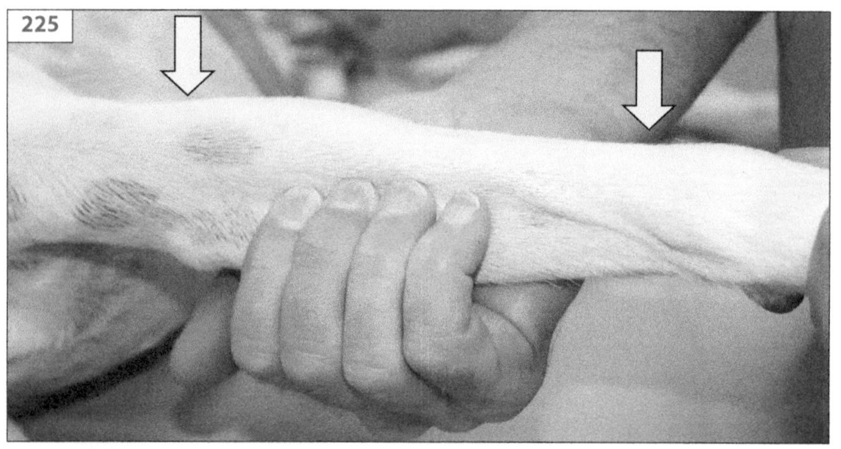

Fig. 225 Digital palpation is made on the anteriomedial aspect of the antebrachium, where there is minimal muscle cover. In the normal dog the elbow joint is parallel to the carpal joint.

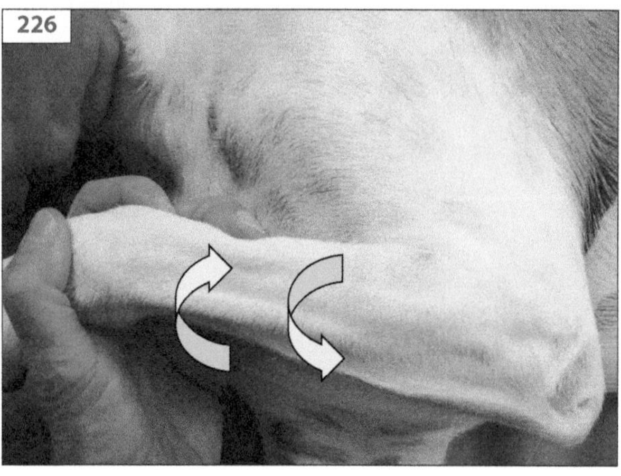

Fig. 226 Examination of the elbow joint includes manipulation through a full range of motion. Pronation and supination should also be performed.

elbow should elicit minimal to no discomfort. Valgus (away from the midline) and varus (toward the midline) stress placed upon the joint are performed to assess integrity of the joint capsule and collateral ligaments/tendons. Joint effusion accompanying disease often distends the joint, palpable by digital placement of the thumb and index finger in the normally concave depression caudal to the distal humeral epicondyles (**Fig. 227**). Common orthopedic diseases of the elbow joint include fragmented coronoid process (FCP), ununited anconeal process (UAP), and OCD, (**Fig. 228**). Palpation of the medial joint, in the area of the medial coronoid, often elicits a painful response in dogs suffering from this condition.

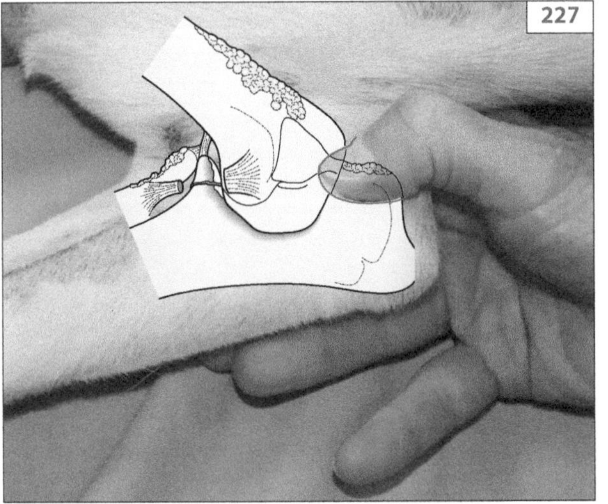

Fig. 227 Fragmented medial coronoid, ununited anconeal process, and osteochondritis are common diseases of the elbow, constituting elbow dysplasia. Patients with any of these pathologies often resent deep digital pressure on the medial aspect of the joint near the affected location. Further, joint capsule distension is common with any of these conditions, and can best be identified by palpation, as with thumb placement in the figure.

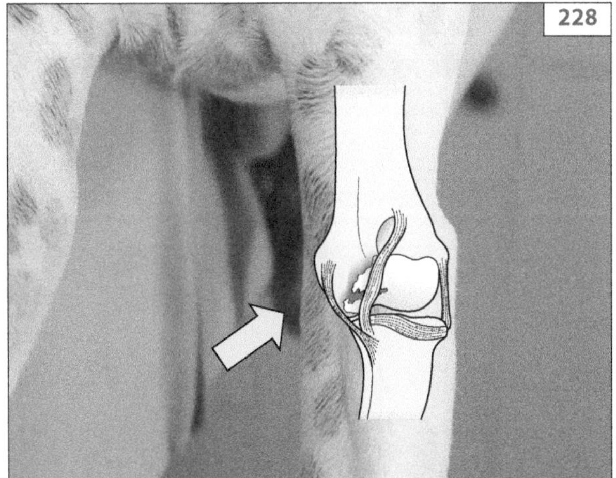

Fig. 228 Osteochondritis dissecans of the elbow most commonly occurs on the distal, medial, humeral condyle.

Less common findings of the elbow, aside from OA, include:

- Subluxations or luxation (can be associated with OA).
- Fractures.
- Radioulnar incongruities (can be associated with OA).
- Inflammatory arthropathies.
- Neoplasia.

Brachium

Osteosarcoma is a common tumor of the forelimb, frequently residing in the proximal humerus (and distal radius/ulna). Deep palpation along the length of the humerus is conducted to reveal evidence of pain and areas of inflammation or swelling. Other abnormal conditions of the brachium (not associated with OA) include:

- Hypertrophic osteodystrophy.
- Fractures.
- Hypertrophic osteopathy.
- Panosteitis.

Shoulder

As with examination of all joints, the shoulder joint should be examined through a full ROM to include flexion (**Fig. 229**), extension, adduction, and abduction as well as internal and external rotation. Of particular note is examination of the shoulder joint in extension. The examiner should be mindful to *avoid placing the forelimb into extension with his/her hand placed caudal or distal to the elbow joint* (**Fig. 230**). Placing the hand behind or distal to the elbow when forcing the shoulder into extension also forces the elbow into extension. A resultant painful response from the patient might actually be from elbow disease rather than shoulder disease. The examiner's hand placed above the elbow allows the elbow to be placed in a neutral position, and avoids this potential complication.

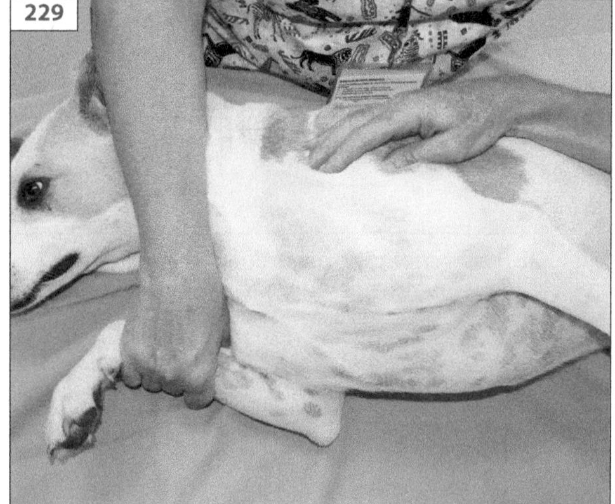

Fig. 229 Examination of the shoulder in flexion. The shoulder joint should also be assessed in abduction and adduction. Note constraint of the patient with the animal health technician's forearm over the patient's neck.

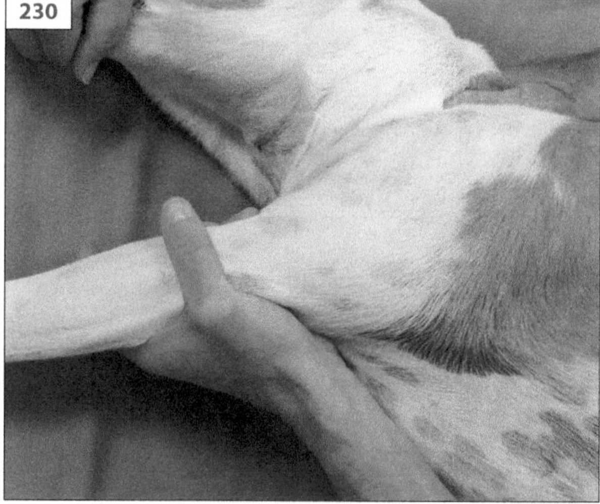

Fig. 230 Avoid placing the forelimb in extension with hand placement caudal to the elbow. This typically causes simultaneous hyperextension of the elbow and may give a false impression that the source of discomfort is in the shoulder joint when it actually resides in the elbow joint.

Painful conditions associated with the shoulder joint include:

- OCD (especially in young animals, which can lead to OA).
- Biceps tenosynovitis.
- Mineralization of the supraspinatus.
- Infraspinatus contracture.
- DJD (of unknown etiology).
- Articular fractures.
- Incomplete ossification of the caudal glenoid process.
- Medial shoulder instability (leading to OA).
- Luxation, either congenital or acquired (leading to OA).

Stabilization of the shoulder joint is maintained by both medial and lateral glenohumeral ligaments, the shape of the articular surfaces (humeral head and glenoid), and musculotendinous units of the rotator cuff: the supraspinatus, infraspinatus, teres minor, and subscapularis. Abnormal excursion of the shoulder joint, with or without pain, suggests involvement of several of these periarticular soft tissue structures. Medial shoulder instability gives rise to abduction greater than approximately 32°, an angle easily measured with a goniometer.

Scapula

The scapula is not a common source of forelimb pain; however, atrophy of scapular muscles is frequently associated with disuse of the forelimb as well as many neurologic conditions. Tumors, acromion fractures, midbody fractures, and scapular luxation from the thoracic wall are commonly seen when pain is localized to the scapular area, so deep palpation and manipulation of the scapula should be performed when this anatomical structure is suspect.

The biceps tendon should be palpated from its origin on the supraglenoid tubercle through its excursion within the intertubercular groove in the proximal humerus (**Fig. 231**). Biceps tenosynovitis frequently results in the patient's painful response to this deep palpation. Another maneuver that may elicit pain is to flex the shoulder joint while simultaneously extending the elbow joint. This places maximal stretch on the biceps tendon and may exacerbate a pain response.

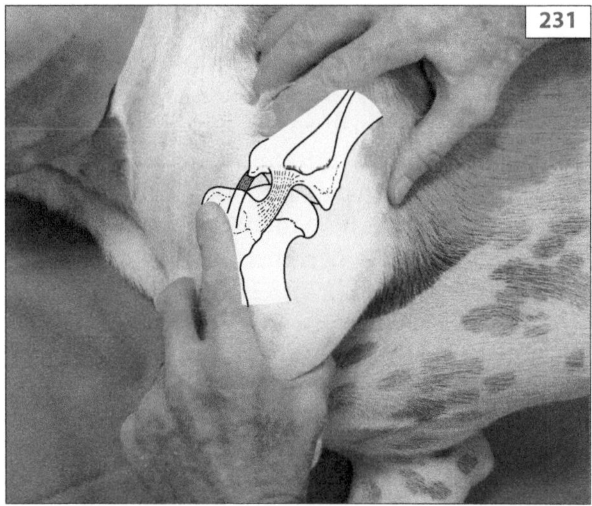

Fig. 231 Examination of the shoulder joint with superimposed arthrology. A 'drawer manipulation' of the shoulder joint should be part of the examination, as well as palpation of the biceps tendon (red) from its origin on the supraglenoid tubercle of the scapula through the intertubercular groove of the humerus.

Spine
Intervertebral disk disease and lumbosacral disease commonly lead to limb dysfunction. Therefore, examination of the patient's spine should be part of a musculoskeletal/neurologic examination. Deep palpation of the paravertebral musculature with the patient in extension of the spine often reveals peripheral neuropathies and spinal pathology (**Fig. 232**). DJD of the spinal articular facets is not uncommon in vertebral disk disease and instability. Further, clinical presentation of distal spinal disease can mimic the pain associated with hip dysplasia.

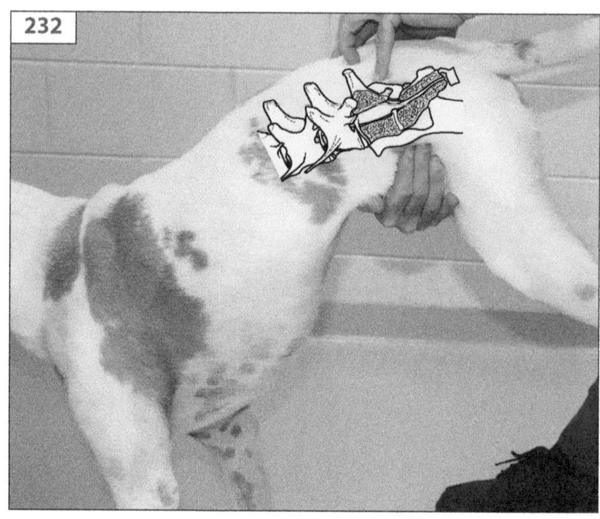

Fig. 232 Lumbosacral (or intervertebral disk) disease can often manifest as hip or limb disease; therefore, palpation of the spine should be included as part of an orthopedic examination.

Rear limb examination
In the *growing dog*, rear limb lameness differentials, most of which reflect abnormal stressors on normal bone or normal stressors on abnormal bone (excluding fractures and minor soft tissue injuries) and include:
- Hip dysplasia.
- Avascular necrosis: femoral head (Legg–Calvé–Perthes)*.
- OCD: stifle.
- Luxating patella complex.
- Genu valgum (knock knee).
- OCD: hock.
- Avulson of long digital extensor*.
- Panosteitis*.
- Hypertrophic osteodystrophy*.

(* Denote pathology/disease conditions which are not considered OA, but often manifest similar clinical presentations.)

Adult dog hind limb lameness differentials, mostly reflect abnormal stressors on normal bone or normal stressors on abnormal bone (excluding fractures and minor soft tissue injuries) and include:
- Arthritis.
- Hip dysplasia.
- OCD: stifle.
- Cruciate/meniscal syndrome.
- Luxating patella complex.
- Genu valgum.
- Avulsion of long digital extensor*.
- Luxation of superficial digital flexor tendon*.
- Inflammatory arthritis.
- Neoplasia*.

(* Denote pathology/disease conditions which are not considered OA, but often manifest similar clinical presentations.)

As with the forelimb, the rear limb can be divided into anatomic regions: paw, tarsus, tibia/fibula, stifle or knee, femur, hip, and pelvis. Cranial cruciate ligament compromise of the stifle and hip dysplasia constitute two of the most common DJD conditions causing pain/lameness in the dog.

Paw
Examination of the rear paws is similar to examination of the front paws. Each individual digit, including the nail and nail bed, should be assessed.

Tarsus
The tarsocrural joint accounts for ROM in flexion and extension (**Fig. 233**, **234**). Popping of the joint, palpated during ROM assessment, may be associated with displacement of the superficial digital flexor tendon following retinaculum tearing. This condition can lead to hyperflexion of the tarsus and digits. Damage to the common

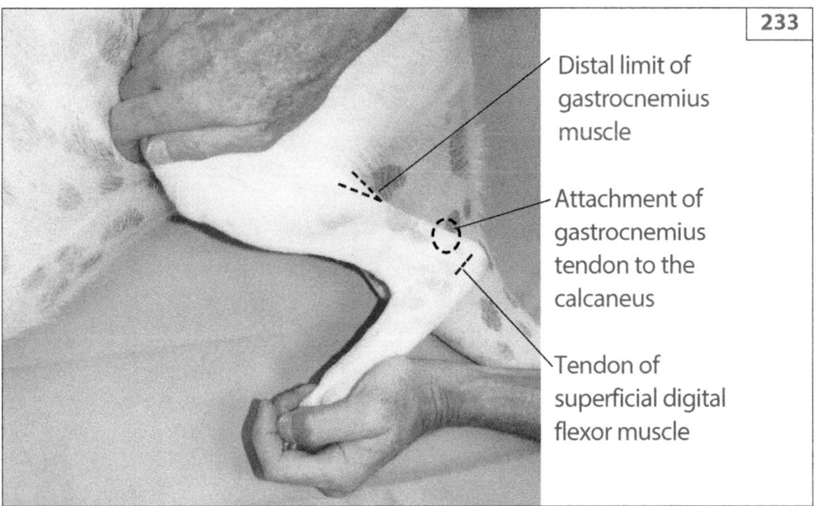

Fig. 233 Examination of the tibiotarsal (hock) joint in flexion. Compromise of the gastrocnemius tendon and superficial digital flexor muscle tendon are best identified with this joint in flexion.

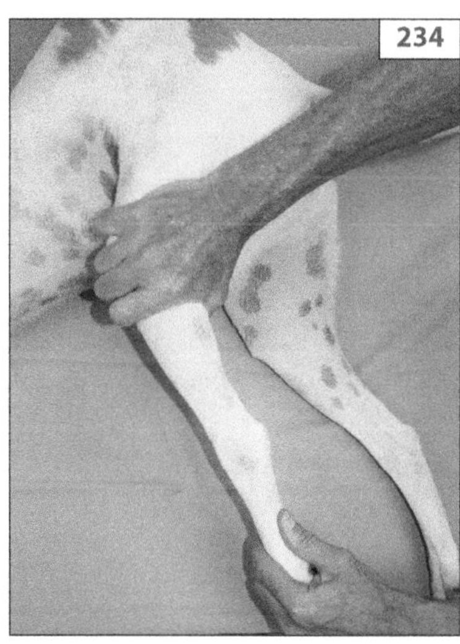

Fig. 234 Examination of the tibiotarsal joint in extension. Examination of this joint should include palpation of the joint capsule, looking for distension.

calcaneal tendon can also lead to tarsal hyperflexion. Assessing this tendon from its insertion on the calcaneus, proximally to the gastrocnemius muscles, should be performed with a clinical presentation of hyperflexion.

The tarsocrural joint can also show instability resulting from trauma. Placing the joint in both varus and valgus stress evaluates the collateral ligaments that maintain the structural integrity of this hinge joint. The tarsocrural joint is also predisposed in some breeds to OCD (both the medial and lateral ridges of the talus). OCD is often accompanied by distention of the joint capsule, palpable on the dorsal as well as the caudomedial and caudolateral joint surfaces.

Tibia and fibula

The medial aspect of the tibia has little soft tissue cover, making the identification of osseous abnormalities relatively easy during palpation. Deep palpation is required on the lateral aspect of the tibia and fibula, where there is considerable proximal muscle mass. Lameness and pain of the tibia and fibula (not considered OA) can arise from:

- Panosteitis.
- Hypertrophic osteodystrophy.
- Physeal fractures (possibly, with associated limb deformity).
- Physeal disturbances.
- Neoplasia.
- Limb deformity (often associated with patella luxation) (which can contribute to OA).
- Fractures.

Stifle

Examination of the stifle is most informative when performed both in the standing and laterally recumbent positions. Both stifles are examined simultaneously by approaching the standing patient caudally and wrapping your fingers from lateral to medial around the patellae. This allows comparison of one limb to the other and easier determination of the presence of a 'medial buttress – a firm swelling medial to the joint, often associated with long-standing cruciate disease. In this same position of examination, both patellae can be manipulated, assessing for luxation (**Fig. 235**). An attempt should be made to luxate each patella through a range of stifle flexion and extension. Most luxating patellae are apparent in extension. Paradoxically, the most severe patella luxations can be the most difficult to detect, because severe (Grade IV) luxations are commonly associated with fibrosis of the patella outside the trochlear groove, giving the false impression that the patella is properly seated because it cannot be displaced. In these cases, the patella may be located by finding the tibial tuberosity, and palpating proximally along the patella ligament until the patella is located. The trochlear groove (if one is present in such cases) may be palpated in the central region of the distal femur and compared with the position of the patella to confirm that it is ectopic.

Osteosarcoma is a common tumor type found in the rear limb, most frequently in the distal femur or proximal tibia. Stretching of the periosteum by expansile tumors sensitizes the periosteum to a painful response with deep palpation.

Examination of the stifle in lateral recumbency begins with assessment of ROM, noting the patient's response to pain. Clicking or popping during this manipulation may indicate meniscal pathology. Assessment of cruciate ligament integrity is made by the cranial tibial thrust maneuver and/or a cranial drawer test (**Figs. 236–238**).

Disease conditions of the stifle include:

- Cruciate ligament disease.
- Meniscal disease.
- Patella luxation.
- OCD.
- Collateral ligament injury.
- Stifle luxation.
- Long digital extensor tendon injury (not associated with OA).

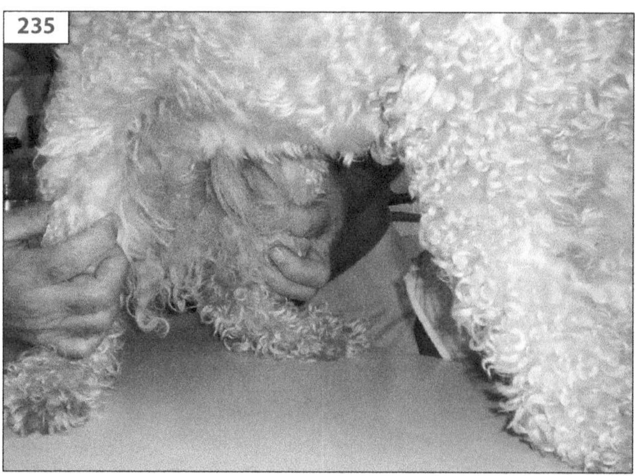

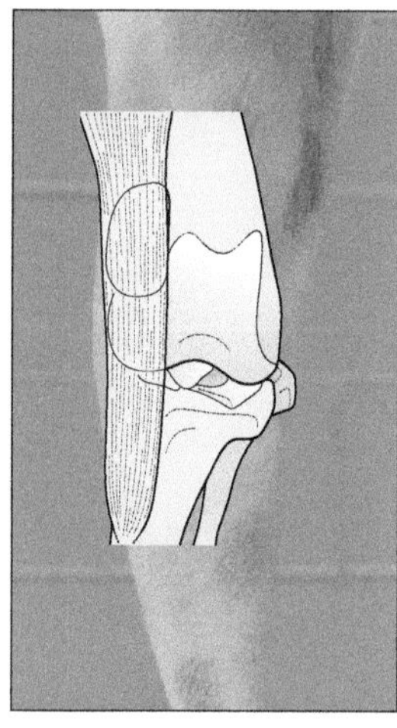

Fig. 235 Bilateral patella assessment should be conducted on each patient, especially small breed dogs. In the more pronounced presentation of medial luxated patella (Grade IV), the patella permanently resides medial to the distal, medial trochlear ridge of the femur. This is often accompanied by a medial rotation of the tibia.

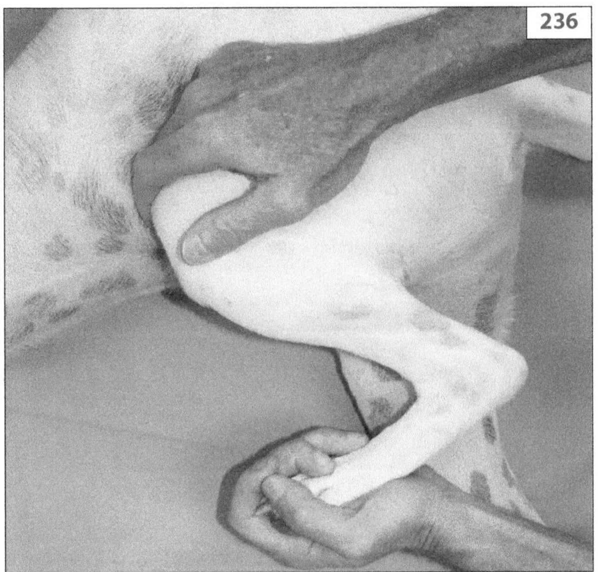

Fig. 236 Examination of the stifle includes range of motion assessment with flexion and extension. During this manipulation the 'tibial thrust' manipulation can be performed to further examine the cranial cruciate ligament. For this test, the index finger of one hand is extended from the patella along the patella tendon to the tibial crest. With the other hand, the hock is flexed until tension of the common calcanean tendon is achieved. If the cranial cruciate ligament is ruptured, the tensed gastrocnemius muscle pushes the tibia forward in relation to the femur, which is palpable by movement of the index finger along the patella tendon.

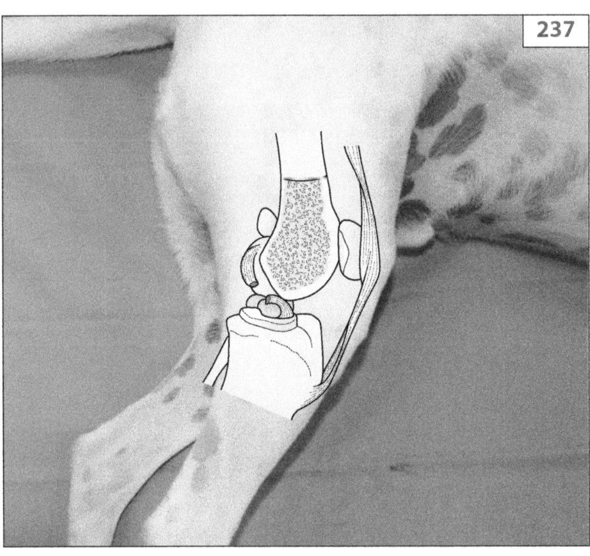

Fig. 237 Anterior cruciate ligament rupture is a common injury to the stifle. Several specific diagnostics help to identify this condition: the 'tibial thrust' manipulation, a firm swelling in the region of the medial collateral stifle ligament, termed 'medial buttress', and the 'drawer' test.

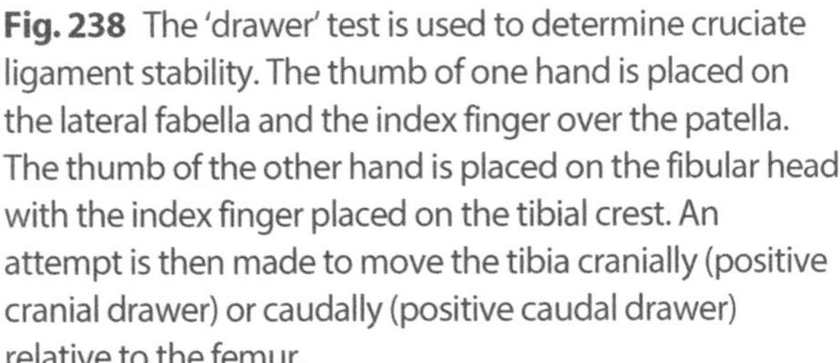

Fig. 238 The 'drawer' test is used to determine cruciate ligament stability. The thumb of one hand is placed on the lateral fabella and the index finger over the patella. The thumb of the other hand is placed on the fibular head with the index finger placed on the tibial crest. An attempt is then made to move the tibia cranially (positive cranial drawer) or caudally (positive caudal drawer) relative to the femur.

§ This insert is a medial view of the joint, yet demonstrates proper hand placement for 'drawer' testing.

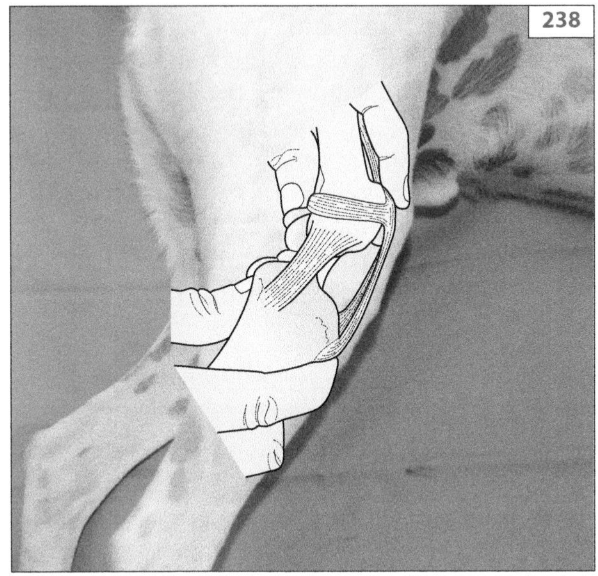

Femur

Palpation along the length of the femur should be performed, searching for swelling and pain. Pathologic conditions of the femur not associated with OA may include:

- Hypertrophic osteopathy.
- Hypertrophic osteodystrophy.
- Panosteitis.
- Neoplasia.
- Fracture.
- Limb deformity (often associated with patella luxation).

Hip

The hip is a common source of pain, especially in older dogs (**Figs. 239**, **240**). Hip dysplasia is a prevalent musculoskeletal disease, particularly in large breeds, and tends to manifest with pain in a biphasic pattern: near skeletal maturity and when the animal enters its 'senior years' (**Fig. 241**).

The most revealing examination technique for hip dysplasia in young dogs is the Ortolani examination, which tests for laxity of the coxofemoral joint (**Fig. 242**). This is best performed under sedation or general anesthesia (so as to yield joint relaxation) with the patient in lateral or dorsal recumbency. The femur is forced in a dorsal, axial direction with one hand on the flexed stifle and the other hand over the hip/pelvis. In the presence of hip laxity, the hand over the pelvis will detect subluxation when the femoral head moves dorsal and lateral 'up and over' the acetabular rim. Maintaining the axial force, the femur is then slowly abducted (away from the midline), allowing the femoral head to once again reduce into the acetabulum. A palpable (and occasionally audible) 'clunk' is detected in the 'positive Ortolani maneuver', confirming coxofemoral laxity.

Digital rectal palpation might further be informative in animals showing signs of pelvic pain.

Other musculoskeletal conditions of the hip, exclusive of OA, include:

- Neoplasia.
- Fractures.
- Inflammatory arthropathies.
- Physeal fractures (e.g. capital physis in skeletally immature dogs).

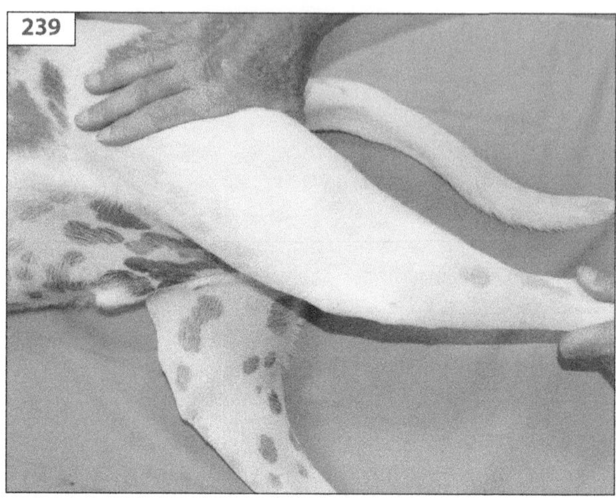

Fig. 239 Examination of the hip joint in extension.

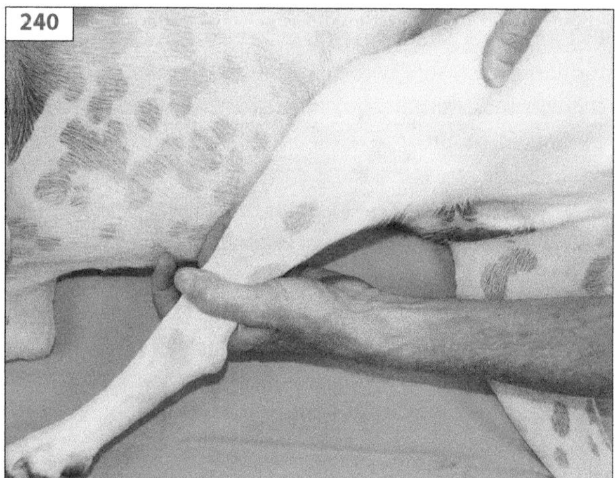

Fig. 240 Examination of the hip joint in flexion.

Tables 87 and *88 (overleaf)* present the normal ROM for canine and feline joints, respectively. Figure **243** shows the use of a goniometer for assessing ROM.

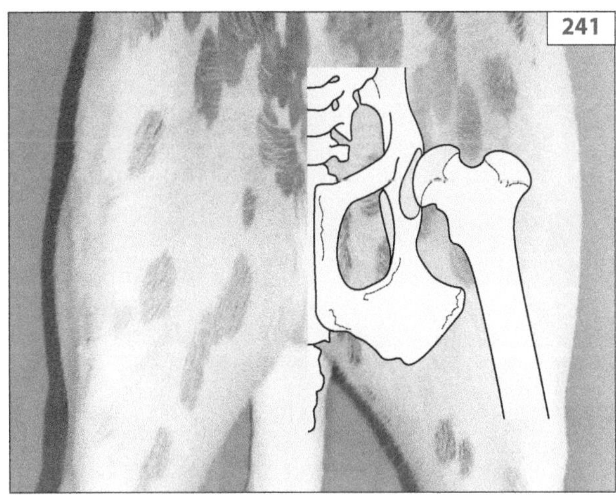

Fig. 241 Ventrodorsal radiographic positioning for assessment of hip dysplasia. The overlay demonstrates subluxation of the coxofemoral joint.

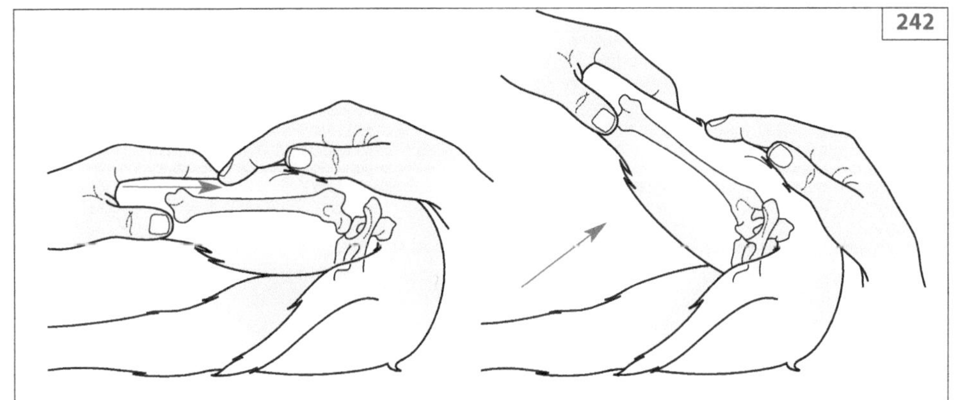

Fig. 242 A positive Ortolani sign is the most revealing diagnostic manipulation for hip dysplasia.

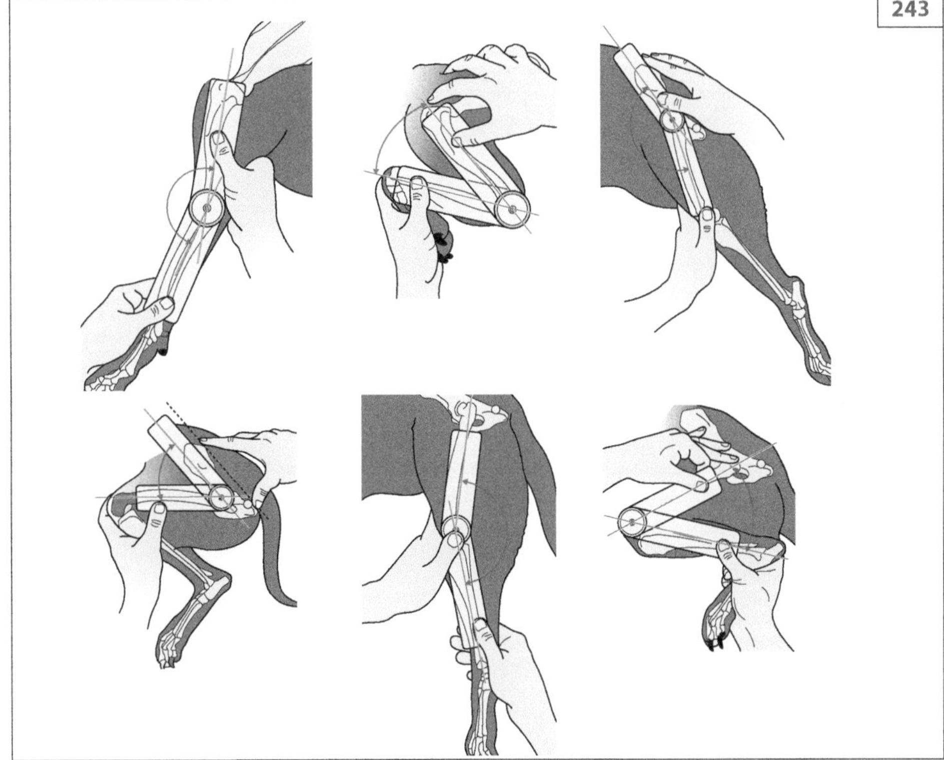

Fig. 243 Joint motion is assessed objectively by lining up the arms of a goniometer with specific anatomic landmarks, then flexing and extending individual joints: elbow, stifle, and hip.

TABLE 87: Normal range of motion for canine joints

Joint	Range of motion*
Shoulder (relative to the spine of the scapula)	Flexion to 57° Extension to 165°
Elbow (relative to the axis of the humerus)	Flexion to 36° Extension to 166°
Carpus (relative to the antebrachium)	Flexion to 32° Extension to 196°
Hip (relative to the axis of the pelvis)	Flexion to 50° Extension to 162°
Stifle (relative to the femur)	Flexion to 41° Extension to 162°
Tarsus (relative to the tibia with the stifle at 90°)	Flexion to 38° Extension to 165°

*These data should be used as a guide, interpreted together with the clinician's experience and comparison with the contralateral joint.
Data from Jaegger G, Marcellin-Little DJ, Levine D (2002)[6].

TABLE 88: Normal range of motion (ROM) for feline joints without sedation, during sedation, and on radiographic evaluation

		Angle measurement for ROM											
		Mean ± SD (°)			95% CI of the mean (°)			CV (%)			Median (°)		
Joint	Position	Non	Sed	Rad	Non	Sed	Rad	Non	Sed	Rad	Non	Sed	Rad
Carpal	Flex	22 ± 2	22 ± 1	21 ± 3	22–23	21–22	19–22	7	6	13	22	22	20
	Ext	198 ± 6	198 ± 5	197 ± 5	196–199	197–199	195–199	3	2	2	198	198	197
	Val	10 ± 2	11 ± 2	11 ± 1	9–10	10–11	11–12	23	19	12	10	10	11
	Var	7 ± 2	7 ± 2	7 ± 1	6–7	6–7	6–8	25	30	20	7	6	7
Elbow	Flex	22 ± 2	22 ± 1	23 ± 2	22–23	22–22	22–24	8	6	9	22	22	23
	Ext	163 ± 4	165 ± 3	167 ± 3	162–164	164–165	166–169	3	2	2	162	164	168
Shoulder	Flex	32 ± 3	32 ± 2	36 ± 6	31–32	31–32	34–39	8	8	16	32	32	36
	Ext	163 ± 6	167 ± 3	162 ± 4	162–165	167–168	160–163	4	2	2	164	168	163
Tarsal	Flex	21 ± 1	22 ± 1	19 ± 1	21–22	21–22	19–20	7	5	7	22	22	19
	Ext	167 ± 4	168 ± 2	169 ± 4	166–168	167–170	167–170	3	1	2	167	168	170
	Val	7 ± 2	7 ± 2	9 ± 3	7–8	7–8	8–11	32	22	32	7	7	8
	Var	10 ± 3	11 ± 3	12 ± 2	10–11	11–12	11–13	26	23	19	10	11	12
Stifile	Flex	24 ± 2	24 ± 3	21 ± 2	24–25	24–25	20–22	9	13	11	24	24	21
	Ext	164 ± 4	164 ± 3	159 ± 9	163–165	164–165	155–163	2	2	6	166	164	162
Hip	Flex	33 ± 3	33 ± 2	36 ± 4	32–33	32–33	34–38	9	7	11	32	33	36
	Ext	164 ± 4	166 ± 4	163 ± 4	163–165	165–167	161–164	2	2	3	164	166	164

CI: Confidence interval; CV: Coefficient of variation; Non: Nonsedated cats; Sed: Sedated cats; Rad: Radiographs; Flex: Flexion; Ext: Extension; Val: Valgus angulation; Var: Varus angulation.
Data from Jaeger GH, Marcellin-Little DJ, DePuy V, *et al.* (2007)[7].

CHARACTERISTICS AND DIAGNOSIS OF OSTEOARTHRITIS

Figs. 244 and **245** show the location of DJD characteristic changes. The diagnosis of OA is made using the methods presented in *Table 89*.

- Characterized by pain and lameness.
- Diagnosis:
  - Physical and orthopedic examination.
  - Radiographs.
  - Arthroscopy.
  - Diagnostic aids.
- Treatment goals:
  - Alleviate discomfort.
  - Retard disease development.
  - Restore near-normal function.
  - Minimize joint instabilities.

While an extremely useful modality, the radiological examination has the following limitations:

- Bony lesions take time to develop.
- Permanent cartilage damage precedes radiographic changes.
- Changes with septic arthritis take 14–17 days.
- Nonerosive immune-mediated arthropathies may show no bony lesions.
- Osteoarthritic changes may obscure neoplasia or infective changes.
- Severity of clinical signs cannot be predicted from radiographs.

Although the diagnosis of OA is not always obvious, especially in the early phases, the most consistent findings include altered activity, gait abnormalities, joint pain, joint effusion, and restricted joint ROM.

Examination of the cat

Examination of the cat is often more challenging than the dog, because cats generally resent being handled. Therefore, feline examination requires more patience and a general appreciation of subtle differences between the dog and cat. An excellent video of feline orthopedic examination conducted by Dr. Duncan Lascelles (North Carolina State University) can be accessed at the Nutramax Laboratories Inc. website: **http://www.nutramaxlabs.com/veterinary-continuing-education**

Access to this video is via registration; however, registration is free and available to licensed veterinarians, veterinary technicians, and students.

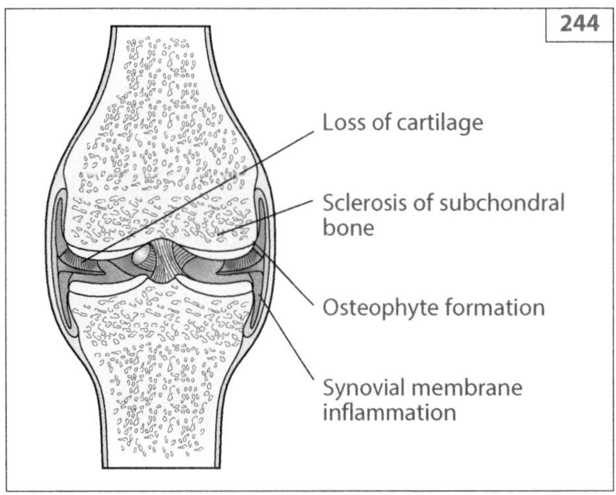

Fig. 244 Location of characteristic degenerative joint disease changes.

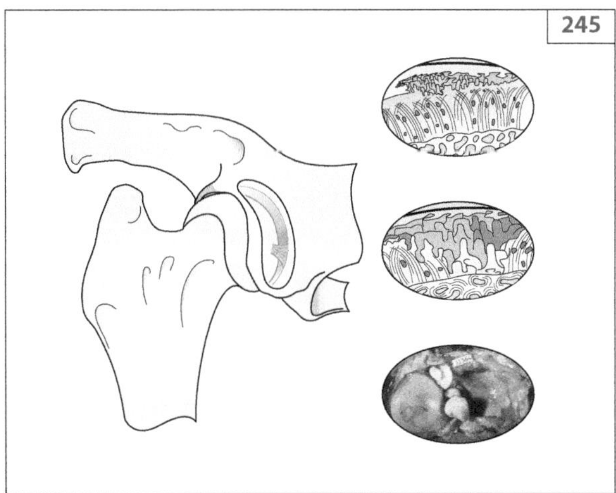

Fig. 245 Degenerative joint disease progresses (top to bottom) from fibrillation of the hyaline cartilage, to deep crevassing, to loss of hyaline cartilage and replacement with inferior (structure and function) fibrocartilage, or loss of fibrocartilage and eburnation of subchondral bone.

TABLE 89: Diagnosis of osteoarthritis

- History
- Distant observation:
  - Assess body conformation
  - Note decrease in weight bearing or altered limb motion
  - Observe for trembling while standing
  - Note asymmetrical joint or soft tissue swelling
  - Discern muscle atrophy
  - Notice digit and joint alignment
- Dogs with tarsocrural OCD tend to be straight legged
- Gait assessment:
  - Chronic lameness often 'disappears' in the exam room
  - Gait is observed at a walk and trot, if necessary
  - Observe ambulation on various surfaces, as well as on inclines and stairs
  - 'Covert lameness' may become apparent with tight circles or stair climbing
  - Gait abnormalities may include:
    - Shortened stride
    - Toe-in/toe-out
    - Stumbling
    - Audible click
    - Leg criss-crossing
    - Dragging toenails
    - Limb circumduction
    - Ataxia
    - Head bob
    - Asymmetrical pelvic motion
    - Weakness
    - Hypermetria
    - Vocalization
- Standing palpation:
  - Examine the contralateral limb simultaneously, looking for asymmetry from:
    - Trauma
    - Degenerative changes
    - Inflammation
    - Congenital defects
    - Neoplasia
  - Palpate for:
    - Swelling
    - Heat
    - Malalignment
    - Crepitus
    - Muscle atrophy
- Recumbent examination
- Diagnostic aids:
  - Arthroscopy
  - Diagnostic imaging:
    - Radiography
    - Fluoroscopy
    - Ultrasonography
    - Nuclear medicine
    - Computed tomography
    - Magnetic resonance imaging
  - Routine laboratory evaluation:
    - Hematology
    - Biochemical profile
    - Urinalysis
    - Arthrocentesis
    - Microbiologic examination
    - Serology

OCD: ostechondrosis dissecans.

Appendix 1

Analgesic Drugs and Premedicants

Various analgesic drugs and premedicants commonly used in the dog and cat are presented in Appendix 1 *Tables 1–7*. These drugs are often used together in multimodal protocols, where they are administered at lower doses.

TABLE 1: Analgesic drugs commonly used in the dog and cat

Opioid	Dose	Species	Route	Duration	Comments
Morphine	0.5–1.0 mg/kg	Canine	IM, SC, IV	3–4 h	Caution with IV administration: histamine release, give slowly
	0.05–0.1 mg/kg	Feline	IM, SC	3–4 h	
	0.2 mg/kg: loading, IM	Canine: 0.1–0.5 mg/kg/h Feline: 0.05–0.1 mg/kg/h	IM then CRI (IV)		
	0.1 mg/kg preservative-free	Canine/Feline	Epidural	12–24 h	
	1–5 mg in 5–10 ml saline	Canine	Intra-articular		
Meperidine	3–5 mg/kg	Canine/Feline	IM, SC	1–2 h	Do NOT give IV (histamine release)
Methadone	0.1–0.5 mg/kg	Canine/Feline	IM, SC, IV	2–4 h	NMDA antagonist activity
Oxymorphone	0.05–0.1 mg/kg 0.03–0.05 mg/kg	Canine Feline	IM, IV, SC IM, SC	3–4 h 3–4 h	Minimal histamine release
Hydromorphone	0.1–0.2 mg/kg	Canine/Feline	IM, IV, SC	2–4 h	Minimal histamine release Hyperthermia may be seen in cats
Fentanyl	5 µg/kg +3–6 µg/kg/h	Canine	IV	Infusion	
	2–3 µg/kg + 2–3 µg/kg/h	Feline	IV	Infusion	
Fentanyl patch	25 µg/h 50 µg/h 75 µg/h	Canine: 3–10 kg Canine: 10–20 kg Canine: 20–30 kg		1–3 days 1–3 days 1–3 days	24 h to reach peak concentrations

(continued)

TABLE 1: Analgesic drugs commonly used in the dog and cat (continued)

Opioid	Dose	Species	Route	Duration	Comments
	100 µg/h 25-50 µg/h	Canine: >30 kg Feline		1–3 days ≤6 days	 6 h to reach peak concentrations
Butorphanol	0.1–0.2 mg/kg	Canine/Feline	IM, IV, SC	1 h: dog, 2–4 h: cat	Low oral bioavailability
(10 mg/ml)	0.2–0.4 mg/kg IV; then 0.1–0.2 mg/kg/h	Canine/Feline	CRI		
Pentazocine	1–3 mg/kg	Canine/Feline	IM, IV, SC	2–4 h	
Nalbuphine	0.03–0.1 mg/kg	Canine/Feline	IM, IV, SC	2–4 h	
Buprenorphine	10–30 µg/kg	Canine/Feline	IM, IV, SC	4–10 h	15–30 min onset Excellent buccal mucosa absorption in cats and dogs
Tramadol	2–10 mg/kg	Canine	PO	12–24 h	Nonscheduled Mu-agonist activity Serotonin and norepinephrine reuptake inhibitor
	5 mg/kg (suggested)	Feline	PO		NMDA antagonist at lower doses, GABA receptor inhibitor at high concentrations
Codeine	1–2 mg/kg	Canine	PO		
α_2-agonist					
Medetomidine/ Dex-medetomidine	2–15 µg/kg	Canine	IM, IV	0.5–1.5 h	Sedation, bradycardia, vomition
	5–20 µg/kg 1.0 mg/ml, 1 µg/kg IV, then 1–2 µg/kg/h 1–5 µg/kg 2–5 µg/kg	Feline Canine/Feline Canine/Feline Canine/Feline	IM, IV CRI Epidural IA	0.5–1.5 h	
Xylazine	0.1–0.5 µg/kg	Canine/Feline	IM, IV	0.5–1.0 h	
(antagonist) yohimbine	0.1 mg/kg IV; 0.3–0.5 mg/kg IM	Canine/Feline			
(antagonist) atipamezol	0.05–0.2 mg/kg IV	Canine/Feline			2–4 times the medetomidine dose
NMDA antagonist					
Ketamine	0.5 mg/kg; IV then 0.1–0.5 mg/kg/h	Canine/Feline	CRI		
Amantadine	3–5 mg/kg	Canine/Feline	PO	24 h	Neuropathic pain
Dextromethorphan	0.5–2 mg/kg	Canine	PO, SC, IV		D-isomer of codeine; weak NMDA antagonist NOT RECOMMENDED due to side-effects
Methadone	0.1–0.5 mg/kg	Canine/Feline	IM, SC	2–4 h	Opioid derivative
Tricyclic antidepressant					
Amitriptyline	1.0 mg/kg 0.5–1.0 mg/kg	Canine Feline	PO PO	12–24 h 12–24 h	Enhanced noradrenergic activity
Ca^{++} channel modulator					
Gabapentin	5–10 mg/kg	Canine/Feline	PO	12–24 h	VDCC

TABLE 1: Analgesic drugs commonly used in the dog and cat (continued)

Opioid	Dose	Species	Route	Duration	Comments
adjunct					
Acepromazine	0.025–0.05 mg/kg	Canine	IM, SC, IV	8–12 h	3 mg maximum total dose; used to potentiate or prolong analgesic drug effect
	0.05–0.2 mg/kg	Feline	IM, SC	8–12 h	
Diazepam	0.1–0.2 mg/kg	Canine/Feline	IV	2–4 h	Used to potentiate or prolong analgesic drug effect
	0.25–1.0 mg/kg	Canine/Feline	PO	12–24 h	
Local anesthetics					
Lidocaine (1–2%)	≤6.0 mg/kg	Canine	Perineural	1–2 h	Onset: 10–15 min Maximum dose: 12 mg/kg (canine); 6 mg/kg (feline)
	≤3.0 mg/kg	Feline	Perineural	1–2 h	
	2–4 mg/kg IV, then 25–80 µg/kg/min	Canine	IV: CRI		
	0.25–0.75 mg/kg slow IV, then 10–40 µg/kg/min	Feline	IV: CRI		NOTE: efficacy and safety are not yet convincing
Bupivacain	0.25–0.5% ≤ 2.0 mg/kg	Canine	Perineural	2–6 h	Onset: 20-30 min. Maximum dose: 2 mg/kg (canine or feline)
	≤1.0 mg/kg	Feline	Perineural	2–6 h	
Mepivacaine (1–2%)	≤6.0 mg/kg	Canine	Perineural	2–2.5 h	
	≤3.0 mg/kg	Feline	Perineural	2–2.5 h	

CRI: constant rate infusion; GABA: γ-aminobutyric acid; NMDA; N-methyl-D-aspartate; VDCC: voltage-dependent Ca^{++} channel inhibitor.

TABLE 2: Premedicants commonly used in dogs and cat

Class	Agent	Dog dose	Cat dose	Comments
Anticholinergic				
	Atropine	0.02–0.04 mg/kg IV, SC, IM	Same	
	Glycopyrrolate	0 005–0.011 mg/kg IV, SC, IM	Same	
α_2-agonists				
	Medetomidine	0.001–0.010 mg/kg IM, IV, SC	Same	Lower dose when used with an opioid and half dose postoperatively as anxiolytic
	Dexmedetomidine			Same volume, but half the dose of medetomidine
NMDA receptor antagonist				
	Ketamine	CRI	5 mg/kg IV	
			CRI	1–2 mg/kg IV, IM or 0.5 mg/kgIV, followed by 2–10 μg/kg/min IV
NSAID				
	Carprofen	1–2 mg/kg or 4 mg/kg SC or PO daily		

(continued)

TABLE 3: USA FDA approved NSAIDs with product details

	Deramaxx®	Rimadyl ®	Previcox®	Metacam®
Company	Novartis	Pfizer	Merial	Boehringer-Ingelheim
Active Ingredient	Deracoxib	Carprofen	Firocoxib	Meloxicam
Formulation	25 mg, 75 mg, 100 mg scored chewable tablets	Caplets/chewable tablets: 25, 75, 100 mg scored caplets or scored chewable tablets SC injectable: 50 mg carprofen/ml	Chewable tablets containing 57 or 227 mg palatability 68%	Liquid suspension: to be squirted on food Injectable: 5 mg/ml, SC or IV
Dosage	For the control of pain and inflammation associated with orthopedic surgery in dogs: 3–4 mg/kg Give prior to surgery for postoperative pain For the control of pain and inflammation associated with OA in dogs: 1–2 mg/kg daily	Oral and injectable: 4.4 mg/kg daily; may be administered once daily or divided as 2.2 mg/kg twice daily For postoperative pain, administer 2 h before the procedure	5 mg/kg oral once daily Tablets are scored and dosage should be calculated in ½ tablet increments	0.2 mg/kg injectable once or oral once; followed by 0.1 mg/kg oral suspension daily Cats: 0.3 mg/kg presurgical one-time dose (contraindicated to follow in cats w/another NSAID or Metacam)
Indications	For the control of pain and inflammation associated with orthopedic surgery in dogs weighing ≤4 lb (1.8kg) For the control of pain and inflammation associated with OA	For the relief of pain and inflammation associated with OA in dogs and the control of postoperative pain in soft tissue and orthopedic surgeries in dogs	For the control of pain and inflammation associated with OA in dogs	Control of pain and inflammation associated with OA in dogs; postoperative pain and inflammation associated with orthopedic surgery, ovariohysterectomy, and castration in cats

TABLE 2: Premedicants commonly used in dogs and cat (continued)

Class	Agent	Dog dose	Cat dose	Comments
	Deracoxib	1–2 mg/kg daily		Note: this is below the labeled perioperative dose
	Meloxicam		0.2 mg/kg SC	Single dose
Opioids				
μ-agonist	Morphine	0.4–1 mg/kg IM, SC	0.05–0.2 mg/kg IM, SC	
	Oxymorphone	0.05–0.1 mg/kg IM, SC, IV	0.05 mg/kg IM, IV, SC	
	Hydromorphone	0.1–0.2 mg/kg IM, IV, SC	0.05–0.1 mg/kg IM, IV, SC	
	Fentanyl	2–5 μg/kg IM, IV, SC	1–2 μg/kg IM, IV, SC	
	Transdermal	4 μg/kg/h	4 μg/kg/h	
	CRI	0.002 mg/kg IV loading; then, 0.001–0.006 mg/kg/h IV infusion	0.001–0.002mg/kg IV loading; then, 0.001–0.004mg/kg/h IV infusion	
Tranquilizers				
	Acepromazine	0.025–0.05 mg/kg SC, IV, IM	Same	Do not exceed 1 mg
	Midazolam	0.2 mg/kg SC, IV, IM	Same	
	Diazepam	0.2 mg/kg IV, IM		

CRI: constant rate infusion; NMDA: N-methyl-D-aspartate; NSAID: nonsteroidal anti-inflammatory drug.

EtoGesic®	Zubrin®	Trocoxil®	Onsior®
Fort Dodge	Schering-Plough	Pfizer	Novartis
Etodolac	Tepoxalin	Mavacoxib	Robenacoxib
150 mg, 300 mg scored tablets	Rapidly-disintegrating tablets of 30, 50, 100, or 200 mg	6, 20, 30, 75 and 95 mg chewable, triangular shaped tablets	Dog: 5, 10, 20, 40 mg tablet (EU: injectable; 20 mg/ml) Cat: 6 mg tablet with NA on one side and AK on the other side (EU: injectable; 20 mg/ml)
10–15 mg/kg once daily (4.5–6.8 mg/lb) Adjust dose until a satisfactory clinical response is obtained reduced to minimum effective dose	10 mg/kg orally or 20 mg/kg on the initial day of treatment, followed by a daily maintenance dose of 10 mg/kg	MONTHLY TREATMENT: initial dose (2 mg/kg), repeated 14 days later, and then monthly dosing for up to a maximum of seven consecutive doses	Dog: 1 mg/kg *sid* Cat: 1 mg/kg *sid* for **maximum of 6 days (EU: 2 mg/kg SC injection both dog and cat)**
For the management of pain and inflammation associated with OA in dogs	Control of pain and inflammation associated with OA in dogs	For the treatment of pain and inflammation in dogs aged 12 months or more associated with degenerative joint disease in dogs in cases where continuous treatment exceeding 1 month is indicated	USA (cat): postoperative pain and inflammation with orthopedic symptoms, ovariohysterectomy, and castration daily for ≤3 days EU (cat): acute pain and inflammation of musculoskeletal disorders EU (dog): pain and inflammation of chronic OA

(continued)

TABLE 3: USA FDA approved NSAIDs with product details (continued)

	Deramaxx®	**Rimadyl ®**	**Previcox®**	**Metacam®**
	For the control of canine postoperative dental pain			when administered prior to surgery
Mechanism of action (MOA)	A coxib class drug that uniquely targets COX-2 while sparing COX-1	Inhibition of COX enzyme; *in vitro* selective against COX-2	Inhibition of COX activity; *in vitro* studies show it to be highly selective for COX-2 in canine blood	MOA not on label; oxicam class NSAID
Maximum concentration (T_{max})	2 h	Oral: C_{max} of 16.9 µg/ml at 0.5–3 h Injectable: C_{max} of 8.0 µg/ml at 1.5–8 h		Dogs: 2.5 h (inj) and 7.5 h (oral) Cats: 1.5 h postinjection
Half-life ($T_{1/2}$)	3 h	8 h in dog	7.8 h	Dogs: 24 h Cats: 15 h after injection
Metabolism and excretion	Metabolism primarily liver; excretion to GI to feces is 75%, urine excretion is 20%	Liver biotransformation 70-80% in feces and 10–20% in urine Some enterohepatic circulation	Primarily hepatic metabolism and fecal excretion	Not on label
Side-effects within licensing studies Serious adverse reactions associated with this drug class can occur without warning and in rare situations result in death	Vomiting, incisional lesions	Black or tarry stools, hypoalbuminemia, dermatologic changes, increased liver enzyme levels, idiosyncratic hepatotoxicosis	Vomiting, diarrhea, decreased appetite (Use of this product at doses above the recommended 5 mg/kg in puppies less than 7 months of age has been associated with serious adverse events, including death)	Vomiting, soft stools, diarrhea, inappetance, epiphora, autoimmune hemolytic anemia, thrombocytopenia, polyarthritis, pyoderma
Packaging	30 count, 90 count	14, 60, 150 count 20 ml bottle of injectable	10 and 30 count blister packs, 60 count bottles	Oral: 1.5 mg/ml: 10, 32 and 100 ml dropper bottles Inj: 5 mg/ml in a 10 ml vial
Marketing status	By prescription only	By prescription only	By prescription only	By prescription only
Protein binding	>90%	>99%	>96%	>99%
Bio-availability	>90%	>90%	38%	Nearly 100%
Concurrent use statement	Concomitant use with any other anti-inflammatory drugs, such as other NSAIDs and corticosteroids, should be avoided or closely monitored	Concomitant use with any other anti-inflammatory drugs, such as other NSAIDs and corticosteroids, should be avoided or closely monitored	Concomitant use with any other anti-inflammatory drugs, such as other NSAIDs and corticosteroids, should be avoided or closely monitored	Concurrent use with potentially nephrotoxic drugs should be carefully approached Concomitant use with other anti-inflammatory drugs, such as NSAIDs and corticosteroids, should be avoided or closely monitored

EtoGesic®	Zubrin®	Trocoxil®	Onsior®
Inhibition of COX activity; inhibits macrophage chemotaxis	COX and LOX inhibitor: 'dual pathway inhibitor of AA metabolism'	A coxib-class NSAID that targets COX-2, while sparing COX-1	A coxib-class NSAID that targets COX-2, while sparing COX-1
1.08–1.6 h	2.3 ± 1.4 h	Increases with exposure (days 1–7)	Dog: <1 h Cat: 1 h
7.6–12 h	2.0 ± 1.2 h Converts to active metabolite with long $T_{1/2}$	16.6 days (range: 7.9–38.8)	Dog: 1.2 h Cat: 1.7 h
Primarily hepatic metabolism and fecal excretion; enterohepatic recirculation	Primarily hepatic with excretion through feces 99%, minor urine	Liver metabolism and excreted primarily in feces	Mainly metabolized in the liver of both cat and dog, similar to its human analogue, lumiracoxib; primarily via oxidation and hydroxylation. Direct glucuronic acid conjugation is relatively minor
Weight loss, fecal abnormalities, hypoproteinemia, small intestine erosions	Vomiting, diarrhea, gastric lesions, decrease in total protein, albumin and calcium, death	Most common side-effects are loss of appetite, diarrhea and vomiting	Dogs: GI adverse events reported very commonly, recovering with treatment Cats: mild and transient diarrhea, soft feces, or vomiting commonly reported
7, 30, and 90 count	Boxes containing 10 foil blisters each	Carton boxes each contain one blister Each blister contains two tablets	Dog: cardboard box containing 1, 2, 4, or 10 blisters,7 tablets per blister Cats: cardboard box containing 1, 2, 5, or 10 blisters,6 tablets per blister
By prescription only	By prescription only	By prescription only	By prescription only
>99%	>98%	Approximately 98%	>99%
Nearly 100%		Approximately 50% when fasted; approximately 90% in fed conditions	Dog: 62% with food; 84% without food Cat: 49% without food
Concomitant use with any other anti-inflammatory drugs, such as other NSAIDs and corticosteroids, should be avoided or closely monitored	Concomitant use with any other anti-inflammatory drugs, such as other NSAIDs and corticosteroids, should be avoided or closely monitored	Concomitant treatments with corticosteroids, anesthetic/analgesic products and tranquilizers could potentially bias efficacy	Do not use concomitantly with corticosteroids or other NSAIDs

(continued)

TABLE 3: USA FDA approved NSAIDs with product details (continued)

	Deramaxx®	Rimadyl ®	Previcox®	Metacam®
Pre-prescription advisement	Thorough history and physical exam; appropriate laboratory tests	Thorough history and physical exam; appropriate laboratory tests	Thorough history and physical exam; appropriate laboratory tests	Thorough history and physical exam; appropriate laboratory tests
Miscellaneous			*In vitro*: showed more COX-2 inhibition than COX-1	Not evaluated for IM injection

AA: arachidonic acid; COX: cyclo-oxygenase; EU: European Union; FDA: Food and Drug Administration; GI: gastrointestinal; LOX: lipoxygenase; NSAID: nonsteroidal anti-inflammatory drug; OA: osteoarthritis.

TABLE 4: Nonsteroidal anti-inflammatory drug (NSAID) pharmacokinetic parameters and dose recommendations for dog and cat

	Dog			Cat				
NSAID	**Half-life (h)**	**Dose/route**	**Ref.**	**Half-life (h)**	**Dose/route**	**Ref.**	**Species difference?**	**Clearance mechanism/s**
Acetaminophen	1.2	100 mg/kg PO	a/b	0.6	20 mg/kg PO	a/b	Cat > dog	Glucuronidation and sulfation
	1.2	200 mg/kg PO	a	2.4	60 mg/kg PO	a		
				4.8	120 mg/kg PO	a		
Aspirin	7.5–12	25 mg/kg PO	b	22	20 mg/kg IV	cd	Cat > dog	Glucuronidation and glycination
Carprofen	5	25 mg PO	e	20	4 mg/kg IV	c	Cat > dog	Glucuronidation and oxidation
	8.6	25 mg *bid* PO 7 days	e	19	4 mg/kg SC, IV	f/g		
	7	25 mg SC	e					
	8.3	25 mg *bid* SC 7 day	e					
Flunixin	3.7	1.1 mg/kg IV	h	1–1.5	1 mg/kg PO, IV	i	Cat < dog	Glucuronidation and active transport
				6.6	2 mg/kg PO	j		
Ketoprofen	1.6 for S-ketoprofen	1 mg/kg PO racemic	k	1.5 for S-ketoprofen	2 mg/kg IV racemic	l	Cat = dog	Glucuronidation and thioesterification
				0.6 for R-ketoprofen	2 mg/kg IV racemic	l		

EtoGesic®	Zubrin®	Trocoxil®	Onsior®
Thorough history and physical exam; appropriate laboratory tests	Geriatric examination; appropriate laboratory tests	Thorough history and physical exam; appropriate laboratory tests Dogs with hepatic disorders should not be treated	Safety not established in cats weighing less than 2.5 kg or under 4 months of age Do not use in cats suffering from GI ulceration or in dogs with GI ulceration or with hepatic disease Safety not established in dogs weighing less than 2.5 kg or under 3 months of age
In vitro: showed more COX-2 inhibition than COX-1	Give with a meal to enhance absorption	May undergo enterohepatic recycling	Inadequate response to treatment was seen in 10–15% of dogs In cats: COX-1/COX-2 ratio = 502[58]

	Dog			Cat				
NSAID	Half-life (h)	Dose/route	Ref.	Half-life (h)	Dose/route	Ref.	Species difference?	Clearance mechanism/s
				0.9 for S-ketoprofen	1 mg/kg PO racemic	l		
				0.6 for R-ketoprofen	1 mg/kg PO racemic	l		
				0.5 for S-ketoprofen	1 mg/kg IV S-ketoprofen	m		
				0.5 for R-ketoprofen	1 mg/kg IV R-ketoprofen	m		
Mavacoxib	16.6 DAYS	2 mg/kg 1Qmo PO (7 dose max)	n	Not approved for cats				
Meloxicam	12 24	0.2 mg/kg PO 0.2 mg/kg PO, SC, IV	k o	15	0.3 mg/kg SC	Label	Cat < dog	Oxidation
Piroxicam	40	0.3 mg/kg PO, IV	p	12	0.3 mg/kg PO, IV	q	Cat < dog	Oxidation
Robenacoxib	1.2	1 mg/kg PO	r	1.7	1 mg/kg PO 6 days max **(EU: 2 mg/kg SC injection both dog and cat)**	s		Believed similar to its analogue lumiracoxib: oxidation and hydroxylation

Correlation to base dosing intervals is undetermined.

EU: European Union.

(continued)

TABLE 4: Nonsteroidal anti-inflammatory drug (NSAID) pharmacokinetic parameters and dose recommendations for dog and cat (continued)

References

a Court MH, Greenbelt DJ (2000). Molecular genetic basis for deficient acetaminophen glucuronidation by cats: UGT1A6 is a pseudogene, and evidence for reduced diversity of expressed hepatic UGT1A isoforms. *Pharmacogenetics* **10**:355–369[97].

b Savides M, Oohed F, Nash S, *et al.* (1984). The toxicity and biotransformation of single doses of acetaminophen in dogs and cats. *Toxicol Appl Pharm* **74**:26–34.

c Dittert LW, Caldwell HC, Ellison T, *et al.* (1968). Carbonate ester prodrugs of salicylic acid. Synthesis, solubility characteristics, *in vitro* enzymatic hydrolysis rates, and blood levels of total salicylate following oral administration to dogs. *J Pharm Sci* **57**:828–831.

d Parton K, Balmer TV, Boyle J, *et al.* (2002). The pharmacokinetics and effects of intravenously administered carprofen and salicylate on gastrointestinal mucosa and selected biochemical measurements in healthy cats. *J Vet Pharmacol Ther* **23**:73–79.

e Davis LE, Westfall BA (1972). Species differences in biotransformation and excretion of salicylate. *Am J Vet Res* **33**:1253–1262.

f Clark TR, Chief C, Huhn JC, *et al.* (2003). The steady-state pharmacokinetics and bioequivalence of carprofen administered orally and subcutaneously in dogs. *J Vet Pharmacol Ther* **26**:187–192[47].

g Taylor PM, Dilator P, Landoni FM, *et al.* (1996). Pharmacodynamics and enantioselectivity pharmacokinetics of carprofen in the cat. *Res Vet Sci* **60**:144–151.

h Hardie EM, Hardee GE, Rawlings CA (1985). Pharmacokinetics of fluxing meglumine in dogs. *Am J Vet Res* **46**:235–237.

i Lees P, Taylor PM (1991). Pharmacodynamics and pharmacokinetics of flunixin in the cat. *Br Vet J* **147**:298–305.

j Horii Y, Eking M, Shimmed M, *et al.* (2004). Pharmacokinetics of fluxing in the cat: enterohepatic circulation and active transport mechanism in the liver. *J Vet Pharmacol Ther* **27**:65–69.

k Montoya L, Ambros L, Krill V, *et al.* (2004). A pharmacokinetic comparison of meloxicam and ketoprofen following oral administration to healthy dogs. *Vet Res Commun* **28**:415–428.

l Lees P, Taylor PM, Landoni FM, *et al.* (2003). Ketoprofen in the cat: pharmacodynamics and chiral pharmacokinetics. *Vet J* **165**:21–35.

m Castro E, Source A, Fogel F, *et al.* (2000). Chiral inversion of R(-) fenoprofen and ketoprofen enantiomers in cats. *J Vet Pharmacol Ther* **23**:265–271.

n Cox SR, Lesman JF, Boucher MJ, *et al.* (2010). The pharmacokinetics of mavacoxib, a long-acting COX-2 inhibitor, in young adult laboratory dogs. *J Vet Pharmacol Ther* **33**(5):461–470[55].

o Busch U, Schmid J, Heinzel G, *et al.* (1998). Pharmacokinetics of meloxicam in animals and the relevance to humans. *Drug Metab Dispose* **26**:576–584.

p Galbraith EA, McKellar QA (1991). Pharmacokinetics and pharmacodynamics of piroxicam in dogs. *Vet Rec* **128**:561–565.

q Hebe HL, Chun R, Koch DE, *et al.* (2003). Single dose pharmacokinetics of piroxicam in cats. *J Vet Pharmacol Ther* **26**:259–263.

r Jung M, Lees P, Seaweed W, *et al.* (2009). Analytical determination and pharmacokinetics of robenacoxib in the dog. *J Vet Pharmacol Ther* **32**:41–48.

s Girdle J, King M, Jeunesse PC, *et al.* (2009). Use of a pharmacokinetic/pharmacodynamic approach in the cat to determine a dosage regimen for the COX-2 selective drug robenacoxib. *J Vet Pharmacol Ther* **32**:18–30.

TABLE 5: Analgesics commonly used for cancer pain in the dog

Drug	Dose (dog)	Remarks
Amantadine	1.0–4.0 mg/kg orally *sid**	Available as tablet and elixir NMDA-antagonist Effective as adjunct with other drug classes Higher doses can produce GI gas and loose stools Caution use with selegiline or sertraline until interactions further elucidated
Amitriptyline	0.5–2.0 mg/kg orally *sid**	Mode of action at (endogenous) descending serotonergic system Moderate to weak analgesic activity Often used as adjunct to NSAID Toxicity in the dog not evaluated

TABLE 5: Analgesics commonly used for cancer pain in the dog (continued)

Drug	Dose (dog)	Remarks
Aspirin	10 mg/kg orally *bid*	NOT approved for use in the dog; toxicities include: GI, renal, and bleeding Better NSAID choices available
Butorphanol	0.2–0.5 mg/kg orally (*sid–tid*)	Poor bioavailability PO Weak analgesic Possible sedation at higher doses May be used as adjunct to NSAID
Codeine	0.5–2.0 mg/kg orally *sid*	Best bioavailability (~20%) among oral opioids Possible sedation at higher doses
Carprofen	2 mg/kg orally *bid*, or 4 mg/kg orally *sid*	COX-2 preferential Available as injectable, but with inferior pharmacokinetics to the tablet
Deracoxib	1–2 mg/kg orally *sid* (extended use)	COX-2-selective coxib-class NSAID May be effective in altering the course of certain types of COX-2 dependent cancer
Etodolac	5–15 mg/kg orally *sid*	COX-1 selective in the dog Associated with canine keratoconjunctivitis sicca
Fentanyl (transdermal)	2–5 μg/kg/h	Short-term use Variable absorption – systemic levels Expensive
Firocoxib	5.0 mg/kg *sid*	COX-2-selective coxib-class NSAID Questionable safety in dogs <7 months old No data in cancer dogs
Gabapentin	3–10 mg/kg orally *sid–bid*	No analgesic data in dogs Anti-seizure effects Efficacy for neuropathic pain Rapidly metabolized in the dog Often used as adjunct with other analgesics
Glucosamine and chondroitin sulfate	Unestablished	Evidence-base is weak Often used as adjunct with other analgesics Product quality is widely variable
Lidocaine (transdermal patch)	One (10 × 14 cm) patch per 20 lb (9.1 kg)	Clinical efficacy and toxicity not determined Duration of effect approximately 3 days Plasma steady state at 12–60 h
Meloxicam	0.2 mg/kg on Day 1, then 0.1 mg/kg *sid*	Preferential COX-2 inhibitor Narrow safety profile Available as elixir and injectable only
Morphine (liquid)	0.2–0.5 mg/kg orally *tid–qid*	Poor bioavailability (<20%) Short duration of action Sedation and constipation may be seen at higher doses
Morphine (sustained release)	0.5–3.0 mg/kg orally *tid–qid*	Doses >0.5–1.0 mg/kg often reported to result in constipation
Pamidronate	1–1.5 mg/kg, diluted in 250 ml saline, slowly IV (Q 1 mo)*	Inhibits osteoclast activity as a bisphosphonate Effective where osteolysis from bone tumor contributes to pain

(*continued*)

TABLE 5: Analgesics commonly used for cancer pain in the dog (continued)

Drug	Dose (dog)	Remarks
Paracetamol (acetaminophen)	10–15 mg/kg orally *tid* for 5 days Long-term: <10 mg/kg *bid**	Lethal in cats Clinical toxicity not established in dogs Analgesic, but not anti-inflammatory
Piroxicam	0.3 mg/kg Q48 h*	Long-standing use as chemotherapeutic agent Narrow safety margin
Prednisolone	0.25–1 mg/kg orally *sid–bid*, taper to Q48 h after 14 days	DO NOT use concurrently with NSAID Most effective in cases with pronounced inflammation
Tepoxalin	10–20 mg/kg orally on Day 1, then 10 mg/kg *sid*	COX and LOX 'dual pathway inhibitor' No data in cancer patients
Tramadol	2–4 mg/kg orally *bid–qid**	Codeine analog Norepinephrine/serotonin reuptake inhibition No efficacy or toxicity data in dogs Often used as adjunct with other analgesics

* empirical dose, based on personal experiences: pending further investigations.
(None have been assessed for dosage or efficacy in cancer, therefore empirical doses and efficacy reflect dose recommendations for osteoarthritic pain. Not all drugs are licensed in all countries.)
COX: cyclo-oxygenase; GI: gastrointestinal; LOX: lipoxygenase; NMDA: N-methyl-D-aspartate; NSAID: nonsteroidal anti-inflammatory drug.

TABLE 6: Analgesics commonly used for cancer pain in the cat

Drug	Dose (cat)	Remarks
Amantadine	3.0 mg/kg orally *sid*	Toxicity studies not available in cats 100 mg capsules require recompounding for cats Often used as adjunct with other analgesics
Amitriptyline	0.5–2.0 mg/kg orally *sid*	Apparently well tolerated for up to 12 months with daily dosing Occasional (<10%) drowsiness Often used as adjunct with other analgesics
Aspirin	10 mg/kg orally Q48h	Associated with significant GI ulcerations
Buprenorphine	0.02 mg/kg transbuccal Q6–7 h	Same dose IV provides similar analgesia Readily accepted by the cat, therefore acceptable for home administration Anorexia may occur after 2–3 days
Butorphanol	0.2–1.0 mg/kg orally *qid*	Weak analgesic May be more effective in visceral pain Limited bioavailability and duration of effect when given orally

TABLE 6: Analgesics commonly used for cancer pain in the cat (continued)

Drug	Dose (cat)	Remarks
Carprofen	Undetermined	Insufficient data on extended use
Etodolac	Undetermined	Insufficient data on extended use
Fentanyl (transdermal patch)	2–5 μg/kg/h	Not suggested for cats <10 lb (4.5 kg) Do not cut or partial-cover patches
Flunixin meglamine	1mg/kg orally as a single dose	Insufficient data on extended use
Gabapentin	3–10 mg/kg orally *sid–bid*	No analgesic data in cats Anti-seizure effects Efficacy for neuropathic pain Rapidly metabolized in the cat Often used as adjunct with other analgesics
Glucosamine/chondroitin sulfate (CS) combinations	Unestablished: approximately 15 mg/kg CS orally *sid–bid*	Evidence base is weak Often used as adjunct with other analgesics Product quality is widely variable
Ketoprofen	1 mg/kg orally *sid* for a maximum of 5 days	Narrow safety range Possible use in 'pulse therapy' with a few 'rest' days between administrations
Lidocaine (transdermal patch)	One (10 × 14 cm) patch for 5–9.1 kg (11–20 lb) cat	Clinical efficacy and toxicity not determined Duration of effect approximately 3 days Plasma steady state at 12–60 hours
Meloxicam	0.2 mg/kg orally on Day 1, then 0.1 mg/kg orally *sid* for 4 days, then 0.05 mg/kg *sid* for 10 days, then 0.025 mg/kg *sid*	Extended use is off label Easy dosing as an elixir Honey base syrup is well accepted
Morphine (oral, liquid)	0.2–0.5 mg/kg orally *tid–qid*	Limited bioavailability and duration of effect Poor palatability
Morphine (oral, sustained release)	Tablets too large for cats	
Paracetamol (acetaminophen)	Contraindicated	Lethal in cats
Piroxicam	0.3 mg/kg *sid*; however many use up to 1 mg/kg orally *sid* for up to 7 days; every other day dosing suggested for long term	Decreased PCV in up to 30% of cats after 2–3 weeks of daily therapy Compounding may decrease drug activity
Prednisolone	0.25–0.5 mg/kg orally *sid*	DO NOT use concurrently with NSAID Most effective in cases with pronounced inflammation
Tolfenamic acid	4 mg/kg orally *sid* for a maximum of 3 days	Not licensed in many countries
Tramadol	4 mg/kg *bid*	Toxicity data not available in cats

(None have been assessed for dosage or efficacy in cancer, therefore empirical doses and efficacy reflect dose recommendations for other painful conditions, and experience of the authors. Not all drugs are licensed in all countries.)

GI: gastrointestinal; NSAID: nonsteroidal anti-inflammatory drug; PVC: packed cell volume.

TABLE 7: Common analgesics used in the USA

Pharmaceutical	USA Trade name
Acetaminophen + codeine	Tylenol
Alendronate	Fosamax
Amtrak	Mitaban, preventic collar
Bupivacaine – extended-release liposome injection formulation	Exparel
Capsaicin 8% patch	Qutenza
Carprofen	Rimadyl
Cimetidine	Tagamet
Clomipramine	Clomicalm
Deracoxib	Deramax
Dexmedetomidine	Dexdomitor
Dirlotapide	Slentrol
Duloxetine	Cymbalta
Esomeprazole	Nexium
Firocoxib	Previcox
Fluoxetine	Reconcile
S-ketamine	Ketanest S
Lamotrigine	Lamicital
Lansoprazole	PrevAcid
Lidocaine patch	Lidoderm
Mavacoxib	Trocoxil
Meloxicam	Metacam
Meloxicam oral spray	OroCAM
Meperidine (pethidine)	Demerol
Misoprostol	Cytotec
Omeprazole	Prilosec
Oxycodone HCl + acetaminophen	Percocet
Pantoprazole	Protonix
Paracetamol + hydrocodone	Vicodin
Phycocyanin	PhyCox
Rabeprazole	AcipHex
Robenacoxib	Onsior
Selegiline	Anipryl
Tapentadol	Nucynta
Tepoxalin	Zubrin
Tramadol + acetaminophen	Ultracet
Xylazine	Rompun

(See also *Tables 28, 55, 56, 69*)

Appendix 2

Case Examples of Multimodal Management

Signalment: 'Sara', a 6-year-old, female spayed, 96 lb (43.6 kg), Labrador Retriever, body conditioning score 4/5.

History/Presentation: diagnosed at 9 mos of age with bilateral hip dysplasia. At 19 mos of age and weight of 100 lb (45.5 kg), Sara underwent surgical repair of a right cranial cruciate ligament rupture. Two years later, a left cranial cruciate ligament rupture was surgically repaired. Following each cruciate rupture surgery a different nonsteroidal anti-inflammatory drug (NSAID) was administered at a 'high-end' dose, but with decreasing efficacy as time progressed. Upon commencing the multimodal protocol, Sara's blood chemistries and urine profiles were unremarkable. Physical examination revealed no abnormalities other than confirmed chronic stifle degenerative joint disease (DJD) and suspected multifocal DJD.

Treatment protocol–implemented simultaneously:

- Regular, controlled, personalized home exercise program: warm towel application and massage; passive range of motion (ROM); slow leash walks, with inclines and declines; sit-to-stand, and balance exercises.
- High eicosapentaenoic acid (EPA) diet only: 2 cups (16 oz [450 g]) (maximum) of dry Hills' J/D diet per day.
- Eight dose protocol (label) of polysulfated glycosaminoglycan (Adequan® Canine).
- Daily NSAID administration: 100 mg deracoxib.

Results:

1. Over the course of 11 weeks, Sara lost approximately 7 lb (3 kg) (**Fig. 246**).

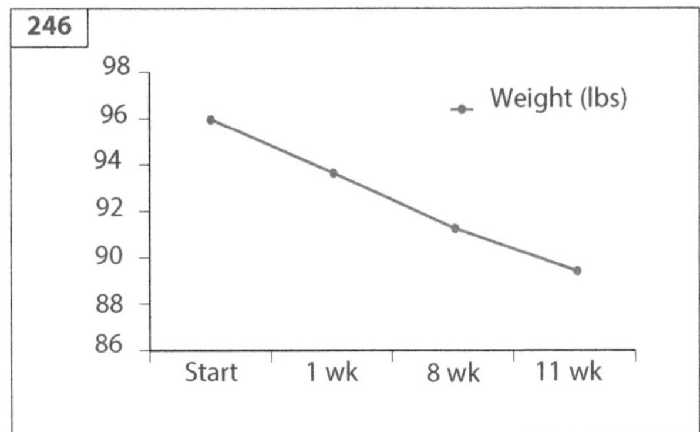

Fig. 246 Weight change with multimodal protocol.

2. Range of motion (ROM) was improved in 79% of the joints, as assessed by goniometer.

Hindlimb	Normal ROM*	Start Left	Start Right	At 11 weeks Left	At 11 weeks Right	Change Left	Change Right
Hip							
Flexion	55°	50	50	60	60	10	10
Extension	160–165°	135	150	160	150	25	NC
Stifle							
Flexion	45°	40	50	60	60	20	10
Extension	160–170°	140	135	160	145	20	10
Tarsus							
Flexion	40°	30	60	45	60	15	NC
Extension	170°	165	160	165	165	NC	5
Forelimb	**Normal ROM**	**Left**	**Right**	**Left**	**Right**	**Left**	**Right**
Shoulder							
Flexion	30–60°	45	30	45	45	NC	15
Extension	160–170°	165	155	160	160	–5	5
Elbow							
Flexion	20–40°	30	30	45	30	15	NC
Extension	160–170°	165	146	165	165	NC	19
		Start	**Start**	**At 11 weeks**	**At 11 weeks**	**Change**	**Change**
Carpus							
Flexion	20–35°	30	30	35	35	5	5
Extension	190–200°	195	195	190	190	–5	–5

Note: The straight joint position is considered to be 180°. *Source: Millis DL, Levine D, Taylor RA (2004). *Canine Rehabilitation and Physical Therapy*. WB Saunders, St. Louis, p.441. ROM estimates may vary, depending on the source.

NC: no change.

3. Force plate gait analysis did not show improved changes as demonstrable as the subjective clinical improvements.

Tekscan® force plate analysis

Foot	Start Peak vertical force (kg/cm²)	Start Vertical impulse (kg*sec)	At 11 weeks Peak vertical force (kg/cm²)	At 11 weeks Vertical impulse (kg*sec)
Right front	25.91	8.018	23.78	8.24
Left front	26.29	8.66	24.12	8.15
Right rear	5.99	1.73	8.66	2.92
Left rear	13.49	4.52	9.12	3.12

Note: Peak force objectively measures the amount of weight the dog is bearing on a particular limb. Impulse (area) represents the total force applied by the limb onto the plate over the entire contact time of the foot onto the plate.

4. Sara's owner was extremely pleased with her dog's improvement resultant from the multimodal protocol, with comments such as, "When Sarah goes outside now, she comes in running like a streak of lightning through the house," and "Sara had another great day!"

Owner's subjective assessment:

Beginning of multimodal protocol

Activity	Observed frequency Not at all	 Some times	 Most times
Difficulty in rising from rest			X
Limping			X
Stiffness			X
Soreness when touched			X
Lagging behind on walks			X
Yelping or whimpering in pain	X		
Aggressive behaviors	X		
Difficulty in running	NA		
Difficulty in walking			X

(continued)

Beginning of multimodal protocol (continued)

Activity	Observed frequency		
	Not at all	**Some times**	**Most times**
Difficulty in climbing stairs			X
Difficulty in jumping		X	
Difficulty in playing	X		
Impaired mobility		X	
Lameness			X
Overall activity level			

At 11 weeks

Activity	Observed frequency			Changes at 11 week exam					
	Not at all	**Some times**	**Most times**	**Dramatically improved**	**Moderately improved**	**Slightly improved**	**About the same**	**Slightly worse**	**Moderately worse**
Difficulty in rising from rest				X					
Limping				X					
Stiffness				X					
Soreness when touched	NA								
Lagging behind on walks		X		X					
Yelping or whimpering in pain	NA								
Aggressive behaviors	NA								
Difficulty in running									
Difficulty in walking		X		X					

	Observed frequency			Changes at 11 week exam					
Activity	**Not at all**	**Some times**	**Most times**	**Dramatically improved**	**Moderately improved**	**Slightly improved**	**About the same**	**Slightly worse**	**Moderately worse**
Difficulty in climbing stairs		X		X					
Difficulty in jumping		X		X					
Difficulty in playing		X		X					
Impaired mobility		X		X					
Lameness		X		X					
Overall activity level				X					

NA: not assessed.

Beginning of multimodal protocol:

Joint	Left	Right	Pain scoring
Hip	2	2	0 = No pain on palpation
Stifle	2	2	1 = Mild pain; palpation completed
Tarsus	0	2	2 = Moderate pain; palpation completed with discomfort
Shoulder	1	0	3 = Severe pain; palpation not completed
Elbow	0	0	4 = Pain too severe; restraint/sedation needed to palpate
Carpus	0	0	

Overall subjective lameness score: 2 out of 5 (severe).

At 11 weeks:

Joint	Left	Right	Pain scoring
Hip	1	1	0 = No pain on palpation
Stifle	1	1	1 = Mild pain; palpation completed
Tarsus	0	0	2 = Moderate pain; palpation completed with discomfort
Shoulder	0	0	3 = Severe pain; palpation not completed
Elbow	0	0	4 = Pain too severe; restraint/sedation needed to palpate
Carpus	0	0	

Overall subjective lameness score: 1 out of 5 (severe).

Gait assessment at beginning:

Lameness at stance = 2.	0 = normal stance 1 = slightly abnormal stance (partial weight bearing) 2 = Moderately abnormal stance (toe-touch weight bearing) 3 = Severely abnormal stance (holds limb off floor) 4 = Unable to stand
Lameness at walk = 3 Lameness at trot = 2	0 = no lameness; full weight bearing on all strides 1 = mild subtle lameness with partial weight bearing 2 = obvious lameness with partial weight bearing 3 = obvious lameness with intermittent weight bearing 4 = full nonweight-bearing lame

Gait assessment at 11 weeks:

Lameness at stance = 1	0 = normal stance 1 = slightly abnormal stance (partial weight bearing) 2 = Moderately abnormal stance (toe-touch weight bearing) 3 = Severely abnormal stance (holds limb off floor) 4 = Unable to stand
Lameness at walk = 0–1 Lameness at trot = 1	0 = no lameness; full weight bearing on all strides 1 = mild subtle lameness with partial weight bearing 2 = obvious lameness with partial weight bearing 3 = obvious lameness with intermittent weight bearing 4 = full non-weight-bearing lame

5. Striving to achieve the 'minimal effective dose' of the NSAID; the NSAID dose was decreased by 50% after 6 weeks on the multimodal protocol, and another 50% (to 25 mg *sid*) after 11 weeks.
6. The patient's blood/chemistry profiles and urine assessments were unchanged over the course of the multimodal treatment protocol.

Signalment: 'Lois', a 13.7-year-old, female spayed, 47 lb (21.3 kg), Labrador Retriever, body condition score 2.8/5.

History/Presentation: at an early age, Lois developed ovariohysterectomy incontinence, which was 'somewhat' successfully being managed with phenylpropanolamine hydrochloride at 50 mg *bid*. At approximately 3 years of age, she was diagnosed with lumbosacral disease, and had received a few, intermittent steroid injections over the lumbosacral area, which provided relief for acute symptoms. Lois' owner attributed her weight loss to a reluctance to walk to the food bowl. Physical examination revealed a stiff gait, poor muscle mass, a wide-based rear limb stance, preference to walk on surfaces with 'good footing', and a painful response to manipulation of the hips and lumbosacral spine. Blood work was normal. Radiographs revealed mild hip dysplasia, a narrowing of the lumbosacral intervertebral disc space and lumbosacral spondylosis.

Treatment protocol: Treatment goal was to manage pain, increase muscle strength, and modify progression of lumbar facet DJD by:

- Daily NSAID administration: 31 mg/day (1.46 mg/kg) for the first 4 days only, then 25 mg (1.17 mg/kg) once daily thereafter.
- Exclusive diet of Hills' dry and canned J/D diet.
- Polysulfated glycosaminoglycan (Adequan® Canine) at 4.4 mg/kg Q4–5 days for eight injections, then Q21 days for two injections, and thereafter Q4–5 weeks as needed.

- Regular leash walks with modest inclines and declines; brisk walking/jogging in grass, and sit-to-stand exercises. Massage of the lower back and hips was encouraged together with warm and cold therapy before and after exercise, respectively.
- Acupuncture was suggested, but declined, and inclusion of tramadol as needed was anticipated.

Results:

1. Over the course of 12 weeks Lois gained approximately 2 lb (0.8 kg).
2. Over the 12 week treatment protocol, increased ROM was noted in all joints of the rear limb.

Hindlimb	Normal ROM*	Start Left	Start Right	At 11 weeks Left	At 11 weeks Right	Change Left	Change Right
Hip							
Flexion	55°	55	44	60	46	5	2
Extension	160–165°	151	148	160	151	9	3
Stifle							
Flexion	45°	35	34	44	44	9	10
Extension	160–170°	145	135	146	161	1	26
Tarsus							
Flexion	40°	51	55	54	57	3	2
Extension	170°	145	140	154	151	9	11
Forelimb	**Normal ROM**	**Left**	**Right**	**Left**	**Right**	**Left**	**Right**
Shoulder							
Flexion	30–60°	56	49	59	55	3	6
Extension	160–170°	145	149	150	159	5	10
Elbow							
Flexion	20–40°	35	40	40	44	5	4
Extension	160–170°	160	160	167	160	7	NC
Carpus							
Flexion	20–35°	45	50	46	41	1	–9
Extension	190–200°	142	148	151	159	9	11

Note: The straight joint position is considered to be 180°. *Source: Millis DL, Levine D, Taylor RA (2004). *Canine Rehabilitation and Physical Therapy.* WB Saunders, St. Louis, p. 441. ROM estimates may vary, depending on the source.

3. Force plate analysis showed an improvement of weight bearing in all limbs excepting the right front. Asymmetry between the rear limbs was reduced from 8% (clinically relevant) to 1% (nonclinical).

Foot	Start Z peak force (kg-sec)	Start Z impulse (area) (kg/cm²)	At 12 weeks Z peak force (kg-sec)	At 12 weeks Z impulse (area) (kg/cm²)
Right front	135.4	16.29	133.71	15.39
Left front	132.7	16.54	142.06	17.52
Right rear	69.0	7.04	74.11	7.57
Left rear	61.5	6.74	72.96	8.93

Note: Peak force objectively measures the amount of weight the dog is bearing on a particular limb. Impulse (area) represents the total force applied by the limb onto the plate over the entire contact time of the foot onto the plate.

4. Lois' owner was not aggressive with therapeutic exercises, not striving for an active pet, but rather, simply to increase Lois' comfort. However, a huge improvement in leash walking was noted. Lois' average walk of only a few hundred feet (<60 m), 3–4 times per day, increased to approximately 1 mile (1.6 km) per day. Further, Lois became more willing and able to go up and down stairs, doing so with clearly greater ease and confidence. Overall improvement was noted immediately upon commencement of treatment and further improvement was seen with time.

Owner's subjective assessment:

Beginning of multimodal protocol

Activity	Observed frequency Not at all	Some times	Most times
Difficulty in rising from rest			X
Limping		X	
Stiffness			X
Soreness when touched		X	
Lagging behind on walks			X
Yelping or whimpering in pain	X		
Aggressive behaviors	X		
Difficulty in running			X

Activity	Observed frequency		
	Not at all	Some times	Most times
Difficulty in walking		X	
Difficulty in climbing stairs			X
Difficulty in jumping			X
Difficulty in playing			X
Impaired mobility			X
Lameness			X
Overall activity level			

At 12 weeks

Activity	Observed frequency			Changes at 12 week exam					
	Not at all	Some times	Most times	Dramatically improved	Moderately improved	Slightly improved	About the same	Slightly worse	Moderately worse
Difficulty in rising from rest			X			X			
Limping		X				X			
Stiffness			X			X			
Soreness when touched	X								
Lagging behind on walks		X				X			
Yelping or whimpering in pain	X								
Aggressive behaviors	X								
Difficulty in running			X		X				
Difficulty in walking		X				X			
Difficulty in climbing stairs			X		X				
Difficulty in jumping			X				X		

(continued)

Beginning of multimodal protocol (continued)

Activity	Observed frequency			Changes at 12 week exam					
	Not at all	Some times	Most times	Dramatically improved	Moderately improved	Slightly improved	About the same	Slightly worse	Moderately worse
Difficulty in playing			X			X			
Impaired mobility			X			X			
Lameness			X			X			
Overall activity level									

Beginning of multimodal protocol:

Joint	Left	Right
Hip	3+	3+
Stifle	0	0
Tarsus	0	0
Shoulder	0	0
Elbow	0	1
Carpus	0	0

Pain scoring
0 = No pain on palpation
1 = Mild pain; palpation completed
2 = Moderate pain; palpation completed with discomfort
3 = Severe pain; palpation not completed
4 = Pain too severe; restraint/sedation needed to palpate

Overall subjective lameness score: 4 out of 5 (severe).

At 12 weeks:

Joint	Left	Right
Hip	1	1
Stifle	1	1
Tarsus	0	0
Shoulder	0	0
Elbow	0	0
Carpus	0	0

Pain scoring
0 = No pain on palpation
1 = Mild pain; palpation completed
2 = Moderate pain; palpation completed with discomfort
3 = Severe pain; palpation not completed
4 = Pain too severe; restraint/sedation needed to palpate

Overall subjective lameness score: 1 out of 5 (severe).

Gait assessment at beginning:
Lameness at stance = 2+/4

0 = normal stance
1 = slightly abnormal stance (partial weight bearing)
2 = Moderately abnormal stance (toe-touch weight bearing)
3 = Severely abnormal stance (holds limb off floor)
4 = Unable to stand

Lameness at walk = 2+
Lameness at trot = 2+

0 = no lameness; full weight bearing on all strides
1 = mild subtle lameness with partial weight bearing
2 = obvious lameness with partial weight bearing
3 = obvious lameness with intermittent weight bearing
4 = full nonweight-bearing lame

Gait assessment at 12 weeks:

Lameness at stance = 0.

0 = normal stance
1 = slightly abnormal stance (partial weight bearing)
2 = Moderately abnormal stance (toe-touch weight bearing)
3 = Severely abnormal stance (holds limb off floor)
4 = Unable to stand

Lameness at walk = 0
Lameness at trot = 1

0 = no lameness; full weight bearing on all strides
1 = mild subtle lameness with partial weight bearing
2 = obvious lameness with partial weight bearing
3 = obvious lameness with intermittent weight bearing
4 = full nonweight-bearing lame

5. The patient's blood/chemistry profiles and urine assessments were unchanged over the course of the multimodal treatment protocol.

Signalment: 'Koda', a 9-year-old, female spayed, 60 lb (30 kg), Labrador Retriever, body conditioning score 3/5.

History/Presentation: Following surgical repair (extracapsular) of bilateral anterior cruciate ligament tears at ages 1 year and 3 years, and normal aging as an active dog, Koda was losing her ability to fully participate in a rural, active lifestyle that included running, hunting, swimming, and rigorous activity with other dogs. Following exercise, she would become stiff and suffer exacerbated lameness for at least 24 hours. Prior to implementing this multimodal protocol, Koda was treated conservatively with weight control and various 'traditional' NSAIDs. Koda's blood chemistries and urine profiles were within normal limits. Physical examination was unremarkable, excepting severe, chronic DJD of both stifles and mild DJD of both coxofemoral joints, each diagnosis confirmed by radiographs. She was taking glucosamine sulfate (750 mg PO *sid*).

Treatment protocol:

- High EPA diet of Hills J/D diet.
- Eight dose protocol (label) of polysulfated glycosaminoglycan (Adequan® Canine).
- Daily NSAID administration: 50 mg deracoxib (decreased to 37 mg, i.e. 1.7 mg/kg to 1.2 mg/kg).
- Nutraceutical: glucosamine sulfate (750 mg *sid*).

Results:

1. Over the course of 11 weeks, Koda gained 3.3 lb (1.5 kg).
2. Only the hip and stifle were assessed for ROM. Extension of both the hips and stifle were improved approximately by 10–13%.

Hindlimb	Normal ROM*	Start Left	Start Right	At 11 weeks Left	At 11 weeks Right	Change Left	Change Right
Hip							
Flexion	55°	65	60	60	60	–5	NC
Extension	160–165°	140	145	160	160	20	15
Stifle							
Flexion	45°	55	65	40	45	–15	–20
Extension	160–170°	150	135	165	160	15	25
Tarsus							
Flexion	40°						
Extension	170°						

Note: The straight joint position is considered to be 180°. *Source: Millis DL, Levine D, Taylor RA (2004). *Canine Rehabilitation and Physical Therapy*. WB Saunders, St. Louis, p. 441. ROM estimates may vary, depending on the source.

ROM: range of motion.

3. Based upon force plate analysis, there appeared to be marked improvement in the left hind limb that is characterized by an increase in peak vertical force (PVF) from 51.49 to 62.7 and an increase in vertical impulse (VI) from 8.19 to 10.22. Improvement in the right hind limb is also noted, but less dramatic: PVF from 38.8 to 43.10, and VI from 5.34 to 6.30 (**Fig. 247**). These observations reflect her clinical assessments. Note: Peak force objectively measures the amount of weight the dog is bearing on a particular limb. Impulse (area) represents the total force applied by the limb onto the plate over the entire contact time of the foot onto the plate.
4. Koda's owner believed that Koda once again had the opportunity to truly enjoy 'a summer on the lake' which she had been unable to do for the past couple of years.

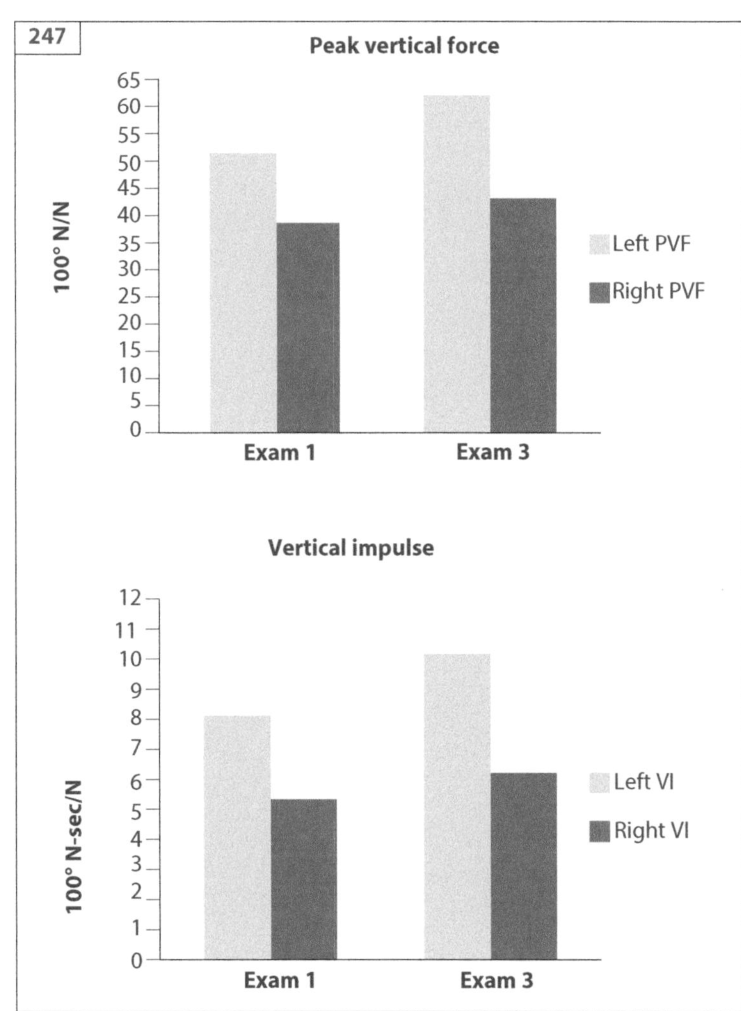

Fig. 247 Force plate analysis of peak vertical force (PVF) and vertical impulse (VI) in the hindlimbs.

Owner's subjective assessment:

Beginning of multimodal protocol

Activity	Observed frequency: Not at all	Some times	Most times
Difficulty in rising from rest		X	
Limping			X
Stiffness			X
Soreness when touched		X	
Lagging behind on walks			X
Yelping or whimpering in pain	X		
Aggressive behaviors	X		
Difficulty in running			X
Difficulty in walking		X	
Difficulty in climbing stairs			X
Difficulty in jumping		X	
Difficulty in playing		X	
Impaired mobility			X
Lameness			X
Overall activity level		X	

At 11 weeks

	Observed frequency			Changes at 11 week exam					
Activity	**Not at all**	**Some times**	**Most times**	**Dramatically improved**	**Moderately improved**	**Slightly improved**	**About the same**	**Slightly worse**	**Moderately worse**
Difficulty in rising from rest	X						X		
Limping		X				X			

(continued)

Beginning of multimodal protocol (continued)

	Observed frequency			Changes at 11 week exam					
Activity	**Not at all**	**Some times**	**Most times**	**Dramatically improved**	**Moderately improved**	**Slightly improved**	**About the same**	**Slightly worse**	**Moderately worse**
Stiffness	X						X		
Soreness when touched	X						X		
Lagging behind on walks	X						X		
Yelping or whimpering in pain	X						X		
Aggressive behaviors	X						X		
Difficulty in running	X					X			
Difficulty in walking	X						X		
Difficulty in climbing stairs		X				X			
Difficulty in jumping	X						X		
Difficulty in playing	X						X		
Impaired mobility	X					X			
Lameness		X				X			
Overall activity level			X				X		

Beginning of multimodal protocol:

Joint	Left	Right
Hip	1	1
Stifle	2	2
Tarsus		
Shoulder		
Elbow		
Carpus		

Pain scoring
0 = No pain on palpation
1 = Mild pain; palpation completed
2 = Moderate pain; palpation completed with discomfort
3 = Severe pain; palpation not completed
4 = Pain too severe; restraint/sedation needed to palpate

Overall subjective lameness score: 4 out of 5 (severe).

At 11 weeks:

Joint	Left	Right	Pain scoring
Hip	0	0	0 = No pain on palpation
Stifle	0	0	1 = Mild pain; palpation completed
Tarsus			2 = Moderate pain; palpation completed with discomfort
Shoulder			3 = Severe pain; palpation not completed
Elbow			4 = Pain too severe; restraint/sedation needed to palpate
Carpus			

Overall subjective lameness score: 1 (none/mild) out of 5 (severe).

Gait assessment at beginning:

Lameness at stance = 2.	0 = normal stance
	1 = slightly abnormal stance (partial weight bearing)
	2 = Moderately abnormal stance (toe-touch weight bearing)
	3 = Severely abnormal stance (holds limb off floor)
	4 = Unable to stand

Lameness at walk = 2	0 = no lameness; full weight bearing on all strides
Lameness at trot = 3	1 = mild subtle lameness with partial weight bearing
	2 = obvious lameness with partial weight bearing
	3 = obvious lameness with intermittent weight bearing
	4 = full nonweight-bearing lame

Gait assessment at 11 weeks:

Lameness at stance = 1	0 = normal stance
	1 = slightly abnormal stance (partial weight bearing)
	2 = Moderately abnormal stance (toe-touch weight bearing)
	3 = Severely abnormal stance (holds limb off floor)
	4 = Unable to stand

Lameness at walk = 1	0 = no lameness; full weight bearing on all strides
Lameness at trot = 1	1 = mild subtle lameness with partial weight bearing
	2 = obvious lameness with partial weight bearing
	3 = obvious lameness with intermittent weight bearing
	4 = full nonweight-bearing lame

5. The NSAID dose was reduced from 1.7 mg/kg to 1.2 mg/kg *sid*.
6. The patient's blood/chemistry profiles and urine assessments were unchanged over the course of the multimodal treatment protocol.

Following this multimodal treatment protocol, the owner has stated, "She (Koda) has been observed running her 'sprints' around the yard, has been on several 2 mile (3.2 km) runs without tiring or becoming lame, has been eager to play fetch, and has actually fought our daughter's 3-year old Labrador for the right to retrieve sticks in the water. It has been wonderful to see her playing tug-of-war with the younger dog! The most impressive change, however, has been the absolute lack of stiffness/lameness the day following vigorous activity at the lake. We attribute this improvement, at least in part, to the NSAID therapy; as when this medication has occasionally been forgotten, stiffness has been particularly noticeable."

Weight management

A 7-year-old, female, spayed Golden Retriever is presented for difficulty rising and climbing steps. Anamnesis suggests a reluctance to exercise. Physical examination is unremarkable, excepting that the patient is obese (*Table 1*). Chemistry and urinary profiles are within normal limits.

What advisement is given to the client regarding the patient's weight (**Fig. 248**)?
What obstacles are inherent with implementing a weight loss program?
How would you structure a weight loss program?

Most owners of obese dogs do not schedule an appointment to explore solutions to the problem of obesity in their pet. It is up to the veterinarian to identify the problem, convince owners of its seriousness, and motivate them to implement a dietary change. Complicating the situation is the finding of Kienzle *et al*., (1989), that owners of obese dogs are often obese (54% versus 28% of owners of normal weight dogs), and are themselves fairly inactive. The owners of obese animals often translate every appeal by the animal as being an appeal for food.

Two challenges face the veterinarian: 1) convince the pet owner of the seriousness associated with obesity, and 2) implementing a program to treat the pet. Two communication approaches are envisaged: positive messages that explain all the advantages of weight reduction for the dog's health, and negative messages explaining all the adverse effects of obesity and associated diseases. Select arguments that most likely appeal to the individual owner, such as longevity, quality of life, and the owner's responsibility to keep the animal in a healthy condition. Perhaps these discussions are best conducted by the registered veterinary technician.

Diseases associated with, or exacerbated by, obesity:

Metabolic alterations:
- Hyperlipidemia
- Insulin resistance
- Glucose intolerance
- Anesthetic complications

Endocrinopathies:
- Hyperadrenocorticism
- Hypothyroidism
- Diabetes mellitus
- Insulinoma
- Hypopituitarism
- Hypothalamic lesions
- Pituitary chromophobe adenoma

TABLE 1: Canine obesity is a common problem in many different countries

	Frequency of obesity in the canine population		
References	**Country**	**Sampling size (number of dogs)**	**Estimation**
Krook *et al.*, 1960	Sweden	10993	9%
Mason, 1970	UK	1000	28%
Anderson, 1973	UK	-	33%
Edney, 1974	UK	1134	34%
Meyer *et al.*, 1978	Germany	266	30%
Steininger, 1981	Austria	-	44%
Edney & Smith, 1986	UK	8268	24%
Armstrong & Lund, 1996	USA	23000	25%
Lund *et al.*, 1999	USA	30517	28%
Royal Canin, survey (2000)	France, UK, Spain, Germany	400 veterinarian respondents	20–22%
Jerico & Scheffer, 2002	Brazil	648	17%
Robertson, 2003	Australia	860	25%

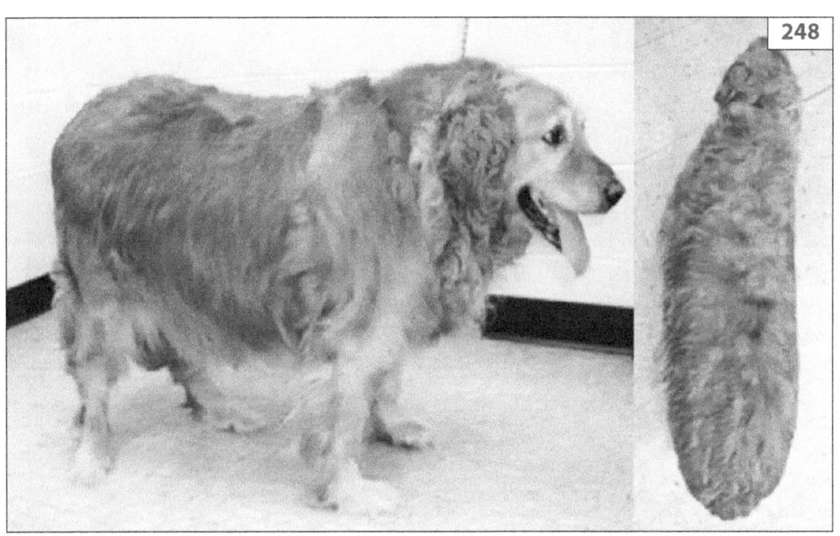

Fig. 248 An obese dog with characteristic body shape.

Functional alterations:
- Joint stress/musculoskeletal pain
- Dyspnea
- Exercise intolerance
- Heat intolerance
- Decreased immune function

Other diseases:
- Degenerative joint and orthopedic disease
- Cardiovascular disease
- Transitional cell carcinoma (bladder)

The core motivation for achieving weight loss should be the owner's desire to improve the quality of the pet's life and avoid paying money to correct problems in the future. Although it is appealing to suggest an owner simply place their pet on a weight reduction diet, success in weight reduction by doing so is usually nil. Weight loss will not occur unless the pet owner recognizes the problem and is willing to take corrective steps.

In motivating for a change, every request for change is accompanied by a reason/request not to change. Prochasta and DiClemente (1984) have created a model for change divided into four steps, which might be helpful in understanding the reluctance to change (**Fig. 249**, *Table 2*).

Step One: absence of awareness

In this precontemplation phase the veterinarian must state the facts of the case: "Your dog is overweight due to …". This step lasts until the pet owner agrees that their pet is too fat.

Step two: contemplation

With the owner aware of the problem, the veterinarian encourages the pet owner to consider change and for what reasons. Pet owners need to realize that the situation presents physiologic risks requiring a change.

Step three: awareness dictating change

A 'roadmap' must be shown to the pet owner, showing how change is achieved. It must be understood that the pleasure of the treat is short-lived, while benefit of the diet is long-lived.

249

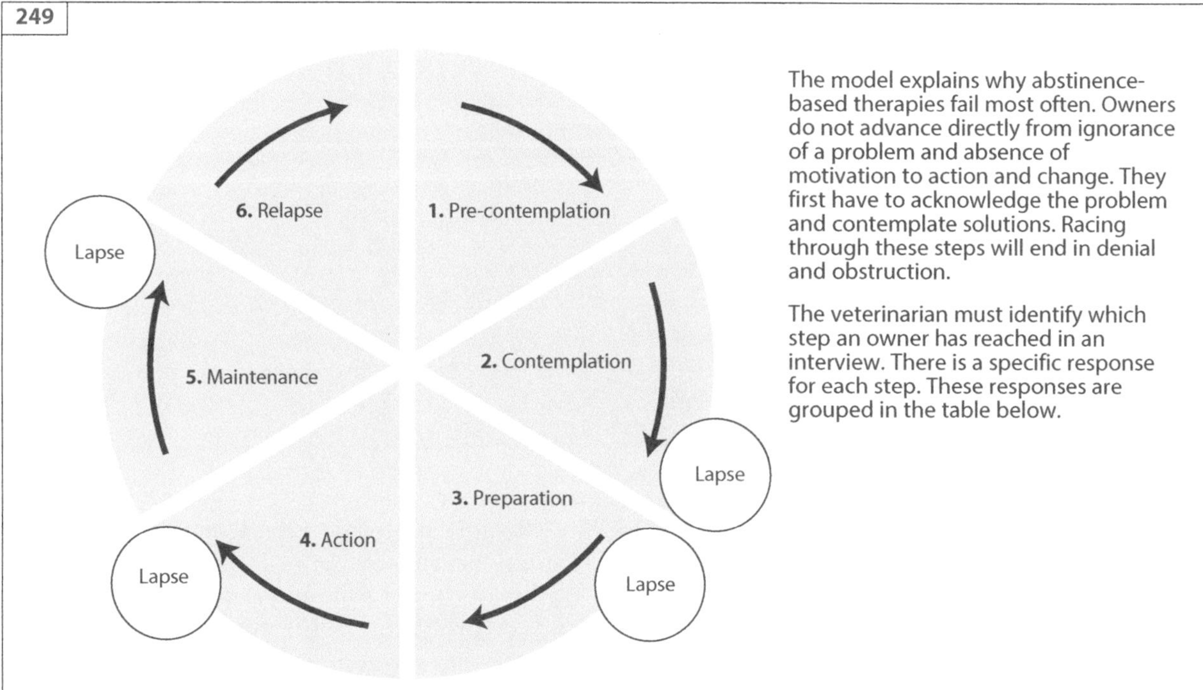

The model explains why abstinence-based therapies fail most often. Owners do not advance directly from ignorance of a problem and absence of motivation to action and change. They first have to acknowledge the problem and contemplate solutions. Racing through these steps will end in denial and obstruction.

The veterinarian must identify which step an owner has reached in an interview. There is a specific response for each step. These responses are grouped in the table below.

1. In 'Pre-contemplation', the person does not see any problem in their current behaviors and has not considered there might be some better alternatives.
2. In 'Contemplation', the person is ambivalent – they are in two minds about what they want to do: should they stay with their existing behaviors and attitudes or should they try changing to something new?
3. In 'Preparation', the person is taking steps to change, usually in the next month or so.
4. In 'Action', they have made the change and living the new set of behaviors is an all-consuming activity.
5. In 'Maintenance', the change has been integrated into the person's life – they are now more 'enterprising'.
6. 'Relapse' is a full return to the old behavior. This is not inevitable, but likely, and should not be seen as failure. Often people will relapse several times before they finally succeed in making a (more or less) permanent change to a new set of behaviors.

Fig. 249 The Prochasta/DiClemente model for change motivation.

Step four: change
The pet owner must be given continual support and not reproached when results are slow in coming.

A successful weight-reduction program is a multi-step process that requires pet owner commitment, a feeding plan, an exercise plan, pet owner communication, and patient monitoring (*Table 2*).

Formulation of a program for achieving weight reduction consists of: 1) setting a goal for the amount of weight to lose, 2) setting an amount for daily caloric intake, 3) selecting a specific food and feeding method, 4) selecting a specific amount of exercise, 5) monitoring the progress of weight loss, 6) adjusting calories, food, and exercise as necessary, and 7) stabilizing caloric intake of the animal at its reduced weight to ensure that weight is not regained.

Relative body weight (RBW) is an animal's current weight divided by its estimated optimal weight. Animals at their optimal weight have a RBW of 1.00 or 100%. Some conservatively suggest obesity begins when an animal is 15% above its optimal weight (RBW of 1.15), while more liberal estimates suggest obesity does not have clinical relevance until the animal is 40% above its optimal weight (RBW of 1.40). A relative weight of 120% is a logical division point between overweight *vs.* obesity until such time as epidemiological data provide greater differentiation between the two.

Body condition score (BCS) is a subjective assessment of an animal's body fat, and to a lesser extent, protein stores, that takes into account the animal's frame size independent of its weight. Systems with either five or nine categories are used most commonly. A 5-point system scored to the nearest half score and a 9-point system scored to the nearest whole score; each have nine total scores for body condition. The most critical division points in a 5-point system are between the scores of 2.0 *vs.* 2.5 and 3.5 *vs.* 4.0, because assignment of a BCS less than 2.5 and greater than 3.5 suggests action should be taken to return the animal's BCS to the optimal range.

Body weight alone does not indicate how appropriate the weight is for an individual animal. Although similar to RBW, BCS uses physical attributes rather than fixed quantities to assess when body condition, and thus weight, is optimal for an individual animal.

Relative weight	80%	90%	100%	110%	120%
Anticipated body condition score	1	2	3	4	5
Anticipated % body fat	<5	5–15	16–25	26–35	>35

Research to assess critically the capability of BCS to predict body composition suggests that body fat changes by 10% for each change in condition score on a 5-point scale.

	Underweight	Ideal	Overweight
5-point scale	1 (very thin)	3	4 (overweight)
	2 (underweight)		5 (obese)
9-point scale	1–3	4–5	6–9

TABLE 2: Overview of the obese dog consultation

	Overview of the obese dog consultation
Step 1	Discussion with the owner, collection of information, identification of risk factors
Step 2	Clinical examination: body weight, body condition score, evaluation of ideal weight; supplementary tests if necessary
Step 3	Convince the owner to introduce a low-calorie diet and regular exercise, if the dog's state of health allows
Step 4	Selection of a low-calorie food and determination of daily quantities
Step 5	Precise written document detailing quantities, mode of rationing and supplementary recommendations (no treats, exercise, etc.); reference weight curve
Step 6	Planning checkups: - weekly weighing - monthly checkup visits at surgery or clinic

Dehydroepiandrosterone administered at a large dose (62 mg/kg/d) reduces the deposition of fatty tissue and has been used as a pharmacologic agent to facilitate weight loss in combination with a low-energy diet in obese dogs. Another, more recent pharmacologic agent is dirlotapide, which blocks the assembly and release of lipoprotein particles into the bloodstream in dogs. The problem with managing obesity with pharmacologic agents is that it does not change the owner's behavior, which is most often predisposing to the weight gain.

TABLE 3: Recommendations of various energy intake levels as part of a low-calorie diet

	Recommendations of various energy intake levels as part of a low-calorie diet					
Excess weight	20–30%		30–40%		>40%	
Fat mass	25–35%		35–45%		>45%	
BCS	7		8		9	
	Loss of 6% of the initial weight per month (approx. –1.5% per week)					
Daily energy intake (kcal/kg IBW$^{0.75}$)	**Male**	**Female**	**Male**	**Female**	**Male**	**Female**
	85	80	75	65	60	55
Probable duration of weight loss	15–18 weeks		18–20 weeks		20–22 weeks (minimum)	
	Loss of 7.5% of the initial weight per month (approx. –2.0% per week)					
Daily energy intake (kcal/kg IBW$^{0.75}$)	**Male**	**Female**	**Male**	**Female**	**Male**	**Female**
	80	75	65	60	55	50
Probable duration of weight loss	9–11 weeks		11–13 weeks		25–17 weeks (minimum)	

BCS: Body condition score on a scale of 1 to 9; IBW: ideal (optimal) body weight; initial weight: weight of the obese dog.

TABLE 4: Calculating the quantities of low-calorie food to be given

Step 1	Determining the optimal weight and the excess weight	Neutered bitch of undetermined breed, BW: 19 kg Estimated ideal weight: 15 kg Excess weight: (19/15) = 27%
Step 2	Selecting the daily energy allocation	Excess weight less than 30%: –80 kcal/kg ideal BW$^{0.75}$, for a loss of 6% of initial weight per month –75 kcal/kg ideal BW$^{0.75}$, for a loss of 7.5% of initial weight per month
Step 3	Calculating the daily energy allocation	Energy allocation = 80 × 15$^{0.75}$ = 610 kcal for a loss of 6% of initial weight per month
Step 4	Determining the daily quantity of food (energy concentration: 3275 kcal/kg)	Daily quantity: 610/3275 = 0.185 kg, spread over two or three meals
Step 5	Estimating the length of the diet based on a loss of 6% per month	Initial weight: 19 kg, quantity to be lost: 4 kg Length of the diet: 4 /(19 × 0.06) = 3.5 months

BW: body weight.

Restriction of energy intake is the only truly valid option for reducing a dog's weight. Restriction of a ration's energy level depends on several criteria, including the degree of weight excess, the animal's sex, and the projected duration of the diet. The first step is to define the ideal weight; the second is setting the energy restriction level. Diets are generally designed to provide 40% (very severe restriction) to 60% or 70% of the energy needed to maintain the optimal weight (*Table 3*). Problems associated with too severe an energy restriction include significant hunger behavior, decreased physical activity, loss of muscle mass, and 'rebound effect' (weight gain at end of diet). Such diets are popular for humans, but ill-advised for pets. Experimental and clinical trial data show that a reasonable objective is to maintain a weight loss of 1–2% of the initial (obese) weight per week, or 4–8% per month (*Table 4*). Spreading the ration over three or four meals per day will increase postprandial thermogenesis.

To initiate weight loss without imposing too severe a restriction immediately the recommended initial energy allocation is:

65% (or 85 kcal/kg IBW 0.75) of the maintenance energy requirement for a male, falling to 55% (or 75 kcal/kg IBW 0.75) if the dog is neutered.

55% (or 75 kcal/kg IBW 0.75) of the maintenance energy requirement for a female, falling to 50% (or 65 kcal/kg IBW 0.75) if the bitch is neutered.

The range in caloric restriction given by various equations or methods for estimating calories appropriate for producing weight loss is evidence that no single method or equation is appropriate for all dogs (and cats). Regardless the level of restriction, the diet must never be deficient in protein, essential amino acids, essential fatty acids, minerals, vitamins, or trace elements. *Table 5* presents reference weights for large breed dogs.

Monitoring is essential for success in a weight loss protocol. During the first visit, an individual weight loss curve should be shared with the pet owner, showing the initial weight and the curves for 1% and 2% of initial weight loss per week. Obese animals should be presented for a checkup no less than monthly; however, weekly weighings at home should be performed at the same time and with the same scales. In practice, the initial weight loss target is rarely achieved, the actual loss generally being lower than 1–2% of initial weight per week (**Fig. 250** *overleaf*).

TABLE 5: Reference weights for large breed dogs

Reference weight variation according to sex in several large breeds

Large breeds	**Average weight of the male (kg)**	**Average weight of the female (kg)**
Irish Setter	26.1 ± 1.9	25.5 ± 4.5
Belgian Sheepdog	27.1 ± 4.5	23.2 ± 2.0
German Pointer	28.5 ± 0.9	24.6 ± 2.3
French Spaniel	29.4 ± 2.1	26.3 ± 3.6
Welmaraner	33.6 ± 3.7	30.5 ± 4.3
Golden Retriever	33.7 ± 3.4	30.4 ± 3.6
Bower	33.9 ± 3.5	28.8 ± 2.4
Labrador	35.5 ± 4.5	30.7 ± 3.4
German Shepherd	35.9 ± 3.6	28.4 ± 2.7
Doberman	39.0 ± 5.5	28.50 ± 50
Glant breeds	**Average weight of the male (kg)**	**Average weight of the female (kg)**
Rottweiler	46.8 ± 4.8	39.7 ± 4.9
Bernese Mountain Dog	59.9 ± 6.9	43.3 ± 6.5
Leonberger	57.0 ± 6.4	49.9 ± 6.8
French Mastiff	58.6 ± 7.3	46.8 ± 7.5
Bullmastiff	58.8 ± 7.5	47.7 ± 6.4
Irish Wolfhound	63.1 ± 1.4	54.3 ± 4.9
Newfoundand	63.5 ± 6.2	51.1 ± 8.6
Great Dane	70.5 ± 8.2	56.6 ± 7.1
St Bemand	81.5 ± 7.2	61.0 ± 8.9
Mastiff	87.0 ± 10.5	71.6 ± 9.2

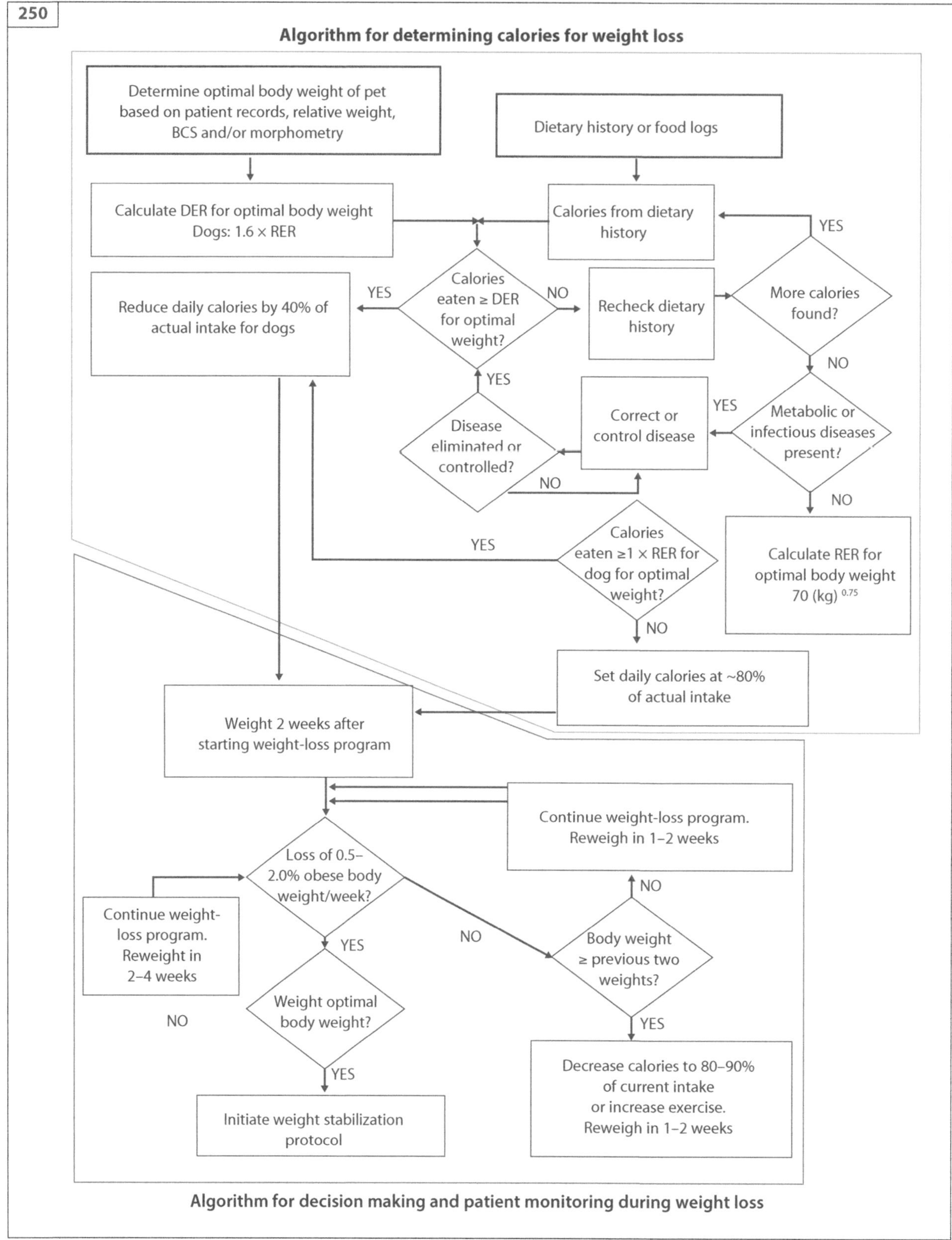

Fig. 250 Algorithm for 1) determining calories for weight loss, and 2) decision making and patient monitoring during weight loss. BCS: body condition score; DER: daily energy requirements; RER: resting energy requirements.

Appendix 3

Selected Patient Conditions and Suggested Physical Rehabilitation

Condition	Physical rehabilitation suggestions
General	
Muscle mass/tone	Neuromuscular electrical stimulation
Pain: chronic, minor	Low-level laser therapy
chronic syndromes	Transcutaneous electrical nerve stimulation, static magnet field
acute (decrease swelling/muscle spasm)	Cryotherapy
lingering (decrease swelling/muscle spasm)	Thermotherapy
Pain reduction/disability	Therapeutic and strengthening exercises: leash walking, rocker platform, exercise balls/rolls, sit-to-stand, stairs/steps, inclines/declines, dancing, wheelbarrowing, treadmill, Cavaletti rails, pole weave, aquatic exercise
Stretching; tendonitis; contracture	US, thermotherapy
Wound healing; analgesia; ROM	Extracorporeal shock wave therapy
Specific	
Shoulder articular fracture	Postop: NSAID, PROM; short leash walks for first few weeks After 8–10 weeks: ROM exercises, stretching, progressive leash walking, aquatic therapy
Bicipital tenosynivitis	NSAID, cryotherapy, pulsed-mode 3-MHz therapeutic US Postop: cryotherapy, PROM, short leash walks; then, gradual strengthening exercises, aquatic therapy, treadmill
Osteochondrosis dissecans	NSAID, chondroprotectant, cryotherapy, rest, PROM Postop: cryotherapy, PROM, short leash walks After 3 weeks: swimming, treadmill, walking At 6 weeks: light jogging

(continued)

Condition	Physical rehabilitation suggestions
Specific	
Infraspinatus muscle contracture	Postop: full weight bearing as soon as possible, pain-free PROM of forelimb joints, followed by cryotherapy With muscle atrophy: progressive walking, wheelbarrowing, aquatic therapy If severe: neuromuscular electrical stimulation
Medial glenohumeral instability	Sling immobilization
	Thereafter: PROM in sagittal plane limited weight-bearing exercises
	Postop: rest, NSAID, cryotherapy, PROM for 3 weeks
	Then: weight-bearing exercises
Pectoral muscle tears	NSAID, cryotherapy, controlled leash walks
	After 1 month: jogging
Scapular fracture	Postop: NSAID, cryotherapy, PROM to glenohumeral joint for first 3–6 weeks Then: 3-plane scapular ROM in increasing amounts ± cross-fiber frictional massage, aquatic therapy, treadmill, walking
Supraspinatus mineralization	Rest, NSAID, cryotherapy, PROM, ± therapeutic US
Elbow articular fracture	Postop to maintain ROM: cryotherapy, NSAID, swimming, underwater treadmill; then Cavaletti rails Active exercise to rebuild atrophied muscle
Elbow luxation	After immobilization: ROM exercises in sagittal plane; minimize varus and valgus stress, and uncontrolled activity until joint healing (8–12 weeks)
Elbow incongruity	NSAID, chondroprotectants, cryotherapy, PROM, progressive leash walks With end-stage OA: PROM, stretching, active ROM, ± neuromuscular electrical stimulation, low-impact exercises, aquatic exercise
Fragmented coronoid process	NSAID, chondroprotectants, low-impact exercises, aquatic exercises, maintain body weight
Ununited anconeal process	Postop attachment: progressive weight bearing over 8–12 weeks using cryotherapy, ROM exercises, aquatic therapy, light leash walks Postop removal: accelerated weight-bearing exercises at pace of patient's tolerance
Medial humeral condyle OCD	As above for OCD
Angular (fore)limb deformity	Postop: NSAID, cryotherapy, stretching, ROM activities, ± therapeutic US
Antebrachium fractures (radius/ulna)	*Caution flexor contraction Stretching, ROM exercises
Carpal hyperextension (luxation)	After arthrodesis and bone healing: weekly cast removal and ROM exercises of normal joints
Distal (fore)limb fractures	Elbow ROM exercises during coaptation and after Remove coaptation weekly to perform ROM exercises Sagittal plane exercises
Flexor tendon contracture	3-MHz therapeutic US or thermotherapy, manual stretching exercises, massage *Caution tearing of tissues

Condition	Physical rehabilitation suggestions
Specific	
Tendon & ligament compromise: tendonitis	NSAID and cryotherapy to decrease inflammation, then 3-MHZ pulsed therapeutic US to stimulate collagen formation Following 3 weeks of coaptation of an avulsion surgery: progressive weight bearing With contracture: 3-MHz continuous mode therapeutic US or thermotherapy followed by stretching
Pelvic fractures	Conservative management: NSAID, cryotherapy, cage rest until weight bearing; then supported weight-bearing exercises Postop: NSAID, cryotherapy, support weight-bearing exercises After 10–12 weeks: treadmill, aquatic exercises, strength building activities
Coxofemoral luxation	Ehmer sling, immobilization for approximately 2 weeks Then: controlled leash walking Avoid external rotation and abduction for about 6 weeks
Hip dysplasia	NSAID, chondroprotectant, ROM exercises, sit-to-stand, aquatic therapy and weight management Postop: NSAID, cryotherapy, PROM, assisted ambulation, controlled therapeutic exercises Then: strengthening exercises Avoid abduction exercises Restrict exercise to leash walks for 8–12 weeks Controlled walking exercises, balance and proprioception exercises After FHO: immediate postoperative PROM, analgesics as needed, NSAID, cryotherapy to avoid fibrosis and loss of motion Encourage limb use
Legg–Calvé–Perthes disease	Same as FHO: aggressive PROM, pain management, NSAID, cryotherapy, aquatic therapy, walking, swimming
Femoral fracture	Postop: NSAID, cryotherapy, PROM, controlled leash walking, treadmill, swimming, stairs added as fracture heals (6–12 weeks) Periarticular fractures require more ROM exercises ± stretching
Rear limb muscle injury	NSAID, cryotherapy, pulsed therapeutic US at about 1 week Following healing: continuous-mode therapeutic US, stretching, swimming, active exercises
ACL extracapsular repair	Postop: within 24 hours: NSAID, cryotherapy, PROM, controlled leash walks, weight bearing encouraged Aquatic therapy after sound healing After 10 days: stair climbing, uphill walking, slow dancing Restrict jumping for 10–12 weeks.
ACL intracapsular repair	Postop: NSAID, cryotherapy, PROM, massage, weight support until toe-touching Then: slow leash walking for 5 minutes 3 times daily followed with 15 minutes of cryotherapy Increase ROM exercises to 3–5 times daily if <60–50° flexion or <120–135° extension May apply heat before exercise
Posterior cruciate ligament compromise	Postop: NSAID, cryotherapy, PROM, controlled leash walks within 24 hours, encourage weight bearing, aquatic therapy at 1 week After 1–2 weeks: strengthening with stair climbing, uphill walks, dancing

(*continued*)

Condition	Physical rehabilitation suggestions
Specific	
Meniscal injury	Following (partial) menisectomy: NSAID, cryotherapy, PROM, progressive leash walks
Collateral ligament injury	± coaptation for no more than 2–4 weeks PROM, stretching, ± therapeutic US, slow leash walking, treadmill, aquatic therapy At 4–6 weeks: strengthening exercises
Patella luxation	Postop: NSAID, cryotherapy, short leash walks for 3 weeks
	Then: strengthening exercises in sagittal plane
Stifle OCD	As above for OCD
Quadriceps contracture (often resultant from femoral fracture)	Prevention is the best treatment! Poor prognosis Postop: NSAID, cryotherapy, massage, slow leash walks, PROM, swimming
Long digital extensor avulsion	Postop: NSAID, cryotherapy, limited weight bearing for 8–10 weeks Then: proprioceptive training and leash weight bearing
Patella ligament rupture	Postop: 2–3 weeks coaptation, followed by: controlled remobilization and 3-MHz pulsed therapeutic US
Stifle articular fractures	As above with elbow fractures
Tibial tuberosity avulsion	Postop: NSAID, cryotherapy, limited weight bearing After 8–12 weeks: increasing weight-bearing activities
Fibrotic myopathy	Cryotherapy, increasing stretching and strengthening exercises

ACL: anterior cruciate ligament; FHO: femoral head (and neck) ostectomy; NSAID: nonsteroidal anti-inflammatory drug; OA: osteoarthritis; OCD: osteochondrosis dissecans; postop: postoperative; PROM: passive range of motion; ROM: range of motion; US: ultrasound.
(Source: Millis DL, Levine D, Taylor RA [2004]. *Canine Rehabilitation and Physical Therapy*. WB Saunders, St. Louis.)

References

CHAPTER 1

1 Dohoo SE, Dohoo IR (1996). Factors influencing the postoperative use of analgesics in dogs and cats by Canadian veterinarians. *Can Vet J* **37**:552–555.

2 Dohoo SE, Dohoo IR (1996). Postoperative use of analgesics in dogs and cats by Canadian veterinarians. *Can Vet J* **37**:546–551.

3 Lascelles BDX, Robertson SA (2004). Use of thermal threshold response to evaluate the antinociceptive effects of butorphanol in cats. *Am J Vet Res* **65**(8):1085–1089.

4 Brock N (1995). Treating moderate and severe pain in small animals. *Can Vet J* **36**:658–660.

5 Taylor PM, Robertson SA (2004). Pain management in cats – past, present, and future. Part 1. The cat is unique. *J Feline Med Surg* **6**:313–320.

6 Hansen BD (1994). Analgesic therapy. *Compend Contin Educ Vet Pract* **16**:868–875.

7 Kyles AE (1995). Clinical pain management. *Perspectives* March/April:6–12.

8 Whipple JK, Lewis KS, Quebbeman EJ, *et al.* (1995). Analysis of pain management in critically ill patients. *Pharmacotherapy* **15**:592–599.

9 Boer C, Treebus AN, Zuurmond WWA, *et al.* (1997). Compliance in administration of prescribed analgesics. *Anaesthesia* **52**:1177–1181.

10 Manias E (2003). Medication trends and documentation of pain management following surgery. *Nurs Health Sci* **5**:85–94.

11 Whipple JK, Lewis KS, Quebbeman EJ, *et al.* (1995). Current patterns of prescribing and administering morphine in trauma patients. *Pharmacotherapy* **15**:210–215.

12 Armitage EA, Wetmore LA, Chan DL, *et al.* (2005). Evaluation of compliance among nursing staff in administration of prescribed analgesic drugs to critically ill dogs and cats. *J Am Vet Med Assoc* **227**:425–429.

13 Hugonnard M, Leblond A, Keroack S, *et al.* (2004). Attitudes and concerns of French veterinarians towards pain and analgesia in dogs and cats. *Vet Anaesth Analg* **31**:154–163.

14 De Rond MEJ, de Wit R, van Dam FSAM, *et al.* (2000). A pain monitoring program for nurses' effect on the administration of analgesics. *Pain* **89**:25–38.

15 Rollins BE (2009). The ethics of pain management. In: *Handbook of Veterinary Pain Management*, 2nd edn. Mosby Elsevier, St Louis, p. 9.

16 ACVA (1998). American College of Veterinary Anesthesiologists' position paper on the treatment of pain in animals. *J Am Vet Med Assoc* **213**:628–630.

17 Hellyer MS, Rodan I, Brunt, *et al.* (2007). AAHA/AAFP pain management guidelines for dogs and cats. *JAAHA* **43**:235–248.

18 Sandlin D (2000). The new Joint Commission Accreditation of Healthcare Organizations' requirements for pain assessment and treatment: a pain in the assessment. *J PeriAnesthesia Nursing* **15**:182–184.

19 Wallace KG, Graham KM, Ventura MR, *et al.* (1997). Lessons learned in implementing a staff education program in pain management in the acute care setting. *J Nurses Staff Dev* **13**:24–31.

20 Resource Center of the American Alliance of Cancer Pain Initiative (2000). *The Wisconsin Resource Manual*, 2nd edn. Building an Institutional Commitment to Pain Management. Madison.

CHAPTER 2

1 No authors listed (2010). Contribution of veterinary technicians to veterinary business revenue, 2007. *J Am Vet Med Assoc* **236**:846.
2 Sharon N (2008). Pain management: the veterinary technician's perspective. In: Mathews KA (ed). Update on Management of Pain. *Vet Clin North Am Small Anim Pract* **38**:1415.
3 Dohoo SE, Dohoo IR (1996). Factors influencing the postoperative use of analgesics in dogs and cats by Canadian veterinarians. *Can Vet J* **37**:552–555.
4 Dohoo SE, Dohoo IR (1996). Postoperative use of analgesics in dogs and cats by Canadian veterinarians. *Can Vet J* **37**:546–551.
5 Capner CA, Lascelles BDX, Waterman-Pearson AE (1999). Current British veterinary attitudes to perioperative analgesia for dogs. *Vet Record* **145**:95–99.
6 Hellyer PW, Frederick C, Lacy M, *et al.* (1999). Attitudes of veterinary medical students, house officers, clinical faculty, and staff toward pain management in animals. *J Am Vet Med Assoc* **214**:238–244.
7 Raekallio M, Heinonen KM, Kuussaari J, *et al.* (2003). Pain alleviation in animals: attitudes and practices of Finnish veterinarians. *Vet J* **165**:131–135.
8 Hugonnard M, Leblond A, Keroack S, *et al.* (2004). Attitudes and concerns of French veterinarians towards pain and analgesia in dogs and cats. *Vet Anaesth Analg* **31**:154–163.
9 Williams VM, Lascelles BD, Robson MC (2005). Current attitudes to, and use of, perioperative analgesia in dogs and cats by veterinarians in New Zealand. *NZ Vet J* **53**:193–202.
10 Vaisanen MAM, Tuomikoski-Alin SK, Brodbelt DC, *et al.* (2008). Opinions of Finnish small animal owners about surgery and pain management in small animals. *J Soc Adm Pharm* **49**:626–632.
11 Tait AR, Voepel-Lewis T, Munro HM, *et al.* (2001). Parents preferences for participation in decisions made regarding their child's anesthetic care. *Paediatr Anaesth* **11**:283–290.
12 Shevde K, Panagopoulos G (1991). A survey of 800 patients' knowledge, attitudes, and concerns regarding anesthesia. *Vet Anaesth Analg* **73**:190–198.
13 Shaw JR (2006). Four core communication skills of highly effective practitioners. *Vet Clin North Am Small Anim Pract* **36**:385–396.
14 Stewart M, Brown JB, Donner A, *et al.* (2000). The impact of patient-centered care on outcomes. *J Fam Pract* **9**:796–804.
15 Peterson MC, Holbrook J, Voin Hales D, *et al.* (1992). Contributions of the history, physical examination and laboratory investigation in making medical diagnoses. *West J Med* **156**: 163–165.
16 Groopman J (2007). *How Doctors Think*. Houghton Mifflin Company, New York.
17 Beckman HB, Markakis KM, Suchman AL, *et al.* (1994). The doctor–patient relationship and malpractice: lessons from plaintiff disposition. *Arch Intern Med* **154**:1365–1370.
18 Braddock CH, Edwards KA, Hasenberg NM, *et al.* (1999). Informed decision making in outpatient practice: time to get back to basics. *J Am Med Assoc* **282**:2313–2320.
19 Bonvicini KA, Cornell KK (2008). Are clients truly informed? Communication tools and risk reduction. *Comp Small Anim Pract* **11**: 572–576.
20 Coe JB, Adams CL, Bonnett BN (2007). A focus group study of veterinarians' and pet owners' perceptions of the monetary aspects of veterinary care. *J Am Vet Med Assoc* **231**:1510–1518.
21 AAHA (2003). *The Path to High-Quality Care: Practical Tips for Improving Compliance*. AAHA Press, Lakewood.
22 Cron WL, Slocum JV Jr, Goodnight DB, *et al.* (2000). Executive summary of the Brakke management and behavior study. *J Am Vet Med Assoc* **217**:332–338.
23 Bell RA, Kravitz RL, Thom D, *et al.* (2002). Unmet expectations for care and the patient–physician relationship. *J Gen Intern Med* **17**: 884–885.
24 Coe JB, Adams CL, Bonnett BN (2008). A focus group study of veterinarians' and pet owners' perceptions of veterinarian–client communication in companion animal practice. *J Am Vet Med Assoc* **233**:1072–1080.
25 Silverman JD, Kurtz SM, Draper J (2005). *Skills for Communicating with Patients*, 2nd edn. Radcliffe Publishing, Oxford, UK.
26 Rhoades DR, McFarland KF, Finch WH, Johnson AO (2001). Speaking and interruptions during primary care office visits. *Fam Med* **33**:528–532
27 Marvel MK, Epstein RM, Flowers K, *et al.* (1999). Soliciting the patient's agenda: have we improved? *J Am Med Assoc* **281**:283–287.
28 Beckman HB, Frankel RM (1984). The effect of physician behaviour on the collection of data. *Ann Intern Med* **101**:692–696.

CHAPTER 3

1 IASP Subcommittee on Taxonomy (1979). Pain terms: a list of definitions and notes on usage. Recommended by the IASP Subcommittee on Taxonomy. *Pain* **6**:249.

2 Zimmerman M (1986). Behavioural investigations of pain in animals. In: Duncan IJH, Malony V (eds). *Assessing Pain in Farm Animals*. European Communities, Luxembourg, pp. 16–27.

3 Fox SM, Mellor DJ, Firth EC, *et al.* (1994). Changes in plasma cortisol concentrations before, during, and after analgesia, anaesthesia and anaesthesia plus ovariohysterectomy in bitches. *Res Vet Sci* **57**:110–118.

4 McQuay H, Moore A (1999). *An Evidence-Based Resource for Pain Relief*. Oxford University Press, New York, p. 191.

5 Mathews KA (2000). Pain assessment and general approach to management. In: Mathews KA (ed). Management of Pain. *Vet Clin North Am Small Anim Pract* **30**(4):732–733.

6 Fox SM, Mellor DJ, Stafford KJ, Lowoko CRO, Hodge H (2000). The effects of ovariohysterectomy plus different combinations of halothane anaesthesia and butorphanol analgesia on behaviour in the bitch. *Res Vet Sci* **68**:265–274.

7 Conzemius MG, Hill GM, Sammarco JL, *et al.* (1977). Correlation between subjective and objective measures used to determine severity of postoperative pain in dogs. *J Am Vet Med Assoc* **210**:1619–1622.

8 Hansen BD, Hardie EM, Carroll GS (1997). Physiological measurements after ovariohysterectomy in dogs: what's normal? *Appl Anim Behav Sci* **51**:101–109.

9 Holton LL, Scott EM, Nolan AM, *et al.* (1998). Relationship between physiological factors and clinical pain in dogs scored using a numerical rating scale. *J Soc Adm Pharm* **39**: 469–474.

10 Mellor DJ, Cook CJ, Stafford KJ (2000). Quantifying some responses to pain as a stressor. In: Moberg GP, Mench JA (eds). *The Biology of Animal Stress – Basic Principles and Implications for Animal Welfare*. CAB International Publishing, Wallingford, UK, pp. 171–198.

11 Fox SM, Mellor DJ, Lawoko CRO, Hodge H, Firth EC (1998). Changes in plasma cortisol concentrations in bitches in response to different combinations of halothane and butorphanol, with or without ovariohysterectomy. *Res Vet Sci* **65**:125–133.

12 Jensen MP, Turner JA, Romano JM (1994). What is the maximum number of levels needed in pain intensity measurement? *Pain* **58**:387–392.

13 Frayers PM, Hand DJ (2002). Causal variables, indicator variables, and measurement scales: an example from quality of life. *J R Stat Soc* (ser A) **165**:233–261.

14 Jensen MP, Karoly P, Braver S (1986). A comparison of six methods. *Pain* **27**:117–126.

15 Bennett D, Morton C (2009). A study of owner observed behavioural and lifestyle changes in cats with musculoskeletal disease before and after analgesic therapy. *J Feline Med Surg* **11**:997–1004.

16 Burton NJ, Owen MR, Colborne GR, *et al.* (2009). Can owners and clinicians assess outcome in dogs with fragmented medial coronoid process? *Vet Comp Orthop Traumatol* **22**:183–189.

17 Firth AM, Haldane SL (1999). Development of a scale to evaluate postoperative pain in dogs. *J Am Vet Med Assoc* **214**:651–659.

18 Hardy JD, Wolff HD, Goodel H (1952). *Pain Sensation and Reaction*. Williams & Wilkins, Baltimore, pp. 86–112.

19 Grossi E, Borghi C, Cerchiari EL, *et al.* (1983). Analogue chromatic continuous scale (ACCS): a new method of pain assessment. *Clin Exp Rheumatol* **1**:337–340.

20 Melzack R, Torgerson WS (1971). On the language of pain. *Anesthesiology* **34**:50–59.

21 Holton L, Reid J, Scott EM, *et al.* (2001). Development of a behaviour-based scale to measure acute pain in dogs. *Vet Rec* **148**: 525–531.

22 Morton CM, Reid J, Scott M, *et al.* (2005). Application of a scaling model to establish and validate an interval level pain scale for assessment of acute pain in dogs. *Am J Vet Res* **66**:2154–2166.

23 Reid J, Nolan AM, Hughes JML, *et al.* (2007). Development of the short-form Glasgow Composite Measure Pain Scale (CMPS-SF) and derivation of an analgesic intervention score. *Anim Welfare* **16**(5):97–104.

24 Wiseman-Orr ML, Nolan AM, Reid J, *et al.* (2004). Development of a questionnaire to measure the effects of chronic pain on health-related quality of life in dogs. *Am J Vet Res* **65**:1077–1084.

25 Wiseman-Orr M, Scott EM, Reid J, *et al.* (2006). Validation of a structured questionnaire as an instrument to measure chronic pain in dogs on the basis of effects on health-related quality of life. *Am J Vet Res* **67**:1826–1836.

26 McMillan FD (2000). Quality of life in animals. *J Am Vet Med Assoc* **216**:1904–1910.

27 Hielm-Björkman AK, Kuusela E, Markkola A, *et al.* (2003). Evaluation of methods for assessment of pain associated with chronic osteoarthritis in dogs. *J Am Vet Med Assoc* **222**:1552–1558.

28 Yazhek KVB, Fantoni DT (2005). Validity of a health-related quality-of-life scale for dogs with signs of pain secondary to cancer. *J Am Vet Med Assoc* **226**:1354–1358.

29 Brown DC, Boston RC, Coyne JC, *et al.* (2007). Development and psychometric testing of an instrument designed to measure chronic pain in dogs with osteoarthritis. *Am J Vet Res* **68**:631–637.
30 Hielm-Bjorkman AK, Rita H, Tulamo R-M (2009). Psychometric testing of the Helsinki chronic pain index by completion of a questionnaire in Finnish by owners of dogs with chronic signs of pain caused by osteoarthritis. *Am J Vet Res* **70**:727–734.
31 Gingerich DA, Strobel JD (2003). Use of client-specific outcome measures to assess treatment effects in geriatric, arthritic dogs: controlled clinical evaluation of a nutraceutical. *Vet Ther* **4**:56–66.
32 Baillie L (1993). Clinical pain management: a review of pain assessment tools. *Nurs Stand* 7:25–29.

CHAPTER 4

1 Gaynor JS, Muir WW (2002). *Handbook of Veterinary Pain Management*, 2nd edn. p. 31.
2 Djouhri L, Bleazard L, Lawson SN (1998). Association of somatic action potential shape with sensory receptive properties in guinea-pig dorsal root ganglion neurons. *J Physiol* **513**: 857–872.
3 Rexed B (1952). The cytoarchitectonic organization of the spinal cord in the cat. *J Comp Neurol* **96**(3):414–495.
4 Melzack R, Wall PD (1965). Pain mechanisms: a new theory. *Science* **150**(699):971–979.
5 Brosseau L, Yonge KA, Robinson V, *et al.* (2008). Transcutaneous electrical nerve stimulation (TENS) for the treatment of rheumatoid arthritis in the hand (Cochrane Review). In: *The Cochrane Library*, Issue 4.
6 Osiri M, Welch V, Brosseau L, *et al.* (2008). Transcutaneous electrical nerve stimulation for knee osteoarthritis (Cochrane Review). In: *The Cochrane Library*, Issue 4.
7 Pelage L, Brosseau L, Casimir L, *et al.* (2008). Electrical stimulation for the treatment of rheumatoid arthritis (Cochrane Review). In: *The Cochrane Library*, Issue 4.
8 DeSantana JM, ad Silva LFS, Sluka KA (2010). Cholecystokinin receptors mediate tolerance to the analgesic effect of TENS in arthritic rats. *Pain* **148**:84–93.
9 Facchinetti F, Sandrini G, Petraglia F, *et al.* (1984). Concomitant increase in nociceptive flexion reflex threshold and plasma opioids following transcutaneous nerve stimulation. *Pain* **19**:295–303.
10 Salar G, Job I, Mingrino S, *et al.* (1981). Effect of transcutaneous electrotherapy on CSF beta-endorphin content in patients without pain problems. *Pain* **10**:169–172.
11 Leonard G, Goffaux P, Marchand S (2010). Deciphering the role of endogenous opioids in high-frequency TENS using low and high doses of naloxone. *Pain* **151**:215–219.
12 La Motte RH, Thalhammer JG, Robinson CJ (1983). Peripheral neural correlates of magnitude of cutaneous pain and hyperalgesia: a comparison of neural events in monkey with sensory judgements in human. *J Neurophysiol* **50**:1–26.
13 Davis KD, Meyer RA, Campbell JN (1993). Chemosensitivity and sensitization of nociceptive afferents that innervate the hairy skin of monkey. *J Neurophysiol* **69**:1071–1081.
14 Woolf CJ, Salter MW (2006). Plasticity and pain: role of the dorsal horn. In: McMahon SB, Koltzenburg M (eds). *Wall and Melzack's Textbook of Pain*. Elsevier, St Louis, pp. 91–105.
15 Woolf CJ (1996). Windup and central sensitization are not equivalent. *Pain* **66**:105–108.
16 Mendell LM (1984). Modifiability of spinal synapses. *Physiol Rev* **64**:260–324.
17 Woolf CJ (1983). Evidence for a central component of post-injury pain hypersensitivity. *Nature* **306**:686–688.
18 Torebjork HE, Lundberg LER, LaMotte RH (1992). Central changes in processing of mechanoreceptor input in capsaicin-induced sensory hyperalgesia in humans. *J Physiol* (Lond.) **448**:765–780.
19 Lei Z, Ruan Y, Yang AN, *et al.* (2006). NMDA receptor-mediated dendritic plasticity in cortical cultures after oxygen-glucose deprivation. *Neurosci Lett* **407**:224–229.
20 Klop EM, Mauton LJ, Holster C (2004). How many spinothalamic tract cells are there? A retrograde tracing study in cat. *Neurosci Lett* **360**:121–124.
21 Katter JT, Burstein R, Gesture GJ (1991). The cells of origin of the spinohypothalamic tract in cats. *J Comp Neurol* **303**:101–112.
22 Wiata K, Fukuoka T, Kondo E, *et al.* (2002). Plastic changes in nociceptive transmission of the rat spinal cord with advancing age. *J Neurophysiol* **87**:1086–1093.
23 Staud R, Robinson ME, Vierek CJ Jr, Price DD (2003). Diffuse noxious inhibitory controls (DNIC) attenuate temporal summation of second pain in normal males but not in normal females or fibromyalgia patients. *Pain* **101**: 167–174.
24 Ruda MA, Bennett GJ, Dubber R (1986). Neurochemistry and neural circuitry in the dorsal horn. *Prog Brain Res* **66**:219–268.
25 Wall P (1988). The prevention of postoperative pain. *Pain* **33**(3):289–290.
26 Dahl JB, Kehlet H (2011). Preventive analgesia. *Curr Opin Anaesthesiol* **24**(3):331–338.

27 Fox SM, Mellor DJ, Firth EC, *et. al.* (1994). Changes in plasma cortisol concentrations before, during and after analgesia, anaesthesia, and anaesthesia plus ovariohysterectomy in bitches. *Res Vet Sci* **57**:110–118.

28 Hansen BD, Hardie EM, Carroll GS (1997). Physiological measurements after ovariohysterectomy in dogs: what's normal? *Appl Anim Behav Sci* **51**:101–109.

29 Shafford HL, Lascelles BDX, Hellyer PW (2001). Preemptive analgesia: managing pain before it begins. *Vet Med* **6**:478–491.

30 Tverskoy M, Oz Y, Isakson A, *et al.* (1994). Preemptive effect of fentanyl and ketamine on postoperative pain and wound hyperalgesia. *Anesth Analg* **78**:205–209.

31 Rockemann MG, Selling W, Bischof C, *et al.* (1996). Prophylactic use of epidural mepivacaine/morphine, systemic diclofenac, and metamizol reduces postoperative morphine consumption after major abdominal surgery. *Anesthesiology* **84**:1027–1034.

32 Lee VC, Rowlingson JC (1995). Pre-emptive analgesia: update on nonsteroidal anti-inflammatory drugs in anesthesia. *Adv Anesth* **12**:69–110.

33 Souter AJ, Fredman B, White PF (1994). Controversies in the perioperative use of nonsteroidal anti-inflammatory drugs. *Anesth Analg* **79**:1178–1190.

34 Malmberg AB, Yaksh TL (1993). Pharmacology of the spinal action of ketorolac, morphine, ST-91, U50488H, and L-PIA on the formalin test and an isobolographic analysis of the NSAID interaction. *Anesthesiology* **79**:211–213.

35 Vaughn C, Ingram SL, Connor MA, *et al.* (1997). How opioids inhibit GABA-mediated transmission. *Nature* **390**:611–614.

36 Emkey R, Rosenthal N, Wu S-C, *et al.* (2004). Efficacy and safety of tramadol/acetaminophen tablets (Ultracet®) as add-on therapy for osteoarthritis pain in subjects receiving a COX-2 nonsteroidal anti-inflammatory drug: a multicenter, randomized, double-blind, placebo-controlled trial. *J Rheumatol* **31**(1):150–156.

37 Edwards JE, McQuay HJ, Moore RA (2002). Combination analgesic efficacy: individual patient data meta-analysis of single-dose oral tramadol plus acetaminophen in acute postoperative pain. *J Pain Symptom Manag* **23**(2):121–130.

38 Gillies GWA, Kenny GNC, Bullingham RES, *et al.* (1987). The morphine sparing effects of ketorolac tromethamine: a study of a new parenteral nonsteroidal anti-inflammatory agent after abdominal surgery. *Anaesthesia* **42**:727–731.

39 Sevarino FB, Sinatra RS, Paige D, *et al.* (1992). The efficacy of intramuscular ketorolac in combination with intravenous PCA morphine for post operative pain relief. *J Clin Anesth* **4**:285–288.

40 Vertosick FT (2000). *Why We Hurt. The Natural History of Pain*. Harcourt, New York.

41 Pogatzki EM, Raja SN (2003). A mouse model of incisional pain. *Anesthesiology* **99**(4): 1023–1027.

42 Ali Z, Meyer RA, Campbell JN (1996). Secondary hyperalgesia to mechanical but not heat stimuli following a capsaicin injection in hairy skin. *Pain* **68**:401–411.

43 Kehlet H, Jensen TS, Woolf CJ (2006). Persistent postsurgical pain: risk factors and prevention. *Lancet* **367**:1618–1625.

44 Drygus KA, McClure S, Goring RL, *et al.* (2011). Prospective evaluation of cold compression therapy on postoperative pain, swelling, range of motion and lameness following tibial plateau leveling osteotomy in dogs. *J Am Vet Med Assoc* **238**(10):1284–1291.

45 Merskey H, Bogduk N (1994). *Classification of Chronic Pain: Descriptions of Chronic Pain Syndromes and Definitions of Pain Terms*, 2nd edn. IASP Press, Seattle, p. 222.

46 Russo CM, Brose WG (1998). Chronic pain. *Annu Rev Med* **49**:123–133.

47 Schaible HG, Richter F (2004). Pathophysiology of pain. *Langerbecks Arch Surg* **389**:237–243.

48 Jacobsen L, Mariano A (2001). General considerations of chronic pain. In: Loeser JD, Butler SH, Chapman SR (eds). *Bonica's Management of Pain*, 3rd edn. Lippincott Williams & Wilkins, Baltimore, pp. 241–254.

49 Cervero F, Laird JM (2003). From acute to chronic pain: peripheral and central mechanisms. In: Bountra C, Munglani R, Schmidt WK (eds). *Pain: Current Understanding, Emerging Therapies, and Novel Approaches to Drug Discovery*. Marcel Kekker, New York, pp. 29–44.

50 Bonica JJ (1991). History of pain concepts and pain theory. *Mt Sinai J Med* **58**:191–202.

51 Cervero F (1994). Sensory innervation of the viscera: peripheral basis of visceral pain. *Physiol Rev* **74**:95–138.

52 Habler HJ, Janig W, Koltzenburg M (1990). Activation of unmyelinated afferent fibers by mechanical stimuli and inflammation of the urinary bladder in the cat. *J Physiol* (Lond) **425**:545–562.

53 Gebhart GF (2000). Pathobiology of visceral pain: molecular mechanisms and therapeutic implications *vs*. central nervous system processing of somatic and visceral sensory signals. *Am J Physiol Gastrointest Liver Physiol* **278**:G834–G838.

54 Cervero F (2000). Visceral hyperalgesia revisited. *Lancet* **356**:1127–1128.
55 Petersen P, Gao C, Arendt-Neielsen K, *et al.* (2003). Pain intensity and biomechanical responses during ramp-controlled distension of the human rectum. *Dig Dis Sci* **48**:1310–1316.
56 McMahon SB, Dmitrieva N, Koltzenberg M (1995). Visceral pain. *Br J Anaesth* **75**:132–144.
57 Unruh AM (1996). Gender variations in clinical pain experience. *Pain* **65**:123–167.
58 Muir WW, Wiese AJ, Wittum TE (2002). Prevalence and characteristics of pain in dogs and cats examined as outpatients at a veterinary teaching hospital. *J Am Vet Med Assoc* **224**: 1459–1463.
59 Holdcroft A, Sapsed-Byrne S, Ma D, *et al.* (2000). Sex and oestrous cycle differences in visceromotor responses and vasopressin release in response to colonic distention in male and female rats anaesthetized with halothane. *Br J Anaesth* **85**:907–910.
60 Kamp EH, Jones RCW, Tillman SR, *et al.* (2003). Quantitative assessment and characterization of visceral nociception and hyperalgesia in mice. *Am J Physiol Gastrointest Liver Physiol* **284**:G434–G444.
61 Mogil JS, Chanda ML (2005). The case for the inclusion of female subjects in basic science studies of pain. *Pain* **117**:1–5.
62 Strigo IA, Bushnell MC, Boivin M, *et al.* (2002). Psychophysical analysis of visceral and cutaneous pain in human subjects. *Pain* **97**:235–246.
63 Sugiura Y, Terui N, Hosoya Y, *et al.* (1993). Quantitative analysis of central terminal projections of visceral and somatic unmyelinated C primary afferent fibers in the guinea pig. *J Comp Neurol* **332**:315–325.
64 Ness TJ, Powell-Boone T, Cannon R, *et al.* (2005). Psychophysical evidence of hypersensitivity in subjects with interstitial cystitis. *J Urology* **173**:1983–1987.
65 Alagiri M, Chottiner S, Ratner V, Slade D, Hanno PM (1997). Interstitial cystitis: unexplained associations with other chronic disease and pain syndromes. *Urology* **49**(Suppl 5A):52–57.
66 Whorwell PJ, McCallum M, Creed FH, Roberts CT (1986). Noncolonic features of irritable bowel syndrome. *Gut* **27**:37–40.
67 Pezzone MA, Liang R, Fraser MO (2005). A model of neural cross-talk and irritation in the pelvis: implications for the overlap of chronic pelvic pain disorders. *Gastroenterology* **128**:1953–1964.
68 Qin C, Foreman RD (2004). Viscerovisceral convergence of urinary bladder and colorectal inputs to lumbosacral spinal neurons in rats. *Neuro Report* **15**:467–471.
69 McMahon SB, Morrison JFB (1982). Two groups of spinal interneurons that respond to stimulation of the abdominal viscera of the cat. *J Physiol* **322**:21–34.
70 Mertz H (2003). Review article: Visceral hypersensitivity. *Aliment Pharmacol Ther* **17**: 623–633.
71 Woolf CJ, Borsook D, Koltzenburg M (2003). Mechanism-based classifications of pain and analgesic drug discovery. In: Bountra C, Munglani R, Schmidt WK (eds). *Pain: Current Understanding, Emerging Therapies, and Novel Approaches to Drug Discovery*. Marcel Kekker, New York, pp. 1–8.

CHAPTER 5

1 Baggot JD (1995). Pharmacokinetics: disposition and fate of drugs in the body. In: Adams HR (ed). *Veterinary Pharmacology and Therapeutics*, 7th edn. Iowa State University Press, Ames, p.36.
2 Martin M, Matifas A, Maldonado R, *et al.* (2003). Acute antinociceptive responses in single and combinatorial opioid receptor knockout mice: distinct mu, delta and kappa tones. *Eur J Neurosci* **17**:701–708.
3 Pfeiffer A, Pasi A, Meraein P, *et al.* (1982). Opiate receptor binding sites in human brain. *Brain Res* **248**:87–96.
4 Jordan B, Devi LA (1998). Molecular mechanisms of opioid receptor signal transduction. *Br J Anaesth* **81**:12–19.
5 Le Bars D, Cozariu M, Cadden S (2001). Animal models of nociception. *Pharmacol Rev* **53**:597–652.
6 Jadad AR, Carroll D, Glynn CJ, *et al.* (1992). Morphine responsiveness of chronic pain: double-blind randomized crossover study with patient controlled analgesia. *Lancet* **339**:1367–1371.
7 Dourish CT, Hawley D, Iversen SD (1988). Enhancement of morphine analgesia and prevention of morphine tolerance in the rat by cholecystokinin antagonist L-364, 718. *Eur J Pharmacol* **147**:469–472.
8 Talbot-Stern J, Paoloni R (2000). Prophylactic metoclopramide is unnecessary with intravenous analgesia in the ED. *Am J Emerg Med* **18**: 653–657.
9 Robertson SA, Hauptan JG, Nachreiner RF, *et al.* (2001). Effects of acetylpromazine or morphine on urine production in halothane-anesthetized dogs. *Am J Vet Res* **62**:1922–1927.
10 Chu LF, Clark DJ, Angst MS (2006). Opioid tolerance and hyperalgesia in chronic pain patients after one month of oral morphine therapy: a preliminary prospective study. *J Pain* **7**:43–48.
11 Mercadante S, Ferrera P, Villari P, *et al.* (2003). Hyperalgesia: an emerging iatrogenic syndrome. *J Pain Symptom Manage* **26**:769–775.

12 Gardell LR, Wang R, Burgess SE, *et al.* (2002). Sustained morphine exposure induces a spinal dynorphin-dependent enhancement of excitatory transmitter release from primary afferent fibers. *J Neurosci* **22**:6747–6755.

13 Ossipov MH, Lai J, King T, *et al.* (2004). Antinociceptive and nociceptive actions of opioids. *J Neurobiol* **61**:126–148.

14 King T, Vardanyan A, Majuta L, *et al.* (2007). Morphine treatment accelerates sarcoma-induced bone pain, bone loss, and spontaneous fracture in a murine model of bone cancer. *Pain* **132**: 154–168.

15 Lee M, Silverman S, Hansen H, *et al.* (2011). A comprehensive review of opioid-induced hyperalgesia. *Pain Physician* **14**:145–161.

16 Kukanich B, Lascelles BD, Aman AM, *et al.* (2005). The effects of inhibiting cytochrome P450 3A, p-glycoprotein, and gastric acid secretion on the oral bioavailability of methadone in dogs. *J Vet Pharmacol Ther* **28**:461–466.

17 Kukanich B, Lascelles BD, Papich MG (2005). Pharmacokinetics of morphine and plasma concentrations of morphine-6-glucuronide following morphine administration to dogs. *J Vet Pharmacol Ther* **28**:371–376.

18 Hansen B (1996). How to prevent and relieve patient pain. *Vet Forum* **8**:34–39.

19 Barnhart MD, Hubbell JAE, Muir WW, *et al.* (2000). Pharmacokinetics, pharmacodynamics, and analgesic effects of morphine after rectal, intramuscular, and intravenous administration in dogs. *Am J Vet Res* **61**:24–28.

20 Egger CM, Duke T, Archer J, *et al.* (1998). Comparison of plasma fentanyl concentrations by using three transdermal fentanyl patch sizes in dogs. *Vet Surg* **27**(2):159–166.

21 Kyles AE, Papich M, Hardie EM (1996). Disposition of transdermally administered fentanyl in dogs. *Am J Vet Res* **57**:715–719.

22 Scherk-Nixon M (1996). A study of the use of a transdermal fentanyl patch in cats. *J Am Anim Hosp Assoc* **32**:19–24.

23 Lee DD, Papich MG, Hardie EM (1998). Pharmacokinetics of intravenously and transdermally administered fentanyl in cats (abstr). *Proceedings ACVS Symposium* 15.

24 Bellei E, Roncada P, Pisoni L, *et al.* (2011). The use of fentanyl-patch in dogs undergoing spinal surgery: plasma concentration and analgesic efficacy. *J Vet Pharmacol Ther* **34**:437–441.

25 Pascoe, PJ (2000). Opioid analgesics. *Vet Clin North Am: Sm Anim Pract* **30**:757–772.

26 Evans HC, Easthope SE (2003). Transdermal buprenorphine. *Drugs* **63**:1999–2010.

27 Andaluz A, Moll X, Abellan R, *et al.* (2009). Pharmacokinetics of buprenorphine after intravenous administration of clinical doses to dogs. *Vet J* **181**:299–304.

28 Andaluz A, Moll X, Ventura R, *et al.* (2009). Plasma buprenorphine concentrations after the application of a 70 µg/h transdermal patch in dogs. Preliminary report. *J Vet Pharmacol Ther* **32**:503–505.

29 Moll X, Fresno L, Garcia F, *et al.* (2011). Comparison of subcutaneous and transdermal administration of buprenorphine for pre-emptive analgesia in dogs undergoing elective ovariohysterectomy. *Vet J* **187**:124–128.

30 Sitti R, Griebinger N, Likar R (2003). Analgesic efficacy and tolerability of transdermal buprenorphine in patients with inadequately controlled chronic pain related to cancer and other disorders: a multicenter, randomized, double-blind, placebo-controlled trial. *Clin Therap* **25**:150–168.

31 Bartholomaus J (2002). Moderne darreichungsformen fur opioide. *Pharmazie in Unserer Zeit* **31**:74–81.

32 Pieper K, Schuster T, Levionnois O, *et al.* (2011). Antinociceptive efficacy and plasma concentrations of transdermal buprenorphine in dogs. *Vet J* **187**:335–341.

33 Boden BP, Fassler S, Cooper S, *et al.* (1994). Analgesic effect of intraarticular morphine, bupivacaine, and morphine/bupivacine after arthroscopic knee surgery. *Arthroscopy* **10**: 104–107.

34 Carroll GW (2008). *Small Animal Anesthesia and Analgesia*, 2nd edn. Blackwell Publishing, Ames.

35 Raffa RB, Friderichs E, Reimann W, *et al.* (1992). Opioid and nonopioid components independently contribute to the mechanism of action of tramadol, an 'atypical' opioid analgesic. *J Pharmacol Exp Ther* **260**:275–285.

36 Novartis Animal Health US, Inc. Over a 2 year period (2006–2007), 34% (99/289) of adverse drug events reported for serious gastric events (perforation and GI bleeding) involved the concurrent use of tramadol together with a NSAID (relationship cause/effect undetermined). (Data on File.)

37 Torring ML, Riis A, Christensen S, *et al.* (2007). Perforated peptic ulcer and short-term mortality among tramadol users. *Br J Clin Pharm* **65**(4):565–572.

38 Garcia-Hernandez L, Deciga-Campos M, Guevara-Lopez U, *et al.* (2002). Coadministration of rofencoxib and tramadol results in additive or sub-additive interaction during arthritic nociception in rat. *Pharm Biochem Behav* **87**:331–340.

39 Abrams TW (2009). Warning Letter to William C. Weldon, Chairman of the Board and Chief Executive Officer, Johnson & Johnson, 5/12/2009.

40 Bianchi M, Broggini M, Balzarini P, *et al.* (2003). Effects of tramadol on synovial fluid concentrations of substance P and interleukin-6 in patients with knee osteoarthritis: comparison with paracetamol. *Int Immunopharm* **3**: 1901–1908.

41 Wu WN, McKown LA, Gauthler AD, *et al.* (2001). Metabolism of the analgesic drug, tramadol hydrochloride, in rat and dog. *Xenobiotica* **31**:423–441.

42 Kukanich B, Papich MG (2004). Pharmacokinetics of tramadol and the metabolite O-desmethyltramadol in dogs. *J Vet Pharmacol Ther* **27**:239–246.

43 Grond S, Meuser T, UraggH, *et al.* (1999). Serum concentrations of tramadol enantiomers during patient-controlled analgesia. *Br J Clin Pharm* **48**:254–257.

44 McMillan CJ, Livingston A, Clark CR, *et al.* (2008). Pharmacokinetics of intravenous tramadol in dogs. *Can J Vet Med* **72**:325–331.

45 Giorgi M, Saccomanni G, Lebkowska-Wienuszewska B, *et al.* (2009). Pharmacokinetic evaluation of tramadol and its major metabolites after single oral sustained tablet administration in the dog: a pilot study. *Vet J* **180**(2): 252–255.

46 Pypendop BH, Ilkiw JE (2007). Pharmacokinetics of tramadol and O-desmethyltramadol in cats. *J Vet Pharmacol Ther* **31**:52–59.

47 Mastrocinque S, Fantoni DT (2003). A comparison of preoperative tramadol and morphine for the control of early postoperative pain in canine ovariohysterectomy. *Vet Anaesth Analg* **30**:220–228.

48 Martins TL, Kahvegian MAP, Noel-Morgan J, *et al.* (2010). Comparison of the effects of tramadol, codeine, and ketoprofen alone or in combination on postoperative pain and on concentrations of blood glucose, serum cortisol, and serum interleukin-6 in dogs undergoing maxillectomy or mandibulectomy. *Am J Vet Res* **71**(9):1019–1026.

49 Armstrong PJ, Bersten A (1986). Normeperidine toxicity. *Anesth Analg* **65**(5):536–538.

50 Robertson SA, Lascelles BDX, Taylor PM, *et al.* (2005). PK-PD modeling of buprenorphine in cats: intravenous and oral transmucosal administration. *J Vet Pharmacol Ther* **28**:453–460.

51 Webb AR, Leong S, Myles PS, *et al.* (2002). The addition of a tramadol infusion to morphine patient-controlled analgesia after abdominal surgery: a double-blinded, placebo-controlled randomized trial. *Anesth Analg* **95**:1713–1718.

52 Tuncer S, Pirbudak L, Balat O, *et al.* (2003). Adding ketoprofen to intravenous patient-controlled analgesia with tramadol after major gynecological cancer surgery: a double-blinded, randomized, placebo-controlled clinical trial. *Eur J Gynaecol Oncol* **24**:181–184.

53 Sindrup SH, Andersen G, Madsen C, *et al.* (1999). Tramadol relieves pain and allodynia in polyneuropathy: a randomized, double-blind, controlled trial. *Pain* **83**(1):85–90.

54 Muir WW, Wiese AJ, March PA (2003). Effects of morphine, lidocaine, ketamine, and morphine-lidocaine-ketamine drug combination on minimum alveolar concentration in dogs anesthetized with isoflurane. *Am J Vet Res* **64**:1155–1160.

55 Virtanen R (1989). Pharmacologic profiles of medetomidine and its antagonist, antipamezole. *Acta Vet Scand* (Suppl) **85**:29–37.

56 Duke T, Cox AM, Remedios AM, *et al.* (1994). The cardiopulmonary effects of placing fentanyl or medetomidine in the lumbosacral epidural space of isoflurane-anesthetized cats. *Vet Surg* **23**:149–155.

57 Pan H-L, Chen S-R, Eisenach JC (1999). Intrathecal clonidine alleviates allodynia in neuropathic rats: interaction with spinal muscarinic and nicotinic receptors. *Anesthesiology* **90**:509–514.

58 Murrell JC, Hellebrekers LJ (2005). Medetomidine and dexmedetomidine: a review of cardiovascular effects and antinociceptive properties in the dog. *Vet Anaesth Analg* **32**: 117–127.

59 Kuusela E, Raekallio M, Anttila M, *et al.* (2000). Clinical effects and pharmacokinetics of medetomidine and its enantiomers in dogs. *J Vet Pharmacol Ther* **23**:15–20.

60 McKusick BC, Westerholm FC, Vaisanen M (2005). Clinical evaluation of dexmedetomidine premedication prior to ketamine anaesthesia in cats (abstr). *Proc Assoc Vet Anaesth* **66**.

61 Granholm M, McKusick BC, Westerholm FC, *et al.* (2006). Evaluation of the clinical efficacy and safety of dexmedetomidine or medetomidine in cats and their reversal with atipamezole. *Vet Anaesth Analg* **22**:214–223.

62 No Author listed (2009). FAQs; Analgesia, sedation, and anesthesia. Making the switch from medetomidine to dexmedetomidine. *Compend Contin Edu Vet* (Suppl) **31**.

63 Grimm IKA, Lemke KA (2007). Preanesthetics and anesthetic adjuncts. In: Thurman JC, Tranquilli WJ (eds). *Lumb & Jones' Veterinary Anesthesia and Analgesia*, 4th edn. Blackwell Publishing, Ames.

64 Dworkin RH, Backonja M, Rowbotham MC, *et al*. (2003). Advances in neuropathic pain diagnosis, mechanisms, and treatment recommendations. *Arch Neurol* **60**: 1524–1534.
65 Pypendop BH, Iikiw JE (2005). Assessment of the hemodynamic effects of lidocaine administered IV in isodlurane-anesthetized cats. *Am J Vet Res* **66**(4):661–668.
66 Devor M, Wall PD, Catalan N (1992). Systemic lidocaine silences ectopic neuroma and DRG discharge without blocking nerve conduction. *Pain* **48**:261–268.
67 Biella G, Sotgiu ML (1993). Central effects of systemic lidocaine mediated by glycine spinal receptors: an iontophoretic study in the rat spinal cord. *Brain Res* **603**:201–206.
68 Chabal C, Jacobson L, Mariano A, *et al*. (1992). The use of oral mexiletine for the treatment of pain after peripheral nerve injury. *Anesthesiology* **76**:513–517.
69 Koppert W, Weigand M, Neumann F, *et al*. (2004). Perioperative intravenous lidocaine has preventive effects on postoperative pain and morphine consumption after major abdominal surgery. *Anesth Analg* **98**:1050–1055.
70 Insler SR, O'Conner RM, Samonte AF, *et al*. (1995). Lidocaine and the inhibition of postoperative pain in coronary artery bypass patients. *J Cardiothorac Vasc Anesth* **9**:541–546.
71 Birch K, Jørgensen J, Chraemmer-Jørgensen B, *et al*. (1987). Effect of i.v. lignocaine on pain and the endocrine metabolic responses after surgery. *Br J Anaesth* **59**:721–724.
72 Cassuto J, Wallin G, HögstrōM S, *et al*. (1985). Inhibition of postoperative pain by continuous low-dose intravenous infusion of lidocaine. *Anesth Analg* **64**:971–974.
73 Sjögren P, Banning AM, Hebsgaarch K, *et al*. (1989). Intravenous lidocaine in the treatment of chronic pain caused by bone metastases. *Ugeskr Laeger* **151**:2144–2146.
74 Elleman K, Sjögren P, Banning AM, *et al*. (1989). Trial of intravenous lidocaine on painful neuropathy in cancer patients. *Clin J Pain* **5**: 291–294.
75 Nagaro T, Shimizu C, Inous H, *et al*. (1995). The efficacy of intravenous lidocaine on various types of neuropathic pain. *Masui* **44**:862–867.
76 Tanelian DL, Brose WG (1991). Neuropathic pain can be relieved by drugs that are use-dependent sodium channel blockers: lidocaine, carbamazepine, and mexiletine. *Anesthesiology* **74**:949–951.
77 Ferrante FM, Paggioli J, Cherukuri S, *et al*. (1996).The analgesic response to intravenous lidocaine in the treatment of neuropathic pain. *Anesth Anal*g **82**:91–97.
78 Galer BS, Miller KV, Rowbotham MC (1993). Response to intravenous lidocaine infusion differs based on clinical diagnosis and site of nervous system injury. *Neurology* **43**: 1233–1235.
79 Wallace MS, Dyck JB, Rossi SS, *et al*. (1996). Computer-controlled lidocaine infusion for the evaluation of neuropathic pain after peripheral nerve injury. *Pain* **66**:69–77.
80 Edmondson SA, Simpson RK Jr., Stubler DK, *et al*. (1993). Systemic lidocaine therapy for poststroke pain. *South Med J* **86**:1093–1096.
81 Rowbotham MC, Reisner-Keller LA, Fields HL (1992). Both intravenous lidocaine and morphine reduce the pain of postherpetic neuralgia. *Neurology* **41**:1024–1028.
82 Sörensen J, Bengtsson A, Bäckman E, *et al*. (1995). Pain analysis in patients with fibromyalgia. Effects of intravenous morphine, lidocaine, and ketamine. *Scand J Rheumatol* **24**:360–365.
83 Bach FW, Jensen TS, Kastrup J, *et al*. (1990). The effect of intravenous lidocaine on nociceptive processing in diabetic neuropathy. *Pain* **40**: 29–34.
84 Ackerman WE, Colclough GW, Juneja MM, *et al*. (1991). The management of oral mexiletine and intravenous lidocaine to treat chronic painful symmetrical distal diabetic neuropathy. *J Ky Med Assoc* **89**:500–501.
85 McGeeney BE (2006). Anticonvulsants. In : de Leon-Casasola OA (ed). *Cancer Pain: Pharmacological, Interventional and Palliative Care Approaches*. Elsevier WB Saunders, Philadelphia.
86 Raymond SA, Steffensen SC, Gugino LD, *et al*. (1989). The role of length of nerve exposed to local anesthetics in impulse blocking action. *Anesth Analg* **68**:563–570.
87 Campoy L, Martin-Flores M, Looney AL, *et al*. (2008). Distribution of a lidocaine-methylene blue solution staining in brachial plexus, lumbar plexus and sciatic nerve blocks in the dog. *Vet Anaesth Analg* **35**:348–354.
88 Chabal C, Russell LC, Burchiel K (1989). The effect of intravenous lidocaine, tocainide, and mexiletine on spontaneously active fibers arising in rat sciatic nerve neuromas. *Pain* **38**:333–338.
89 Devers A, Galer BS (2000). Topical lidocaine patch relieves a variety of neuropathic pain conditions: an open label study. *Clin J Pain* **16**:205–208.
90 Klein J, Fernandes D, Gazarian M, *et al*. (1994). Simultaneous determination of lidocaine, prilocaine and the prilocaine metabolite 0-toluidine in plasma by high-performance liquid chromatography. *J Chromatogr B Biomed Sci Appl* **655**:83–88.

91 Erkert RS, MacAllister CG (2005). Use of a eutectic mixture of lidocaine 2.5% and prilocaine 2.5% as a local anesthetic in animals. *J Am Vet Med Assoc* **226**:1990–1992.
92 Paoli F, Darcourt G, Corsa P (1960). Note preliminaire sur l'action de l'imipramine dans les états douloureux. *Rev Neurol* **2**:503–504.
93 Arsenault A, Sawynok J (2009). Perisurgical amitriptyline produces a preventive effect on afferent hypersensitivity following spared nerve injury. *Pain* **146**:308–314.
94 Hall H, Ögren S-O (1981). Effects of antidepressant drugs on different receptors in the brain. *Eur J Pharmacol* **70**:393–407.
95 Nelson KA, Park KM, Robinovitz E, *et al*. (1997). High-dose oral dextromethorphan versus placebo in painful diabetic neuropathy and postherpetic neuralgia. *Neurology* **48**:1212–1218.
96 Sato J, Perl ER (1991). Adrenergic excitation of cutaneous pain receptors induced by peripheral nerve injury. *Science* **251**:1608–1611.
97 Pancrazio JJ, Kamatchi GL, Roscoe AK, *et al*. (1998). Inhibition of neuronal Na+ channels by antidepressant drugs. *J Pharmacol Exp Ther* **284**:208–214.
98 Sindrup SH, Jensen TS (1999). Efficacy of pharmacological treatments of neuropathic pain: an update and effect related to mechanism of drug action. *Pain* **83**:389–400.
99 Mogil JS (1999). The genetic mediation of individual differences in sensitivity to pain and its inhibition. *Proc Nat Acad Sci* **96**:7744–7751.
100 Ash G, Dickens CM, Creed FH, *et al*. (1999). The effects of dothiepin on subjects with rheumatoid arthritis and depression. *Rheumatology* (Oxford) **38**:959–967.
101 Sindrup SH, Brosen K, Gram LF (1992). The mechanism of action of antidepressants in pain treatment: controlled cross-over studies in diabetic neuropathy. *Clin Neuropharmacol* **15**(Suppl 1 part A):380A–381A.
102 Max M, Culnane M, Schafer S, *et al*. (1987). Amitriptyline relieves diabetic neuropathy pain in patients with normal or depressed mood. *Neurology* **37**:589–596.
103 Chapel AS, Oscine MJ, iLu-Seifert H, *et al*. (2009). Duloxetine, a centrally acting analgesic, in the treatment of patients with osteoarthritis knee pain: a 13-week, randomized, placebo-controlled trial. *Pain* **146**:253–260.
104 Sudoh Y, Cahoon EE, Gerner P, *et al*. (2003). Tricyclic antidepressants as long-acting local anesthetics. *Pain* **103**:49–55.
105 Schroder W, Tzschentke TM, Terlinden R, *et al*. (2011). Synergistic interaction between the two mechanisms of action of tapentadol in analgesia. *J Pharmacol Exp Ther* **337**(1):312–320.
106 Nossaman VE, Ramadhyani U, Kadowitz PJ, *et al*. (2010). Advances in perioperative pain management: use of medications with dual analgesic mechanisms, tramadol and tapentadol. *Anesthesiol Clin* **28**(4):647–666.
107 Schroder W, Vry JD, Tzschentke TM, *et al*. (2010). Differential contribution of opioid and noradrenergic mechanisms of tapentadol in rat models of nociceptive and neuropathic pain. *Eur J Pain* **14**(8):814–821.
108 Basile AS, Janowsky A, Golembiowska K, *et al*. (2007). Characterization of the antinociceptive actions of bicifadine in models of acute, persistent, and chronic pain. *J Pharmacol Exp Ther* **321**(3):1208–1225.
109 Hoyer D, Martin G (1997). 5-HT receptor classification and nomenclature: towards a harmonization with the human genome. *Neuropharmacology* **36**:419–428.
110 Lesch KP, Wolozin BL, Murphy DL, *et al*. (1993). Primary structure of the human platelet serotonin uptake site: identity with the brain serotonin transporter. *J Neurochem* **60**: 2319–2322.
111 Skop BP, Brown TM (1996). Potential vascular and bleeding complications of treatment with selective serotonin reuptake inhibitors. *Psychosomatics* **37**:12–16.
112 De Abajo FJ, Montero D, Garcia Rodriguez LA, *et al*. (2006). Antidepressants and risk of upper gastrointestinal bleeding. *Basic Clin Pharmacol Toxicol* **98**:304–310.
113 Martesson B, Wagner A, Beck O, *et al*. (1991). Effects of clomipramine treatment on cerebrospinal fluid monoamine metabolites and platelet ^{3}H-imipramine binding and serotonin uptake and concentration in major depressive disorder. *Acta Psychiatr Scand* **83**:125–133.
114 Crowell-Davis SL, Pogglagliolmi S (2008). Serotonin syndrome. *Compend Contin Edu Sm Anim Pract* September: 490–493.
115 White HS (1999). Comparative anticonvulsant and mechanistic profile of the established and newer antiepileptic drugs. *Epilepsia* **40** (Suppl 5):S2–10.
116 Tremont-Lukats IW, Megeff C, Backonja MM (2001). Anticonvulsants for neuropathic pain syndromes: mechanisms of action and place in therapy. *Drugs* **60**:1029–1052.

117 Fields HL, Rowbotham MC, Devor M (1997). Excitability blockers: anticonvulsants and low concentration local anesthetics in the treatment of chronic pain. In: Dickenson AH, Besson JM (eds). *Handbook of Experimental Pharmacology*. Springer-Verlag, Berlin.

118 Bedouin A, Utahan BM, Sackellares C (1995). Gabapentin: pharmacokinetics, efficacy and safety. *Clin Neuropharmacol* **18**:469–481.

119 Taylor CP, Gee NS, Su TZ, *et al*. (1998). A summary of mechanistic hypotheses of gabapentin pharmacology. *Epilepsy Res* **29**:233–249.

120 Rock DM, Kelly KM, Macdonald RL (1993). Gabapentin actions on ligand- and voltage-gated responses in cultured rodent neurons. *Epilepsy Res* **16**:89–98.

121 Shimoyama N, Shimoyama M, Davis AM, *et al*. (1997). Spinal gabapentin is antinociceptive in the rat formalin test. *Neurosci Lett* **222**:65–67.

122 Field MJ, Oles RJ, Lewis AS, *et al*. (1997). Gabapentin (Neurontin) and S-(+)-3-isobutylgaba represent a novel class of selective antihyperalgesic agents. *Br J Pharmacol* **121**:1513–1522.

123 Houghton AK, Lu Y, Westlund KN (1988). S-(+)-3-Isobutylgaba and its stereoisomer reduces the amount of inflammation and hyperalgesia in an acute arthritis model in the rat. *J Pharmacol Exp Ther* **285**:533–538.

124 Lu L, Westlund KN (1999). Gabapentin attenuates nociceptive behaviors in an acute arthritis model in rats. *J Pharm Exp Ther* **290**:214–219.

125 Field MJ, Holloman EF, McCleary S, *et al*. (1997). Evaluation of gabapentin and S-(+)-isobutylgaba in a rat model of postoperative pain. *J Pharmacol Exp Ther* **282**:1242–1246.

126 Hyashida K, Degors S, Curry R, Eisenach JC (2007). Gabapentin activates spinal noradrenergic activity in rats and humans and reduces hypersensitivity after surgery. *Anesthesiology* **106**(3):557–562.

127 Hanesch U, Pawlak M, McDougall JJ (2003). Gabapentin reduces the mechanosensitivity of fine afferent nerve fibres in normal and inflamed rat knee joints. *Pain* **104**:363–366.

128 Ivanavicius SP, Ball AD, Heapy CG, *et al*. (2007). Structural pathology in a rodent model of osteoarthritis is associated with neuropathic pain: increased expression of ATF-3 and pharmacological characterization. *Pain* **128**:272–282.

129 Maneuf YP, Hughes J, McKnight AT (2001). Gabapentin inhibits the substance P-facilitated K(+)-evoked release of [(3)H]glutamate from rat caudal trigeminal nucleus slices. *Pain* **93**:191–196.

130 Boileau C, Martel-Pelletier J, Brunet J, *et al*. (2005). Oral treatment with PD-0200347, an α2δ ligand, reduces the development of experimental osteoarthritis by inhibiting metalloproteinases and inducible nitric oxide synthase gene expression and synthesis in cartilage chondrocytes. *Arthritis Rheum* **52**:488–500.

131 Wagner AE, Mich PM, Uhrig SR, *et al*. (2010). Clinical evaluation of perioperative administration of gabapentin as an adjunct for postoperative analgesia in dogs undergoing amputation of a forelimb. *J Am Vet Med Assoc* **236**(7):751–756.

132 Boel A, Fransson KE, Peck JK, *et al*. (2002). Transdermal absorption of a liposome encapsulated formulation of lidocaine following topical administration in cats. *Am J Vet Res* **63**(9):1309–1312.

133 Woolf CJ, Thompson SWN (1991). The induction and maintenance of central sensitization is dependent on N-methyl-D-aspartic acid receptor activation; implications for the treatment of post-injury pain hypersensitivity states. *Pain* **44**:293–299.

134 Dambisya YM, Lee TL (1995). Antinociceptive effects of ketamine-opioid combinations in the mouse tail flick test. *Meth Find Exp Clin Pharmacol* **16**:179–184.

135 Mather LE, Edwards SR (1998). Chirality in anaesthesia—ropivacaine, ketamine and thiopentone. *Curr Opin Anaesthesiol* **11**: 383–390.

136 Scheller M, Bufler J, Hertle I, *et al*. (1996). Ketamine blocks currents through mammalian nicotinic acetylcholine receptor channels by interaction with both the open and the closed state. *Anesth Analg* **83**:830–836.

137 Hirota K, Lambert DG (1996). Ketamine: its mechanism(s) of action and unusual clinical uses. *Br J Anaesth* **77**:441–444.

138 Tverskoy M, Oz Y, lsakson A, Finger J, Bradley EL Jr, Kissin I (1994). Preemptive effect of fentanyl and ketamine on postoperative pain and wound hyperalgesia. *Anesth Analg* **78**(2):205–209.

139 Slingsby LS, Waterman-Pearson AE (2000). The post-operative analgesic effects of ketamine after canine ovariohysterectomy—a comparison between pre- or post-operative administration. *Res Vet Sci* **69**:147–152.

140 Van Pragg H (1990). The role of glutamate in opiate descending inhibition of nociceptive spinal reflexes. *Brain Res* **524**:101–105.

141 Backonja M, Arndt G, Gombar KA, *et al*. (1994). Response of chronic neuropathic pain syndromes to ketamine: a preliminary study. *Pain* **56**:51–57.

142 Eide PK, Stubhaug A, Øye I, *et al.* (1995). Continuous subcutaneous administration of the N-methyl-D-aspartic acid (NMDA) receptor antagonist ketamine in the treatment of post-herpetic neuralgia. *Pain* **61**:221–228.

143 Hoffmann V, Copperjans H, Vercauteren M, *et al.* (1994). Successful treatment of post-herpetic neuralgia with oral ketamine. *Clin J Pain* **10**:240–242.

144 Eisenberg E, Pud D (1998). Can patients with chronic neuropathic pain be cured by acute administration of the NMDA receptor antagonist amantadine? *Pain* **74**:337–339.

145 Pud D, Eisenberg E, Spitzer A, *et al.* (1998). The NMDA receptor antagonist amantadine reduces surgical neuropathic pain in cancer patients: a double blind, randomized, placebo controlled trial. *Pain* **75**:349–354.

146 Kleinbohl D, Gortelmeyer R, Bender HJ, *et al.* (2006). Amantadine sulfate reduces experimental sensitization and pain in chronic back pain patients. *Anesth Analg* **102**: 840–847.

147 Lascelles BDX, Gaynor JS, Smith SC, *et al.* (2008). Amantadine in a multimodal analgesic regimen for alleviation of refractory osteoarthritis pain in dogs. *J Vet Intern Med* **22**:53–59.

148 Lascelles BDX, Gaynor JS (2007). Cancer patients. In: Tranquilli WJ, Thurmon JC, Grimm KA (eds). *Lumb & Jones Veterinary Anesthesia and Analgesia*, 4th edn. Blackwell Publishing, Ames.

149 Cevc G, Blume G (2001). New, highly efficient formulation of diclofenac for the topical, transdermal administration in ultradeformable drug carriers. Transfersomes. *Biochem Biophys Acta* **1514**:191–205.

150 Chen X, Gallar J, Belmonte C (1997). Reduction by anti-inflammatory drugs of the response of corneal sensory nerve fibers to chemical irritation. *Invest Ophthalmic Vis Sci* **38**:1944–1953.

151 Dong X, Svensson P, Cairns BE (2009). The analgesic action of topical diclofenac may be mediated through peripheral NMDA receptor antagonism. *Pain* **147**:36–45.

152 Enarson MC, Hays H, Woodroffe MA (1999). Clinical experience with oral ketamine. *J Pain Symptom Manage* **17**:384–386.

153 Siao KT, Pypendop BH, Stanley SD, *et al.* (2011). Pharmacokinetics of amantadine in cats. *J Vet Pharmacol Ther* **14**:599–604.

154 Eisenberg E, Pud D (1988). Can patients with chronic neuropathic pain be cured by acute administration of NMDA receptor antagonist amantadine? *Pain* **74**:337–339.

155 Kukanich B, Papich MG (2004). Plasma profile and pharmacokinetics of dextromethorphan after intravenous and oral administration in healthy dogs. *J Vet Pharmacol Ther* **27**: 337–341.

156 Finnerup NB, Sindrup SH, Jensen TS (2010). The evidence for pharmacological treatment of neuropathic pain. *Pain* **150**:573–581.

157 Weinstein RS, Robertson PK, Manolagas SC (2009). Giant osteoclast formation and long-term oral bisphosphonate therapy. *N Engl J Med* **360**:53–62.

158 Luger NM, Honore P, Sabino MA, *et al.* (2001). Osteoprotegerin diminishes advanced bone cancer pain. *Cancer Res* **61**:4038–4047.

159 Honore P, Luger NM, Sabino MA, *et al.* (2000). Osteoprotegerin blocks bone cancer-induced skeletal destruction, skeletal pain and pain-related neurochemical reorganization of the spinal cord. *Nat Med* **6**:521–528.

160 Fan TM, de Lorimier LP, Carney SC, *et al.* (2005). Evaluation of intravenous pamidronate administration in 33 cancer-bearing dogs with primary or secondary bone involvement. *J Vet Intern Med* **19**:74–80.

161 Abe Y, Iba K, Takada J, *et al.* (2011). Improvement of pain and regional osteoporotic changes in the foot and ankle by low-dose bisphosphonate therapy for complex regional pain syndrome type I. *J Med Case Rep* **5**(349):1–12.

162 Anand P, Bley K (2011). Topical capsaicin for pain management. *Br J Anaesth* **107**(4): 490–502.

163 Karai L, Brown DC, Mannes AJ, *et al.* (2004). Deletion of vanilloid receptor 1-expressing primary afferent neurons for pain control. *J Clin Invest* **113**:1344–1352.

164 Caterina MJ, Rosen TA, Tominaga M, *et al.* (1999). A capsaicin-receptor homologue with a high threshold for noxious heat. *Nature* **398**:436–441.

165 Brown DC, Iadarola MJ, Perkowski SZ, *et al.* (2005). Physiologic and antinociceptive effects of intrathecal resiniferatoxin in a canine bone cancer model. *Anesthesiology* **103**:1052–1059.

166 Grimm KA, Tranquilli WJ, Thurmon JC, Benson GJ (2000). Duration of nonresponse to noxious stimulation after intramuscular administration of butorphanol, medetomidine, or a butorphanol-medetomidine combination during isoflurane administration in dogs. *Am J Vet Res* **61**(1):42–47.

167 Gomez de Segura iIA, Criado AB, Santos M, Tendillo FI (1998). Aspirin synergistically potentiates isoflurane minimum alveolar concentration reduction produced by morphine in the rat. *Anesthesiology* **89**(6):1489–1494.

CHAPTER 6

1 Wallace JL, Keenan CM, Gale D, *et al.* (1992). Exacerbation of experimental colitis by nonsteroidal anti-inflammatory drugs is not related to elevated leukotriene B4 synthesis. *Gastroenterology* **102**(1):18 27.

2 Lascelles BDX, Blikslager AT, Fox SM, *et al.* (2005). Gastrointestinal tract perforations in dogs treated with a selective cyclooxygenase-2 inhibitor: 29 cases (2002–2003). *J Am Vet Med Assoc* **227**(7):1112–1117.

3 Dow SW, Rosychuk RA, McChesney AE, *et al.* (1990). Effects of flunixin and flunixin plus prednisone on the gastrointestinal tract of dogs. *Am J Vet Res* **51**:1131–1138.

4 Boston SE, Moens NM, Kruth SA, *et al.* (2003). Endoscopic evaluation of the gastroduodenal mucosa to determine the safety of short-term concurrent administration of meloxicam and dexamethasone in healthy dogs. *Am J Vet Res* **64**:1369–1375.

5 De Leon-Casasola OA (ed) (2006). *Cancer Pain. Pharmacologic, Interventional, and Palliative Approaches*. WB Saunders, Philadelphia, p. 284.

6 Hemler M, Lands WE (1976). Purification of the cyclooxygenase that forms prostaglandins. Demonstration of two forms of iron in the holoenzyme. *J Biol Chem* **251**:5575–5579.

7 Vane JR, Botting RM (1995). A better understanding of anti-inflammatory drugs based on isoforms of cyclooxygenase (COX-1 and COX-2). *Adv Prostaglandin Thromboxane Leukot Res* **23**:41–48.

8 Warner TD, Mitchell JA (2004). Cyclooxygenases: new forms, new inhibitors, and lessons from the clinic. *FASEB J* **18**:790–804.

9 Kay-Hungerford, Benn SJ, Lamar J, *et al.* (2000). *In vitro* effects of nonsteroidal anti-inflammatory drugs on cyclooxygenase activity in dogs. *Am J Vet Res* **61**:802–810.

10 Brideau C, Van Staden C, Chan CC (2001). *In vitro* effects of cyclooxygenase inhibitors in whole blood of horses, dogs, and cats. *Am J Vet Res* **62**:1755–1760.

11 Streppa HK, Jones CJ, Budsberg SC (2002). Cyclooxygenase selectivity of nonsteroidal antiinflammatory drugs in canine blood. *Am J Vet Res* **63**:91–94.

12 Li J, Lynch MP, Demerol KL, *et al.* (2005). *In vitro* and *in vivo* profile of 2-(3-id-fluoromethyl-5-phenylpyrazol-1-yl)-5-methanesulfonylpyridine, a potent, selective, and orally active canine COX-2 inhibitor. *Bioorg Med Chem* **13**:1805–1809.

13 Warner TD, Mitchell JA (2002). Cyclooxygenase-3 (COX-3): filling in the gaps toward a COX continuum? *Proc Natl Acad Sci USA* **99**:13371–13373.

14 Singh G, Fort JG (2006). Celecoxib versus naproxen and diclofenac in osteoarthritis patients: SUCCESS-I Study. *Am J Med* **119**:255–288.

15 Liu SK, Tilley LP, Tappe JP, *et al.* (1986). Clinical and pathologic findings in dogs with atherosclerosis: 21 cases (1970–1983). *J Am Vet Med Assoc* **189**(2):227–232.

16 Trepanier LA (2004). Idiosyncratic toxicity associated with potentiated sulfonamides in the dog. *J Vet Pharmacol Ther* **27**:129–138.

17 Agnello KA, Reyolds LR, Budsberg SC (2005). *In vivo* effects of tepoxalin, an inhibitor of cyclooxygenase and lipoxygenase, on prostanoid and leukotriene production in dogs with chronic osteoarthritis. *Am J Vet Res* **66**:966–972.

18 Papich MG (2008). An update on nonsteroidal anti-inflammatory drugs (NSAIDs) in small animals. *Vet Clin North Am: Small Anim Pract* **38**:1243–1266.

19 Dahl G, Dahlinger L, Ekenved G, *et al.* (1982). The effect of buffering of acetylsalicylic acid on dissolution, absorption, gastric pH and faecal blood loss. *Int J Pharm* **10**:143–151.

20 Phillips BM (1973). Aspirin-induced gastrointestinal microbleeding in dogs. *Toxicol Appl Pharmacol* **24**:182–189.

21 Singh G, Triadafilopoulos G (1999). Epidemiology of NSAID-induced GI complications. *J Rheumatol* **26**(Suppl):18–24.

22 Morton DJ, Knottenbelt DC (1989). Pharmacokinetics of aspirin and its application in canine veterinary medicine. *J S Afr Vet Assoc* **60**(4):191–194.

23 Price AH, Fletcher M (1990). Mechanisms of NSAID-induced gastroenteropathy. *Drugs* **40**(Suppl 5):1–11.

24 Christoni A, Lapressa F (1909). Richerche farmalologiche sull asspirinia. *Arch Farmarol* **8**:63. Cited by Ghross M, Greenburg LA (1948). *The Salicylates*. Hillhouse Press, New Haven.

25 Boulay JP, Lipowitz AJ, Klausner JS (1986). The effect of cimetidine on aspirin-induced gastric hemorrhage in dogs. *Am J Vet Res* **47**:1744–1746.

26 Hurley JW, Crandall LA (1964). The effects of salicylates upon the stomachs of dogs. *Gastroenterology* **46**:36–43.

27 Taylor LA, Crawford LM (1968). Aspirin-induced gastrointestinal lesions in dogs. *J Am Vet Med Assoc* **152**(6):617–619.

28 Lipowitz AJ, Boulay JP, Klausner JS (1986). Serum salicylate concentrations and endoscopic evaluation of the gastric mucosa in dogs after oral administration of aspirin-containing products. *Am J Vet Res* **47**(7):1586–1589.

29 Nap RC, Breen DJ, Lam TJ, De Bruyne JJ (1990). Gastric retention of enteric-coated aspirin tablets in beagle dogs. *J Vet Pharmacol Ther* **13**(2):148–153.

30 Fiorucci S, Santucci L, Wallace JL, *et al.* (2003). Interaction of a selective cyclooxygenase-2 inhibitor with aspirin and NO-releasing aspirin in the human gastric mucosa. *Proc Natl Acad Sci USA* **100**(19):10937–10941.

31 Cotran RS (1999). Inflammation historical perspectives. In: Gallin JI, Snyderman R, Fearon DT, Haynes BF, Nathan C (eds). *Inflammation; Basic Principles and Clinical Correlates*, 3rd edn. Lippincott Williams & Wilkins, Philadelphia, pp. 5–10.

32 Wallace JL (1997). Nonsteroidal anti-inflammatory drugs and gastroenteropathy: the second hundred years. *Gastroenterology* **112**:1000–1016.

33 Colgen SP, Serhan CN, Parkos CA, *et al.* (1993). Lipoxin A_4 modulates transmigration of human neutrophils across intestinal epithelial monolayers. *J Clin Invest* **92**:75–82.

34 Wallace JL, Fiorucci S (2003). A magic bullet for mucosal protection…and aspirin is the trigger! *Trends Pharmacol Sci* **24**(7):323–326.

35 Fiorucci S, Santucci L, Gresele P, *et al.* (2003). Celecoxib exacerbates gastrointestinal damage induced by aspirin but not by NO-aspirin (NCX-4016): a randomized, parallel group, blind-observer endoscopic study. *Gastroenterology* **124**:A93.

36 Weissmann G, Smolen JE, Korchak HM (1980). Release of inflammatory mediators from stimulated neutrophils. *N Engl J Med* **303**:27–34.

37 Perez, HD (1994). Chemoattractant receptors. *Curr Opin Hematol* **1**:40–44.

38 Savides M, Oehme F, Nash S, *et al.* (1984). The toxicity and biotransformation of single doses of acetaminophen in dogs and cats. *Toxicol Appl Pharmacol* **74**:26–34.

39 Romsing J, Mountie S, Dahl JB (2002). Rectal and parenteral paracetamol, and paracetamol in combination with NSAIDs, for postoperative analgesia. *Br J Anaesth* **88**:215–226.

40 Nikles CJ, Yelland M, Del Mar C, *et al.* (2005). The role of paracetamol in chronic pain: an evidence-based approach. *Am J Ther* **12**:80–91.

41 Godfrey L, Bailey I, Toms NJ, *et al.* (2007). Paracetamol inhibits nitric oxide synthesis in murine spinal cord slices. *Eur J Pharmacy* **562**:68–71.

42 Bannwarth B, Netter P, Lapicque F, *et al.* (1992). Plasma and cerebrospinal fluid concentrations of paracetamol after a single intravenous dose of propacetamol. *Br J Clin Pharmacy* **34**:79–81.

43 Bonnefont J, Chapuy E, Clottes E, *et al.* (2005). Spinal 5-HT1A receptors differentially influence conceptive processing according to the nature of the noxious stimulus in rats: effect of WAY-100635 on the antinociceptive activities of paracetamol, venlafaxine and 5-HT. *Pain* **114**:482–490.

44 Mallet C, Eschalier A (2010). Pharmacology and mechanism of action of acetaminophen. In: Beaulieu P, Lussier D, Porreca F, *et al.* (eds). *Pharmacology of Pain*. IASP Press, Seattle, pp. 65–85.

45 Boutaud O, Aronoff DM, Richardson JH, *et al.* (2002). Determinants of the cellular specificity of acetaminophen as an inhibitor of prostaglandin H2 syntheses. *Proc Natl Acad Sci USA* **99**:7130–7135.

46 Lascelles BDX (2007). Supportive care for the cancer patient. In: Withrow SJ, Vail DM, (eds). *Withrow & McAllen's Small Animal Clinical Oncology*, 4th edn. Elsevier, St. Louis.

47 Clark TP, Chieffo C, Huhn JC, *et al.* (2003). The steady-state pharmacokinetics and bioequivalence of carprofen administered orally and subcutaneously in dogs. *J Vet Pharmacol Ther* **26**(3):187–192.

48 Hodge TM, Wahlstrom T (2000). Three years (1997–1999) of US clinical experience with Rimadyl® (carprofen). Pfizer Technical Bulletin, Dec.

49 Brant CE, Farnfield BA, Janicke HJ (2003). Evaluation of the ability of carprofen and flunixin meglumine to inhibit activation of nuclear factor kappa B. *Am J Vet Res* **64**:211–216.

50 Sessions JK, Agnello KA, Reynolds LR, *et al.* (2005). *In vivo* effects of carprofen, deracoxib and etodolac on whole blood, gastric mucosal and synovial fluid prostaglandin synthesis in dogs with osteoarthritis. *Am J Vet Res* **66**: 812–817.

51 McCann ME, Anderson DR, Zhang D, *et al.* (2004). *In vitro* effects and *in vivo* efficacy of a novel cyclooxygenase-2 inhibitor in dogs with experimentally induced synovitis. *Am J Vet Res* **65**:503–512.

52 Millis DL, Conzemius MG, Wells KL *et al.* (2002). A multi-center clinical study on the effects of deracoxib, a COX-2 selective drug, on post-operative analgesia associated with cranial cruciate ligament stabilization in dogs. Proceedings VOS, VOS, Salt Lake City, Utah.

53 Johnston SA, Conzemius MG, Cross AR, *et al.* (2001). A multi-center clinical study of the effects of deracoxib, a COX-2 selective drug, on chronic pain in dogs with osteoarthritis. *Vet Surg* **30**(5): abstract #42, p. 497.

54 Bienhoff SE, Smith ES, Roycroft LM, *et al.* (2011). Efficacy and safety of deracoxib for the control of postoperative pain and inflammation associated with dental surgery in dogs. ISRN *Vet Sci* **2011**, Article ID 593015, DOI: 10.5402/2011/593015.

55 McMillan SK, Moore GE, Widmer WR, *et al.* (2011). Antitumor effects of deracoxib treatment in 26 dogs with transitional cell carcinoma of the urinary bladder. *J Am Vet Med Assoc* **239**(8): 1084–1089.

56 Lees P, Cheng Z, Keef, TJ, *et al.* (2012). Bioequivalence in dogs of a meloxicam formulation administered as a transmucosl oral mist with an orally administered pioneer suspension product. *J. Vet Pharmacol Ther* DOI: 10.1111/j.1365-2885.2012.01402.x.

57 Cox SR, Lesman SP, Boucher JF, *et al.* (2010). The pharmacokinetics of mavacoxib, a long-acting COX-2 inhibitor, in young adult laboratory dogs. *J Vet Pharmacol Ther* **33**:461–470.

58 King JN, Dawson J, Esser RE, *et al.* (2009). Preclinical pharmacology of robenacoxib: a novel selective inhibitor of cyclooxygenase-2. *J Vet Pharmacol Ther* **32**:1–17.

59 Jung M, Lees P, Seewald W, *et al.* (2009). Analytical determination and pharmacokinetics of robenacoxib in the dog. *J Vet Pharmacol Ther* **32**:41–48.

60 Giraudel JM, King JN, Jeunesse EC, *et al.* (2009). Use of a pharmacokinetic/pharmacodynamics approach in the cat to determine a dosage regimen for the COX-2 selective drug robenacoxib. *J Vet Pharmacol Ther* **32**:18–30.

61 Giraudel JM, Toutain PL, King JN, *et al.* (2009). Differential inhibition of cyclooxygenase isoenzymes in the cat by the NSAID robenacoxib. *J Vet Pharmacol Ther* **32**:31–40.

62 Schmid VB, Spreng DE, Seewald W, *et al.* (2009). Analgesic and anti-inflammatory actions of robenacoxib in acute joint inflammation in dog. *J Vet Pharmacol Ther* **33**:118–131.

63 Schmid VB, Seewald W, Lees P, *et al.* (2010). *In vitro* and *ex vivo* inhibition of COX isoforms by robenacoxib in the cat: a comparative study. *J Vet Pharmacol Ther* **33**:444–452.

64 Giraudel JM, Gruet P, Alexander DG, *et al.* (2010). Evaluation of orally administered robenacoxib versus ketoprofen for treatment of acute pain and inflammation associated with musculoskeletal disorders in cats. *Am J Vet Res* **71**:710–719.

65 Gruet P, Seewald W, King JN (2011). Evaluation of subcutaneous and oral administration of robenacoxib and meloxicam for the treatment of acute pain and inflammation associated with orthopedic surgery in dogs. *Am J Vet Res* **72**:184–193.

66 Hampshire VA, Doddy FM, Post LO, *et al.* (2004). Adverse drug event reports at the United States Food and Drug Administration Center for Veterinary Medicine. *J Am Vet Med Assoc* **225**:533–536.

67 Menguy R, Masters YF (1963). Effect of cortisone on mucoprotein secretion by gastric antrum of dogs: pathogenesis of steroid ulcer. *Surgery* **54**:19–28.

68 Sessions JK, Reynolds LR, Budsberg SC (2005). *In vivo* effects of carprofen, deracoxib, and etodolac on prostanoid production in blood, gastric mucosa, and synovial fluid in dogs with chronic osteoarthritis. *Am J Vet Res* **66**: 812–817.

69 Jones CJ, Streppa HK, Harmon BG, *et al.* (2002). *In vivo* effects of meloxicam and aspirin on blood, gastric mucosal, and synovial fluid prostanoid synthesis in dogs. *Am J Vet Res* **63**:1527–1531.

70 Wooten JG, Blikslager AT, Ryan KA, *et al.* (2008). Cyclooxygenase expression and prostanoid production in pyloric and duodenal mucosae in dogs after administration of nonsteroidal anti-inflammatory drugs. *Am J Vet Res* **69**:457–464.

71 Blikslager AT, Zimmel DN, Young KM, *et al.* (2002). Recovery of ischaemic injured porcine ileum: evidence for a contributory role of COX-1 and COX-2. *Gut* **50**:615–623.

72 Punke JP, Speas AL, Reynolds LR, *et al.* (2008). Effects of firocoxib, meloxicam, and tepoxalin on prostanoid and leukotriene production by duodenal mucosa and other tissues of osteoarthritic dogs. *Am J Vet Res* **69**:1203–1209.

73 Novartis Animal Health US (2005). Deracoxib: 3 Year Adverse Drug Event Report. Data on file.

74 Cheng HF, Harris RC (2005). Renal effects of non-steroidal anti-inflammatory drugs and selective cyclooxygenase-2 inhibitors. *Curr Pharm Res* **11**:1795–1804.

75 Cohen HJ, Marsh DJ, Kayser B (1983). Autoregulation in vasa recta of the rat kidney. *Am J Physiol* **245**:F32–F40.

76 Pages JP (2005). Nephropathies dues aux anti-inflammatores non steroidiens (AINS) chez le chat: 21 observations (1993–2001). *Prat Med Chir Anim Comp* **40**:177–181.

77 Harvey JW, Kaneko JJ (1976). Oxidation of human and animal haemoglobins with ascorbate, acetylphenylhydraxine, nitrite, and hydrogen peroxide. *Br J Haematol* **32**:193–203.

78 Fox SM, Gorman MP (1998). New study findings and clinical experiences enhance understanding of Rimadyl® (carprofen). Pfizer Animal Health Technical Bulletin, August.

79 Boelsterli UA, Zimmerman HJ, Kretz-Rommel A (1995). Idiosyncratic liver toxicity of nonsteroidal anti-inflammatory drugs: molecular mechanisms and pathology. *Crit Rev Toxicol* **25**:207–235.

80 Boelsterli UA (2002). Xenobiotic acyl glucuronides and acyl CoA thioesters as protein-reactive metabolites with the potential to cause idiosyncratic drug reactions. *Curr Drug Metab* **3**:439–450.

81 Bailey MJ, Dickinson RG (2003). Acyl glucuronide reactivity in perspective: biological consequences. *Chem Biol Interact* **145**:117–137.

82 Dowers KL, Uhrig SR, Mama KR, *et al.* (2006). Effect of short-term sequential administration of nonsteroidal anti-inflammatory drugs on the stomach and proximal portion of the duodenum in healthy dogs. *Am J Vet Res* **67**(10):1794–1801.

83 Williams JT (1997). The painless synergism of aspirin and opium. *Nature* **390**:557–559.

84 Lee A, Cooper MC, Craig JC, *et al.* (2004). Effects of nonsteroidal anti-inflammatory drugs on postoperative renal function in adults with normal renal function. *Cochrane Database Syst Rev* (2):CD002765.

85 Radi ZA, Khan NK (2005). Review: Effects of cyclooxygenase inhibition on bone, tendon, and ligament healing. *Inflamm Res* **54**:358–366.

86 Quinn MM, Keuler NS, Lu Y, *et al.* (2007). Evaluation of agreement between numerical rating scales, visual analogue scoring scales, and force plate gait analysis in dogs. *Vet Surg* **36**: 360–367.

87 Millis DL (2006). A multimodal approach to treating osteoarthritis. Western Veterinary Conference Symposium Proceedings.

88 Franks JN, Boothe HW, Taylor L, *et al.* (2000). Evaluation of transdermal fentanyl patches for analgesia in cats undergoing onychectomy. *J Am Vet Med Assoc* **217**:1013–1020.

89 Lascelles BDX, Hansen BD, Thomson A, *et al.* (2008). Evaluation of a digitally integrated accelerometer-based activity monitor for the measurement of activity in cats. *Vet Anaesth Analg* **35**:173–183.

90 Rostom A, Dube C, Lewin G, *et al.* (2007). Nonsteroidal anti-inflammatory drugs and cyclooxygenase-2 inhibitors for primary prevention of colorectal cancer: a systematic review prepared for the US Preventive Services Task Force. *Ann Inter Med* **146**:376–389.

91 Page GG, Blakely WP, Ben-Eliyahu S (2001). Evidence that postoperative pain is a mediator of the tumor-promoting effects of surgery in rats. *Pain* **90**(1-2):191–199.

92 Zweifel BS, Davis TW, Ornberg RL, *et al.* (2002). Direct evidence for a role of cyclooxygenase-2-derived prostaglandin E2 in human head and neck xenograft tumors. *Cancer Res* **62**:6706–6711.

93 Raegg C, Dormond O (2001). Suppression of tumor angiogenesis by nonsteroidal anti-inflammatory drugs: a new function for old drugs. *Scientific World J* **1**:808–811.

94 Ohno R, Yoshinaga K, Fujita T, *et al.* (2001). Depth of invasion parallels increased cyclooxygenase-2 levels in patients with gastric carcinoma. *Cancer* **91**:1876–1881.

95 Boria PA, Biolsi SA, Greenberg CB, *et al.* (2003). Preliminary evaluation of deracoxib in canine transitional cell carcinoma of the urinary bladder. *Vet Cancer Soc Proc* **17**.

96 Wise JK, Heathcott BL, Gonzales ML (2002). Results of the AVMA survey on companion animal ownership in US pet-owning households. *J Am Vet Med Assoc* **221**:1572–1573.

97 Lascelles BDX, Court MH, Hardie EM, *et al.* (2007). Nonsteroidal anti-inflammatory drugs in cats: a review. *Vet Anaesth Analg* **34**:228–250.

98 Hardie EM, Roe SC, Martin FR (2002). Radiographic evidence of degenerative joint disease in geriatric cats: 100 cases (1994–1997). *J Am Vet Med Assoc* **220**:628–632.

99 Court MH, Greenblatt DJ (2000). Molecular genetic basis for deficient acetaminophen glucuronidation by cats: UGRT1A6 is a pseudogene, and evidence for reduced diversity of expressed hepatic UGT1A isoforms. *Pharmacogenetics* **10**:355–369.

100 Thoulon F, Narbe R, Johnston L, *et al.* (2009). Metabolism and excretion of oral meloxicam in the cat (abstract). *J Vet Intern Med* **23**:695.

101 Gunew MN, Menrath VH, Marshall RD (2008). Long-term safety, efficacy and palatability of oral meloxicam at 0.01–0.03 mg/kg for treatment of osteoarthritic pain in cats. *J Feline Med Surg* **10**(3): 235–241.

102 Lascelles B, Robertson S (2010). DJD-associated pain in cats: what can we do to promote patient comfort? *J Feline Med Surg* **12**:200–212.

103 Lascelles B, Hansen B, Roe S, *et al.* (2007). Evaluation of client-specific outcome measures and activity monitoring to measure pain relief in cats with osteoarthritis. *J Vet Intern Med* **21**: 410–416.

104 Lascelles B, Henderson A, Hackett I (2001). Evaluation of the clinical efficacy of meloxicam in cats with painful locomotor disorders. *J Small Anim Pract* **42**:587–593.

105 Lascelles B (2010). Feline degenerative joint disease. *Vet Surg* **39**:2–13.

106 Allan G (2000). Radiographic features of feline joint diseases. *Vet Clin North Am: Small Anim Pract* **30**:281–302.

107 Hardie E, Roe S, Martin F (2002). Radiographic evidence of degenerative joint disease in geriatric cats:100 cases (1994–1997). *J Am Vet Med Assoc* **220**:628–632.

108 Clarke S, Bennett D (2006). Feline osteoarthritis: a prospective study of 28 cases. *J Small Anim Pract* **47**:439–445.

109 Clarke S, Mellor D, Clements D, *et al*. (2005). Prevalence of radiographic signs of degenerative joint disease in a hospital population of cats. *Vet Rec* **157**:793–799.

110 Bennett D, Morton C (2009). A study of owner observed behavioural and lifestyle changes in cats with musculoskeletal disease before and after analgesic therapy. *J Feline Med Surg* **11**:997–1004.

111 Slingerland L, Hazewinkel H, Meij B, *et al*. (2011). Cross-sectional study of the prevalence and clinical features of osteoarthritis in 100 cats. *Vet J* **187**(3):304–309.

112 Beam S, Rassnick K, Moore A, *et al*. (2003). An immunohistochemical study of cyclooxygenase-2 expression in various feline neoplasms. *Vet Pathol* **40**: 496–500.

113 Dibernardi L, Dore M, Davis J, *et al*. (2007). Study of feline oral squamous cell carcinoma: potential target for cyclooxygenase inhibitor treatment. *Prostaglandins Leukot Essent Fatty Acids* **76**:245–250.

114 Hayes A, Scase T, Miller J, *et al*. (2006). COX-1 and COX-2 expression in feline oral squamous cell carcinoma. *J Comp Pathol* **135**:93–99.

115 Hayes A, Adams V, Scase T, *et al*. (2007). Survival of 54 cats with oral squamous cell carcinoma in United Kingdom general practice. *J Small Anim Pract* **48**:394–399.

116 Millis DL (2010). Dasuquin's efficacy may be similar to that of NSAIDs in dogs. Joint Health: a roundtable discussion. Supplement. *Vet Med* **105**(11):10.

117 Millis DL (2005). Effects of feeding omega-3 fatty acids on force plate gait analysis in dogs with osteoarthritis, 3-month feeding study, 2003. Hill's Clinical Evidence Report.

CHAPTER 7

1 Theodosakis J (1997). *The Arthritis Cure*. St Martin's Press, New York.

2 Consumer Reports (2002). January p. 18.

3 Animal Pharm Report (2005). October; www.animalpharmreports.com

4 Innes J (2005). Diet and disease: exploring the link through nutrigenomics. *Vet Rev* July.

5 Hardy G (2000). Nutraceuticals and functional foods: Introduction and meaning. *Nutrition* **16**:688–698.

6 Diplock AT, Charleux JL, Crozier-Willi G, *et al*. (1998). Functional food science and defence against reactive oxidative species. *Br J Nutr* **80**:S77–112.

7 Lascelles BDX, Blikslager AT, Fox SM, *et al*. (2005). Gastrointestinal tract perforations in dogs treated with a selective cyclooxygenase-2 inhibitor: 29 cases (2002–2003). *J Am Vet Med Assoc* **227**(7):1112–1117.

8 Dingle JT (1999). The effect of nonsteroidal anti-inflammatory drugs on human articular cartilage glycosaminoglycan synthesis. *Osteoarthr Cartil* **7**:313–314.

9 Goldring MB (2000). Osteoarthritis and cartilage: the role of cytokines. *Curr Rheumatol Rep* **2**(6):459–465.

10 Billinghurst RC, Dahlberg L, Ionescu M, *et al*. (1997). Enhanced cleavage of type II collagen by collagenases in osteoarthritic articular cartilage. *J Clin Invest* **99**:1534–1545.

11 Mengshol JA, Mix KS, Brinckerhoff CE (2002). Matrix metalloproteinases as therapeutic targets in arthritic diseases: bull's-eye or missing the mark? *Arthritis Rheum* **46**:13–20.

12 Reboul P, Pelletier JP, Tardif G, *et al*. (1996). The new collagenase, collagenase 3, is expressed and synthesized by human chondrocytes but not by synovial fibroblasts: a role in osteoarthritis. *J Clin Invest* **97**:2011–2019.

13 Sandy JD, Verscharen C (2001). Analysis of aggrecan in human knee cartilage and synovial fluid indicates that aggrecanase (ADAMTS) activity is responsible for the catabolic turnover and loss of whole aggrecan whereas other protease activity is required for C-terminal processing *in vivo*. *Biochem J* **358**:615–626.

14 Pelletier JP, McCollum R, Cloutier JM, *et al*. (1995). Synthesis of metalloproteases and interleukin 6 (IL6) in human osteoarthritic synovial membrane is an IL-1 mediated process. *J Rheumatol* **22**:109–114.

15 Pelletier JP, DiBattista JA, Roughley P, *et al*. (1993). Cytokines and inflammation in cartilage degradation. *Rheum Dis Clin North Am* **19**: 545–568S.

16 Basleer C, Rovati L, Franchimont P (1998). Stimulation of proteoglycan production by glucosamine sulfate in chondrocytes isolated from human osteoarthritis articular cartilage *in vitro*. *Osteoarthr Cartil* **6**:427–434.

17 Ronca F, Palmieri L, Panicucci P, *et al.* (1998). Anti-inflammatory activity of chondroitin sulfate. *Osteoarthr Cartil* **6**(Suppl A):14–21.

18 Dodge GR, Hawkins D, Boesier E, *et al.* (1998). Production of cartilage oligomeric matrix protein (COMP) by cultured human dermal and synovial fibroblasts. *Osteoarthr Cartil* **6**(6):435–440.

19 Setnikar I, Palumbo R, Canali S, Zanolo G (1993). Pharmacokinetics of glucosamine in man. *Arzneimittelforschung* **43**(10):1109–1113.

20 Setnikar I, Rovati LC (2001). Absorption, distribution, metabolism and excretion of glucosamine sulfate. A review. *Arzneimittelforschung* **51**(9):699–725.

21 Fenton JL, Chlebek-Brown KA, Caron JP, Orth MW (2002). Effect of glucosamine on interleukin-1-conditioned articular cartilage. *Equine Vet J Suppl* **34**(2):19–23.

22 Gouze JN, Bianchi A, Becuwe P, *et al.* (2002). Glucosamine modulates IL-1-induced activation of rat chondrocytes at a receptor level, and by inhibiting the NF-kappa B pathway. *FEBS Lett* **510**(3):166–170.

23 Largo R, Alverez-Soria MA, Diez-Ortego I, *et al.* (2003). Glucosamine inhibits IL-1β-induced NFκB activation in human osteoarthritic chondrocytes. *Osteoarthr Cartil* **11**:290–298.

24 Chan PS, Caron JP, Rosa GJ, Orth MW (2005). Glucosamine and chondroitin sulfate regulate gene expression and synthesis of nitric oxide and prostaglandin E(2) in articular cartilage explants. *Osteoarthr Cartil* **13**(5):387–394.

25 Chan PS, Caron JP, Orth MW (2005). Effect of glucosamine and chondroitin sulfate on regulation of gene expression of proteolytic enzymes and their inhibitors in interleukin-1-challenged bovine articular cartilage explants. *Am J Vet Res* **66**(11):1870–1876.

26 Neil KM, Orth MW, Coussens PM, *et al.* (2005). Effects of glucosamine and chondroitin sulfate on mediators of osteoarthritis in cultured equine chondrocytes stimulated by use of recombinant equine interleukin-1 beta. *Am J Vet Res* **66**(11):1861–1869.

27 Sandy JD, Gamell D, Thompson V, Verscharen C (1998). Chondrocyte-mediated catabolism of aggrecan: aggrecanase-dependent cleavage induced by interleukin-1 or retinoic acid can be inhibited by glucosamine. *Biochem J* **335** (1):59–66.

28 Bucsi L, Poor G (1998). Efficacy and tolerability of oral chondroitin sulfate as a symptomatic slow-acting drug for osteoarthritis (SYSADOA) in the treatment of knee osteoarthritis. *Osteoarthr Cartil* **6**(Suppl A):31–36.

29 Verbruggen G, Goemaere S, Veys EM (1998). Chondroitin sulfate: S/DMOAD (structure/disease modifying anti-osteoarthritis drug) in the treatment of finger joint OA. *Osteoarthr Cartil* **6** (Suppl A):37–38.

30 Lippiello L, Woodward J, Karpman R, *et al.* (2000). *In vivo* chondroprotection and metabolic synergy of glucosamine and chondroitin sulfate. *Clin Orthop Relat Res* **381**:229–240.

31 Lippiello L (2004). Glucosamine and chondroitin sulfate: biological response modifiers of chondrocytes under simulated conditions of joint stress. *Osteoarthr Cartil* **11**(5):335–342.

32 Paroli E, Antonilli L, Biffoni M (1991). A pharmacological approach to glycosaminoglycans. *Drugs Exp Clin Res* **17**(1): 9–19.

33 Bartolucci C, Cellai L, Corrandini C, *et al.* (1991). Chondroprotective action of chondroitin sulfate. Competitive action of chondroitin sulfate on the digestion of hyaluranan by bovine testicular hyaluronidase. *Int J Tissue React* **13**(6):311–317.

34 Adebowale AO, Cox DS, Liang Z, *et al.* (2000). Analysis of glucosamine and chondroitin sulfate content in marketed products and the Caco-2 permeability of chondroitin sulfate raw materials. *J Am Nutraceutical Assoc* **3**:33–44.

35 Volpi N (2003). Oral absorption and bioavailability of ichthyic origin chondroitin sulfate in healthy male volunteers. *Osteoarthr Cartil* **11**:433–441.

36 Volpi N (2002). Oral bioavailability of chondroitin sulfate (Chondrosulf) and its constituents in healthy male volunteers. *Osteoarthr Cartil* **10**:768–777S.

37 Liau YH, Horowitz MI (1974). Desulfation and depolymerization of chondroitin-4-sulfate and its degradation products by rat stomach, liver and small intestine. *Proc Soc Exp Biol Med* **146**: 1037–1043.

38 King M (2007). Equine joint treatments and applications. *Vet Prac News* July:38.

39 Dobenecker B, Beetz Y, Kienzle E (2002). A placebo-controlled double-blind study on the effect of nutraceuticals (chondroitin sulphate and mussel extract) in dogs with joint diseases as perceived by their owners. *J Nutr* **132**:1690S–1691S.

40 Platt D (2001). The role of oral disease-modifying agents glucosamine and chondroitin sulphate in the management of equine degenerative joint disease. *Equine Vet Educ* **3**:262–272.

41 Fenton JI, Chlebek-Brown KA, Peters TL, *et al.* (2000). The effects of glucosamine derivatives on equine articular cartilage degradation in explant culture. *Osteoarthr Cartil* **8**:444–451.

42 Hoffer LJ, Kaplan LN, Hamadeh MT, *et al.* (2001). Sulfate could mediate the therapeutic effect of glucosamine sulfate. *Metabolism* **50**: 767–770.

43 Dodge GR, Hawkins JF, Jimenez SA (1999). Modulation of aggrecan, MMP1 and MMP3 productions by glucosamine sulfate in cultured human osteoarthritis articular chondrocytes. *Arthritis Rheum* **42S**:253.

44 Rovati LC (1997). Clinical development of glucosamine sulfate as selective drug in osteoarthritis. *Rheumatol Eur* **26**:70.

45 Houpt JB, McMillan R, Wein C, *et al.* (1999). Effect of glucosamine hydrochloride in the treatment of pain of osteoarthritis of the knee. *J Rheumatol* **26**:2413–2430.

46 Russell AS, Aghazadeh-Habashi A, Jamali F (2001). Active ingredient consistency of commercially available glucosamine sulfate products. *J Rheumatol* **29**:2407–2409.

47 Persiani S, Rotini R, Trisolino G, *et al.* (2007). Synovial and plasma glucosamine concentrations in osteoarthritic patients following oral crystalline glucosamine sulphate at therapeutic dose. *Osteoarthr Cartil* **15**:764–772.

48 Cordoba F, Nimni ME (2003). Chondroitin sulfate and other sulfate containing chondroprotective agents may exhibit their effects by overcoming a deficiency of sulphur amino acids. *Osteoarthr Cartil* **11**:228–230.

49 Piepoli T, Zanelli T, Letari O, *et al.* (2005). Glucosamine sulfate inhibits IL1β-stimulated gene expression at concentrations found in humans after oral intake (Abstract). *Arthritis Rheum* **52** (9 Suppl):1326.

50 Bond M, Baker AH, Newby AC (1999). Nuclear factor κB is essential for matrix metalloproteinase-1 and -3 upregulation in rabbit dermal fibroblasts. *Biochem Biophys Res Commun* **264**:561–567.

51 Kuroki K, Cook JL, Stoker AM (2005). Evaluation of chondroprotective nutriceuticals in an *in vitro* osteoarthritis model. Poster. 51st Annual Meeting of the Orthopaedic Research Society.

52 Ramey DW (2005). Skeptical of treatment with glucosamine and chondroitin sulfate. (editorial) *J Am Vet Med Assoc* **226**:1797–1799.

53 Adebowale A, Du J, Liang Z, *et al.* (2002). The bioavailability and pharmacokinetics of glucosamine hydrochloride and low molecular weight chondroitin sulfate after single and multiple doses to beagle dogs. *Biopharm Drug Dispos* **23**:217–225.

54 McAlindon T (2003). Why are clinical trials of glucosamine no longer uniformly positive? *Rheum Dis Clin North Am* **29**:789–801.

55 Hochberg MC (2006). Nutritional supplements for knee osteoarthritis. Still no resolution (editorial). *N Engl J Med* **354**:858–860.

56 McCarthy G, O'Donovan J, Jones B, *et al.* (2007). Randomized double-blind, positive-controlled trial to assess the efficacy of glucosamine/chondroitin sulfate for the treatment of dogs with osteoarthritis. *Vet J* **174**:54–61.

57 Leffler CT, Philippi AF, Leffler SG, *et al.* (1999). Glucosamine, chondroitin, and manganese ascorbate for degenerative joint disease of the knee or low back: a randomized, double-blind, placebo-controlled pilot study. *Mil Med* **164**: 85–91.

58 Forsyth RK, Brigden CV, Northrop AJ (2006). Double blind investigation of the effects of oral supplementation of combined glucosamine hydrochloride (GHCL) and chondroitin sulphate (CS) on stride characteristics of veteran horses. *Equine Vet J* (Suppl) **36**:622–625.

59 Davidson G (2000). Glucosamine and chondroitin sulfate. *Comp Contin Educ Pract Vet* **22**:454–458.

60 Lenox CE, Lunn KF (2010). Effects of glucosamine-chondroitin sulfate supplementation on serum fructosamine concentration in healthy dogs. *J Am Vet Med Assoc* **236**:183–186.

61 Clegg DO, Reda DJ, Harris CL, *et al.* (2006). Glucosamine, chondroitin sulphate, and the two in combination for painful knee osteoarthritis. *New Eng J Med* **354**:795–808.

62 Hazewinkel HAW, Frost-Christensen LFN (2006). Disease-modifying drugs in canine osteoarthritis. 13th ESVOT Congress, Munich, 7–10 September:5054.

63 Aragon CL, Hofmeister EH, Budsberg SC (2007). Systematic review of clinical trials of treatments for osteoarthritis in dogs. *J Am Vet Med Assoc* **230**:514–521.

64 Horstman J (1999). *The Arthritis Foundation's Guide to Alternative Therapies*. The Arthritis Foundation, Atlanta, Georgia, pp. 179–180.

65 Chan P-S, Caron JP, Orth MW (2007). Effects of glucosamine and chondroitin sulfate on bovine cartilage explants under long-term culture conditions. *Am J Vet Res* **68**:709–715.

66 Henrotin YE, Labasse AH, Jaspar JM, *et al.* (1998). Effects of three avocado/soybean unsaponifiable mixtures on metalloproteinases, cytokines and prostaglandin E_2 production by human articular chondrocytes. *Clin Rheumatol* **17**:31–39.

67 Maheu E, Mazieres B, Valat JP, *et al.* (1998). Symptomatic efficacy of avocado/soybean unsaponifiables in the treatment of osteoarthritis of the knee and hip. A prospective randomized, double-blind, placebo-controlled multicenter clinical trial with six-month treatment period and a two-month follow-up demonstrating a persistent effect. *Arthritis Rheum* **41**:81–91.

68 Henrotin YE, Sanchez C, Deberg MA, *et al.* (2003). Avocado/soybean unsaponifiables increase aggrecan synthesis and reduce catabolic and proinflammatory mediator production by human osteoarthritic chondrocytes. *J Rheumatol* **30**:1825–1834.

69 Boileau C, Martel-Pelztier J, Caron J, *et al.* (2009). Protective effects of total fraction of avocado/soybean unsaponifiables on the structural changes in experimental dog osteoarthritis: inhibition of nitric oxide synthase and matrix metalloproteinase-13. *Arthritis Res Ther* **11**:R41:1–9.

70 Au RY, Al-Talbi TK, Au AY, *et al.* (2007). Avocado soybean unsaponifiables (ASU) suppress TNF-α, IL-1β, COX-2, iNOS gene expression, and prostaglandin E_2 and nitric oxide production in articular chondrocytes and monocyte/macrophages. *Osteoarthr Cartil* **15**:1249–1255.

71 Heinecke LF, Grazia MW, Au AY, *et al.* (2010). Inhibition of cyclooxygenase-2 expression and prostaglandin E_2 production in chondrocytes by avocado soybean unsaponifiables and epigallocatechin gallate. *Osteoarthr Cartil* **18**:220–227.

72 Hilal G, Martel-Pelletier J, Pelletier JP, *et al.* (1998). Osteoblast-like cells from human subchondral osteoarthritic bone demonstrate an altered phenotype *in vitro*: possible role in subchondral bone sclerosis. *Arthritis Rheum* **41**:891–899.

73 Hillal G, Massicotte F, Martel-Pelletier J, *et al.* (2001). Endogenous prostaglandin E2 and insulin-like growth factor 1 can modulate the levels of parathyroid hormone receptor in human osteoarthritic osteoblasts. *J Bone Miner Res* **16**:713–721.

74 Henrotin YE, Deberg MA, Crielaard JM, *et al.* (2006). Avocado/soybean unsaponifiables prevent the inhibitory effect of osteoarthritis subchondral osteoblasts on aggrecan and type II collagen synthesis by chondrocytes. *J Rheumatology* **33**:1668–1678.

75 Imhof H, Breitenseher M, Kainberger F, *et al.* (1999). Importance of subchondral bone to articular cartilage in health and disease. *Top Magn Reson Imaging* **10**:180–192.

76 Kawcak CE, Frisbie DD, McIlwraith W, *et al.* (2007). Evaluation of avocado and soybean unsaponifiable extracts for treatment of horses with experimentally induced osteoarthritis. *Am J Vet Res* **68**:598–604.

77 Altinel L, Saritas ZK, Kose KC, *et al.* (2007). Treatment with unsaponifiable extracts of avocado and soybean increases TGF-β_1 and TGF-β_2 levels in canine joint fluid. *J Exp Med* **211**:181–186.

78 Grimaud E, Heymann D, Redini F (2002). Recent advances in TGF-beta effects on chondrocyte metabolism. Potential therapeutic roles of TGF-beta in cartilage disorders. *Cytokine Growth Factor Rev* **13**:241–257.

79 Millis DL (2010). Dasuquin's efficacy may be similar to that of NSAIDs in dogs. Joint Health: a roundtable discussion. Supplement. *Vet Med* **105**(11):10.

80 Wang CT, Lin J, Chang CJ, *et al.* (2004). Therapeutic effects of hyaluronic acid on osteoarthritis of the knee. A meta-analysis of randomized controlled trials. *J Bone Joint Surg Am* **86**-A(3):538–545.

81 Frizziero L, Govoni E, Bacchini P (1998). Intra-articular hyaluronic acid in the treatment of osteoarthritis of the knee: clinical and morphological study. *Clin Exp Rheumatol* **16**:441–449.

82 Smith MM, Ghosh P (1987). The synthesis of hyaluronic acid by human synovial fibroblasts is influenced by the nature of the hyaluronate in the extracellular environment. *Rheumatol Int* **7**(3): 113–122.

83 Creamer P, Sharif M, George E, *et al.* (1994). Intra-articular hyaluronic acid in osteoarthritis of the knee: an investigation into mechanisms of action. *Osteoarthr Cartil* **2**:133–140.

84 Marshall KW (2000). Intra-articular hyaluronan therapy. *Curr Opin Rheumatol* **12**:468–474.

85 Takahashi K, Hashimoto S, Kubo T, *et al.* (2001). Hyaluronan suppressed nitric oxide production in the meniscus and synovium of rabbit osteoarthritis model. *J Orthop Res* **19**: 500–503.

86 Yasui T, Akatsuka M, Tobetto K, *et al.* (1992). The effect of hyaluronan on interleukin-1-alpha-induced prostaglandin E2 production in human osteoarthritic synovial cells. *Agents Actions* **37**:155–156.

87 DeVane CL (2001). Substance P: a new era, a new role. *Pharmacotherapy* **21**:1061–1069.

88 Moore AR, Willoughby DA (1995). Hyaluronan as a drug delivery system for diclofenac: a hypothesis for mode of action. *Int J Tissue React* **17**:153–156.

89 Pozo MA, Balazs EA, Belmonte C (1997). Reduction of sensory responses to passive movements of inflamed knee joints by hylan, a hyaluronan derivative. *Exp Brain Res* **116**:3–9.

90 Reddy CM, Bhat VB, Kiranmai G, *et al*. (2000). Selective inhibition of cyclooxygenase-2 by C-phycocyanin, a biliprotein from *Spirulina platensis*. *Biochem Biophys Res Comm* **277**:599–603.

91 Romay C, LedÓn N, Gonzalez R (1998). Further studies on anti-inflammatory activity of phycocyanin in some animal models of inflammation. *Inflamm Res* **47**:334–338.

92 Cherng S, Cheng S, Tarn A, *et al*. (2007). Anti-inflammatory activity of c-phycocyanin in lipopolysaccharide-stimulated RAW 264.7 macrophages. *Life Sci* **81**:1431–1435.

93 Caterson B (2005). Cartilage physiology: unique aspects of canine cartilage. Proceedings Symposium on Nutritional Management of Chronic Canine Osteoarthritis. North American Veterinary Conference, Orlando Florida.

94 Caterson, B, Little CV, Cramp J, *et al*. (2005). The modulation of canine articular cartilage degradation by omega-3 (n-3) polyunsaturated fatty acids. Proceedings of the 77th Western Veterinary Conference, Las Vegas, Nevada.

95 Soeken KL, Lee WL, Bausell RB, *et al*. (2002). Safety and efficacy of S-adenosylmethionine (SAMe) for osteoarthritis. *J Fam Pract* **51**: 425–430.

96 Konig B (1987). A long-term (two years) clinical trial with S-adenosinemethionine for the treatment of osteoarthritis. *Am J Med* **83**: 78–80.

97 Center SA (2000). S-adenosylmethionine (SAMe): an antioxidant and anti-inflammatory nutraceutical. Proceedings of the 18th American College of Veterinary Internal Medicine Conference, Seattle, Washington, pp. 549–552.

98 Steinmeyer J, Burton-Wurster N (1992). Effects of three antiarthritic drugs on fibronectin and keratin sulfate synthesis by cultured canine articular cartilage chondrocytes. *Am J Vet Res* **53**:2077–2083.

99 Harmand MF, Jana JV, Maloche E, *et al*. (1987). Effects of S-adenosylmethionine on human articular chondrocyte differentiation. *Am J Med* **83**:48–54.

100 Lippiello L, Prudhomme A (2005). Advantageous use of glucosamine combined with S-adenosylmethionine in veterinary medicine: preservation of articular cartilage in joint disorders. *Intern J Appl Res Vet Med* **3**:6–12.

101 Bui LM, Bierer TL (2003). Influence of green lipped mussels (*Perna canaliculus*) in alleviating signs of arthritis in dogs. *Vet Ther* **4**:397–407.

102 Hielm-Bjorkman, Tulamo R-M, Salonen H, *et al*. (2009). Evaluating complementary therapies for canine osteoarthritis part I: green-lipped mussel (*Perna canaliculus*). *Evid Based Complement Alternat Med* **6**(3):365–373.

103 Dobenecker B, Beetz Y, Kienzle E (2002). A placebo-controlled double-blind study on the effect of nutraceuticals (chondroitin sulfate and mussel extract) in dogs with joint diseases as perceived by their owners. *J Nutr* **132**: 1690S–1691S.

104 Pollard B, Guilford WG, Ankerbauer-Perkins KL, *et al*. (2006). Clinical efficacy and tolerance of an extract of green-lipped mussel (*Perna canaliculus*) in dogs presumptively diagnosed with degenerative joint disease. *NZ Vet J* **54**:114–118.

105 Sackett DL, Straus SE, Richardson SW, *et al*. (2000). *Evidence-Based Medicine: How to Practice and Teach EBM*. Churchill Livingstone, Edinburgh.

106 Oke SL (2009). Indications and contraindications for the use of orally administered joint health products in dogs and cats. *J Am Vet Med Assoc* **234**:1393–1397.

107 Budsberg SC, Bartges JW (2006). Nutrition and osteoarthritis in dogs: Does it help? *Vet Clin North Am Small Anim Pract* **36**:1307–1323, vii.

108 Servet E, Biourge V, Marniquet P (2006). Dietary intervention can improve clinical signs in osteoarthritic dogs. *J Nutr* **136**:1995S–1997S.

109 Hansen RA, Harris MA, Pluhar GE, *et al*. (2008). Fish oil decreases matrix metalloproteinases in knee synovia of dogs with inflammatory joint disease. *J Nutr Biochem* **19**:101–108.

110 LeBlanc CJ, Horohov DW, Bauer JE, *et al*. (2008). Effects of dietary supplementation with fish oil on *in vivo* production of inflammatory mediators in clinically normal dogs. *Am J Vet Res* **69**:486–493.

111 Bierer TL, Bui LM (2002). Improvement of arthritic signs in dogs fed green-lipped mussel (*Perna canaliculus*). *J Nutr* **132**:1634S–1636S.

112 Bui LM, Bierer RL (2001). Influence of green lipped mussels (*Perna canaliculus*) in alleviating signs of arthritis in dogs. *Vet Ther* **2**:101–111.

113 Yamka RM, Friesen KG, Lowry SR, *et al*. (2006). Measurement of arthritic and bone serum metabolites in arthritic, non-arthritic, and geriatric cats fed wellness foods. *Int J Appl Res Vet Med* **4**:265–273.

114 Lascelles BDX, Depuy A, Thomson B, *et al.* (2010). Evaluation of a therapeutic diet for feline degenerative joint disease. *J Vet Intern Med* **24**:487–495.

115 Letters to the Editor (2010). More on accidental overdosing of joint supplements. *J Am Vet Med Assoc* **236**:1061–1062.

116 Innes JF, Caterson B, Little CB, *et al.* (2006). Effect of omega-3 fatty acids on canine cartilage: using an *in vitro* model to investigate therapeutic mechanisms. In 13th ESVOT Congress, Munich, 7–10 September.

117 Dodge GR, Jiminez SA (2003). Glucosamine sulfate modulates the levels of aggrecan and matrix metalloproteinase-3 synthesized by cultured human osteoarthritis articular chondrocytes. *Osteoarthr Cartil* **11**(6):424–432.

CHAPTER 8

1 Kehlet H, Dahl JB (1993). The value of 'multimodal' or 'balanced analgesia' in postoperative pain treatment. *Anesth Analg* 77:1048–1056.

2 Penning JP, Yaksh TL (1992). Interaction of intrathecal morphine with bupivacaine and lidocaine in the rat. *Anesthesiology* **77**: 1186–2000.

3 Grimm KA, Tranquilli WJ, *et al.* (2000). Duration of nonresponse to noxious stimulation after intramuscular administration of butorphanol, medetomidine, or a butorphanol-medetomidine combination during isoflurane administration in dogs. *Am J Vet Res* **61**(1): 41–47.

4 Skinner HB (2004). Multimodal acute pain management. *Am J Orthop* **33**:5–9.

5 Rockemann MG, Seeling W, Bischof C, *et al.* (1996). Prophylactic use of epidural mepivacaine/morphine, systemic diclofenac, and metamizole reduces postoperative morphine consumption after major abdominal surgery. *Anesthesiology* **84**:1027–1034.

6 American Pain Society (2002). Guideline for the management of pain in osteoarthritis, rheumatoid arthritis, and juvenile chronic arthritis. *Clin Pract Guide* **2**.

7 Muir WW, Woolf CJ (2001). Mechanisms of pain and their therapeutic implications. *J Am Vet Med Assoc* **219**:1346–1356.

8 American Society of Anesthesiologist (ASA) (2011). Annual Meeting: Abstract 1178. Presented October 18, 2011.

9 Lascelles BDX, Gaynor JS, Smith ES, *et al.* (2008). Amantadine in a multimodal analgesic regimen for alleviation of refractory osteoarthritis pain in dogs. *J Vet Intern Med* **22**:53–59.

10 Ko JCH, Abbo LA, Weil AB, *et al.* (2008). Effect of orally administered tramadol alone or with an intravenously administered opioid on minimum alveolar concentration of sevoflurane in cats. *J Am Vet Med Assoc* **232**(12):1834–1840.

11 Martins TL, Kahvegian MAP, Noel-Morgan J, *et al.* (2010). Comparison of the effects of tramadol, codeine, and ketoprofen alone or in combination on postoperative pain and on concentrations of blood glucose, serum cortisol, and serum interleukin-6 in dogs undergoing maxillectomy or mandibulectomy. *Am J Vet Res* **71**(9):1019–1026.

12 Brondani JT, Luna SPL, Beier SL, *et al.* (2009). Analgesic efficacy of perioperative use of vedaprofen, tramadol or their combination in cats undergoing ovariohysterectomy. *J Feline Med Surg* **11**:420–429.

13 Roudebush P, Schoenherr WD, Delaney SJ (2008). An evidence based review of the use of therapeutic foods, owner education, exercise, and drugs for the management of obese and overweight pets. *J Am Vet Med Assoc* **233**(5): 717–725.

14 *An Animated Guide to the Multimodal Management of Canine Osteoarthritis* (2007). Novartis Animal Health USA, Inc.

15 McQuay HJ, Moore A (2006). NSAIDS and Coxibs: clinical use. In: McMahon SB, Koltzenburg M. (eds). *Wall and Melzack's Textbook of Pain*, 5th edn. Elsevier, Philadelphia, p. 474.

16 Scarda RT, Tranquilli WJ (2007). Local anesthetics. In: Tranquilli WJ, Thurmon JC, Grimm KA, (eds). *Lumb and Jones' Veterinary Anesthesia and Analgesia*, 4th edn. Blackwell, Ames, pp. 395–419, 561–604.

17 Feldman HS, Arthur GR, Covino BG (1989). Comparative systemic toxicity of convulsant and supraconvulsant doses of intravenous ropivacaine, bupivacaine, and lidocaine in the conscious dog. *Anesth Analg* **69**:794–801.

18 Liu PL, Feldman HS, Giasi R, *et al.* (1983). Comparative CNS toxicity of lidocaine, etidocaine, bupivacaine, and tetracaine in awake dogs following rapid intravenous administration. *Anesth Analg* **62**:375–379.

19 Patronek GJ (2001). Assessment of claims of short- and long-term complications associated with onychectomy in cats. *J Am Vet Med Assoc* **219**:932–937.

20 Cambridge AJ, Tobias KM, Newberry RC, *et al.* (2000). Subjective and objective measurements of postoperative pain in cats. *J Am Vet Med Assoc* **217**:685–690.

21 Curcio K, Bidwell LA, Boohart GV, *et al*. (2006). Evaluation of signs of postoperative pain and complications after forelimb onychectomy in cats receiving buprenorphine alone or with bupivacaine administered as a four-point regional nerve block. *J Am Vet Med Assoc* **228**:65–68.

22 Conzemius MG, Brockman DJ, King LG, *et al*. (1994). Analgesia in dogs after intercostal thoracotomy: a clinical trial comparing intravenous buprenorphine and interpleural bupivacaine. *Vet Surg* **23**:291–298.

23 Dhokarikar P, Caywood DD, Stobie D, *et al*. (1996). Effects of intramuscular or interpleural administration of morphine and interpleural administration of bupicacaine on pulmonary function in dogs that have undergone median sternotomy. *Am J Vet Res* **57**:375–380.

24 Lemke KA, Dawson SD (2000). Local and regional anesthesia. In: Mathews KA (ed). Management of Pain. *Vet Clin North Am Small Anim Pract* **30**(4):849.

25 Carpenter RE, Wilson DV, Evans AT (2004). Evaluation of intraperitoneal and incisional lidocaine or bupivacaine for analgesia following ovariohysterectomy in the dog. *Vet Anesth Analg* **31**:46–52.

26 Thompson SE, Johnson JM (1991). Analgesia in dogs after intercostal thopracotomy. A comparison of morphine, selective intercostal nerve block, and intrapleural regional analgesia with bupivacaine. *Vet Surg* **20**(1):73–77.

27 Stobie D, Caywood DD, Rozaski EA, *et al*. (1995). Evaluation of pulmonary function and analgesia in dogs after intercostal thoracotomy and use of morphine administered intramuscularly or intrapleurally and bupivacaine administered intrapleurally. *Am J Vet Res* **56**(8):1098–1109.

28 Lemke KA, Creighton CM (2008). Paravertebral blockade of the brachial plexus in dogs. *Vet Clin North Am Small Anim Pract* **38**:1231–1241.

29 Møiniche S, Mikkelsen S, Wetterslev J, *et al*. (1999). A systematic review of intra-articular local anesthesia for postoperative pain relief after arthroscopic knee surgery. *Reg Anesth Pain Med* **24**:430–437.

30 Sammarco JL, Conzemius MG, Perkowski SZ, *et al*. (1996). Postoperative analgesia for stifle surgery: a comparison of intra-articular bupivacaine, morphine, or saline. *Vet Surg* **25**:59–69.

31 Yaksh TL, Rudy TA (1976). Analgesia mediated by a direct spinal action of narcotics. *Science* **192**:1357–1358.

32 Valverde A, Dyson DH, McDonell WN (1989). Epidural morphine reduces halothane MAC in the dog. *Can J Anaesth* **36**:629–632.

33 Wetmore LA, Glowaski MM (2000). Epidural analgesia in veterinary critical care. *Clin Tech Small Anim Pract* **15**:177–188.

34 Mahler SP, Adogwa AO (2008). Anatomical and experimental studies of brachial plexus, sciatic, and femoral nerve-location using peripheral nerve stimulation in the dog. *Vet Anaesth Analg* **35**(1):80–89.

35 Mahler SP, Reece JLM (2007). Electrical nerve stimulation to facilitate placement of an indwelling catheter for repeated brachial plexus block in a traumatized dog. *Vet Anaesth Analg* **34**(5):365–370.

36 Wenger S (2004). Brachial plexus block using electrolocation for pancarpal arthrodesis in a dog. *Vet Anaesth Analg* **31**(4):272–275.

37 Portela D, Melanie P, Briganti A, *et al*. (2008). Nerve-stimulator guided paravertebral lumbar plexus anaesthesia in dogs. *Vet Res Commun* **32**(Suppl 1):S307–S310.

38 Marhofer P, Greher M, Kapral S (2005). Ultrasound guidance in regional anaesthesia. *Br J Anaesth* **94**:7–17.

39 Campoy L, Bezuidenhour A, Gleed RD, *et al*. (2010). Ultrasound-guided approach for axillary brachial plexus, femoral nerve, and sciatic nerve blocks in dogs. *Vet Anaesth Analg* **37**:144–153.

40 Costa-Farre C, Blanch XS, Cruz JI, *et al*. (2011). Ultrasound guidance for the performance of sciatic and saphenous nerve blocks in dogs. *Vet J* **187**:221–224.

41 Myrna KE, Bentley E, Sdmith IJ (2010). Effectiveness of injection of local anesthetic into the retrobulbar space for postoperative analgesia following eye enucleation in dogs. *J Am Vet Med Assoc* **237**:174–177.

42 Barber FA, Herbert MA (2002). The effectiveness of an anesthetic continuous-infusion device on postoperative pain control. *Arthroscopy* **18**:76–81.

43 Wolfe TM, Bateman SW, Cole LK (2006). Evaluation of a local anesthetic delivery system for the postoperative analgesic management of canine total ear canal ablation – a randomized, controlled, double-blinded study. *Vet Anaesth Analg* **33**:328–339.

44 Radlinsky MG, Mason DE, Roush JK, *et al*. (2005). Use of a continuous, local infusion of bupivacaine for postoperative analgesia in dogs undergoing total ear canal ablation. *J Am Vet Med Assoc* **227**:414–419.

45 Davis KM, Hardie EM, Martin FR, *et al*. (2007). Correlation between perioperative factors and successful outcome in fibrosarcoma resection in cats. *Vet Rec* **161**:199–200.

46 Robertson SA, Lascelles BDX, Taylor PM, *et al.* (2005). Pk-Pd modeling of buprenorphine in cats: intravenous and oral transmucosal administration. *J Vet Pharmacol Ther* **28**:453–460.

47 World Health Organization (2002). *WHO Traditional Medicine Strategy 2002–2005*. World Health Organization, Geneva.

48 Bache F (1826). Cases illustrative of the remedial effects of acupuncture. *North Am Med Surg J* **2**:311–321.

49 Scarda RT, Glowaski M (2007). Acupuncture. In: Tranquilli WJ, Thurman JC, Grimm KA (eds). *Lumb and Jones' Veterinary Anesthesia and Analgesia*, 4th edn. Blackwell, Ames, pp. 683–697.

50 Ma Y-T, Ma M, Cho ZH (2005). *Biomedical Acupuncture for Pain Management: an Integrative Approach*. Elsevier, St. Louis.

51 Helms JM (1997). *Acupuncture Energetics: A Clinical Approach for Physicians*. Medical Acupuncture Publishers, Berkeley, CA.

52 Poneranz B, Chiu D (1976). Naloxone blockade of acupuncture analgesia. Endorphin implicated. *Life Sci* **19**:1757–1762.

53 American Cancer Society (2000). *American Cancer Society's Guide to Complementary and Alternative Cancer Methods*. American Cancer Society, Atlanta.

54 Lee A, Done ML (1999). The use of nonpharmacologic techniques to prevent postoperative nausea and vomiting. A Meta-analysis. *Anesth Analg* **88**:1362–1369.

55 Kukanich B, Papich MG (2004). Plasma profile and pharmacokinetics of dextromethorphan after intravenous and oral administration in healthy dogs. *J Vet Pharmacol Ther* **27**:337–341.

56 Baker JF, Byrne DP, Walsh PM, Mulhall KJ (2011). Human chondrocyte viability after treatment with local anesthetic and/or magnesium: Results from an *in vitro* study. Arthroscopy **27**(2):213–217.

57 Baker JF, Mulhall KJ (2012). Local anaesthetics and chondrotoxicty: What is the evidence? *Knee Surgery, Sports Traumatology, Arthroscopy* **20**(11):2294–2301.

58 Chu CR, Coyle CH, Chu CT, *et al.* (2010). *In vivo* effects of single intra-articular injection of 0.5% bupivacaine on articular cartilage. *J Bone Joint Surg* Series A **92**(3):599–608.

59 Grishko V, Xu M, Wilson G, Pearsall IV AW (2010). Apoptosis and mitochondrial dysfunction in human chondrocytes following exposure to lidocaine, bupivacaine, and ropivacaine. *J Bone Joint Surg* Series A **92**(3):609–618.

60 Syed HM, Green L, Bianski B, Jobe CM, Wongworawat MD (2011). Bupivacaine and triamcinolone may be toxic to human chondrocytes: a pilot study. *Clin Orthop Relat Res* **469**(10):2941–2947.

CHAPTER 9

1 Fleming JM, Creevy KE, Promislow DEL (2011). Mortality in North American dogs from 1984 to 2004: an investigation into age-, size-, and breed-related causes of death. *J Vet Intern Med* **25**:187–198.

2 Johnston SA (1997). Osteoarthritis. Joint anatomy, physiology and pathobiology. *Vet Clin North Am Small Anim Pract* **27**:699–723.

3 Millis DL (2006). Nonsteroidal anti-inflammatory drugs, disease-modifying drugs, and osteoarthritis. A multimodal approach to treating osteoarthritis. Western Veterinary Conference, Symposium Proceedings.

4 Millis DL, Weigel JP, Moyers T, *et al.* (2002). Effect of deracoxib, a new COX-2 inhibitor, on the prevention of lameness induced by chemical synovitis in dogs. *Vet Ther* **24**:7–18.

5 Vasseur PB, Johnson AL, Budsberg SC, *et al.* (1995). Randomized, controlled trial of the efficacy of carprofen, a nonsteroidal anti-inflammatory drug, in the treatment of osteoarthritis in dogs. *J Am Vet Med Assoc* **206**:807–811.

6 Peterson KD, Keef TJ (2004). Effects of meloxicam on severity of lameness and other clinical signs of osteoarthritis in dogs. *J Am Vet Med Assoc* **225**:1056–1060.

7 Lust G, Williams AJ, Burton-Wurster N, *et al.* (1992). Effects of intramuscular administration of glycosaminoglycan polysulfates on signs of incipient hip dysplasia in growing pups. *Am J Vet Res* **53**:1836–1843.

8 De Haan JJ, Goring RL, Beale BS (1994). Evaluation of polysulfated glycosaminoglycan for the treatment of hip dysplasia in dogs. *Vet Surg* **23**:177–181.

9 Sevalla K, Todhunter RJ, Vernier-Singer M, *et al.* (2000). Effect of polysulfated glycosaminoglycan on DNA content and proteoglycan metabolism in normal and osteoarthritic canine articular cartilage explants. *Vet Surg* **29**:407–414.

10 Millis DL, Korvick D, Dean D, *et al.* (1999). 45th Meetingg ORS, p. 792.

11 Kukanich B, Papich MG (2004). Pharmacokinetics of tramadol and the metabolite O-desmethyltramadol in dogs. *J Vet Pharmacol Ther* **27**:239–246.

12 Emkey R, Rosenthal N, Wu SC, *et al.* (2004). Efficacy and safety of tramadol/acetaminophen tablets (Ultracet) as add-on therapy for osteoarthritis pain in subjects receiving a COX-2 nonsteroidal antiinflammatory drug: a multicenter, randomized, double-blind, placebo-controlled trial. *J Rheum* **31**:150–156.

13 Bennett GJ (2000). Update on the neurophysiology of pain transmission and modulation: focus on the NMDA receptor. *J Pain Symptom Manage* (www.hosppract.com) (discontinued).

14 Kealy RD, Lawler DF, Ballam JM, *et al*. (2000). Evaluation of the effect of limited food consumption on radiographic evidence of osteoarthritis in dogs. *J Am Vet Med Assoc* **217**(11):1678–1680.

15 Kealy RD, Lawler DF, Ballam JM, *et al*. (2002). Effects of diet restriction on life span and age-related changes in dogs. *J Am Vet Med Assoc* **220**:1315–1320.

16 Kealy RD, Olsson SE, Monti KL, *et al*. (1992). Effects of limited food consumption on the incidence of hip dysplasia in growing dogs. *J Am Vet Med Assoc* **201**:857–863.

17 Kealy RD, Lawler DF, Ballam JM, *et al*. (1997). Five-year longitudinal study on limited food consumption and development of osteoarthritis in coxofemoral joints of dogs. *J Am Vet Med Assoc* **210**(2):222–225.

18 Impellizeri JA, Tetrick MA, Muir P (2000). Effect of weight reduction on clinical signs of lameness in dogs with hip osteoarthritis. *J Am Vet Med Assoc* **216**(7):1089–1091.

19 Burkholder WJ, Taylor L, Hulse DA (2000). Weight loss to optimal body condition increases ground reaction forces in dogs with osteoarthritis. Purina Research Report.

20 Johnston SA, Budsberg SC, Marcellin-Little D, *et al*. (2005). Canine osteoarthritis: overview, therapies, & nutrition. NAVC Clinician's Brief, April; Supplement.

21 Waldron M (2004). The role of fatty acids in the management of osteoarthritis. Nestlé Purina Clinical Edge, Oct, pp. 14–16.

22 IAMS (2003). Nutrition plays a key role in joint health. Study finds that proactive nutrition can minimize use of NSAIDs. IAMS Partners for Health, July; V1,No.3.

23 Laflamme DP (2006). Fatty acids in health and disease. Nestlé Purina Research Report 10(2).

24 Bauer JE (2007). Responses of dogs to dietary omega-3 fatty acids. *J Am Vet Med Assoc* **231**:1657–1661.

25 Innes JF, Caterson B, Little CB, *et al*. (2006). Effect of omega-3 fatty acids on canine cartilage: using an *in vitro* model to investigate therapeutic mechanisms. 13th ESVOT Congress, Munich.

26 Levine D, Millis DL, Marcellin-Little D (2005). Introduction to veterinary physical rehabilitation. *Vet Clin North Am Small Anim Pract* **35**:1247–1254.

27 Millis DL, Levine D, Brumlow M, *et al*. (1997). A preliminary study of early physical therapy following surgery for cranial cruciate ligament rupture in dogs. VOS, Big Sky MT.

28 Marcellin-Little D (2007). Multimodal management of osteoarthritis in dogs. Symposium: a multimodal approach to treating osteoarthritis. Western Veterinary Conference, Las Vegas.

29 Millis DL, Levine D, Taylor RA (eds) [2004]. *Canine Rehabilitation & Physical Therapy*. WB Saunders St. Louis.

30 Sanderson RO, Beata C, Flipo R-M, *et al*. (2009). Systematic review of the management of canine osteoarthritis. *Vet Rec* **164**:418–424.

31 Aragon CL, Hofmeister EH, Budsberg SC (2007). Systematic review of clinical trials of treatments for osteoarthritis in dogs. *J Am Vet Med Assoc* **230**:514–521.

32 Lascelles BDX, Blikslager AT, Fox SM, *et al*. (2002). Gastrointestinal tract perforations in dogs treated with a selective cyclooxygenase-2 inhibitor: 29 cases (2002–2003). *J Am Vet Med Assoc* **227**(7):1112–1117.

33 Novartis Animal Health (2007). 3-Year Deramaxx Update. DER 060058A 35618.

34 Cook RJ, Sackett DL (1995). The number needed to treat: a clinically useful measure of treatment effect. *Br Med J* **310**: 452–454.

35 Edwards JE, McQuay HJ, Moore RA (2002). Combination analgesic efficacy: individual patient data meta-analysis of single-dose oral tramadol plus acetaminophen in acute postoperative pain. *J Pain Symptom Manage* **23**:121–130.

36 Millis DL (2010). Dasuquin's efficacy may be similar to that of NSAIDs in dogs. Joint Health: a roundtable discussion. Supplement. *Vet Med* **105**(11):10.

37 Millis DL (2005). Effects of feeding omega-3 fatty acids. Hill's Clinical Evidence Report.

38 Millis DL (2005). Clinician's update™, Supplement to NAVC Clinician's Brief®. April.

39 Novartis Animal Health (2004). Pharmacovigilance summary: Clinical experience with Deramaxx (deracoxib) since its US launch. Advisor for the Practicing Veterinarian. DER 030103A.

40 Lascelles BDX, McFarland JM (2004). Guidelines for safe and effective use of non-steroidal anti-inflammatory drugs in dogs. Technical Bulletin, Pfizer Animal Health.

41 Lascelles BDX, Blikslager AT, Fox SM, *et al*. (2005). Gastrointestinal tract perforations in dogs treated with a selective cyclooxygenase-2 inhibitor: 29 cases (2002–2003). *J Am Vet Med Assoc* **227**(7):1112–1117.

42 Dow SW, Rosychuk RA, McChesney AE, *et al.* (1990). Effects of flunixin and flunixin plus prednisone on the gastrointestinal tract of dogs. *Am J Vet Res* **51**:1131–1138.

43 Boston SE, Moens NM, Kruth SA, *et al.* (2003). Endoscopic evaluation of the gastroduodenal mucosa to determine the safety of short-term concurrent administration of meloxicam and dexamethasone in healthy dogs. *Am J Vet Res* **64**:1369–1375.

44 De Leon-Casasola OA (ed) (2006). *Cancer Pain. Pharmacologic, Interventional, and Palliative Approaches*. WB Saunders, Philadelphia, p. 284.

45 Hampshire VA, Doddy FM, Post LO, *et al.* (2004). Adverse drug event reports at the United States Food and Drug Administration Center for Veterinary Medicine. *J Am Vet Med Assoc* **225**: 533–536.

46 Williams JT (1997). The painless synergism of aspirin and opium. *Nature* **390**:557–559.

47 Lee A, Cooper MC, Craig JC, *et al.* (2004). Effects of nonsteroidal anti-inflammatory drugs on postoperative renal function in adults with normal renal function. *Cochrane Database Syst Rev* **2**:CD002765.

48 Burkhardt D, Ghosh P (1987). Laboratory evaluation of antiarthritic drugs as potential chondroprotective agents. *Sem Arthr Rheum* **17**(2) Suppl 1:3–34.

49 Baici A, Salgram P, Fehr K, *et al.* (1980). Inhibition of human elastase from polymorphonuclear leukocytes by a glycosaminoglycan polysulfate (Arteparon). *Biochem Pharmacol* **29**:1723–1727.

50 Stephens RW, Walton EA, Ghosh P, *et al.* (1980). A radioassay for proteolytic cleavage of isolated cartilage proteoglycan: inhibition of human leukocyte elastase and cathepsin G by anti-inflammatory drugs. *Arzneimittelforschung* **30**:2108–2112.

51 Stancikova M, Trnavsky K, Keilova H (1977). Effects of antirheumatic drugs on collagenolytic activity of cathepsin B1. *Biochem Pharmacol* **26**:2121–2124.

52 Egg D (1983). Effects of glycosaminoglycan polysulfate and two nonsteroidal anti-inflammatory drugs on prostaglandin E2 synthesis in Chinese hamster ovary cell cultures. *Pharm Res Commun* **15**:709–717.

53 Nishikawa H, Mori I, Umemoto J (1985). Influences of sulfated glycosaminoglycans on biosynthesis of hyaluronic acid in rabbit knee synovia. *Arch Biochem Biophys* **240**: 146–148.

54 Ghosh P (1991). The pathobiology of osteoarthritis and the rationale for the use of pentosan polysulfate for its treatment. *Sem Arthr Rheum* **28**:211–267.

55 Ghosh P, Hatadilok N (1996). Interactions of pentosan polysulfate with cartilage matrix proteins and synovial fibroblasts derived from patients with osteoarthritis. *Osteoarthr Cartil* **4**:43–53.

56 Rogachefsky RA, Dean DD, Howell DS, *et al.* (1994). Treatment of canine osteoarthritis with sodium pentosan polysulfate and insulin-like growth factor-1. *Ann NY Acad Sci* **6**:392–394.

57 Budsberg SC, Bergh MS, Reynolds LR, *et al.* (2007). Evaluation of pentosan polysulfate sodium in the postoperative recovery from cranial cruciate injury in dogs: a randomized, placebo-controlled clinical trial. *Vet Surg* **36**: 234–244.

58 Hannon RL, Smith JG, Cullis-Hill D, *et al.* (2003). Safety of Cartrophen Vet in the dog: review of adverse reaction reports in the UK. *J Soc Adm Pharm* **44**:202–208.

59 Heidrich JE, Fox SM, Vander Jagt RR, *et al.* (2008). Fluorescein-labeled polysulfated glycosaminoglycan in a feline acute traumatic knee model. VOS annual meeting, March, Big Sky MT.

60 McQuay HJ, Moore A (2006). NSAIDs and coxibs: clinical use. In: McMahon SB, Koltzenburg M (eds). *Wall and Melzack's Textbook of Pain*, 5th edn. Elsevier Churchill Livingston, Philadelphia, pp. 471–480.

61 Bianchi M, Broggini M, Balzarini P, *et al.* (2003). Effects of tramadol on synovial fluid concentrations of substance P and interleukin-6 in patients with knee osteoarthritis: comparison with paracetamol. *Int Immunopharm* **3** (13–14):1901–1908.

62 American College of Rheumatology Subcommittee on Osteoarthritis (2000). Recommendations for the medical management of osteoarthritis of the hip and knee. *Arthritis Rheum* **43**:1905–1915.

63 American Medical Directors Association (1999). *Chronic Pain Management in the Long-Term Care Setting: Clinical Practice Guideline*. American Medical Directors Association, Baltimore, i-32.

64 Torring ML, Riis A, Christensen S, *et al.* (2007). Perforated peptic ulcer and short-term mortality among tramadol users. *Br J Clin Pharm* **65**:565–572.

65 Garcia-Hernandez L, Deciga-Campos M, Guevara-Lopez U, *et al.* (2007). Co-administration of rofecoxib and tramadol results in additive or sub-additive interaction during arthritic nociception in rat. *Pharm Bio Behav* **87**:331–340.

66 Muller M, Kersten S (2003). Nutrigenomics: Goals and strategies. *Nature Rev* **4**:315–322.

67 Vester BM, Swanson K (2007). Nutrient-gene interactions: application to pet nutrition and health. *Vet Focus* **17**:25–32.

68 Eisele I, Wood IS, German AJ, *et al.* (2005). Adipokine gene expression in dog adipose tissues and dog white adipocytes differentiated in primary culture. *Horm Metabol Res* **37**: 474–481.

69 Trayhurn P, Wood IS (2004). Adipokines: inflammation and the pleiotropic role of white adipose tissue. *Br J Nutr* **92**:347–355.

70 Wander RC, Hall JA, Gradin JL, *et al.* (1997). The ratio of dietary (n-6) to (n-3) fatty acids influences immune system function, eicosanoids metabolism, lipid peroxidation and vitamin E status in aged dogs. *J Nutr* **127**:1198–1205.

71 Schwab JM, Serhan CN (2006). Lipoxins and new lipid mediators in the resolution of inflammation. *Curr Opin Pharmacol* **6**:414–420.

72 Serhan CN (2005). Novel omega-3-derived local mediators in anti-inflammation and resolution. *Pharmacol Ther* **105**:7–21.

73 Henrotin Y (2006). Nutraceuticals in the management of osteoarthritis: an overview. *J Vet Pharmacol Ther* **29**(Suppl 1): 201–210.

74 Henrotin YE, Deberg MA, Crielaard JM, *et al.* (2006). Avocado/soybean unsoponifiables prevent the inhibitory effect of osteoarthritic subchondral osteoblasts on aggrecan and Type II collagen synthesis by chondrocytes. *J Rheumatol* **33**:1668–1678.

75 Schaffler A, Buchler C (2007). Concise review: adipose tissue-derived stem cells – basic and clinical implications for novel cell-based therapies. *Stem Cells* **25**:818–827.

76 Parker A, Katz A (2006). Adipose-derived stem cells for the regeneration of damaged tissues. *Expert Opin Biol Ther* **6**:567–578.

77 Luyten FP (2004). Mesenchymal stem cells in osteoarthritis. *Curr Opin Rheumatol* **16**(5): 599–603.

78 Ortiz LA, DuTreil M, Fattman C, *et al.* (2007). Interleukin 1 receptor antagonist mediates the anti-inflammatory and antifibrotic effect of mesenchymal stem cells during lung injury. *Proc Natl Acad Sci USA* **104**:11002–11007.

79 Arend W, Malyak M, Guthridge C, *et al.* (1998). Interleukin-1 receptor antagonist: role in biology. *Annu Rev Immunol* **16**:27–55.

80 Kilroy G, Foster S, Wu X, *et al.* (2007). Cytokine profile of human adipose-derived stem cells: expression of angiogenic, hematopoietic, and pro-inflammatory factors. *J Cell Physiol* **212**: 702–709.

81 Jorgensen C, Gordeledze J, Noel D (2004). Tissue engineering through autologous mesenchymal stem cells. *Curr Opin Biotechnol* **15**:406–410.

82 Dominici M, Le Blanc K, Mueller I, *et al.* (2006). Minimal criteria for defining multipotent mesenchymal stromal cells. The International Society for Cellular Therapy position statement. *Cytotherapy* **8**:315–317.

83 Toghraie FS, Chenari N, Gholipour MA, *et al.* (2011). Treatment of osteoarthritis with infrapatellar fat pad derived mesenchymal stem cells in rabbit. *The Knee* **18**(2):71–75.

84 Black L, Gaynor J, Gahring D, *et al.* (2007). Effect of adipose-derived stem and regenerative cells in dogs with chronic osteoarthritis of the coxofemoral joints: a randomized, double-blinded multicenter controlled trial. *Vet Ther* **8**:272–284.

85 Black L, Gaynor J, Adams C, *et al.* (2008). Effect of intraarticular injection of autologous adipose-derived mesenchymal stem and regenerative cells on clinical signs of chronic osteoarthritis of the elbow joint in dogs. *Vet Ther* **9**:192–200.

86 Sampson S, Gerhardt M, Mandelbaum B (2012). Platelet rich plasma injection grafts for musculoskeletal injuries: a review. *Curr Rev Musculoskelet Med* DOI 10.1007/s12178-008-9032-5.

87 Fahie Ma, Ortolano G, Guercio V, *et al.* (2012). Clinical outcome using canine platelet enhancement therapy (C-PET). Veterinary Orthopedic Society 39th Annual Conference. March 3–10, 2012. Crested Butte, CO.

FURTHER READING

American Cancer Society (2000). *American Cancer Society's Guide to Complementary and Alternative Cancer Methods*. American Cancer Society, Atlanta.

Bache F (1826). Cases illustrative of the remedial effects of acupuncture. *North Am Med Surg J* **2**:311–321.

Helms JM (1997). *Acupuncture Energetics: A Clinical Approach for Physicians*. Medical Acupuncture Publishers, Berkeley.

Kienzle E, Bergler R, Mandernach A (1998). Comparison of the feeding behavior and the man-animal relationship in owners of normal and obese dogs. *J Nutr* **128**:2779S–2782S.

Lee A, Done ML (1999). The use of nonpharmacologic techniques to prevent postoperative nausea and vomiting. A Meta-analysis. *Anesth Analg* **88**:1362–1369.

Ma Y-T, Ma M, Cho ZH (2005). *Biomedica Acupuncture for Pain Management: an Integrative Approach*. Elsevier, St. Louis.

Poneranz B, Chiu D (1976). Naloxone blockade of acupuncture analgesia. Endorphin implicated. *Life Sci* **19**:1757–1762.

Prochaska J, DiClemente C (1984). *The Transtheoretical Approach: Crossing Traditional Boundaries of Therapy*. Dow Jones-Irwin, Homewood.

Skarda RT, Glowaski M (2007). Acupuncture. In: Tranquilli WJ, Thurman JC, Grimm KA (eds). *Lumb and Jones' Veterinary Anesthesia and Analgesia*, 4th edn. Blackwell, Ames, pp. 683–697.

World Health Organization (2002). *WHO Traditional Medicine Strategy 2002–2005*. World Health Organization, Geneva.

CHAPTER 10

1 Zhang W, Moskowitz RW, Nuki G, *et al*. (2007). OARSI recommendations for the management of hip and knee osteoarthritis, part 1: critical appraisal of existing treatment guidelines and systematic review of current research evidence. *Osteoarthr Cartil* **15**:981–1000.

2 McMaster W (1977). A literary review on ice therapy in injuries. *Am J Sports Med* **5**:124–126.

3 Olson J, Stravino V (1972). A review of cryotherapy. *Phys Ther* **62**:840–853.

4 Hayes K (1993). Cryotherapy. In: *Physical Agents*, 4th edn. Appleton & Lange, Norwalk, CT, pp. 9–15.

5 Millis DL (2002). Physical therapy and rehabilitation in dogs. In: Gaynor JS, Muir WM (eds). *Handbook of Veterinary Pain Management*, 2nd edn. Mosby Elsevier, St. Louis, p. 508.

6 Drez D, Faust DC, Evans JP (1981). Cryotherapy and nerve palsy. *Am J Sports Med* **9**:256–257.

7 Bassett FH III, Kirkpatrick JS, Englehardt DL, *et al*. (1992). Cryotherapy-induced nerve injury. *Am J Sports Med* **20**:516–518.

8 Nadler SF, Weingand KW, Stitik TP, *et al*. (2001). Pain relief runs hot and cold. *Biomechanics* **8**:1.

9 Myrer JW, Measom G, Fellingham GW (1998). Temperature change in the human leg during and after two methods of cryotherapy. *J Athletic Training* **33**:25–29.

10 Zemke JE, Andersen JC, Guion WK, *et al*. (1998). Intramuscular temperature responses in the human leg to two forms of cryotherapy: ice massage and ice bag. *J Orthop Sports Phys Ther* **27**:301–307.

11 Ho SS, Coel MN, Kajawa R, *et al*. (1994). The effects of ice on blood flow and bone metabolism in knees. *Am J Sports Med* **22**:537–540.

12 Brosseau L, Yonge KA, Robinson V, *et al*. (2003). Thermotherapy for treatment of osteoarthritis. *Cochrane Database Syst Rev* 4, Art. No.: CD004522. DOI: 10.1002/14651858.CD004522.

13 Howatson G, Van Someren KA (2003). Ice massage, effects on exercise-induced muscle damage. *J Sports Med Phys Fitness* **43**:500–505.

14 Moeller JL, Monroe J, McKeag DB (1997). Cryotherapy-induced common peroneal nerve palsy. *Clin J Sport Med* **7**:212–216.

15 Saxena A (1994). Achilles peritendinosis: an unusual case due to frostbite in an elite athlete. *J Foot Ankle Surg* **33**:87–90.

16 Sallis R, Chassay CM (1999). Recognizing and treating common cold-induced injury in outdoor sports. *Med Sci Sport Exerc* **31**:1367–1373.

17 Vannatta ML, Millis DL, Adair S, *et al*. (2004). Effects of cryotherapy on temperature change in caudal thigh muscles of dogs. In: Marcellin-Little DJ (ed). *Proceedings of the Third International Symposium on Rehabilitation and Physical Therapy in Veterinary Medicine* (abstr). Department of Continuing Education, NC State College of Veterinary Medicine, Raleigh, p.205.

18 Drygas KA, McClure S, Goring RL, *et al*. (2011). Prospective evaluation of cold compression therapy on postoperative pain, swelling, range of motion and lameness following tibial plateau leveling osteotomy in dogs. *J Am Vet Med Assoc* **238**(10):1284–1291.

19 Petrov R, McDoonald MH, Tesch AM, *et al*. (2003). Influence of topically applied cold treatmen on core temperature and cell viability in equine superficial digital flexor tendons. *Am J Vet Res* **64**:835–844.

20 Cameron MH (1999). Thermal agents: physical principles, cold and superficial heat. In: *Physical Agents in Rehabilitation: From Research to Practice*. WB Saunders, Philadelphia,, pp. 149–175.

21 Reid RW, Foley JM, Prior BM, *et al*. (1999). Mild topical heat increases popliteal blood flow as measured by MRI. *Med Sci Sports Exer* **31**:S208.

22 Erasala GN, Rubin JM, Tuthill TA, *et al*. (2001). The effect of topical heat treatment on trapezius muscle blood flow using power Doppler ultrasound. *Phys Ther* **81**:A5.

23 Davis KD, Kwan CL, Crawley AP, *et al*. (1998). Functional MRI study of thalamic and cortical activations evoked by cutaneous heat, cold, and tactile stimuli. *J Neurophysiol* **80**:1533–1546.

24 Nadler SF, Steiner DJ, Erasala GN, *et al*. (2002). Continuous low level heat wrap therapy provides more efficacy than ibuprofen and acetaminophen for acute low back pain. *Spine* **27**:1012–1014.

25 Markovic M, Stuhlmeier KM (2006). Short-term hyperthermia prevents activation of proinflammatory genes in fibroblast-like synoviocytes by blocking the activation of the transcription factor NF-kappaB. *J Mol Med* **84**:821–832.

26 Levine D, Marcellin-Little DJ, Millis DL, *et al.* (2010). Effects of partial immersion in water on vertical ground reaction forces and weight distribution in dogs. *Am J Vet Res* **71**:1413–1416.

27 Templeton MS, Booth DL, O'Kelly WD (1996). Effects of aquatic therapy on joint flexibility and functional ability in subjects with rheumatic disease. *J Orthop Sports Phys Ther* **23**:376–381.

28 Enwemeka CS, Rodriguez O, Mendosa S (1990). The biomechanical effects of low-intensity ultrasound on healing tendons. *Ultrasound Med Biol* **16**:801–807.

29 Saini NS, Roy KS, Bansal PS, *et al.* (2002). A preliminary study on the effect of ultrasound therapy on the healing of surgically severed Achilles tendons in five dogs. *J Vet Med A Physiol Pathol Clin Med* **49**:321–328.

30 Loonam JE, Millis DL (2002). The effect of therapeutic ultrasound on tendon healing and extensibility. In: *Proceedings of the 30th Annual Conference of the Veterinary Orthopedic Society*, Veterinary Orthopedic Society, Newmarket NH, p. 69.

31 Dyson M, Pond JB, Joseph J, *et al.* (1968). The stimulation of tissue regeneration by means of ultrasound. *Clin Sci* **35**:273–285.

32 Warden SJ (2003). A new direction for ultrasound therapy in sports medicine. *Sports Med* **33**:95–107.

33 Melzack R, Wall PD (1965). Pain mechanisms: a new theory. *Science* **150**:971–979.

34 Walsh DM (1997). *TENS: Clinical Application and Related Theory*. Churchill Livingstone, New York.

35 Garrison DW, Foreman RD (1996). Effects of transcutaneous electrical nerve stimulation (TENS) on spontaneous and noxiously evoked dorsal horn cell activity in cats with transected spinal cords. *Neurosci Lett* **216**:125–128.

36 Sluka KA, Deacon M, Stibal A, *et al.* (1999). Spinal blockade of opioid receptors prevents the analgesia produced by TENS in arthritic rats. *J Pharmacol Exp Ther* **289**:840–846.

37 Chandran P, Sluka KA (2003). Development of opioid tolerance with repeated transcutaneous electrical nerve stimulation administration. *Pain* **102**:195–201.

38 Osiri M, Welch V, Brosseau L, *et al.* (2000). Transcutaneous electrical nerve stimulation for knee osteoarthritis. *Cochrane Database Syst Rev* **4**. Art. No.: CD002823. DOI: 10.1001/14651858.CD002823.

39 Levine D, Johnston KD, Price MN, *et al.* (2002). The effect of TENS on osteoarthritic pain in the stifle of dogs. *Proceedings of the 2nd International Symposium on Rehabilitation and Physical Therapy in Veterinary Medicine*. University of Tennessee Knoxville, p.199.

40 Millis DL, Francis D, Adamson C (2005). Emerging modalities in veterinary rehabilitation. In: Levine D, Millis DL, Marcellin-Little DJ, *et al.* (eds). Rehabilitation and Physical Therapy. *Vet Clin North Am Small Anim Pract* **35**(6):1344.

41 Stelian J, Gil I, Habot B, *et al.* (1991). Laser therapy is effective for degenerative osteoarthritis: improvement of pain and disability in elderly patients with degenerative osteoarthritis of the knee treated with narrow-band light therapy. *J Am Geriatr Soc* **40**:23–26.

42 Djavid GE, Mortazavi SMJ, Basirnia A, *et al.* (2003). Low level laser therapy in musculoskeletal pain syndromes: pain relief and disability reduction. *Lasers Surg Med* **152**:43.

43 Gur A, Cosut A, Sarac AJ, *et al.* (2003). Efficacy of different therapy regimes of low-power laser in painful osteoarthritis of the knee: a double-blind and randomized-controlled trial. *Lasers Surg Med* **33**:330–338.

44 Tascioglu F, Armagan O, Tabak Y, *et al.* (2004). Low power laser treatment in patients with knee osteoarthritis. *Swiss Med Wkly* **134**:254–258.

45 Guzz GA, Tigani D, Torricelli P, *et al.* (2001). Low-power diode laser stimulation of surgical osteochondral defects: results after 24 weeks. *Artif Cells Blood Substit Immobil Biotechnol* **29**:235–244.

46 Fung DT, Ng GY, Leung MC, Tay DK (2002). Therapeutic low energy laser improves the mechanical strength of repairing medial collateral ligament. *Lasers Surg Med* **31**:91–96.

47 Mester E, Spiry T, Szende B, *et al.* (1971). Effect of laser rays on wound healing. *Am J Surg* **122**:532–538.

48 Enwemeka CS, Parker JC, Dowdy DS, *et al.* (2004). The efficacy of low-power lasers in tissue repair and pain control: a meta-analysis study. *Photomed Laser Surg* **22**:323–329.

49 Barber A, Luger JE, Karpf A, *et al.* (2001). Advances in laser therapy for bone repair. *Laser Ther* **29**:80–85.

50 Bjordal JM, Couppé C, Chow R, *et al.* (2003). A systematic review of low level laser therapy with location-specific doses for pain from chronic joint disorders. *Aust J Physiother* **49**: 107–116.

51 Thiel M (2001). Application of shock waves in medicine. *Clin Orthop* **387**:18–21.

52 Ogden JA, Alvarez RG, Levitt R, *et al.* (2001). Shock wave therapy (Orthotripsy) in musculoskeletal disorders. *Clin Orthop* **387**:22–40.

53 Wand CJ, Wand FS, Yang KD, *et al.* (2003). Shock wave therapy induces neovascularization at the tendon-bone junction: a study in rabbits. *J Orthop Res* **21**:984–989.

54 Wang FS, Yang KD, Kuo YR, *et al*. (2003). Temporal and spatial expression of bone morphogenetic proteins in extracorporeal shock wave-promoted healing of segmental defect. *Bone* **32**:387–396.
55 Francis DA, Millis DL, Evans M, *et al*. (2004). Clinical evaluation of extracorporeal shockwave therapy for the management of canine osteoarthritis of the elbow and hip joints. In: *Proceedings of the 31st Veterinary Orthopedic Society*. Veterinary Orthopedic Society, Okemos MI.
56 Adamson CP, Taylor RA (2003). Preliminary functional outcomes of extracorporeal shockwave therapy on ten dogs with various orthopaedic conditions. *Vet Comp Orthop Traumatol* **3**:A11.
57 Towle JM, Fleck T (2004). Clinical results of radial shockwave therapy for the treatment of ostoarthritis in dogs. *Proceedings of the 56th Convention of the Canadian Veterinary Association*, Quebec City, PQ, Canada.
58 Bockstahler B (2004). Extracorporeal shock wave therapy (ESWT) for hip osteoarthritis. Proceedings of the 12th ESVOT Congress, Munich, Germany, pp. 21–22.
59 http://nccam.nih.gov/health/magnet/magnetsforpain.htm. Accessed 12/12/12.
60 Markov MS, Pilla AA (1997). Weak static magnetic field modulation of myosin phosphorylation in a cell-free preparation: calcium dependence. *Bioelectrochem Bioenerg* **43**:233–238.
61 McKay JC, Prato FS, Thomas AW (2007). A literature review: the effects of magnetic field exposure on blood flow and blood vessels in the microvasculature. *Bioelectromagnetics* **28**:81–98.
62 Taniguchi N, Kanai S, KawamotoM, *et al*. (2004). Study on application of static magnetic field for adjuvant arthritis rats. *Evid Based Complement Alternat Med* **1**:187–191.
63 Xu S, Tomita N, Ikeuchi K, *et al*. (2007). Recovery of small-sized blood vessels in ischemic bone under static magnetic field. *Evid Based Complement Alternat Med* **4**:59–63.
64 Morris CE, Skalak TC (2007). Chronic static magnetic field exposure alters microvessel enlargement resulting from surgical intervention. *J Appl Physiol* **101**:629–636.
65 Steyn PD, Ramey DW, Kirschvink J, *et al*. (2000). Effect of a static magnetic field on blood flow to the metacarpus of horses. *J Am Vet Med Assoc* **217**:874–878.
66 Colbert AP, Wahbeh H, Harling N, *et al*. (2007). Static magnetic field therapy: a critical review of treatment parameters. *eCAM* DOI:10.1093/ecam/nem131.
67 Black LL, Gaynor J, Adams C, *et al*. (2008). Effect of intra-articular injection of autologous adipose derived mesenchymal stem and regenerative cells on clinical signs of chronic osteoarthritis of the elbow joint in dogs. *Vet Ther* **9**:192–200.
68 Black LL, Gaynor J, Gathering D, *et al*. (2007). Effect of adipose-derived mesenchymal stem and regenerative cells on lameness in dogs with chronic osteoarthritis of the coxofemoral joint: a randomized, double-blind, multicenter, controlled trial. *Vet Ther* **8**:272–284.

CHAPTER 11

1 Steinbeck J (1939). *The Grapes of Wrath*. Viking Press–James Lloyd.
2 Vertosick FT (2000). *Why We Hurt: the Natural History of Pain*. Harcourt, New York.
3 Merskey H, Bogduk N (eds) (1994). *Classification of Chronic Pain*, 2nd edn. IASP Press, Seattle.
4 Ventafridda V, Caracen A (1991). Cancer pain classification: a controversial issue. *Pain* **46**:1–2.
5 Caraceni A, Weinstein S (2001). Classification of cancer pain syndromes. *Oncology* **15**:1627–1640.
6 Twycross R (1997). Cancer pain classification. *Acta Anaesthesiol Scand* **41**:141–145.
7 Verstappen C, Heimans J, Hoekman K, *et al*. (2003). Neurotoxic complications of chemotherapy in patients with cancer: clinical signs and optimal management. *Drugs* **63**:1549–1563.
8 Portenoy R (1992). Cancer pain: Pathophysiology and syndromes. *Lancet* **339**:1026–1031.
9 Stute P, Soukup, Menzel M (2003). Analysis and treatment of different types of neuropathic cancer pain. *J Pain Symptom Manage* **26**:1123–1130.
10 Portenoy R, Foley K, Intumisi C (1990). The nature of opioid responsiveness and its implications for neuropathic pain: New hypotheses derived from studies of opioid infusions. *Pain* **43**:273–286.
11 Chong M, Bajwa Z (2003). Diagnosis and treatment of neuropathic pain. *J Pain Symptom Manage* **25**:S4–S11.
12 Caraceni A, Zecca E, Martini C, *et al*. (1999). Gabapentin as an adjuvant to opioid analgesia for neuropathic cancer pain. *J Pain Symptom Manage* **17**:441–445.
13 Martin L, Hagen N (1997). Neuropathic pain in cancer patients: Mechanism syndromes and clinical controversies. *J Pain Symptom Manage* **14**:99–117.
14 Tasker R (1987). The problem of deafferentation pain in the management of the patient with cancer. *J Palliat Care* **2**:8–12.

15 England J, Happel L, Kline D, *et al.* (1996). Sodium channel accumulation in humans with painful neuromas. *Neurology* **47**:272–276.

16 Ashby M, Fleming B, Brooksbank M, *et al.* (1992). Description of a mechanistic approach to pain management in advanced cancer. Preliminary report. *Pain* **51**:273–282.

17 World Health Organization (1986). *Cancer Pain Relief.* Geneva, World Health Organization.

18 Ashby M, Fleming B, Brooksbank M, *et al.* (1992). Description of a mechanistic approach to pain management in advanced cancer. Preliminary report. *Pain* **51**:153–161.

19 Dorn CR, Taylor DON, Frye FL, *et al.* (1968). Survey of animal neoplasms in Alameda and Contra Costa Counties, California 1. Methodology and description of cases. *J Natl Cancer Inst* **40**:295–305.

20 Bronson RT (1982). Variation in age at death of dogs of different sexes and breeds. *Am J Vet Res* **43**:2057–2059.

21 Larue F, Colleau SM, Breasseur L, *et al.* (1995). Multicenter study of cancer pain and its treatment in France. *Br Med J* **310**:1034–1037.

22 Wagner G (1984). Frequency of pain in patients with cancer. *Rec Results in Cancer Res* **89**:64–71.

23 Capner CA, Lascelles BD, Waterman-Pearson AE (1999). Current British veterinary attitudes to perioperative analgesia for dogs. *Vet Rec* **145**: 95–99.

24 Dohoo SE, Dohoo IR (1996). Postoperative use of analgesics in dogs and cats by Canadian veterinarians. *Can Vet J* **37**:546–551.

25 Portenoy RK, Lesage P (1999). Management of cancer pain. *Lancet* **353**:1695–1700.

26 Lascelles BDX (2003). Relief of chronic cancer pain. In: Dobson JM, Lascelles BDX (eds). *BSAVA Manual of Canine and Feline Oncology*. BSAVA, Quedgeley, UK, pp. 137–151.

27 Miguel RV (2006). Initial approach to the patient with cancer pain. In: de Leon-Casasola OA (ed.). *Cancer Pain: Pharmacology, Interventional and Palliative Care Approaches*. WB Saunders, Philadelphia, p. 26.

28 Yazbek KVB, Fantoni DT (2005). Validity of a health-related quality-of-life scale for dogs with signs of pain secondary to cancer. *J Am Vet Med Assoc* **226**:1354–1358.

29 Conzemius MG, Hill CM, Sammarco JL, *et al.* (1997). Correlation between subjective and objective measures used to determine severity of postoperative pain in dogs. *J Am Vet Med Assoc* **210**:1619–1622.

30 Fox SM, Mellor DJ, Lawoko CRO, *et al.* (1998). Changes in plasma cortisol concentrations in bitches in response to different combinations of halothane and butorphanol, with or without ovariohysterectomy. *Res Vet Sci* **65**: 125–133.

31 Fox SM, Mellor DJ, Stafford, KJ, *et al.* (2000). The effects of ovariohysterectomy plus different combinations of halothane anaesthesia and butorphanol analgesia on behaviour in the bitch. *Res Vet Sci* **68**:265–274.

32 Hardie EM, Hansen BD, Carroll GS (1997). Behavior after ovariohysterectomy in the dog: what's normal? *Appl Anim Behav Sci* **51**:111–128.

33 Hunt SP, Mantyh PW (2001). The molecular dynamics of pain control. *Nat Rev Neurosci* **2**:83–91.

34 Hunt SP, Pini A, Evan G (1987). Induction of c-fos-like protein in spinal cord neurons following sensory stimulation. *Nature* **328**:632–634.

35 Dubois RN, Radhika A, Reddy BS, *et al.* (1996). Increased cyclooxygenase-2 levels in carcinogen-induced rat colonic tumors. *Gastroenterology* **110**:1259–1262.

36 Kundu N, Yang QY, Dorsey R, *et al.* (2001). Increased cyclooxygenase-2 (COX-2) expression and activity in a murine model of metastatic breast cancer. *Int J Cancer* **93**:681–686.

37 Masferrer JL, Leahy KM, Koki AT, *et al.* (2000). Antiangiogenic and antitumor activities of cyclooxygenase-2 inhibitors. *Cancer Res* **60**:1306–1311.

38 Moore BC, Simmons DL (2000). COX-2 inhibition, apoptosis, and chemoprevention by non-steroidal anti-inflammatory drugs. *Curr Med Chem* 7:1131–1144.

39 Dempke W, Rie C, Grothey A, *et al.* (2001). Cyclooxygenase-2: a novel target for cancer chemotherapy? *J Cancer Res Clin Oncol* **127**: 411–417.

40 Khan KN, Knapp DW, Denicola DB, *et al.* (2000). Expression of cyclooxygenase-2 in transitional cell carcinoma of the urinary bladder in dogs. *Am J Vet Res* **61**:478–481.

41 Khan KN, Stanfield KM, Trajkovic D, *et al.* (2001). Expression of cyclooxygenase-2 in canine renal cell carcinoma. *Vet Pathol* **38**:116–119.

42 Pestili de Almeida EM, Piche C, Sirois J, *et al.* (2001). Expression of cyclo-oxygenase-2 in naturally occurring squamous cell carcinomas in dogs. *J Histochem Cytochem* **49**:867–875.

43 Tremblay C, Dore' M, Bochsler PN, *et al.* (1999). Induction of prostaglandin G/H synthase-2 in a canine model of spontaneous prostatic adenocarcinoma. *J Natl Cancer Instit* **91**:1398–1403.

44 McEntee MF, Cates JM, Neilsen N (2002). Cyclooxygenase-2 expression in spontaneous intestinal neoplasia of domestic dogs. *Vet Pathol* **39**:428–436.

45 Borzacchiello G, Paciello O, Papparella S (2004). Expression of cyclooxygenase-1 and -2 in canine nasal carcinomas. *J Comp Path* **131**:70–76.

46 Mullins MN, Lana SE, Dernell WS, *et al.* (2004). Cyclooxygenase-2 expression in canine appendicular osteosarcoma. *J Vet Intern Med* **18**:859–865.
47 Heller DA, Clifford CA, Goldschmidt MH, *et al.* (2005). Cycloxygenase-2 expression is associated with histologic tumor type in canine mammary carcinoma. *Vet Pathol* **42**:776–780.
48 Mohammed SI, Khan KNM, Sellers RS, *et al.* (2004). Expression of cyclooxygenase-1 and 2 in naturally-occuring canine cancer. *Prostaglandins, Leukot Essent Fatty Acids* **70**:479–483.
49 Beam SL, Rassnick KM, Moore AS, *et al.* (2003). An immunohistochemical study of cyclooxygenase-2 expression in various feline neoplasms. *Vet Pathol* **40**:496–500.
50 Pomonis JD, Rogers SD, Peters CM, *et al.* (2001). Expression and localization of endothelin receptors: Implication for the involvement of peripheral glia in nociception. *J Neurosci* **21**:999–1006.
51 Kurbel S, Kurbel B, Kovacic D, *et al.* (1999). Endothelin-secreting tumors and the idea of the pseudoectopic hormone secretion in tumors. *Med Hypotheses* **52**:329–333.
52 Nelson JB, Hedican SP, George DJ, *et al.* (1995). Identification of endothelin-1 in the pathophysiology of metastatic adenocarcinoma of the prostate. *Nature Med* **1**:944–999.
53 Julius D, Basbaum AL (2001). Molecular mechanisms of nociception. *Nature* **413**: 203–210.
54 Delaisse J-M, Vales G (1992). Mechanism of mineral solubilization and matrix degradation in osteoclastic bone resorption. In: Rifkin BR, Gay CV (eds). *Biology and Physiology of the Osteoclast*. CRC, Ann Arbor.
55 Honore P, Menning PM, Rogers SD, *et al.* (2000). Neurochemical plasticity in persistent inflammatory pain. *Prog Brain Res* **129**:357–363.
56 Mannix K, Ahmedazai SH, Anderson H, *et al.* (2000). Using bisphosphonates to control the pain of bone metastases: Evidence based guidelines for palliative care. *Palliat Med* **14**: 455–461.
57 Honore P, Rogers SD, Schwei MJ, *et al.* (2000). Murine models of inflammatory, neuropathic and cancer pain each generates a unique set of neurochemical changes in the spinal cord and sensory neurons. *Neuroscience* **98**:585–598.
58 Koltzenburg M (1999). The changing sensitivity in the life of the nociceptor. *Pain* (Suppl 6); S93–102.
59 Boucher TJ, McMahon SB (2001). Neurotrophic factors and neuropathic pain. *Curr Opin Pharmacol* **1**:66–72.
60 Schwei MJ, Honore P, Rogers SD, *et al.* (1999). Neurochemical and cellular reorganization of the spinal cord in a murine model of bone cancer pain. *Neuroscience* **19**:10886–10897.
61 Ripamonti C, Dickerson ED (2001). Strategies for the treatment of cancer pain in the new millennium. *Drugs* **61**:955–977.
62 Honore P, Schwei J, Rogers SD, *et al.* (2000). Cellular and neurochemical remodeling of the spinal cord in bone cancer pain. *Prog Brain Res* **129**:389–397.
63 National Institutes Health (2002). State-of-the-Science Conference Statement: Symptom management in cancer: Pain, depression, and fatigue. *J Natl Cancer Inst* **95**:1110–1117.
64 Quasthoff S, Hartung H (2002). Chemotherapy-induced peripheral neuropathy. *J Neurol* **249**: 9–17.
65 Mangioni C, Bolis G, Pecorelli, *et al.* (1989). Randomized trial in advanced ovarian cancer comparing cisplatin and carboplatin. *J Natl Cancer Inst* **81**:1464–1471.
66 Rowinsky EK, Donehower RS (1995). Paclitaxel (Taxol). *N Engl J Med* **332**:1004–1013.
67 Verwei J, Clavel M, Chevalier B (2003). Paclitaxel (Taxol™) and docetaxel (Taxotere™): not simply two of a kind. *Ann Oncol* **5**:495–505.
68 Hamers FPT, Gispen WH, Neijt JP (1991). Neurotoxic side-effects of cisplatin. *Eur J Cancer* **27**:372–376.
69 Gurney H, Crowther D, Anderson H, *et al.* (1990). Five year follow-up and dose delivery analysis of cisplatin, iroplatin or carbopolatin combination with cyclophosphamide in advanced ovarian carcinoma. *Ann Oncol* **1**:427–433.
70 Swenerton K, Jeffrey J, Stuart G, *et al.* (1992). Cisplatin-cyclophosphamide versus carboplatin-cyclophosphamide in advanced ovarian cancer: A randomized phase III study of the national cancer institute of Canada clinical trial group. *J Clin Oncol* **10**:718–726.
71 Forman AD (1990). Peripheral neuropathy in cancer patients: Clinical types, etiology, and presentation. *Oncology* **4**:85–89.
72 Tuxen MK, Hansen SW (1994). Complications of treatment: Neurotoxicity secondary to antineoplastic drugs. *Cancer Treat Rev* **20**: 191–214.
73 McBride WH, Withers HR (2002). Biological basis of radiation therapy. In: Perez CA (ed). *Principles and Practice of Radiation Oncology*. Lippincott, Philadelphia, pp. 96–136.
74 Kerr JF, Winterford CM, Harmon BV (1994). Apoptosis: Its significance in cancer and cancer therapy. *Cancer* **13**:2013–2026.

75 Azinovic I, Calvo FA, Puebla F (2001). Long-term normal tissue effects of intraoperative electron radiation therapy (IOERT): Late sequelae, tumor recurrence, and second malignancies. *Int J Radiat Oncol Bio Phys* **49**: 597–604.

76 Carsten RE, Hellyer PW, Bachand AM, *et al.* (2008). Correlations between acute radiation scores and pain scores in canine radiation patients with cancer of the forelimb. *Vet Anaes Analg* **35**:355–362.

77 DeWys WD, Begg C, Lavin PT, *et al.* (1980). Prognostic effect of weight loss prior to chemotherapy in cancer patients. *Am J Med* **69**:491.

78 Langer CI, Hoffman JP, Ottery FD (2001). Clinical significance of weight loss in cancer patients: rationale for the use of anabolic agents in the treatment of cancer-related cachexia. *Nutrition* **17**:S1.

79 Michel KE, Sorenmo K, Shofer FS (2004). Evaluation of body condition and weight loss in dogs presented to a veterinary oncology service. *J Vet Intern Med* **18**:692–695.

80 Rotat C, Lhoest E, Istasse L, *et al.* (2010). Influence of a liquid nutritional supplement on water intake in experimental beagle dogs. Viyo Publications (www.viyoveterinary.com).

81 Mauldin GE (2007). Nutritional management of the cancer patient. In: Withrow SJ, Vail DM (eds). *Small Animal Clinical Oncology*, 4th edn. WB Saunders Elsevier, St. Louis.

82 Eisenberg E, Marinangeli F, Birkhahn J, *et al.* (2005). Time to modify the WHO analgesic ladder? *Pain: Clinical Updates* **13**(5):1–4.

CHAPTER 12

1 Bernstein P (2005). The human-cat relationship. In: Rochlitz (ed). *The Welfare of Cats*. Springer, Dordrecht, pp.47–89.

2 Scott HW, McLaughlin R (2007). *Feline Orthopedics*. Manson Publishing, London, pp. 10–16.

3 Lascelles BD, Capner CA, Waterman-Pearson AE (1999). A survey of current British veterinary attitudes to peri-operative analgesia for cats and small mammals. *Vet Rec* **145**:601–604.

4 Taylor PM, Robertson SA (2004). Pain management in cats – past, present, and future. Part 1. The cat is unique. *J Feline Med Surg* **6**:313–320.

5 Waran N, Best L, Williams V, *et al.* (2007). A preliminary study of behavior-based indicators of pain in cats. *Anim Welf* **16**(S):105–108.

6 Lascelles D, Waterman A (1997). Analgesia in cats. *In Practice* **19**:203–213.

7 Brondani JT, Luna SP, Padovani CR (2011). Refinement and initial validation of a multidimensional composite scale for use in assessing acute postoperative pain in cats. *Am J Vet Res* **72**(2):174–183.

8 Bennett D, Morton C (2009). A study of owner observed behavioural and lifestyle changes in cats with musculoskeletal disease before and after analgesic therapy. *J Feline Med Surg* **11**:997–1004.

9 Lascelles BD, Hansen BD, Roe S, *et al.* (2007). Evaluation of client-specific outcome measures and activity monitoring to measure pain relief in cats with osteoarthritis. *J Vet Intern Med* **21**: 410–416.

10 Klepstad P, Dale O, Skorpen F, *et al.* (2005). Genetic variability and clinical efficacy of morphine. *Acta Anaesthesiol Scand* **49**(7):902–908.

11 FDA (1994). NADA 141-047 Torbugesic-SA (butorphanol) veterinary injection – original approval.

12 Wegner K, Robertson SA (2007). Dose-related thermal antinociceptive effects of intravenous hydromorphone in cats. *Vet Anaesth Analg* **34**(2):132–138.

13 Robertson S, Wegner K, Lascelles BDX (2009). Antinociceptive and side-effects of hydromorphone after subcutaneous administration in cats. *J Feline Med Surg* **11**(2):76–81.

14 Taylor PM, Robertson SA, Dixon MJ, *et al.* (2001). Morphine, pethidine and buprenorphine disposition in the cat. *J Vet Pharmacol Ther* **24**(6):391–398.

15 Dobbins S, Brown NO, Shofer FS (2002). Comparison of the effects of buprenorphine, oxymorphone hydrochloride, and ketoprofen for postoperative analgesia after onychectomy or onychectomy and sterilization in cats. *J Am Anim Hosp Assoc* **38**(6):507–514.

16 Briggs SL, Sneed K, Sawyer DC (1998). Antinociceptive effects of oxymorphone-butorphanol-acepromazine combination in cats. *Vet Surg* **27**(5):466–472.

17 Niedfeldt RL, Robertson SA (2006). Post-anesthetic hyperthermia in cats: a retrospective comparison between hydromorphone and buprenorphine. *Vet Anesth Analg* **33**(6):381–389.

18 Posner LP, Gleed RD, Erb HN, *et al.* (2007). Post-anesthetic hyperthermia in cats. *Vet Anaesth Analg* **34**(1):40–47.

19 Lascelles BD, Robertson SA (2004). Use of thermal threshold response to evaluate the antinociceptive effects of butorphanol in cats. *Am J Vet Res* **65**(8):1085–1089.

20 Mandsager RE, Raffe MR (1991). Evaluation of periosteal nociception in the cat. *Prog Vet Neurol* **2**:237–242.

21 Robertson SA, Taylor PM, Lascelles BD, *et al.* (2003). Changes in thermal threshold response in eight cats after administration of buprenorphine, butorphanol and morphine. *Vet Rec* **153**(15):462–465.

22 Robertson SA, Lascelles BD, Taylor PM, *et al.* (2005). PK-PD modeling of buprenorphine in cats: intravenous and oral transmucosal administration. *J Vet Pharmacol Therap* **28**: 453–460.

23 Stanway G, Taylor P, Brodbelt D (2002). A preliminary investigation comparing preoperative morphine and buprenorphine for postoperative analgesia and sedation in cats. *Vet Anaesth Analg* **29**:23–35.

24 Murrell JC, Robertson SA, Taylor PM, *et al.* (2007). Use of a transdermal matrix patch of buprenorphine in cats: preliminary pharmacokinetic and pharmacodynamics data. *Vet Rec* **160**(17):578–583.

25 Robertson SA, Taylor PM, Sear JW, *et al.* (2005). Relationship between plasma concentrations and analgesia after intravenous fentanyl and disposition after other routes of administration in cats. *J Vet Pharmacol Ther* **28**:1–7.

26 Riviere JE, Papich MG (2001). Potential and problems of developing transdermal patches for veterinary applications. *Adv Drug Deliv Rev* **50**(3):175–203.

27 Lee DD, Papich MG, Hardie EM (2000). Comparison of pharmacokinetics of fentanyl after intravenous and transdermal administration in cats. *Am J Vet Res* **61**(6):672–677.

28 Kukanich B, Lascelles BD, Aman AM, *et al.* (2005). The effects of inhibiting cytochrome P450 3A, p-glycoprotein, and gastric acid secretion on the oral bioavailability of methadone in dogs. *J Vet Pharmaol Ther* **28**(5):461–466.

29 Mollenhoff A, Nolte I, Kramer S (2005). Anti-nociceptive efficacy of carprofen, levomethadone and buprenorphine for pain relief in cats following major orthopaedic surgery. *J Vet Med A Physiol Pathol Clin Med* **52**(4):186–198.

30 Ferreira TH, Rezende ML, Mama KR, *et al.* (2011). Plasma concentrations and behavioral, antinociceptive, and physiologic effects of methadone after intravenous and oral transmucosal administration in cats. *Am J Vet Res* **72**:764–771.

31 Pypendop BHG, Siao KT, Likiw JE (2009). Effects of tramadol hydrochloride on the thermal threshold in cats. *Am J Vet Res* **70**:1465–1470.

32 Brondani JT, Luna SP, Marcello GC, *et al.* (2009). Perioperative administration of vedaprofen, tramadol or their combination does not interfere with platelet aggregation, bleeding time and biochemical variables in cats. *J Feline Med Surg* **11**:503–509.

33 Lamont LA (2002). Feline perioperative pain management. *Vet Clin North Am Small Anim Pract* **32**:747–763.

34 Brodbelt DC, Pfeiffer DU, Young LE, *et al.* (2007). Risk factors for anaesthetic-related death in cats: results from the confidential enquiry into perioperative small animal fatalities (CEPSAF). *Br J Anaesth* **99**(5):617–623.

35 Slingsby LS (2006). Efficacy of buccal compared to intramuscular dexmedetomidine for antinociception to a thermal nociceptive stimulus in the cat. 9th World Congress of Vet Anaesth, Santos, Brazil.

36 Slingsby LS, Taylor PM (2008). Thermal antinociception after dexmedetomidine administration in cats: a dose-finding study. *J Vet Pharmacol Ther* **31**:135–142.

37 Slingsby LS, Lane EC, Mears ER, *et al.* (1998). Postoperative pain after ovariohysterectomy in the cat: a comparison of two anaesthetic regimens. *Vet Rec* **143**(21):589–590.

38 Gaynor JS, Muir WW (2009). *Handbook of Veterinary Pain Management*, 2nd edn. Mosby Elsevier, St. Louis, p. 267.

39 Eisenberg E, Pud D (1988). Can patients with chronic neuropathic pain be cured by acute administration of NMDA receptor antagonist amantadine? *Pain* **74**:337–339.

40 Chew DJ, Buffington CA, Kendall MS, *et al.* (1998). Amitriptyline treatment for severe recurrent idiopathic cystitis in cats. *J Am Vet Med Assoc* **213**(9):1282–1286.

41 Robertson S, Lascelles BDX (2010). Long-term pain in cats. How much do we know about this important welfare issue? *J Feline Med Surg* **12**:188–199.

42 Brandt KD, Braunstein EM, Visco DM, *et al.* (1991). Anterior (cranial) cruciate ligament transection in the dog: a bona fide model of osteoarthritis, not merely of cartilage injury and repair. *J Rheumatol* **18**:436–446.

43 Suter E, Herzog W, Leonard TR, *et al.* (1998). One-year changes in hindlimb kinematics, ground reaction forces and knee stability in an experimental model of osteoarthritis. *J Biomech* **31**:511–551.

44 Maitland ME, Leonard TR, Frank CB, *et al.* (1998). Longitudinal measurement of tibial motion relative to the femur during passive displacements and femoral nerve stimulation in the ACL-deficient cat model of osteoarthritis. *J Orthop Res* **16**:484–454.

45 Tashman S, DuPre K, Goitz H, *et al*. (1995). A digital radiographic system for determining 3D joint kinematics during movement. 19th Annual Meeting, Am Soc Biomech, pp. 249–250.

46 Korvick DL, Pijanowski GJ, Schaeffer DJ (1994). Three-dimensional kinematics of the intact and cranial cruciate ligament-deficient siffle of dogs. *J Biomech* **27**:77–87.

47 Clarke SP, Mellor D, Clements DN, *et al*. (2005). Prevalence of radiographic signs of degenerative joint disease in a hospital population of cats. *Vet Rec* **157**:793–799.

48 Godfrey DR (2005). Osteoarthritis in cats: a retrospective radiological study. *J Small Anim Pract* **46**:425–429.

49 Hardie EM, Roe SC, Martin FR (2002). Radiographic evidence of degenerative joint disease in geriatric cats: 100 cases (1994–1997). *J Am Vet Med Assoc* **220**:628–632.

50 Freire M, Robertson I, Bondell HD, *et al*. (2008). Cross-sectional study evaluating the radiographic prevalence of feline degenerative joint disease. ACVS Annual Meeting, San Diego.

51 Lascelles BDX, Thomson Sumrell A, Henry JB III, *et al*. (2010). Cross-sectional study evaluating the prevalence of radiographic degenerative joint disease in domesticated cats. *Vet Surg* **39**:535–544.

52 Clarke SP, Bennett D (2006). Feline osteoarthritis: a prospective study of 28 cases. *J Small Anim Pract* **47**:439–445.

53 Gunew MN, Menrath VH, Marshall RD (2008). Long-term safety, efficacy and palatability of oral meloxicam at 0.01–0.03mg/kg for treatment of osteoarthritic pain in cats. *J Feline Med Surg* **10**:235–241.

54 Lascelles BD, Henderson AJ, Hackett IJ (2001). Evaluation of the clinical efficacy of meloxicam in cats with painful locomotor disorders. *J Small Anim Pract* **42**:587–593.

55 Freire M, Robertson I, Bondell HD, *et al*. (2011). Radiographic evaluation of feline appendicular degenerative joint disease vs. macroscopic appearance of articular cartilage. *Vet Radiol Ultrasound* **52**(3):239–247.

56 Stampler C (2008). Osteoarthritis in cats: A more common disease than you might expect. *FDA Veterinarian* **23**(2):6–7.

57 Lascelles BDX, DePuy V, Thomson A, *et al*. (2010). Evaluation of a therapeutic diet for feline degenerative joint disease. *J Vet Intern Med* **24**:487–495.

CHAPTER 13

1 Wilson DG, Vanderby R Jr (1995). An evaluation of fiberglass cast application techniques. *Vet Surg* **24**:118–121.

2 Scott HW, McLaughlin R (2007). *Feline Orthopedics*. Manson Publishing, London.

CHAPTER 14

1 Johnston SA (1997). Osteoarthritis: joint anatomy, physiology and pathobiology. *Vet Clin North Am Small Anim Pract* **27**:699–723.

2 Hadler N (1998). Why does the patient with osteoarthritis hurt? In: Brandt KD, Doherty M, Lohmander LS (eds). *Osteoarthritis*. Oxford University Press, New York, pp. 255–261.

3 Kellgren JH, Samuel EP (1950). The sensitivity and innervation of the articular capsule. *J Bone Joint Surg* **4**:193–205.

4 Reimann I, Christensen SB (1977). A histological demonstration of nerves in subchondral bone. *Acta Orthop Scand* **48**:345–352.

5 Arnoldi CC, Djurhuus JC, Heerfordt J, *et al*. (1980). Intraosseous phlebography, intraosseus pressure measurements and 99mTc polyphosphate scintigraphy in patients with painful conditions in the hip and knee. *Acta Orthop Scand* **51**:19–28.

6 Jaegger G, Marcellin-Little DJ, Levine D (2002). Reliability of goniometry in Labrador retrievers. *Am J Vet Res* **63**:979–986.

7 Jaegger GH, Marcellin-Little DJ, DePuy V, *et al*. (2007). Validity of goniometric joint measurements in cats. *Am J Vet Res* **68**(8): 822–826.

FURTHER READING

Beale SB, Hulse DA, Schulz KS, *et al*. (eds) (2003). *Small Animal Arthroscopy*. WB Saunders, Philadelphia.

Brandt KD, Fife RS, Braunstein EM, *et al*. (1991). Radiographic grading of the severity of knee osteoarthritis: Relation of the Killgren and Lawrence grade to a grade based on joint space narrowing, and correlation with arthroscopic evidence of articular cartilage degeneration. *Arthritis Rheum* **34**:1381–1386.

Cicuttini FM, Baker J, Hart DJ, *et al*. (1996). Association of pain with radiological changes in different compartments and views of the knee joint. *Osteoarthr Cartil* **4**:143–147.

Hadler NM (1998). Why does the patient with osteoarthritis hurt? In: Brandt KD, Doherty M, Lohmander LS (eds). *Osteoarthritis*. Oxford University Press, New York, pp. 255–261.

Leach RE, Gregg T, Siber FJ (1970). Weight-bearing radiography in osteoarthritis of the knee. *Radiology* **97**:265–268.

Lozier SM, Menard M (1998). Arthrocentesis and synovial fluid analysis. In: Bojrab MJ (ed). *Current Techniques in Small Animal Surgery*, 4th edn. Williams & Wilkins, Baltimore, p. 1057.

Morgan JP (1969). Radiological pathology and diagnosis of degenerative joint disease in the stifle joint of the dog. *J Soc Adm Pharm* **10**:541–544.

Moskowitz R (1999). Bone remodeling in osteoarthritis: subchondral and osteophytic responses. *Osteoarthr Cartil* 7:323–324.

Suter PF (1984). Normal radiographic anatomy and radiographic examination. In: *Thoracic Radiography: Thoracic Disease of the Dog and Cat*. Wettswil, Switzerland, p. 2.

Index

Note: Page numbers in *italic* refer to tables and boxes; those in **bold** refer to figures

D

Q

R

For Product Safety Concerns and Information please contact our EU representative GPSR@taylorandfrancis.com Taylor & Francis Verlag GmbH, Kaufingerstraße 24, 80331 München, Germany

T - #0075 - 160425 - C416 - 261/194/22 [24] - CB - 9781840761832 - Gloss Lamination